Pharmacology

A 2-in-1 Reference for Nurses

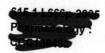

Pharmacology

A 2-in-1 Reference for Nurses

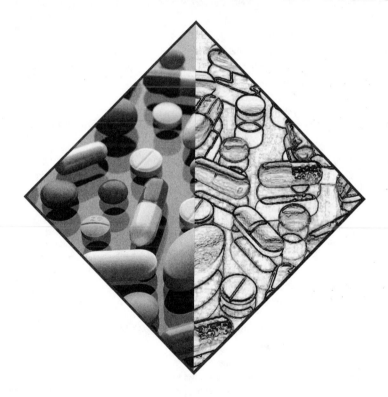

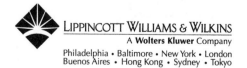

LIPPINCOTT WILLIAMS & WILKINS
A **Wolters Kluwer** Company
Philadelphia • Baltimore • New York • London
Buenos Aires • Hong Kong • Sydney • Tokyo

STAFF

Executive Publisher
Judith A. Schilling McCann, RN, MSN

Editorial Director
William J. Kelly

Clinical Director
Joan M. Robinson, RN, MSN

Senior Art Director
Arlene Putterman

Art Director
Elaine Kasmer

Clinical Manager
Eileen Cassin Gallen, RN, MSN

Drug Information Editor
Melissa M. Devlin, PharmD

Editorial Project Manager
Christiane L. Brownell

Editors
Nancy Priff, Catherine Harold

Clinical Editors
Lisa M. Bonsall, RN, MSN, CRNP; Christine
M. Damico, RN, MSN, CPNP; Kimberly A.
Zalewski, RN, MSN

Copy Editors
Kimberly Bilotta (supervisor),
Heather Ditch, Dona Hightower Perkins

Designers
PubTech, LLC

Digital Composition Services
Diane Paluba (manager), Joyce Rossi Biletz,
Joe Clark, Donna S. Morris

Manufacturing
Patricia K. Dorshaw (director),
Beth Janae Orr

Editorial Assistants
Carol A. Caputo, Tara L. Carter-Bell, Arlene
P. Claffee

Indexer
Barbara Hodgson

Pharm2in1- D
06 05 04   10 9 8 7 6 5 4 3 2

**Library of Congress
Cataloging-in Publication Data**

Pharmacology: a 2-in-1 reference for nurses.
   p. ; cm.
Includes index.
  1. Pharmacology 2. Nursing. I. Lippincott
Williams & Wilkins.
  [DNLM: 1. Pharmacology—methods—Nurses'
Instruction. 2. Drug Therapy—nursing. 3.
Pharmaceutical Preparations—administration &
dosage. QV 4 P53608 2004]
RM300.P5175 2004
615'.1—dc22
ISBN 1-58255-320-3 (alk. paper)   2003027064

Contents

Contributors and consultants

Tricia M. Berry, PharmD, BCPS
Associate Professor of Pharmacy
  Practice
St. Louis College of Pharmacy

Lawrence P. Carey, PharmD
Assistant Professor, Physician Assistant
  Studies
Philadelphia University

Mary Milano Carter, RNC, MS, ANP, BC
North Shore Pain Services
North Shore University Hospital
Syosset, N.Y.

Brenda Denson, PharmD
Pharmacy Clinical Coordinator
Children's Health System
Birmingham, Ala.

Jennifer Faulkner, PharmD, BCPP
Clinical Pharmacy Specialist, Psychiatry
Central Texas Veterans Health Care
  System
Temple

Christopher A. Fausel, PharmD,
  BCPS, BCOP
Clinical Pharmacist, Adult Hematology,
  Oncology, Bone Marrow Transplant
Indiana University Hospital
Indianapolis

Tatyana Gurvich, PharmD
Clinical Pharmacologist
Glendale (Calif.) Adventist Family
  Practice Residency Program

Michelle Kosich, PharmD
Pharmacy Clinical Coordinator
Mercy Fitzgerald Hospital
Darby, Pa.

Nicole M. Maisch, PharmD
Assistant Clinical Professor
St. John's University
College of Pharmacy and Allied Health
  Professions
Jamaica, N.Y.

Molly J. Moran, APRN, MS, BC
Clinical Nurse Specialist
Arthur G. James Cancer Hospital and
  Richard J. Solove Research Institute
Columbus, Ohio

Christine K. O'Neil, PharmD, BCPS,
  FCCP, GCP
Associate Professor
Mylan School of Pharmacy
Duquesne University
Pittsburgh

Steven G. Ottariano, RPh
Clinical Herbal Specialist
Veteran's Administration Medical
  Center
Manchester, N.H.

Susan Sard, PharmD
Clinical Pharmacist
Anne Arundel Medical Center
Annapolis, Md.

Dominique A. Thuriere, MD
Chief, Mental Health and Behavioral
  Sciences
Bay Pines (Fla.) Veteran's
  Administration Medical Center

Joanne Whitney, RPh, PharmD, PhD
Associate Clinical Professor; Director,
  Drug Product Services
University of California
San Francisco

Barbara S. Wiggins, PharmD, BCPS
Pharmacy Clinical Specialist,
  Cardiology
University of Virginia Medical Center
Charlottesville

Lei Xi, MD
Instructor of Medicine
Virginia Commonwealth University
Richmond

Foreword

Take a moment to consider these questions. How much can you call to mind about drugs in general, why drugs of a certain class act the way they do, which related drugs might cause similar interactions or adverse effects, and which assessment, monitoring, and follow-up steps you should pursue if your patient's regimen includes less-familiar drugs?

The demands and hectic pace of everyday practice requires you to work efficiently; time management is essential. That's why I'm pleased to recommend *Pharmacology: A 2-in-1 Reference for Nurses*. Whether you need a minor memory booster or a complete refresher course, this book has it.

Ingenious format

The first thing you'll notice about *Pharmacology: A 2-in-1 Reference for Nurses* is its ingenious two-column format. The inner two-thirds of each page contains a full narrative on drugs and their classes. The outer third of each page contains abbreviated, bulleted information that's perfect for quick scanning. The full effect of this two-part design is that you can skip the information you already know, quickly review anything you want to clarify or update, and easily go in-depth whenever you choose—all in the same book, often on the same page.

For example, if you're pressed for time or you just want a quick refresher, skim the narrow column on the outside edge of each page. Here you'll find all the most pertinent points of each drug class and many individual drugs in convenient bulleted form. If you want a more extensive review, simply shift your eyes over to the main column, where you'll find a more expanded version of the same topic. The information is still concise and clear, just more detailed.

Practical approach

And here's an important distinction. It isn't just the flexible format that sets this book apart. It's the content itself.

For one thing, it's grouped in the most practical way possible: by therapeutic use. You'll find individual chapters on the most important drug groups, such as cardiovascular drugs, respiratory drugs, GI drugs, anti-infectives, antineoplastics, neurologic drugs, and much more. You'll also find full chapters on drug classes of increasing scope and importance, such as immunomodulating drugs, psychotropic drugs, and endocrine drugs.

For another thing, drug information is organized to follow a consistent, practical order: pharmacokinetics, pharmacodynamics, pharmacotherapeutics, interactions, adverse reactions, and nursing considerations.

You'll also find chapters on equally practical matters, such as essential dosage calculations, step-by-step drug administration techniques, best drug-error sidesteps, and the must-know pharmacologic fundamentals.

A final practical aspect of this flexible book is its special logo features. These targeted short pieces call your attention to selected major topics and offer concise, scan-and-go information. Look for these helpful boxes and illustrations throughout the text:

♦ *Eye on drug action:* Illustrations to help you visualize—and remember—the often complicated ways drugs work.

♦ *Lifespan:* Considerations to carefully care for pregnant, breast-feeding, pediatric, or geriatric patients.

♦ *Warning:* Highlighted information about dangerous, hazardous, or life-threatening developments and how to avoid them.

♦ *Anatomy & physiology:* Illustrations of body systems and functions to refresh your memory.

♦ *Patient teaching:* Important points to tell patients about a drug class or a particular drug.

♦ *Clinical alert:* A colored logo to draw your attention to vitally important information in the main body of the text.

Every nurse knows that a sound understanding of pharmacology goes hand in hand with safe drug administration. *Pharmacology: A 2-in-1 Reference for Nurses* gives you as quick a review as you want and as complete a reference as you need, all in a surprisingly practical package. I recommend it enthusiastically.

Lisa A. Salamon, RNC, MSN, CNS, ETN
Clinical Nurse Specialist
Cleveland (Ohio) Clinic Foundation

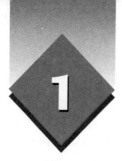

Fundamentals of clinical pharmacology

Before you can calculate dosages and give drugs safely, you need to understand the fundamental principles of pharmacology. Besides being aware of how drugs are named and made, you need to know their pharmacokinetics, pharmacodynamics, and pharmacotherapeutics, which include drug interactions and adverse reactions. You also need to consider the unique needs of pregnant, breast-feeding, pediatric, and geriatric patients.

DRUG NAMES AND CLASSES

Nearly every drug has three different names. Its *chemical* name is the scientific name that precisely describes its atomic and molecular structure. Its *generic*, or *nonproprietary*, name typically is an abbreviation of its chemical name. Its *trade* name, which is also called the *brand* or *proprietary* name, is selected by the drug manufacturer. Trade names are protected by copyright.

To avoid confusion, refer to a drug by its generic name because any drug can have many trade names. For example, use the generic name diltiazem when discussing this drug, instead of Cardizem, Tiazac, or any of its other trade names.

Every drug also belongs to at least two classes: a pharmacologic class and a therapeutic class. Drugs with similar chemical characteristics, such as beta blockers, fall into the same pharmacologic class. Drugs used to treat the same disorder fall into the same therapeutic class. For example, all drugs used to treat hypertension are part of the antihypertensive therapeutic class, even if they belong to different pharmacologic classes.

DRUG SOURCES

Traditionally, drugs were derived from natural sources, such as plants, animals, and minerals. Today, most drugs are produced in laboratories and can be natural, synthetic, or a combination of the two.

The three names of most drugs
+ Chemical
+ Generic
+ Trade

The two classes of every drug
+ Pharmacologic
+ Therapeutic

Plants

The earliest drugs used all parts of the plants, including the leaves, roots, bulb, stem, seeds, buds, and blossoms. Because of this, harmful substances commonly found their way into the mixture.

As the understanding of plants as drug sources became more sophisticated, researchers tried to isolate and intensify active components while avoiding harmful ones. Several types of active components vary in their character and effects.

◆ *Alkaloids,* the most active component in plants, react with acids to form a salt that dissolves readily in body fluids. The names of alkaloids and their salts usually end in *–ine,* such as atropine, caffeine, and nicotine.

◆ *Glycosides* also appear in plants. Their names usually end in *–in* like digoxin.

◆ *Gums,* usually in the form of polysaccharides, produce viscous solutions and allow products to attract and hold water. An example is psyllium, which is found in over-the-counter (OTC) laxatives. The laxative effect is probably due to the swelling of the psyllium as it absorbs water. This absorption increases stool bulk and stimulates peristalsis.

◆ *Resins,* primarily from pine tree sap, can be used for their actions as local irritants, laxatives, and caustic agents.

◆ *Oils,* which are thick and sometimes greasy liquids, may be volatile or fixed. Volatile oils, which evaporate easily, include peppermint, spearmint, and juniper. Fixed oils, including the laxative castor oil, don't evaporate easily.

Animals

Body fluids and glands of animals also can serve as drug sources. Drugs obtained from animal sources include:

◆ *hormones* such as insulin

◆ *oils* and *fats* such as cod-liver oil

◆ *enzymes,* which are produced by living cells and act as catalysts, such as pancreatin and pepsin

◆ *vaccines,* which are suspensions of killed, modified, or attenuated microorganisms.

Minerals

Metallic and nonmetallic minerals provide inorganic material that isn't available from plants or animals. Minerals may be used as they occur in nature or may be combined with other ingredients. Some drugs that contain minerals are iodine and epsom salts.

Synthetic drugs

Today, researchers blend traditional knowledge with modern chemistry to develop synthetic drugs. One advantage of synthetic drugs is that they're free from the impurities found in natural substances.

Another advantage is that drug developers can manipulate a drug's molecular structure slightly to make it more effective. Researchers commonly do this with antibiotics to make them effective against different organisms. For example, an organism cultured in seawater produced first-generation cephalosporins, which were effective against *Streptococcus, Staphylococcus, Escherichia coli, Proteus mirabilis,* and *Shigella.* Changes to the drugs' chemical structure resulted in second-generation cephalosporins, which effectively treated infections caused by *Bacteroides fragilis* and *Haemophilus influenzae,* and then in third-generation drugs, which were effective against *Pseudomonas.* Over time, bacteria developed resistance to those drugs, which prompted the development of fourth-generation cephalosporins. These

---

Active components of plants

◆ Alkaloids
◆ Glycosides
◆ Gums
◆ Resins
◆ Oils

Drugs from animal sources

◆ Hormones
◆ Oils
◆ Fats
◆ Enzymes
◆ Vaccines

Advantages of synthetic drugs

◆ They're free from impurities found in natural substances
◆ Their molecular structure can be manipulated

Phases of new drug development

Before the Food and Drug Administration (FDA) approves the application for a new drug, the drug undergoes clinical evaluation divided into three phases. The fourth phase isn't required for approval but is often done to make sure the drug is working properly in a clinical setting.

Phase I: The drug is tested on healthy volunteers.

Phase II: The drug is tested on people who have the disease for which the drug is thought to be effective.

Phase III: The drug is given to large numbers of patients in medical research centers. This larger sampling provides information about infrequent or rare adverse reactions. If phase III studies are satisfactory, the FDA approves the new drug application.

Phase IV: This voluntary phase involves postmarket surveillance of the drug's therapeutic effects. The pharmaceutical company receives reports from prescribers about the drug's therapeutic and adverse effects. Drugs that are found to be toxic are removed from the market.

drugs, which are active against a broad spectrum of gram-negative and gram-positive organisms, are powerful tools for fighting serious, life-threatening infections.

Recombinant deoxyribonucleic acid (DNA) research has led to the combination of natural and synthetic sources of drugs. For example, by reordering genetic information, scientists have developed bacteria that produce insulin.

NEW DRUG DEVELOPMENT

In the past, drugs were found by trial and error. Now, they're developed primarily by systematic scientific research. The Food and Drug Administration (FDA) carefully monitors new drug development, which can take many years.

First, the FDA reviews extensive animal studies and data on the safety and effectiveness of the proposed drug. Then it approves an application for an investigational new drug (IND). Next, the drug goes through four phases of clinical testing in humans to obtain information on its purity, bioavailability, potency, efficacy, safety, and toxicity. Depending on the test results, the studies can be stopped at any phase. (See *Phases of new drug development.*)

The three types of INDs are an Investigator IND, an Emergency Use IND, and a Treatment IND.

✦ An *Investigator IND* is submitted by the physician who initiates and conducts the investigation. The investigational drug must be administered or dispensed under his immediate direction. The study may involve an unapproved drug or an approved drug that's being tested for use in a new indication or patient population.

✦ An *Emergency Use IND* authorizes the use of an experimental drug in emergencies when time doesn't allow for IND submission according to established guidelines. It also may be used when patients don't meet the criteria of an existing study protocol or when an approved study protocol doesn't exist.

✦ A *Treatment IND* applies to an experimental drug that shows promise in clinical testing and is desperately needed to treat a serious or immediately life-threatening illness. This IND can be used while researchers complete the final clinical work and the FDA reviews the data.

Sponsors of drugs that reach phase II or III clinical trials can apply for FDA approval of Treatment IND status. When the IND is approved, the sponsor supplies the drug to prescribers whose patients meet appropriate criteria.

Three types of investigational new drugs

✦ Investigator IND
✦ Emergency Use IND
✦ Treatment IND

Difference between labeled and unlabeled uses

✦ Labeled uses are FDA-approved indications for which phase II and III clinical studies have shown safety and effectiveness.
✦ Unlabeled uses are indications that aren't FDA-approved but that the drug effectively treats in clinical use.

What is pharmacokinetics?

✦ A drug's actions as it moves through the body

The two types of transport mechanisms

✦ In passive transport, a drug moves from an area of higher concentration to one of lower concentration, which requires no cellular energy.
✦ In active transport, a drug moves from an area of lower concentration to one of higher concentration, which requires cellular energy.

LABELED AND UNLABELED USES

When approving a new drug, the FDA accepts it only for the indications for which phase II and III clinical studies have shown it to be safe and effective. These indications are approved, or labeled; all others are unapproved, or unlabeled.

For example, the FDA may approve a new drug to treat hypertension if phase II and III studies show that it's safe and effective in patients with hypertension. If the drug also works well as an antianginal, the FDA can't approve it for this indication unless formal studies in patients with angina pectoris are completed successfully. Such a drug is unapproved for treatment of angina pectoris, yet it may be used for this unlabeled indication, based on empirical evidence.

Here's how a drug can start being used for an unlabeled indication. After ordering a new drug approved to treat hypertension, a prescriber may discover that it also decreases the patient's angina. The prescriber may share this finding with colleagues in medical journals or at meetings, and they may prescribe it for unlabeled uses, too.

The FDA recognizes that a drug's labeling doesn't always contain the most current information about its use. Therefore, after the FDA approves a drug for one indication, a prescriber legally may order it, a pharmacist may dispense it, and a nurse may give it to a patient for any labeled — or unlabeled — indication.

Although prescribers may prescribe, dispense, and give a drug for an unlabeled use, the FDA forbids the manufacturer from promoting a drug for any unlabeled indications. That's why drug package inserts and the *Physicians' Desk Reference* contain no information about unlabeled uses and why pharmaceutical sales representatives can't discuss such uses.

Many drugs are commonly prescribed for unlabeled uses, which later become approved uses. Tretinoin (Retin-A) is an example. Once only prescribed for acne, it was noted to help eliminate wrinkles. Thus, the drug was prescribed for wrinkles. Although tretinoin now has FDA approval for this use, it continues to have off-label uses for certain skin cancers and dermatologic conditions.

PHARMACOKINETICS

Kinetics refers to movement. Pharmacokinetics refers to a drug's actions as it moves through the body. Specifically, pharmacokinetics describes how a drug is absorbed into, distributed through, metabolized within, and excreted from the body. This branch of pharmacology also reflects the drug's onset of action, peak level, and duration of action.

ABSORPTION

Drug absorption covers a drug's progress from the time it's given, through the time it moves into tissues, until it becomes available for use by the body. At the cellular level, drug absorption depends primarily on transport mechanisms.

Transport mechanisms

Two mechanisms are responsible for the absorption of most drugs: passive and active transport. Passive transport requires no cellular energy because the drug moves from an area of higher concentration to one of lower concentration. It occurs when small molecules diffuse across membranes. Diffusion is complete when the drug concentration on both sides of the membrane is equal.

Active transport requires cellular energy to move the drug from an area of lower concentration to one of higher concentration. Active transport is used to absorb electrolytes, such as sodium and potassium, as well as some drugs, such as levodopa.

Pinocytosis is a unique form of active transport that happens when a cell engulfs a drug particle. During pinocytosis, the drug doesn't need to be dissolved because the cell forms a vesicle for drug transport across the cell membrane and into the inner cell. Pinocytosis commonly occurs to transport fat-soluble vitamins, such as vitamins A, D, E, and K.

What affects absorption

The administration route plays a key role in absorption. When only a few cells separate the drug from systemic circulation, absorption takes place rapidly and the drug quickly reaches a therapeutic level in the body. Typically, absorption occurs within seconds or minutes when a drug is given by the sublingual, I.V., or inhalation route.

Absorption occurs more slowly when a drug is given by the oral, I.M., or subcutaneous (S.C.) route because the complex membranes of GI mucosa, muscles, and skin delay drug passage. With rectal or sustained-release drugs, absorption occurs even more slowly, taking several hours or days to reach a peak level.

Other factors can affect the rate of drug absorption. First, most oral drug absorption takes place in the small intestine. If a large portion of a patient's small intestine has been surgically removed, drug absorption decreases because of the reduced surface area and intestinal transit time.

Second, a drug absorbed by the small intestine travels to the liver before circulating to the rest of the body. The liver can perform a first-pass effect, metabolizing much of the drug to an inactive form before it enters the circulation and reaches its site of action. If the first-pass effect significantly reduces the amount of active drug released into the systemic circulation, the patient will need a higher drug dosage to obtain the desired effect. This explains why a drug's oral dose may be much higher than its I.V. dose for the same indication.

Third, increased blood flow to an absorption site improves drug absorption and leads to a quicker onset of drug action. Conversely, reduced blood flow decreases absorption and leads to a more gradual onset. For faster absorption of an I.M. drug, for example, the deltoid muscle is a good choice because blood flows faster through the deltoid muscle than through the gluteal muscle. The gluteal muscle, however, can accommodate a larger volume of drug than the deltoid muscle.

Fourth, pain and stress can decrease the amount of drug absorbed. This effect may result from altered blood flow, reduced GI motility, or gastric retention triggered by the autonomic nervous system's response to pain.

Fifth, high-fat meals and solid foods slow the rate at which the contents of the stomach enter the intestines. This, in turn, delays intestinal absorption of a drug.

Sixth, the drug formulation (such as tablets, capsules, liquids, sustained-release forms, inactive ingredients, and coatings) affects the drug absorption rate and the time needed to reach a peak level.

Finally, combining one drug with another or with food or an herbal preparation can cause interactions that increase or decrease drug absorption.

DISTRIBUTION

Drug distribution is the process by which a drug is delivered to body tissues and fluids. After a drug is absorbed, its distribution is influenced by blood flow, its solubility and ability to bind with proteins, and the volume of distribution.

Factors affecting drug absorption
+ Administration route
+ Intestinal surface area and transit time
+ First-pass effect
+ Blood flow to the absorption site
+ Pain and stress
+ GI motility
+ Drug formulation
+ Interactions with other drugs, food, or herbs
+ High-fat and solid food

What is distribution?
+ Process that allows drug delivery to tissues and fluid

Factors affecting drug distribution

+ Blood flow
+ Drug solubility
+ Protein-binding capability
+ Volume of distribution

Low-volume distribution

+ Is caused by high water solubility
+ Is caused by high protein-binding
+ Results in a higher drug level

High-volume distribution

+ Is caused by high lipid solubility
+ Is caused by high tissue-binding
+ Results in a lower drug level

Blood flow and drug solubility

Once a drug reaches the bloodstream, its distribution depends on blood flow. A drug is distributed rapidly to organs with a large blood supply, such as the heart, liver, and kidneys. It's distributed more gradually to other internal organs, skin, fat, and muscle.

Solubility also helps determine distribution. A drug's ability to cross a cell membrane depends on whether it's soluble in fats (lipids) or water. A lipid-soluble drug easily crosses cell membranes, whereas a water-soluble drug doesn't.

Protein binding

The degree of protein binding influences the distribution and storage of a drug. When distributed in the vascular or lymphatic system, a drug comes in contact with proteins. There, it remains free (unbound) or it binds to a plasma carrier protein, storage tissue protein, or receptor protein. As soon as a drug binds to a plasma carrier protein or storage tissue protein, it becomes inactive, which means it can't bind to a receptor protein or exert any therapeutic activity. However, a bound drug can free itself rapidly to maintain a balance between the amounts of free and bound drug. Only the free drug remains active.

The percentage of drug that remains free and available for activity depends on the amount of protein available for binding. The major source for carrier protein binding is plasma albumin.

The percentage of free drug differs widely among drugs. For example, a highly protein-bound drug, such as warfarin, is more than 80% bound to protein. A poorly protein-bound drug, such as cimetidine, may be less than 20% bound to protein.

The amount of free drug in the plasma also differs among patients, depending on their health status. For example, a patient with malnutrition typically has less protein and plasma albumin in his body. His decreased plasma albumin level — and number of protein-binding sites — can boost the amount of free drug in his plasma, which may be undesirable. That's why you should note changes in the patient's health status that could alter the percentage of free drug in his plasma.

Volume of distribution

Volume of distribution isn't actual volume, but a measure of the size of a compartment, such as blood, total body water, or fat, that would be filled by the amount of drug in the same concentration as that found in the blood or plasma. Keep in mind, however, that a drug's volume of distribution is unrelated to its effectiveness or duration of action.

A highly water-soluble drug possesses a small volume of distribution and has a high blood concentration level. In contrast, a highly lipid-soluble drug possesses a large volume of distribution and has a low blood concentration level. Factors that tend to keep a drug in circulation, such as high water solubility and high protein binding, result in a lower volume of distribution and a higher level. Conversely, factors that promote drug movement from the blood to other compartments, such as high lipid solubility (promoting storage of the drug in fat) and high tissue binding, result in a higher volume of distribution and a lower blood concentration level.

A drug's ability to cross barriers, such as the blood-brain barrier, can influence a drug's volume of distribution. The blood-brain barrier refers to a network of capillary endothelial cells in the brain. These cells have no pores and are surrounded by a sheath of glial connective tissue that makes them impermeable to water-soluble drugs. The network excludes most ionized drug molecules, such as dopamine, from the brain. However, it allows nonionized, unbound drug molecules, such as barbiturates, to pass readily and enter the brain.

Don't assume that a drug is well distributed throughout the body. Abscesses, exudates, glands, and tumors can adversely affect drug distribution. Also, variable drug concentrations among different organs and tissues within a single organ can complicate drug distribution. The differences in drug levels in tissues result from such factors as a tissue's affinity for the drug, blood flow, and protein-binding sites.

METABOLISM

Drug metabolism, or biotransformation, refers to the body's ability to change a drug from its original form to a more or less active form that can then be excreted. Through metabolism, the body detoxifies and disposes of foreign substances such as drugs. In most cases, enzymes increase the drug's water solubility so that the kidneys can excrete the drug. For some drugs, enzymes may alter their lipid solubility so that the end products enter into and are excreted in bile. Using the kidneys or biliary system for disposal, the body usually transforms the drug into a readily eliminated, pharmacologically inactive substance. Usually, the resulting product, called a metabolite, is an inactive form of the original drug. For some drugs, however, one or all of the metabolites may have some drug activity. These are called active metabolites. All metabolites, active or inactive, may undergo further metabolism or may be excreted from the body unchanged.

Some drugs are given as prodrugs (inactive drugs that don't become active until they're metabolized). After oral administration, intestinal and hepatic enzymes rapidly convert this type of drug to its active form. For example, the prodrug valganciclovir is metabolized into the active drug ganciclovir.

What affects metabolism

Not all drugs are metabolized to the same extent or by the same mechanisms. Some drugs, such as aminoglycosides, aren't metabolized; they pass through the body and are excreted unchanged. Other drugs, such as barbiturates, stimulate or induce enzyme metabolic activity, thus reducing the amount of active drug in the body.

In contrast, some drugs inhibit or compete for enzyme metabolism, which may cause other drugs to accumulate. Accumulation increases the risk of adverse reactions and drug toxicity. Before interpreting a drug response or adjusting therapy because of an inappropriate level of an active drug, check for drug-induced changes in drug metabolism.

Disease-induced changes can interfere with drug metabolism. When end-stage cirrhosis damages the liver enough to reduce liver blood flow, the supply of a drug to liver enzyme metabolic sites decreases. When heart failure decreases cardiac output, drug metabolism decreases because the drug delivery to liver metabolic sites becomes inefficient. Genetics also may play a part in drug metabolism. Certain ethnic groups are slow or fast acetylators, which refers to their rate of sulfamethazine acetylation (a common metabolic process) for such drugs as isoniazid, hydralazine, and many sulfa drugs. Slow acetylators may be at increased risk for toxicity because of increased exposure to a drug. Fast acetylators may metabolize a drug too rapidly, minimizing its therapeutic effects. (See *Predicting the effects of genetics on drug metabolism*, page 8.)

Developmental changes also can affect drug metabolism. For instance, infants have immature livers that reduce the rate of metabolism. Geriatric patients experience a decline in liver size, blood flow, and enzyme production that also slows metabolism.

What is metabolism?

+ Alters a drug to a more active or less active form
+ Helps convert the drug to a more water soluble form, facilitating excretion

Factors affecting metabolism

+ Drugs that induce enzyme activity
+ Drugs that inhibit enzyme activity
+ Disease, such as cirrhosis and heart failure
+ Genetics
+ Age-related differences

Ways to evaluate drug acetylation

- Check the patient's ethnicity.
- Monitor the drug level.
- Assess for therapeutic and adverse drug effects.

Routes of excretion

- Kidneys via urine
- Liver via bile and into feces
- Lungs via exhaled air
- Saliva, sweat, and tears

What is half-life?

- The time needed for the total amount of a drug in the body to decrease by 50%

The importance of five half-lives

- A drug that's given only once is eliminated almost completely after five half-lives.
- A drug that's given regularly reaches a steady-state level after five half-lives.

Predicting the effects of genetics on drug metabolism

Certain percentages of different ethnic groups may be slow acetylators. The table below can help you predict which patients may have this altered metabolism. However, the only way to determine a patient's acetylation rate is to monitor the drug level in his blood and to assess him for therapeutic and adverse effects.

ETHNIC GROUP	PERCENTAGE OF SLOW ACETYLATORS	ETHNIC GROUP	PERCENTAGE OF SLOW ACETYLATORS
Black	40% to 70%	Indian	60%
Canadian Indian	10%	Italian	55%
Caucasian	40% to 70%	Japanese	10%
Chinese	20%	Korean	10%
Egyptian	80%	Spanish	55%
German	50%	Thai	25%

EXCRETION

Drug excretion refers to the elimination of drugs from the body. Most drugs are excreted by the kidneys and leave the body through urine. Drugs also can be excreted through the lungs, exocrine (sweat, salivary, or mammary) glands, skin, and intestines via bile and feces.

Half-life

Knowing how long a drug remains in the body helps determine how frequently a drug should be given. Usually, a drug's rate of loss from the body can be estimated by determining its half-life (the time required for the total amount of a drug in the body to diminish by half). A drug's half-life can be determined from a drug concentration-time curve, which plots the drug's concentration level on the vertical axis and the elapsed time in hours on the horizontal axis.

If a patient receives a single dose of a drug with a half-life of 7 hours, the total amount of the drug in his body would diminish by half after 7 hours. The drug amount would continue to decrease accordingly with each subsequent half-life. Most drugs essentially are eliminated after five half-lives because the amount remaining is too low to exert any beneficial or adverse effect.

Although a drug that's given only once is eliminated almost completely after five half-lives, a drug that's given regularly reaches a steady concentration, or steady state, after about five half-lives. Steady state occurs when the amount of drug given equals the amount of drug excreted.

After reaching a steady state, the drug level will fluctuate above and below the average level. This means that, although the drug was once at steady state, its concentration level doesn't remain uniform. Rather, it increases, peaks, and declines within a constant range.

For some drugs, the time required to reach a therapeutic level may be too long to treat an acute problem. For example, digoxin has a half-life of 1½ to 2 days. It could take up to 10 days to achieve a steady-state level to control a life-threatening arrhythmia, such as atrial fibrillation. To reach the desired therapeutic level more rapidly, the patient initially should receive one or more large doses, called loading doses. He can then receive smaller maintenance doses daily to replace the amount of drug eliminated since the last dose. These smaller doses maintain a therapeutic level in the body at all times.

ONSET, PEAK, AND DURATION

Besides absorption, distribution, metabolism, and excretion, three other factors play important roles in a drug's pharmacokinetics: onset of action, peak level, and duration of action.

Onset of action refers to the time period from a drug's administration to the beginning of its therapeutic effect. The rate of onset varies with the administration route and the drug's pharmacokinetics.

The peak level occurs when the body absorbs more drug, the level rises in the blood, and more drug reaches the site of action. Because some drugs require several doses to reach peak level, it isn't necessarily associated with therapeutic response.

As soon as the drug begins to circulate in the blood, it also begins to be eliminated. Eventually, drug elimination exceeds drug absorption because less of the dose remains to be absorbed. At this point, the drug's level and effects begin to decline. When the level falls below the minimum needed to produce an effect, drug action stops although some drug remains in the blood. Therefore, the duration of action is the length of time that the drug level is sufficient to produce a therapeutic response.

PHARMACODYNAMICS

Pharmacodynamics is the study of the mechanisms of drug action that produce biochemical or physiologic changes in the body. Drug action — the interaction between a drug and cellular components, such as complex proteins in cell membranes, enzymes, and target receptors — results in the response known as the drug effect.

DRUG ACTION

A drug can modify cell function or the rate of function, but it can't impart a new function to a cell or target tissue. Therefore, the drug effect depends on what the cell is supposed to do. A drug can only modify what a cell does by altering the cell's physical or chemical environment or by interacting with its receptors.

Many drugs work by stimulating or blocking drug receptors. A drug can be classified as selective (binding with only one type of receptor) or nonselective (binding with various types of receptors). A nonselective drug can cause many widespread effects.

When a drug binds with and stimulates a receptor, it acts as an agonist, which means that it activates a response. A drug's ability to initiate a response after binding with the receptor is referred to as intrinsic activity. When a drug binds with but doesn't stimulate a receptor, it acts as an antagonist, which means it displays no intrinsic activity and, therefore, prevents a response from occurring.

Antagonists can be competitive or noncompetitive. A competitive antagonist competes with the agonist for receptor sites. Because this type of drug binds reversibly with receptor sites, giving larger doses of an agonist can overcome the antagonist's effects. A noncompetitive antagonist binds with receptor sites and always blocks the effects of the agonist no matter how large its dose. Giving larger doses of the agonist can't reverse this type of antagonist's action.

What are onset, peak, and duration?

+ Onset of action is the time between when drug is given and when therapeutic effects begin.
+ The peak level is the maximum drug level achieved through absorption.
+ Duration of action is the length of time a drug produces therapeutic effects.

What is pharmacodynamics?

+ The study of the mechanisms by which a drug produces biochemical and physiologic changes in the body

How a drug acts

+ Changes cell environment physically or chemically
+ Acts as an agonist, binding with and stimulating receptors, which creates a response
+ Acts as an antagonist, binding with but not stimulating receptors, which prevents a response

Dose-response and potency

✦ If one drug produces the same response as a second drug but at a lower dose, then the first drug is more potent.

Understanding beta receptors

✦ Beta$_1$ receptors act mainly on the heart.
✦ Beta$_2$ receptors act mainly on smooth muscle in the lungs.

Defining potency

✦ The relative amount of a drug needed for a desired response

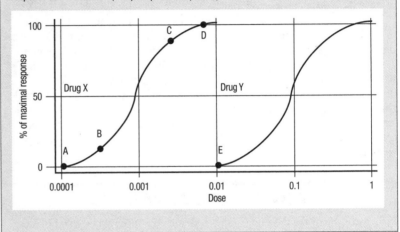

Understanding dose-response curves

This graph shows the dose-response curve for two drugs. As you can see, at low doses of each drug, a dose increase results in only a small increase in drug response, as illustrated by the curve between points A and B.

At higher doses, a dose increase produces a much greater response, as illustrated by the curve between points B and C. As the dosage continues to climb, an increase in dosage produces a very slight increase in response, as illustrated by the curve between points C and D.

This graph also shows that drug X is more potent than drug Y because it results in the same response at a lower dose (compare point A to point E).

Drug receptors are classified by their specific effects. For example, beta receptors typically produce increased heart rate and bronchial relaxation as well as other systemic effects. Beta receptors can be further divided into beta$_1$ receptors (which act primarily on the heart) and beta$_2$ receptors (which act primarily on smooth muscle and gland cells, especially in the lungs). Giving a nonselective beta blocker, such as propranolol, to a patient with tachycardia will decrease his heart rate. Because propranolol is nonselective, however, it also will block beta$_2$ receptors, which could precipitate an asthma attack in a susceptible patient. Giving a selective beta$_1$ blocker, such as metoprolol or atenolol, will decrease heart rate without affecting pulmonary function.

Epinephrine is a nonselective beta agonist used to treat acute asthmatic episodes. When administered S.C., it interacts with beta$_1$ and beta$_2$ receptors and further increases the asthmatic patient's accelerated heart rate. Therefore, the patient may benefit from receiving a drug that's selective for beta$_2$ receptors.

DRUG POTENCY

Drug potency, the relative amount of a drug required to produce a desired response, is helpful in comparing drugs. If drug X produces the same response as drug Y but at a lower dose, then drug X is more potent than drug Y.

As its name implies, a dose-response curve graphically represents the relationship between the dose of a drug and the response it produces. (See *Understanding dose-response curves.*)

On a dose-response curve, a low dose usually corresponds with a low response. From this low level, an increase in dose produces only a slight increase in response.

With further increases in dose, the drug response rises markedly. After a certain point, an increase in dose yields little or no increase in response. At this point, the drug has reached its maximum effectiveness.

Most drugs produce several effects. The relationship between a drug's desired therapeutic effects and its adverse effects is called the drug's therapeutic index, or margin of safety.

The therapeutic index measures the safety of the drug, designating the difference between a toxic dose for 50% of the patients treated and the minimum dose at which therapeutic effects occur. A narrow therapeutic index means that the range between an effective dose and a lethal one is small. Some drugs with narrow therapeutic indices are used to treat life-threatening disorders. Because of their narrow therapeutic index, these drugs increase the risk of serious adverse reactions and typically require blood tests to monitor the drug level. A drug with a wide therapeutic index has a large margin of safety and reduces the risk of toxic effects.

Therapeutic index

✦ A narrow therapeutic index means that the range between effective and dangerous drug doses is small.
✦ A wide therapeutic index means that the range between effective and dangerous drugs doses is large.

PHARMACOTHERAPEUTICS

Pharmacotherapeutics is the use of drugs to treat disease. When choosing a drug to treat a disorder, a prescriber must consider the drug's effectiveness and other factors, such as the type of therapy the patient needs and potential drug interactions and adverse reactions.

TYPES OF THERAPY

For any patient, the type of therapy depends on the severity, urgency, and prognosis of his disorder. Types of therapies include acute, maintenance, supportive, palliative, empiric, and supplemental or replacement.

✦ Acute therapy is for a critically ill patient who requires acute intensive care.
✦ Maintenance therapy is for a patient with a chronic condition who needs to maintain his level of well-being while preventing disease progression.
✦ Supportive therapy doesn't treat the cause of the disease but maintains threatened body systems until the patient's condition resolves.
✦ Palliative therapy is for a patient with an end-stage or terminal disease to make him as comfortable as possible.
✦ Empiric therapy is based on practical experience rather than on pure scientific data, for example, when a hospitalized patient with a fever receives empiric antibiotic therapy while waiting for the results of culture and sensitivity tests.
✦ Supplemental or replacement therapy replenishes or substitutes for missing substances in the patient's body.

A patient's overall health and other factors can alter his response to a drug. When selecting drug therapy, the prescriber must consider the patient's medical conditions and lifestyle factors. (See *Influences on drug response,* page 12.)

Also, the prescriber must remember that certain drugs have a tendency to create drug tolerance and dependence. Drug tolerance develops when a patient's response to a drug decreases over time. Then he requires larger doses to produce the same response. Drug dependence develops when a patient displays a physical or psychological need for the drug. When the drug is stopped, physical dependence produces withdrawal symptoms; psychological dependence results in a craving for the drug.

Types of drug therapy

✦ Acute
✦ Maintenance
✦ Supportive
✦ Palliative
✦ Empiric
✦ Supplemental or replacement

Influences on drug response

Because no two people are alike physiologically or psychologically, a patient's response to a drug may vary greatly, depending on these factors:

✦ Age	✦ Enzyme induction	✦ Lactation
✦ Albumin concentration	✦ Exercise	✦ Occupational exposure
✦ Alcohol intake	✦ Gender	✦ Pregnancy
✦ Barometric pressure	✦ Genetic constitution	✦ Renal function
✦ Body temperature	✦ GI function	✦ Smoking
✦ Cardiovascular function	✦ Hepatic function	✦ Stress level
✦ Circadian variations	✦ Hypersensitivity	✦ Sunlight
✦ Diet	✦ Infection	✦ Trauma
✦ Disease	✦ Immunization	
✦ Drug interactions	✦ Immunologic function	

Sources of drug interactions

- ✦ Other drugs
- ✦ Food or beverages
- ✦ Herbal medicines
- ✦ Lifestyle factors, such as smoking, alcohol or illicit drug use, and exposure to the sun

Effects of drug interactions

- ✦ When two drugs have an additive effect, combining them at reduced doses produces an effect equal to a higher dose of either drug given alone.
- ✦ When two drugs have a synergistic effect, combining them produces an effect greater than that produced by either drug given alone.
- ✦ When two drugs have an antagonistic effect, combining them produces an effect less than that produced by either drug given alone.

INTERACTIONS

Interactions can occur between two drugs or between a drug and a food, herbal product, or lifestyle factor. Interactions may alter drug effects, skew laboratory test results, or produce physical or chemical incompatibilities. The more drugs a patient takes, the greater the chances are that a drug interaction will occur.

Drug-drug interactions

Interactions between drugs can cause additive effects, synergistic effects, antagonistic effects, and decreased or increased absorption, distribution, metabolism, or excretion.

An additive effect occurs when a patient receives two drugs with similar actions and is equal to the effect of either drug given alone at a higher dose. Causing an additive effect, such as by giving two different analgesics, allows the use of lower doses of each drug, which decreases the risk of adverse reactions. It also provides greater pain control than could be produced by one drug (probably because of different mechanisms of action).

A synergistic effect, or potentiation, happens if two drugs with the same effect produce a greater response when given together than when taken alone. In this type of interaction, one drug enhances the effect of the other.

An antagonistic effect develops when the combined response of two drugs is less than the response produced by either drug alone. For example, if levodopa is prescribed to decrease a patient's stiffness, rigidity, and other symptoms of Parkinson's disease, pyridoxine (vitamin B_6) can interfere with (or antagonize) levodopa's effects.

Two drugs given together can change the absorption of one or both drugs. A drug that alters stomach acidity can affect a second drug's ability to dissolve in the stomach. Some drugs can interact to form an insoluble compound that can't be absorbed. After a drug is absorbed, the blood distributes it throughout the body as a free drug or protein-bound drug. When given together, two drugs can compete for protein-binding sites. This may increase the effects of one drug if it's displaced from the protein and becomes free, or unbound. For example, the oral anticoagulant warfarin is more than 97% protein bound, and the anticonvulsant drug phenytoin successfully competes with warfarin for protein-binding sites. Combining these two drugs increases the amount of free warfarin, which significantly increases the risk of bleeding.

Toxic drug levels can occur when one drug inhibits another's metabolism and excretion. For example, the antibiotic erythromycin may decrease hepatic metabolism of cyclosporine, resulting in a high cyclosporine level and nephrotoxicity. Changes in hepatic blood flow from drug interactions or disease also may affect drug metabolism and excretion. Decreased hepatic blood flow affects drugs whose metabolism and excretion depend more on blood flow than on enzyme activity. Conversely, drugs whose metabolism and excretion depend on intrinsic enzyme activity generally aren't affected by changes in hepatic blood flow. Some drug interactions affect excretion only. For example, the interaction between penicillin and the uricosuric drug probenecid can produce therapeutic effects. Probenecid decreases the renal excretion of penicillin, which increases its half-life and level.

CLINICAL ALERT A patient who's discharged from an acute care setting may run a higher risk of developing drug-drug interactions. Before discharge, a patient's regular drug regimen is likely to undergo changes, such as dosage changes and the addition of one or more new drugs. These changes may lead to interactions that may go unnoticed by the prescriber or unreported by the patient at home. To prevent problems, carefully review the patient's drugs before discharge, inform him of any potential interactions, and advise him to call the prescriber if they become bothersome.

Drug-food interactions

Interactions between drugs and food can alter a drug's therapeutic effect and impair vitamin and mineral absorption in several ways. Food can alter the rate and amount of a drug absorbed from the GI tract, affecting bioavailability (the amount of a drug dose available to the systemic circulation). For example, a high-fat meal can increase the bioavailability of the antifungal griseofulvin. A low-protein, high-carbohydrate diet can increase the bioavailability of theophylline.

Some drugs can stimulate enzyme production, increasing the metabolic rate and the demand for vitamins that are enzyme cofactors (substances that unite with the enzyme and allow it to function).

Other dangerous interactions can happen. For instance, when a patient eats tyramine-rich food during therapy with a monoamine oxidase (MAO) inhibitor, hypertensive crisis can occur. (See *Avoiding food interactions with MAO inhibitors,* page 14.) When a patient takes grapefruit juice with a 3-hydroxy-3-methylglutaryl coenzyme A (HMG-CoA) reductase inhibitor, cyclosporine, or amprenavir, drug toxicity may occur. Grapefruit juice also may delay the onset, decrease the absorption, or have other adverse effects on a drug. (See *Preventing interactions between drugs and grapefruit juice,* page 15.)

Drug-herb interactions

Drug-herb interactions are a growing concern as more patients buy and use herbal products, usually without reporting them to their prescriber. Herbal products, such as evening primrose oil, can lower the seizure threshold and shouldn't be used during anticonvulsant therapy. When used with warfarin, gingko may increase the risk of bleeding, and ginseng may decrease warfarin's anticoagulant effect. St. John's wort may decrease the therapeutic effects of protease inhibitors such as indinavir; nonnucleoside reverse transcriptase inhibitors such as nevirapine; digoxin; and cyclosporine. This herb also may cause additive effects when used with a selective serotonin reuptake inhibitor (SSRI), such as sertraline, or other antidepressants,

Effects of drug interactions *(continued)*

✦ When a drug affects stomach pH, it may alter the absorption of other drugs.
✦ When two drugs are highly protein-bound, they may compete for receptor sites, allowing more free drug to exert effects.
✦ When one drug induces or inhibits the hepatic metabolism of a second drug, it may increase or decrease the level of the second drug

Discharge: Avoiding drug interactions

✦ Review the patient's drugs.
✦ Explain possible interactions.
✦ Urge the patient to tell the prescriber about disturbing effects.

Effects of food interactions

✦ Altered rate of absorption
✦ Altered amount of absorption
✦ Induced enzyme production
✦ Drug toxicity

Effects of herb interactions

✦ Depending on their actions, some herbal products can interfere with the therapeutic effects of some drugs. Question all patients about their use of herbal products.

Signs and symptoms of hypertensive crisis

+ Sudden sharp increase in blood pressure
+ Severe headache
+ Abrupt changes in vision
+ Dizziness

WARNING

Avoiding food interactions with MAO inhibitors

In a patient taking a monoamine oxidase (MAO) inhibitor, foods that contain tyramine may produce a hypertensive crisis, which is characterized by a sudden severe increase in blood pressure, severe headache, sudden vision changes, and dizziness. To prevent this dangerous drug-food interaction, teach the patient which foods to avoid during treatment. Foods with a high tyramine content should be avoided completely, those with a moderate content may be eaten occasionally, and those with a low tyramine content are allowable in limited quantities.

Foods with a high tyramine content
+ Aged cheese, such as blue, cheddar, and Swiss
+ Aged or smoked meats, such as corned beef, herring, and sausage
+ Beer
+ Fava or broad beans such as Italian green beans
+ Liver, such as chicken and beef liver
+ Red wines, such as burgundy and Chianti
+ Yeast extracts such as brewer's yeast

Foods with a moderate tyramine content
+ Meat extracts such as bouillon
+ Ripe avocados
+ Ripe bananas
+ Sour cream
+ Yogurt

Foods with a low tyramine content
+ American, mozzarella, cottage, and cream cheese
+ Chocolate
+ Distilled spirits, such as gin, vodka, and scotch
+ Figs
+ White wines

Drugs that don't mix with alcohol

+ Barbiturates
+ Benzodiazepines
+ Drugs that cause drowsiness or sedation
+ Drugs that impair psychomotor skills
+ Drugs that depress the CNS

possibly leading to serotonin syndrome, a serious, sometimes fatal reaction whose symptoms include myoclonus rigidity, mental status changes, hyperthermia, autonomic nervous system instability, rapid fluctuations in vital signs, delirium, and coma.

 CLINICAL ALERT Although herbal products may be all-natural, they can be harmful. To help avoid dangerous interactions, always ask your patient whether he uses any herbal products or dietary supplements.

Drug-lifestyle interactions

Lifestyle factors may interfere with a drug's therapeutic effects. For example, alcohol depresses the central nervous system (CNS), leading to sedation and drowsiness. If a patient combines alcohol with a drug that also depresses the CNS, the interaction enhances the drug's sedative effect and impairs the patient's psychomotor skills. That's why you should caution a patient to avoid alcohol during therapy with a barbiturate, benzodiazepine, or other drug that causes drowsiness or sedation.

WARNING

Preventing interactions between drugs and grapefruit juice

When taken with certain drugs, grapefruit juice can significantly alter absorption, onset, blood level, excretion, and effects. To prevent these drug-food interactions, explain them to your patient and recommend that he avoid grapefruit juice during therapy.

Delayed absorption
+ indinavir
+ itraconazole
+ quinidine

Delayed onset or increased effects
+ midazolam
+ triazolam

Increased level
+ amlodipine
+ buspirone
+ carbamazepine
+ cyclosporine
+ dextromethorphan
+ diltiazem
+ erythromycin

Increased level *(continued)*
+ felodipine
+ lovastatin
+ nicardipine
+ nisoldipine
+ saquinavir
+ sildenafil
+ simvastatin
+ verapamil

Decreased level
+ etoposide
+ fexofenadine

Delayed excretion
+ atorvastatin

Smoking may increase corticosteroid release, requiring higher dosages of these drugs. Heavy smoking can increase haloperidol metabolism, possibly necessitating a dosage adjustment. It also increases theophylline elimination, which decreases the drug's therapeutic effects.

 CLINICAL ALERT A smoker who is stable on a dose of theophylline may be at risk for adverse reactions if he quits smoking without informing his prescriber. The former smoker may be receiving a higher-than-needed dose of theophylline, which may lead to toxicity.

Drug interactions and diagnostic tests
Drug interactions can alter laboratory tests. For example, a patient may undergo a test that measures creatinine level by using a colorimetric method. Many cephalosporins, such as cefazolin and cefoxitin, contain chromogens that aren't creatinine but can't be differentiated by the colorimetric method. As a result, the laboratory test may overestimate the patient's creatinine level, possibly leading to inadequate drug dosages.

Guaiac tests of feces to detect occult blood can show false-positive results in a patient who takes large amounts of iron supplements.

Blood glucose testing is the preferred method of monitoring diabetes. However, some diabetic patients monitor their glucose level with a urine test. Drugs that interfere with urine glucose testing include cephalothin, isoniazid, levodopa, probenecid, and large amounts (1 to 2 g daily) of ascorbic acid. False-positive results indi-

Drugs that may disrupt urine glucose tests
+ Cephalothin
+ Isoniazid
+ Levodopa
+ Probenecid
+ Ascorbic acid

cating a high glucose level could cause a patient to decrease his food intake or to increase his insulin doses when, in fact, the glucose level is stable.

Some drugs visibly affect electrocardiogram (ECG) tracings. For example, class IA and III antiarrhythmics can prolong the QT interval, as can antihistamines, antibiotics, antifungals, antidepressants, and antipsychotics. Prolonging the QT interval can lead to torsades de pointes, ventricular fibrillation, and death. No one knows why these drugs prolong the QT interval; nevertheless, you should ask about a history of syncope or cardiac arrest before giving these drugs. Also obtain a detailed family history of syncope, sudden death at a young age, or congenital deafness because a family history of these disorders suggests a predisposition for prolonged QT interval.

ADVERSE REACTIONS

A drug that produces a desired effect or expected therapeutic response can also cause an undesirable harmful response or adverse drug reaction. Adverse reactions can range from mild ones that disappear when the drug is stopped to debilitating diseases that become chronic. The severity of some adverse reactions may decrease over time.

Adverse reactions can be classified as dose-related or patient sensitivity–related. Most adverse reactions result from a drug's known pharmacologic effects and are dose-related. In most cases, these reactions can be predicted. Less common adverse reactions are unrelated to dose and result from a patient's unusual sensitivity to a drug or its components.

Dose-related adverse reactions

Dose-related reactions include secondary effects, hypersusceptibility, overdose, and iatrogenic effects. A drug typically produces not only therapeutic effects but also secondary effects that can be adverse or beneficial. For example, the analgesic morphine can lead to two adverse secondary effects: constipation and respiratory depression. The antihistamine diphenhydramine commonly causes sedation as a secondary effect, which makes the drug beneficial as a sleep aid.

A patient can be hypersusceptible to a drug's pharmacologic actions. Even when a drug is given in a usual therapeutic dose, a hypersusceptible patient can experience an excessive therapeutic response or secondary effects. Hypersusceptibility typically results from altered pharmacokinetics, which leads to a higher-than-expected drug level. It also may stem from increased receptor sensitivity, which can increase the drug's therapeutic or adverse effects.

When a patient intentionally or accidentally takes an excessive dose (overdose), he may have a toxic drug reaction. It results in an exaggerated response to the drug, which can lead to transient, minor changes or more serious, sometimes irreversible reactions, such as respiratory depression, cardiovascular collapse, or death. To avoid such toxic reactions, give lower drug doses to chronically ill or geriatric patients. These patients may have reduced renal clearance of the drug, which predisposes them to toxicity.

Iatrogenic effects can mimic disorders. For example, such drugs as antineoplastics, aspirin, corticosteroids, and indomethacin commonly cause GI irritation and bleeding, which can be mistaken for signs of peptic ulcer disease or GI tumor. Other iatrogenic effects include propranolol-induced asthma, methicillin-induced nephritis, and gentamicin-induced deafness.

Determining types of allergic reactions

Allergies to drugs and other allergens are categorized into four basic types.

TYPE	RESPONSE	EXAMPLES
I	Immediate reactions to stings and drugs	Anaphylaxis, urticaria, angioedema
II	Drug-induced autoimmune disorders	Sulfonamide-induced granulocytopenia, quinidine-induced thrombocytopenic purpura, hydralazine-induced systemic lupus erythematosus
III	Reactions to penicillins, sulfonamides, iodides; antibody targeted against tissue antigens	Urticarial skin eruptions, arthralgia, lymphadenopathy, fever
IV	Reexposure to an antigen	Poison ivy and its resulting contact dermatitis

Types of allergic reactions

✦ Type I: Immediate reaction to stings and drugs
✦ Type II: Drug-induced autoimmune disorder
✦ Type III: Reaction to penicillin, sulfonamide, or iodide in which antibody is targeted against tissue antigens
✦ Type IV: Re-exposure to an antigen

Patient sensitivity–related adverse reactions

Less common than dose-related reactions, patient sensitivity–related adverse reactions result from a patient's unusual and extreme sensitivity to a drug. They arise from a unique tissue response rather than from an exaggerated pharmacologic action. Extreme patient sensitivity can take the form of a drug allergy or an idiosyncratic response.

A drug allergy develops when a patient's immune system identifies a drug, a drug metabolite, or a drug contaminant as a dangerous foreign substance that must be neutralized or destroyed. Previous exposure to the drug or to one with a similar chemical makeup sensitizes the patient's immune system. Then reexposure causes an allergic reaction. Such a reaction directly injures cells and tissues. It also produces broader systemic damage by triggering cells to release vasoactive and inflammatory substances. An allergic reaction can vary in intensity from a mild, itchy rash to an immediate, life-threatening anaphylactic reaction with circulatory collapse and swelling of the larynx and bronchioles. (See *Determining types of allergic reactions.*)

Some sensitivity-related reactions don't result from a drug's pharmacologic properties or an allergic response, yet are specific to the individual. The cause of these distinctive responses isn't fully understood, but experts believe genetics play an important role.

CLINICAL ALERT Many common adverse reactions, such as nausea, diarrhea, dizziness, and dry mouth, don't usually endanger a patient's health. However, they can threaten his compliance with drug therapy. To help prevent this, be sure to teach your patient about potential adverse effects and ways to cope with them. Suggest that he talk to his prescriber if they become too bothersome. Also tell him not to discontinue therapy or self-treat adverse effects with OTC drugs until he speaks with his prescriber.

Teaching topics related to adverse reactions

✦ Potential adverse reactions
✦ Coping techniques
✦ When to contact prescriber
✦ Not to discontinue drug or self-treat reactions

Defining pregnancy risk categories

- ✦ **A:** Studies failed to show a risk to the fetus.
- ✦ **B:** Either animal studies showed no risk to the fetus and no human studies have been done, or animal studies showed a risk unconfirmed by evidence in humans.
- ✦ **C:** Either animal studies showed a risk to the fetus and no human studies have been done, or no studies exist in animals or humans.
- ✦ **D:** The drug may put the fetus at risk and should be given only if benefits outweigh risks.
- ✦ **X:** The drug may cause fetal abnormalities and is contraindicated in pregnant women.
- ✦ **NR:** The drug hasn't been rated.

LIFESPAN

Pregnancy risk categories

This list summarizes the Food and Drug Administration risk-factor categories for drugs used during pregnancy.

Category A: Controlled studies in women didn't show a risk to the fetus in the first trimester with no evidence of a risk in later trimesters. The possibility of harm to the fetus seems unlikely.

Category B: Either animal reproduction studies haven't shown a risk to the fetus and no controlled studies have been completed in pregnant women, or the animal reproduction studies have shown an adverse effect other than decreased fertility that wasn't confirmed in controlled studies with women in their first trimester and no evidence of a risk in later trimesters exists.

Category C: Either animal studies show adverse effects to the fetus and no controlled studies in women exist, or no studies in women or animals exist. The drug should be given only if the potential benefit to the woman justifies the potential risk to her fetus.

Category D: The drug may cause risk to the fetus but use in pregnant women may be acceptable despite the risk (for example, if the drug is needed in a life-threatening situation or if safer drugs can't be used or are ineffective for a serious disease).

Category X: Studies in animals or women show fetal abnormalities, or evidence of risk to the fetus exists based on studies in pregnant women, or both, and the risk clearly outweighs any possible benefit. The drug is contraindicated in women who are or may become pregnant.

Category NR: No rating available.

SPECIAL CONSIDERATIONS

Four types of patients need special consideration with drug therapy: pregnant, breast-feeding, pediatric, and geriatric patients. In these patients, developmental changes or immature or declining body systems can cause pharmacokinetic and pharmacodynamic differences that make drug effects less predictable than in the usual adult patients. Keep these differences in mind when giving a drug to a patient with these lifespan considerations.

PREGNANT WOMEN

Based on clinical and preclinical information, the FDA assigns a pregnancy risk category to systemically absorbed drugs. The five categories (A, B, C, D, and X) reflect a drug's potential to cause birth defects. Although a pregnant woman should avoid drugs, this rating system permits rapid assessment of the risk-benefit ratio if drugs become necessary for her. Drugs in category A generally are safe to use during pregnancy; drugs in category X generally are contraindicated. (See *Pregnancy risk categories.*)

Several pregnancy-related changes and structures can alter a drug's absorption, distribution, metabolism, and excretion. The fetus also can significantly influence drug distribution and disposition.

Because a pregnant woman may become a breast-feeding mother, the safety of a drug to the mother should be considered for her breast-fed infant as well.

Absorption

During pregnancy, GI tone and motility decrease, probably because of increased progesterone production and a decreased level of motilin (a hormone that increases intestinal motility and stimulates pepsin secretion). These effects prolong gastric emptying and intestinal transit. Hydrochloric acid formation in the stomach also decreases. All these factors delay the absorption of oral drugs that require an acidic environment or that are absorbed in the small intestine.

Parenteral drug absorption also may change during pregnancy. Because of peripheral vasodilation, drugs given by the S.C., I.M., or intradermal route may be absorbed more rapidly.

Distribution

The physiologic changes of pregnancy also alter drug distribution. Influencing factors include increased interstitial and cellular water and increased blood volume, elevated nearly 45% by the end of gestation. These increases change the ratios of blood constituents that affect drug distribution. For example, the ratio of albumin to water decreases during pregnancy, altering protein-binding capacity.

During pregnancy, estrogen and progesterone levels also rise, as do those of free fatty acids (triglycerides, cholesterol, and phospholipids) from increased fatty tissue metabolism. These effects are accompanied by increased competition for protein-binding sites. With fewer binding sites, a larger percentage of a drug remains free to move to receptor sites or across the placenta.

The term "placental barrier" can be misleading because it implies that the placenta protects the fetus from drug effects. In fact, most drugs taken by a pregnant woman will cross the placenta and reach her fetus. Although some drugs, such as insulin, don't cross the placenta, many do when given at a therapeutic level. Placental transport of substances to and from the fetus begins around the fifth week of gestation. Later in pregnancy when the placenta thins, drugs with high lipid solubility or low protein-binding ability pass more easily through the placenta.

Long-term adverse effects may occur in the child of a mother who was given certain drugs during pregnancy. Maternal use of diethylstilbestrol has been noted as a cause of vaginal adenocarcinoma in young girls, a disease that had previously been considered rare in this population.

Metabolism

Because the placenta is metabolically active, it can affect drug disposition. The placenta may perform several enzymatic reactions that can reduce the potency of a drug's metabolites. Conversely, these reactions may produce a more potent and toxic metabolite, thereby increasing danger to the fetus.

Excretion

Many pregnancy-induced changes in the urinary system can affect drug excretion. The glomerular filtration rate (GFR) and renal plasma flow increase early in pregnancy; the increased GFR persists until delivery. Because of the increased renal plasma flow, drugs that normally are excreted easily may be eliminated even more rapidly.

The fetus has slower drug clearance than the adult, and drugs persist longer in the fetus's tissues and blood than in the mother's.

Absorption-altering effects of pregnancy

+ Decreased GI tone
+ Decreased GI motility
+ Prolonged gastric emptying
+ Decreased formation of hydrochloric acid
+ Prolonged intestinal transit
+ Peripheral vasodilation

Distribution-altering effects of pregnancy

+ Increased interstitial water
+ Increased cellular water
+ Increased blood volume
+ Increased competition for protein-binding sites

Metabolism-altering effects of pregnancy

+ Metabolic activity of placenta

Excretion-altering effects of pregnancy

+ Increased GFR
+ Increased renal plasma flow
+ Increased rate of excretion

Influences on drug transfer during breast-feeding

+ Infant sucking behavior
+ Amount of milk consumed per feeding
+ Frequency of feeding

How to reduce infant exposure to drugs

+ Avoid breast-feeding during the drug's peak level.
+ Take the drug before the infant's longest sleep period.
+ Pump and discard breast milk if the drug has a short half-life.

Factors affecting absorption in children

+ Gastric pH (P.O.)
+ Shortness of intestine (P.O.)
+ Diarrhea (P.O.)
+ Decreased transit time (P.O.)
+ Vasomotor instability (I.M.)
+ Decreased muscle tone (I.M.)
+ Underdeveloped epidermis (S.C.)
+ Increased skin hydration (S.C.)

BREAST-FEEDING WOMEN

Breast-feeding confers many health benefits on the infant, such as decreased incidence of diarrhea, bacterial infections, tooth decay, and allergies. However, a woman who breast-feeds during drug therapy may subject her infant to the drug's effects. Unlike a fetus, an infant can't depend on the placenta to metabolize and excrete maternally ingested drugs. Therefore, although few drugs require a woman to stop breast-feeding entirely, the prescriber must consider which ones offer the greatest safety for the infant.

Infant sucking behavior, the amount consumed per feeding, and the frequency of breast-feeding affect the amount of drug ingested. In an infant, low gastric acidity and a slow absorption rate affect the amount of drug absorbed. Changes in protein binding in an infant may alter the drug level at receptor sites. Also, drugs that are metabolized insufficiently and excreted with difficulty by immature body systems may accumulate, increasing the risk of toxicity.

To help minimize the infant's exposure to a drug that reaches a detectable level in breast milk, you should teach the mother how to help protect her infant. Because these steps may vary with the drug used, consult a pharmacist as needed before the teaching session. To ensure success, cover these simple steps and suggest ways to accommodate daily routines and minimize disruptions.

+ Avoid breast-feeding during times of peak concentration in milk by feeding at the end of a dosing interval or by taking the drug immediately after breast-feeding.
+ Take the drug before the infant's longest sleep period to allow sufficient time for the drug to clear from the milk before the next feeding. This is especially useful for a drug that readily diffuses into breast milk.
+ Pump and discard breast milk if the drug has a short half-life. (This step isn't appropriate for drugs with a long half-life.)

PEDIATRIC PATIENTS

A child's age, physiologic state, body composition, immature organ function, and other factors can affect his drug absorption, distribution, metabolism, and excretion.

Absorption

A young child's gastric pH is higher, or less acidic, than an adult's. As the child develops, gastric pH decreases, acidity increases, and drug absorption is altered. For example, an infant absorbs nafcillin and penicillin G better than an adult because of lower gastric acidity. Milk and formula also can affect gastric pH and may alter absorption. Therefore, unless otherwise indicated, plan to give a drug when the child's stomach is empty.

Other factors can influence drug absorption from the GI tract and make absorption less predictable or less efficient in a child younger than age 2. The shortness of the intestine and the presence of diarrhea can reduce the amount of time a drug is available for absorption. Decreased transit time through the GI tract also can decrease drug absorption.

Absorption of an I.M. drug may be unpredictable in an infant because of vasomotor instability and decreased muscle tone. Percutaneous absorption of an S.C. drug is increased in an infant because of an underdeveloped epidermal barrier and increased skin hydration.

LIFESPAN

Recognizing gray baby syndrome

New, safer antibiotics have dramatically reduced the use of chloramphenicol in infants. However, if an infant must receive chloramphenicol, be alert for signs and symptoms of gray baby syndrome, which usually appear 2 to 9 days after treatment begins and may develop in this order:

◆ Vomiting
◆ Refusal to suck
◆ Loose green stools
◆ Hypotension

◆ Cyanosis
◆ Hypothermia
◆ Cardiovascular collapse
◆ Death

Distribution

A drug's distribution is affected by the drug's dilution in the body. The higher percentage of water in neonates and infants dilutes water-soluble drugs, reducing their levels in the blood. That's why a neonate or infant may require a higher mg/kg dosage to achieve a therapeutic drug level.

Body composition affects the distribution and effects of water-soluble drugs. Most drugs travel through extracellular fluid to reach their receptors. Because children have a higher percentage of fluid in their bodies, their distribution area is proportionately greater than an adult's.

To a lesser degree, body composition also affects the distribution of lipid-soluble drugs. As the percentage of body fat increases with age, so does the distribution of lipid-soluble drugs. Therefore, distribution of these drugs is more limited in children than in adults.

An infant's immature liver may affect drug distribution by decreasing plasma protein formation, which results in a lower plasma protein level and a higher fluid volume than in an adult. This reduces the number of plasma proteins for drugs to bind with. Because only unbound, or free, drugs produce pharmacologic effects, an infant's decreased protein binding can intensify drug effects and possibly cause toxicity.

Several disorders, such as nephrotic syndrome and malnutrition, may decrease the plasma protein level and increase the unbound drug concentration, intensifying the drug's effects or producing toxicity.

Metabolism

An infant's immature liver may inefficiently metabolize drugs. As the liver matures during the first year of life, drug metabolism improves. This consideration guides the choice of drugs and dosages for a child. For example, the antibiotic chloramphenicol is used in adults to treat gram-positive and gram-negative bacterial infections. However, it shouldn't be prescribed for neonates, especially premature ones, because it can be fatal. In neonates, the liver doesn't have the enzymes needed for appropriate metabolism. So the drug accumulates, causing toxicity known as gray baby syndrome. (See *Recognizing gray baby syndrome*.) I.V. drugs and flush solutions that contain the preservative benzyl alcohol also shouldn't be given to neonates because their inability to metabolize it properly can also lead to toxicity.

Factors affecting drug distribution in infants
◆ Higher percentage of water
◆ Less body fat
◆ Immature liver
◆ Disorders that decrease protein levels

Effects of children's higher percentage of water
◆ Reduced level of water-soluble drugs
◆ Greater distribution area for water-soluble drugs
◆ Limited distribution of lipid-soluble drugs

Factors affecting drug metabolism and excretion in infants
◆ Immature organs
◆ Lack of liver enzymes
◆ Slow renal excretion
◆ Low blood flow to biliary system

Excretion

Because most drugs are excreted in the urine, the degree of renal development can affect drug excretion and, ultimately, dosage requirements for a child.

At birth, the kidneys are immature, renal excretion is slow, and drug dosages must be adjusted carefully. As the kidneys mature during the first few months after birth, renal excretion of drugs increases, although the rate of increase is slow for a premature neonate.

Some drugs, such as nafcillin, are excreted by the biliary tract into the intestines. In the first few days after birth, however, biliary blood flow is low, which can prolong the drug's effects.

GERIATRIC PATIENTS

Aging is usually accompanied by a decline in organ function, which can profoundly affect drug distribution and clearance, among other things. This physiologic decline is likely to be exacerbated by a disease or chronic disorder. Such a combination can significantly increase the geriatric patient's risk of drug toxicity and adverse reactions.

Absorption

Several age-related changes in the GI system can alter drug absorption. Decreased gastric acidity may affect drug solubility and alter drug absorption. Reduced blood flow to the GI tract and the decreased number of cells available for absorption also can delay drug absorption. However, because the GI transit time is slowed, drugs remain in the system longer, which increases absorption. Overall, the effects of aging slow the absorption rate, but allow absorption to be as complete as in a younger patient.

Distribution

Proportions of fat, lean tissue, and water in the body change with age. Total body mass and lean body mass, for example, decrease with age. These changes lead to a relative increase in body fat and decrease in body water, altering the distribution of most drugs. Highly lipid-soluble drugs, such as diazepam, have an increased volume of distribution and prolonged distribution, leading to a longer half-life and duration of action. Highly water-soluble drugs, such as gentamicin, aren't distributed to fat cells. Because an elderly patient has relatively less lean tissue than a younger patient, more drug remains in the older patient's bloodstream and increases the risk of a toxic reaction.

Factors affecting absorption in geriatric patients

- ◆ Decreased gastric acidity
- ◆ Reduced GI blood flow
- ◆ Fewer cells available for absorption
- ◆ Slowed GI transit time

Factors affecting distribution in geriatric patients

- ◆ Decreased total and lean body mass
- ◆ Increased body fat
- ◆ Decreased body water
- ◆ Decreased albumin level
- ◆ Smaller body size

Aging also reduces the level of albumin, a blood protein that binds with and transports many drugs. As a result, more unbound drugs may circulate, which typically increases the effects of drugs that are highly protein-bound.

Other factors can alter drug distribution. (See *Common characteristics affecting drug distribution in geriatric patients.*) Perhaps the most significant factor is size: Geriatric patients are typically smaller than younger patients. So if a geriatric patient receives the same dose as a younger patient, the older patient's smaller volume may result in a higher drug level.

Metabolism

Aging reduces the liver's ability to metabolize drugs. Liver disease may further compromise its functioning. So may other diseases that reduce hepatic blood flow such as heart failure.

Drug metabolism depends primarily on two processes: hepatic blood flow and metabolic enzyme action. Because aging decreases hepatic blood flow, a smaller amount of the drug is delivered to the liver for metabolism to inactive compounds. Hepatic enzymes metabolize drugs in two major phases. Aging reduces the efficiency of both phases, but phase I reactions (oxidation, reduction, or hydrolysis of drug molecules) are affected more than phase II reactions (coupling of the drug or its metabolite with an acid to produce an inactive compound). Aging leads to different effects, depending on whether a drug is metabolized in phase I, phase II, or both.

Excretion

With aging, glomerular filtration and tubular secretion decline progressively. Also, dehydration and cardiovascular and renal diseases may cause renal impairment. Keep in mind that a geriatric patient has a smaller renal reserve than a younger patient, even if his blood urea nitrogen and creatinine levels appear normal.

When a geriatric patient receives a drug that isn't metabolized, monitor him for signs of toxicity because drug excretion may be delayed. Be particularly cautious with potentially nephrotoxic drugs, such as the aminoglycoside gentamicin, because they may cause severe nephrotoxicity quickly in a geriatric patient.

Drug receptors

Aging reduces the efficiency of many drug receptors and the density of beta-adrenergic receptors. As a result, geriatric patients show diminished response to drugs, such as isoproterenol, and increased toxicity from beta blockers, such as propranolol. With age comes a decline in parasympathetic control, which enhances the effects of anticholinergic drugs. Aging also reduces the number of neurotransmitters, particularly dopamine and acetylcholine, which may affect drugs such as phenothiazines and chlorpromazine.

Adverse drug reactions

Geriatric patients experience adverse drug reactions two to seven times more frequently than younger patients. Age-related physiologic changes account for many of these adverse reactions.

Age-related CNS changes may cause drug-related problems. These changes include increased sensitivity to depressants and decreased cerebral blood flow, which increase the risk of sedation and diminished cognitive function during drug therapy. Other CNS changes may include deterioration of the blood-brain barrier, which may allow a greater concentration in the CNS for some drugs and may account for many drug-induced behavioral changes in geriatric patients. One such change,

Factors affecting metabolism in geriatric patients
+ Decreased liver function
+ Decreased hepatic blood flow
+ Decreased hepatic enzyme function

Factors affecting adverse drug reactions in geriatric patients
+ Increased sensitivity to CNS depressants
+ Decreased cerebral blood flow
+ Deterioration of the blood-brain barrier

Factors affecting adverse drug reactions in geriatric patients
(continued)
+ Decreased cardiac output
+ Increased TPR
+ Increased norepinephrine level
+ Decreased efficiency of baroreceptors
+ Decreased glucose tolerance
+ Decreased thyroid function
+ Decreased respiratory function
+ Decreased GI motility
+ Musculoskeletal changes

Risk factors for adverse reactions in geriatric patients
+ Advanced age
+ Small physique
+ Multiple illnesses
+ Multi-drug therapy
+ Types of drugs taken
+ Previous adverse reactions
+ Living alone
+ Malnutrition

paradoxical excitement, can happen with the use of sedatives and anxiety-relieving drugs.

Age-related cardiovascular changes that may affect drug response include decreased cardiac output, increased total peripheral resistance (TPR), increased circulating norepinephrine, and decreased sensitivity and function of baroreceptors. These changes may contribute to adverse reactions, such as orthostatic hypotension and heart failure.

Several endocrine changes may influence drug therapy in geriatric patients. For example, a decline in glucose tolerance may cause greater hyperglycemia in response to a thiazide diuretic. Reduced response to hypoglycemia may cause a geriatric patient to delay seeking treatment until the hypoglycemia worsens. Reduced thyroid function may decrease body metabolism, which can slow drug metabolism.

Age-related changes in the respiratory, GI, urinary, and musculoskeletal systems also may cause adverse reactions in a geriatric patient. For example, decreased respiratory function may lead to increased sensitivity to respiratory depressants, such as opioids and barbiturates. Decreased GI motility and activity may cause constipation and greater sensitivity to the effects of anticholinergic drugs.

 CLINICAL ALERT Adverse reactions can easily be mistaken for signs and symptoms of aging. Be sure to ask your patient or his caregiver when such symptoms as confusion, fatigue, and urinary dysfunction began. If they first appeared *after* he started taking a particular drug, their cause may be the drug—not the aging process.

Several risk factors help identify geriatric patients who are prone to adverse reactions. These risk factors include advanced age, small physique, multiple illnesses, use of multiple drugs, type of drugs prescribed (such as CNS depressants), previous adverse reactions, living alone, and malnutrition. By identifying high-risk geriatric patients, you can help protect them by monitoring them closely, preventing errors, identifying drug-related problems promptly, and intervening as needed.

Autonomic nervous system drugs

A wide range of drugs affects the autonomic nervous system (ANS). To understand how these drugs act, you need to know about the nervous system. This body system, which controls and coordinates many body functions, has two major divisions: the central and peripheral nervous systems. The central nervous system (CNS) contains the brain and spinal cord. The peripheral nervous system contains afferent, or sensory, neurons that carry information to the CNS and efferent, or motor, neurons that carry information from the CNS. The peripheral nervous system mediates between the CNS and the external and internal environments. It's subdivided into the somatic nervous system and the ANS.

ANATOMY AND PHYSIOLOGY

Different neurons of the ANS innervate smooth and cardiac muscles, glands, and other viscera. Unlike the somatic nervous system, the autonomic nervous system is subdivided into the sympathetic nervous system (adrenergic) and the parasympathetic nervous system (cholinergic).

The sympathetic and parasympathetic nervous systems have two types of neurons (rather than one, like the somatic nervous system) that carry information to target sites. The cell bodies of the first type of neuron, like those of the somatic nervous system, originate in the CNS, but the neurons of the sympathetic and parasympathetic originate in different parts of the CNS. For example, the neurons of the sympathetic nervous system originate in the thoracic and lumbar regions of the spinal cord while those of the parasympathetic nervous system originate in the brain stem or the sacral region of the spinal cord. The two systems are known as the thoracolumbar and craniosacral divisions, respectively.

Axons from the first type of neurons leave the CNS and travel to ganglia where they synapse with a second type of neuron that travels to the target site. Because of the intervening ganglia, the axons of the first type of neurons are called preganglionic fibers; those of the second neurons, postganglionic fibers.

Reviewing the autonomic nervous system
(continued)

effector organs: preganglionic and postganglionic.
+ The ANS includes the sympathetic (adrenergic) and parasympathetic (cholinergic) nervous systems.

Sources of sympathetic stimulation

+ Neurotransmitters, such as norepinephrine, epinephrine, dopamin, and ACh
+ Drugs, such as adrenergics and adrenergic blockers

ANATOMY & PHYSIOLOGY

How the sympathetic division works

The sympathetic branch of the autonomic nervous system has two neurons that carry information to effector organs. Neurons originate from the thoracolumbar region in the central nervous system. Preganglionic and postganglionic fibers transmit nerve impulses. Preganglionic fibers are short, terminating in ganglia that lie adjacent to the spinal cord or a short distance from it. The preganglionic fiber that directly innervates the adrenal medulla without synapsing at a ganglion causes the release of norepinephrine and epinephrine directly into the circulation. Postganglionic fibers are long and travel some distance through effector cells to reach effector organs. Chemicals called neurotransmitters carry out this transmittal. Major neurotrans-

mitters are norepinephrine, epinephrine and, to a lesser extent, dopamine and acetylcholine (ACh).

Major physiologic effects are alpha and beta adrenergic: vasoconstriction; vasodilation; increased heart rate, force of contraction, and conduction velocity; bronchial smooth muscle relaxation; GI tract smooth muscle relaxation; GI sphincter contraction; urinary system smooth muscle relaxation; sphincter contraction; pupillary dilation and ciliary muscle relaxation; sweat gland secretion increase; pancreatic secretion decrease; and thick salivary secretions.

Drugs that influence these functions include adrenergics and adrenergic blockers.

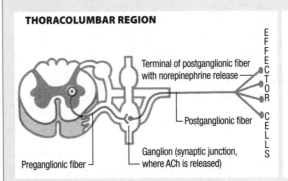

THORACOLUMBAR REGION

Terminal of postganglionic fiber with norepinephrine release

Postganglionic fiber

Ganglion (synaptic junction, where ACh is released)

Preganglionic fiber

EFFECTOR ORGANS
+ Heart
+ Bronchial smooth muscle
+ Blood vessels
+ GI tract
+ Urinary system
+ Eyes
+ Glands (sweat, pancreas, salivary)

EFFECTOR CELLS

The preganglionic fibers of the sympathetic nervous system are short, terminating in ganglia adjacent to the spinal cord (paravertebral chain) or a short distance from the cord (such as the celiac ganglion). The preganglionic fiber that innervates the adrenal medulla is an exception. It goes directly from the spinal cord to special cells in the adrenal medulla without synapsing. The adrenal medulla is like a sympathetic postganglionic neuron, in that its secretory cells originate in nervous tissue, and it releases norepinephrine and epinephrine directly into the circulation. Postganglionic fibers travel some distance to reach their target sites. (*See How the sympathetic division works.*)

In contrast, most preganglionic fibers of the parasympathetic nervous system are long and travel to ganglia close to or inside of the walls of their target sites. The postganglionic fibers of the parasympathetic nervous system are short. The unique distribution of preganglionic and postganglionic fibers allows the two systems to produce contrasting effects. The characteristics of the sympathetic nervous system permit a more generalized, widespread effect; those of the parasympathetic nervous

How the parasympathetic division works

The parasympathetic branch of the autonomic nervous system has two neurons that carry information to the cells of effector organs. Neurons originate in the craniosacral region of the central nervous system. Preganglionic and postganglionic fibers transmit nerve impulses. Most preganglionic fibers are long and travel to ganglia located close to or in the walls of the effector organs. In contrast, the postganglionic fibers are short. The major neurotransmitter is acetylcholine (Ach).

Stimulation of these nerve fibers causes vasodilation of salivary glands; decreased heart rate, force of contraction, and conduction velocity; bronchial smooth muscle constriction; increased GI tract tone and peristalsis with sphincter relaxation; urinary system sphincter relaxation and increased bladder tone; pupil constriction; and increased pancreatic, salivary, and lacrimal secretions.

Drugs that influence these functions include cholinergic agonists, anticholinesterases, and anticholinergics.

CRANIOSACRAL REGION

Terminal of postganglionic fibers (ACh release)

Postganglionic fibers

Ganglia (synaptic junction, where ACh is released)

Preganglionic fiber

EFFECTOR ORGANS

EFFECTOR CELLS

- ✦ Smooth muscle
- ✦ Glands (salivary, pancreatic, lacrimal)
- ✦ Heart
- ✦ Bronchial smooth muscle
- ✦ GI tract
- ✦ Urinary system
- ✦ Eyes

Sources of parasympathetic stimulation

- ✦ Neurotransmitters such as ACh
- ✦ Drugs, such as cholinergic agonists, anticholinesterases, and anticholinergics

Comparing sympathetic and parasympathetic stimulation

- ✦ The sympathetic nervous system helps the body cope with external stimuli and stress by triggering the fight-or-flight response.
- ✦ The parasympathetic nervous system works to save energy, aid digestion, and support resting, restorative body functions.

system permit a more discrete, localized effect. (See *How the parasympathetic division works.*)

Usually, both systems send information to the same target sites. Exceptions include the adrenal medulla, sweat glands, spleen, and hair follicles, which are innervated by the sympathetic nervous system only. Because the physiologic functions of the two systems usually are opposite, dual innervation balances the physiologic effects. Drug therapy sometimes disrupts this critical balance. For example, it may block the parasympathetic nervous system but allow the usual function of the sympathetic nervous system.

The physiologic effects of the subdivisions of the autonomic nervous system are much more complex than those of the somatic nervous system, which initiates a single activity, such as skeletal muscle contraction. In general, however, the sympathetic nervous system can be viewed as an activity-response system, and the parasympathetic nervous system as a homeostatic system.

Stimulation of the sympathetic nervous system increases the heart and respiratory rates, metabolic rate, and fat and glycogen breakdown; produces pupillary dilation, smooth muscle vasoconstriction, and skeletal muscle vasodilation; and decreases GI activity. These effects sometimes are called the fight-or-flight responses because they prepare the body to face or run from a threat.

Conversely, stimulation of the parasympathetic nervous system decreases the heart and respiratory rates, causes pupil constriction and enhanced accommodation, increases digestion and elimination, enhances GI tone, and relaxes sphincter tone. These activities conserve energy and are homeostatic.

NEUROTRANSMITTERS

The nervous system communicates via chemicals called neuroregulators (neurotransmitters) that transmit neuron information between adjacent cells. In the motor limb of the peripheral nervous system, the major neurotransmitters are acetylcholine, norepinephrine, epinephrine and, to a lesser extent, dopamine.

Acetylcholine

Acetylcholine is released from all preganglionic neurons of the autonomic nervous system, from all postganglionic neurons of the parasympathetic nervous system, from some postsynaptic neurons of the sympathetic nervous system, and at neuromuscular junctions in the somatic nervous system. Degraded rapidly by the enzyme acetylcholinesterase, acetylcholine has a short duration of action.

Norepinephrine and epinephrine

Norepinephrine and epinephrine are released from the adrenal medulla, and norepinephrine is also released from the postganglionic adrenergic fibers of the sympathetic nervous system. The norepinephrine and epinephrine released from the adrenal medulla have effects similar to direct adrenergic neuronal stimulation, but can reach and stimulate target sites that don't receive direct innervation from adrenergic fibers.

The duration of action of norepinephrine released at the synapse is extremely short because it rapidly re-enters the neuron from which it was released, diffuses from the area, or is degraded by the enzymes monoamine oxidase (MAO) or catechol-*O*-methyltransferase (COMT). The duration of action of norepinephrine and epinephrine released from the adrenal medulla, however, may be 10 times longer because removal from the circulation is slower than removal from neuronal synapses. This slower removal from the circulation emphasizes the potential difference between the effects of administered drugs and substances produced by the body.

Dopamine

Dopamine is a precursor to norepinephrine. It can interact with dopaminergic as well as alpha- and beta-adrenergic receptors and can stimulate the release of norepinephrine from adrenergic fibers.

RECEPTORS

The major classes of receptors in the motor limb of the peripheral nervous system include alpha-adrenergic, beta-adrenergic, dopaminergic, muscarinic, and nicotinic receptors. Target tissues may have one or more of these receptors. A drug's effects depend on its receptor specificity and on the numbers of each receptor in target tissue.

The catecholamines norepinephrine and epinephrine exert their effects by interacting with alpha- and beta-adrenergic receptors. Each has two subtypes: alpha$_1$ and alpha$_2$, and beta$_1$ and beta$_2$. Norepinephrine affects alpha$_1$, alpha$_2$, and beta$_1$ receptors more than beta$_2$ receptors. Epinephrine affects alpha- and beta-adrenergic receptors equally. That's why epinephrine can exert greater metabolic, vasodilatory, and bronchodilatory effects than norepinephrine can.

Dopamine can interact with dopaminergic as well as alpha- and beta-adrenergic receptors, depending on its concentration. Dopamine, given in doses of less than 5 mcg/kg/min, stimulates dopaminergic receptors, causing renal, mesenteric, and coronary dilation. Doses of 5 to 10 mcg/kg/min stimulate beta$_2$ effects, which increase cardiac contractility and heart rate. Doses higher than 10 mcg/kg/min stimulate alpha effects, which cause arterial vasoconstriction and increase blood pressure. Alpha-adrenergic receptors that regulate sympathetic transmission to the cardiovascular system also exist in the CNS. Therefore, all drugs that act on receptors in the CNS can influence the peripheral nervous system.

Acetylcholine exerts its effects by interacting with nicotinic and muscarinic receptors. Muscarinic receptors are found at the synapses of the postsynaptic fibers of the parasympathetic nervous system, on some postsynaptic fibers of the sympathetic nervous system, and in the CNS. Nicotinic receptors are located in the autonomic ganglia, which are located between presynaptic and postsynaptic fibers of the autonomic nervous system, in the motor end plates (the branching terminals at the end of the motor nerve axon) at the neuromuscular junction of the somatic nervous system, and in the CNS. Nicotinic receptors in skeletal muscles have different properties than those in autonomic ganglia.

Presynaptic receptors

Neuroregulators and presynaptic receptors on neurons control the amount of a neurotransmitter released from a neuron. Presynaptic alpha-adrenergic receptors are alpha-adrenergic$_2$ receptors.

Presynaptic receptors impact a drug's effect. For example, an adrenergic blocker that nonselectively blocks alpha$_1$ and alpha$_2$ receptors will block the contraction of vascular smooth muscle (alpha$_1$) and the negative feedback to adrenergic fibers (alpha$_2$). The negative feedback block will release more norepinephrine that can stimulate the heart's beta receptors and cause tachycardia.

Receptor regulation

Changes in the environment can change receptor number or density (up or down regulation) or change a receptor's affinity for an agonist or antagonist (uncoupling). Therapeutic effects and withdrawal effects are related to receptor number or affinity. For instance, long-term use of a beta agonist can decrease the density of beta receptors and reduce the drug's effects. In contrast, long-term use of a beta antagonist (beta blocker) can increase receptor density and the response to sudden withdrawal of a beta blocker.

Disorders such as diabetes mellitus, hypothyroidism, and hyperthyroidism can affect receptor density or affinity.

Nonspecificity

Drugs can't be directed to a select body area or tissue site. Rather, they act on all receptors to which they have access and can bind. Because the CNS contains receptors for acetylcholine, norepinephrine, and epinephrine, drugs given to affect acetylcholine in the peripheral neurons can exert unwanted CNS effects if they cross the blood-brain barrier.

What influences receptors?

+ Environmental changes
+ Therapeutic drug effects
+ Withdrawal effects
+ Certain diseases, such as diabetes and thyroid disorders

Understanding nonspecificity

+ A drug can't be directed to a specific site. Rather, it acts on all receptors to which it has access and can bind.

DRUG SELECTION AND CLASSES

Drugs affect neural transmission in several ways. For example, they may imitate a neurotransmitter's action, block its effect at a receptor site, or enhance or inhibit its synthesis, storage, release, or breakdown. Drugs may also alter the ability of post-synaptic target cells to recover from stimulation.

Drug selection is based on mechanism of action and clinical objectives. For example, if hypertension treatment is aimed at lowering the norepinephrine level to minimize vasoconstriction, the prescriber will consider a drug that inhibits norepinephrine's effects. Drug selection also is based on target tissue specificity, efficacy, adverse effects, toxicity, and cost. The cost must be evaluated in dollars and effects on the patient's physical and psychological functioning.

Drugs that influence the somatic or autonomic nervous systems can be classified by the location of their primary effect; their primary effect, such as promotion or inhibition of sympathetic or parasympathetic effects; and the receptor with which they interact.

Drug classes that produce effects similar to acetylcholine include cholinergics, parasympathomimetics, cholinesterase inhibitors, muscarinic agents, and nicotinic agents. Drugs that inhibit the sympathetic nervous system may also permit acetylcholine's activity in the parasympathetic nervous system.

Drug classes that inhibit the effects of acetylcholine include anticholinergics, parasympatholytics, antimuscarinics, ganglionic blockers, and neuromuscular blockers. Drugs that promote sympathetic nervous system activity may also antagonize acetylcholine's effects.

Drug classes that produce effects similar to norepinephrine and epinephrine include adrenergics (catecholamines or noncatecholamines that are alpha-adrenergic, beta-adrenergic, dopaminergic, or nonselective), sympathomimetics, and MAO inhibitors. Drugs that inhibit the parasympathetic nervous system may also allow sympathetic nervous system activity.

Drug classes that inhibit the effects of norepinephrine and epinephrine include sympatholytics, adrenergic blockers, and ganglionic blockers, which block the sympathetic and parasympathetic nervous systems at the preganglionic level. Drugs that promote parasympathetic activity also indirectly may antagonize the effects of norepinephrine and epinephrine.

CHOLINERGICS

Cholinergics promote the action of the neurotransmitter acetylcholine. They're also called parasympathomimetics because they produce effects that imitate parasympathetic nerve stimulation. Cholinergics fall into two major classes: cholinergic agonists, which mimic acetylcholine's action, and anticholinesterases, which inhibit acetylcholine destruction at cholinergic receptors. (See *How cholinergics work*.)

CHOLINERGIC AGONISTS

By directly stimulating cholinergic receptors, cholinergic agonists mimic the action of acetylcholine. These drugs include acetylcholine, bethanechol, carbachol, cevimeline, and pilocarpine.

Acetylcholine is rarely given because it can act on nicotinic and muscarinic receptors, causing unpredictable effects, and because it's rapidly destroyed by acetylcholinesterase. Although the other cholinergic agonists resist breakdown by acetylcholinesterase, they also lack specificity of action. They're given for their effects on the eyes, intestines, and bladder; however, their widespread parasympathomimetic actions can produce many adverse effects.

Criteria for drug selection

+ Drug mechanism of action
+ Clinical objectives
+ Target tissue specificity
+ Drug efficacy
+ Adverse effects
+ Toxicity
+ Cost

Features of cholinergic agonists

+ Directly stimulate cholinergic receptors
+ Mimic the action of acetylcholine
+ Used for their effects on the eyes, intestines, and bladder

EYE ON DRUG ACTION

How cholinergics work

Cholinergics fall into one of two major classes: cholinergic agonists and anticholinesterases. Here's how these drugs achieve their effects.

CHOLINERGIC AGONISTS
When a neuron in the parasympathetic nervous system is stimulated, the neurotransmitter acetylcholine is released. Acetylcholine crosses the synapse and interacts with receptors in an adjacent neuron. Cholinergic agonists work by stimulating cholinergic receptors, mimicking the action of acetylcholine.

ANTICHOLINESTERASES
After acetylcholine stimulates the cholinergic receptor, it's destroyed by the enzyme acetylcholinesterase. Anticholinesterases produce their effects by inhibiting acetylcholinesterase. Acetylcholine isn't broken down and begins to accumulate; therefore, its effects are prolonged.

Actions of cholinergics
✦ Cholinergic agonists stimulate cholinergic receptors, mimicking the action of acetylcholine.
✦ Anticholinesterases inhibit acetylcholinesterase, which prolongs the effects of acetylcholine by preventing its breakdown.

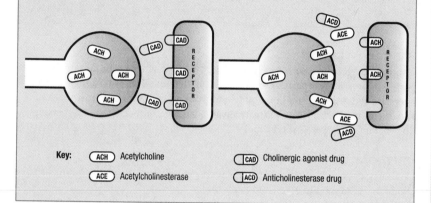

Key:
(ACH) Acetylcholine
(ACE) Acetylcholinesterase
(CAD) Cholinergic agonist drug
(ACD) Anticholinesterase drug

Pharmacokinetics
The action and metabolism of cholinergic agonists vary widely. Because acetylcholine poorly penetrates the CNS, its effects are primarily peripheral and widespread. The drug is rapidly destroyed in the body.

Cholinergic agonists rarely are given I.M. or I.V. because they're almost immediately broken down by cholinesterases in interstitial spaces and in blood vessels. Also, their rapid action can lead to cholinergic crisis. (See *Identifying signs and symptoms of cholinergic crisis*, page 32.)

Usually, cholinergic agonists are given topically as eye drops, orally, or subcutaneously. Compared to oral doses, subcutaneous (S.C.) injections act more rapidly and may produce a more effective response. All cholinergic agonists are metabolized by cholinesterases at muscarinic and nicotinic receptors in the plasma and liver and excreted by the kidneys.

Pharmacodynamics
Cholinergic agonists work by mimicking the action of acetylcholine on the neurons of target organs. When they bind with receptors on the cell membranes of target organs, they stimulate muscles and cause salivation, bradycardia, vasodilation, bronchoconstriction, increased GI tract activity, increased tone and contraction of bladder muscles, and pupil constriction.

Conditions that call for cholinergic agonists

+ Atonic bladder, as in post-operative or postpartum urine retention
+ GI disorders such as GI atony
+ Glaucoma
+ Salivary gland hypofunction

Possible drug interactions

+ Ambenonium
+ Atropine
+ Belladonna
+ Edrophonium
+ Homatropine
+ Methantheline
+ Methscopolamine
+ Neostigmine
+ Physostigmine
+ Propantheline
+ Pyridostigmine
+ Quinidine
+ Scopolamine

Adverse reactions to watch for

+ Belching, nausea, vomiting
+ Intestinal cramps, diarrhea
+ Blurred vision, decreased accommodation
+ Hypotension
+ Increased salivation or sweating
+ Shortness of breath
+ Urinary frequency

WARNING

Identifying signs and symptoms of cholinergic crisis

During cholinergic therapy, be alert for cholinergic crisis and provide appropriate treatment promptly. Without immediate intervention, the crisis may lead to cardiac arrest, respiratory paralysis, pulmonary edema, and death. Signs and symptoms of cholinergic crisis may include:

+ Blurred vision
+ Bradycardia
+ Bronchospasm
+ Cardiac sphincter spasm
+ Diarrhea
+ Excessive salivation and sweating

+ Hypotension
+ Incoordination
+ Increased bronchial secretions
+ Muscle cramps
+ Nausea
+ Paralysis

+ Pupil constriction
+ Tachycardia
+ Tearing
+ Vomiting
+ Weakness

Pharmacotherapeutics

Cholinergic agonists are used to treat atonic (weak) bladder conditions, including postoperative and postpartum urine retention; to treat GI disorders, such as postoperative abdominal distention and GI atony; to reduce eye pressure in glaucoma and during eye surgery; and to treat salivary gland hypofunction caused by radiation therapy or Sjögren's syndrome.

Interactions

Cholinergic agonists interact in specific ways with different drugs, including other cholinergics, anticholinergics, and quinidine.

+ Other cholinergics, particularly anticholinesterases such as ambenonium, edrophonium, neostigmine, physostigmine, and pyridostigmine, boost the effects of cholinergic agonists and increase the risk of cholinergic toxicity.

+ Anticholinergics, such as atropine, belladonna, homatropine, methantheline, methscopolamine, propantheline, and scopolamine, reduce the effects of cholinergic agonists.

+ Quinidine also reduces the effectiveness of cholinergic agonists.

Adverse reactions

Adverse reactions to cholinergic agonists usually stem from the drug's effects in the parasympathetic nervous system. Typically, these drugs bind with receptors in the parasympathetic nervous system, creating undesirable parasympathomimetic effects outside the target organ. For example, the use of bethanechol to reduce urine retention also will increase GI motility, which may cause nausea, belching, vomiting, intestinal cramps, and diarrhea. The drug's effects on the eyes may include blurred vision and decreased accommodation. With high doses, it may cause such cardiovascular responses as vasodilation, decreased heart rate, and decreased force of cardiac contraction, which may cause hypotension. Salivation or sweating may increase greatly. The drug's bronchoconstrictor effect may produce shortness of breath. Even the desired effect on the bladder may cause problems if urinary frequency replaces urine retention. Usually, the greater the dose, the greater the generalized parasympathomimetic effect.

Teaching a patient about cholinergic agonists

Whenever a cholinergic agonist is prescribed, teach the patient and his family the drug's name, dose, frequency, action, and adverse effects, such as headache, dizziness, and decreased night vision. Also take the following action.

✦ Instruct the patient to take the cholinergic agonist 1 hour before or 2 hours after meals to minimize adverse reactions.
✦ Show the patient how to instill an ophthalmic preparation.
✦ Advise the patient that his vision may blur and his accommodation may decrease.
✦ Tell the patient to notify the prescriber if adverse reactions occur.

Cholinergic overstimulation can result from patient hypersensitivity, drug overdose or, rarely, S.C. administration. This overstimulation may cause circulatory collapse, resulting in hypotension, shock, and cardiac arrest.

Nursing considerations
✦ Monitor the patient for adverse reactions.
✦ Keep respiratory support equipment readily available.
✦ Observe the patient for 30 to 60 minutes after giving S.C.; have a syringe of atropine available to use as an antidote.
✦ Check vital signs and auscultate for breath sounds during therapy.
✦ Give on an empty stomach to minimize nausea and vomiting.
✦ Tell the prescriber if the patient has been taking a different cholinergic or an anticholinergic.
✦ Notify the prescriber if the patient shows signs that the drug is becoming less effective.
✦ Monitor urine output in a patient receiving the drug for acute urine retention. Make sure the patient urinates within 1 hour of receiving the drug. If not, the patient should be catheterized.

 CLINICAL ALERT Don't confuse acetylcholine with acetylcysteine. Also, don't confuse neostigmine vials with etomidate vials, which may look alike.

✦ Teach the patient about the prescribed drug. (See *Teaching a patient about cholinergic agonists.*)

ANTICHOLINESTERASES

Anticholinesterases inhibit the action of the enzyme acetylcholinesterase at cholinergic receptors, preventing the breakdown of acetylcholine. This allows acetylcholine to build up and continue to stimulate cholinergic receptors.

Anticholinesterases are categorized as reversible and irreversible. Reversible anticholinesterases have a short duration of action. They include ambenonium, demecarium, donepezil, edrophonium, galantamine, guanidine, neostigmine, physostigmine, pyridostigmine, rivastigmine, and tacrine. Irreversible anticholinesterase drugs have long-lasting effects and are used primarily in toxic insec-

Key nursing actions
✦ Watch patient for 30 to 60 minutes after S.C. injection; keep atropine available.
✦ Check vital signs and breath sounds.
✦ Make sure the patient has an empty stomach.
✦ Monitor urine output.

Features of anticholinesterases
✦ Inhibit the enzyme acetylcholinesterase, causing acetylcholine to build up
✦ May be reversible (short duration of action) or irreversible (long duration of action)

Treating cholinergic crisis caused by nerve gas

Nerve gas is an irreversible anticholinesterase that may be used as a chemical weapon. When inhaled, the gas permanently binds with acetylcholinesterase, resulting in cholinergic crisis. The resulting respiratory paralysis often leads to death.

To prevent this, use pyridostigmine to pretreat the patient before nerve gas exposure. At the first sign of exposure, however, discontinue this drug. To reverse nerve gas toxicity, promptly give two parenteral antidotes: atropine and pralidoxime.

If nerve gas exposure produces eye pain, treat it with a mild, mydriatic-cycloplegic ophthalmic solution, such as 0.5% tropicamide.

ticides, pesticides, and nerve gas for chemical warfare. (See *Treating cholinergic crisis caused by nerve gas.*)

Only one, echothiophate, has therapeutic usefulness.

Pharmacokinetics

Most anticholinesterases are readily absorbed from the GI tract, subcutaneous tissue, and mucous membranes. One exception is neostigmine, which is poorly absorbed from the GI tract and requires higher doses when the patient takes it orally. However, the patient doesn't need to take it as frequently because the oral drug acts longer. When rapid effects are needed, the drug should be given I.M. or I.V.

Physostigmine and rivastigmine can cross the blood-brain barrier. Donepezil is highly bound to plasma proteins. Tacrine is about 55% bound to plasma proteins, rivastigmine is 40% bound, and galantamine is 18% bound. Most anticholinesterases are metabolized by enzymes in the plasma and are excreted in the urine. Donepezil, galantamine, and tacrine are metabolized in the liver.

Pharmacodynamics

Like cholinergic agonists, anticholinesterases promote acetylcholine's action at receptor sites. Depending on the site and the drug's dose and duration of action, they can produce stimulant or depressant effects on cholinergic receptors.

Reversible anticholinesterases block the breakdown of acetylcholine for minutes to hours. Irreversible anticholinesterases produce blocking effects that last for days to weeks.

Pharmacotherapeutics

Anticholinesterases have various therapeutic uses. They're used to reduce eye pressure in glaucoma and during eye surgery, to increase bladder tone, and to improve GI tone and peristalsis in patients with reduced motility and paralytic ileus. They're also used to promote muscle contractions in patients with myasthenia gravis, and neostigmine and edrophonium aid in diagnosing myasthenia gravis. Anticholinesterases can serve as antidotes to anticholinergics, tricyclic antidepressants, belladonna alkaloids, and opioids. They're also used to treat mild to moderate dementia in Alzheimer's disease. (See *Contraindications and precautions for anticholinesterases.*)

Interactions

A number of interactions can occur with anticholinesterases.

Uses of anticholinesterases

- To reduce eye pressure
- To increase bladder tone
- To improve GI tone and peristalsis
- To promote muscle contractions and help diagnose myasthenia gravis
- To act as an antidote to anticholinergics, tricyclic antidepressants, belladonna alkaloids, opioids
- To treat mild to moderate dementia in Alzheimer's disease

Contraindications and precautions for anticholinesterases

Anticholinesterases are contraindicated in patients with mechanical intestinal and urinary obstructions.

Use these drugs cautiously in patients with bronchial asthma, seizure disorder, bradycardia, recent coronary occlusion, vagotonia, hyperthyroidism, arrhythmias, or peptic ulcer. Cardiac and respiratory arrest, possibly vagotonic effects, may occur.

✦ Other cholinergics, particularly cholinergic agonists (such as bethanechol, carbachol, and pilocarpine), can increase the risk of toxic effects when taken with an anticholinesterase drug.
✦ Carbamazepine, dexamethasone, phenobarbital, phenytoin, and rifampin may increase donepezil's rate of elimination.
✦ Aminoglycoside antibiotics, anesthetics, anticholinergics (such as atropine, belladonna, propantheline, and scopolamine), antiarrhythmics (such as procainamide and quinidine), corticosteroids, and magnesium can reduce the effects of an anticholinesterase drug and can mask early signs of cholinergic crisis.

Adverse reactions

Adverse reactions to anticholinesterases almost always result from the increased action of acetylcholine at parasympathetic, motor, and CNS receptors. These reactions are difficult to control, particularly at high doses.

Parasympathomimetic effects are common. In the eyes, they include blurred vision, decreased accommodation, and miosis; in the skin, increased sweating; in the GI system, increased salivation, belching, nausea, vomiting, intestinal cramps, and diarrhea. The bronchoconstrictor effect may lead to shortness of breath, wheezing, or tightness in the chest. Vasodilation, decreased cardiac rate, and decreased cardiac contraction can result in hypotension, although this effect is offset partially by decreased acetylcholine metabolism at preganglionic receptors in the sympathetic nervous system. At the motor end plate, hyperpolarization of skeletal muscles reduces effective contractions. Adverse CNS reactions include irritability, anxiety or fear, and seizures.

Reactions to anticholinesterases are difficult to predict in a patient with myasthenia gravis. The therapeutic dose varies from day to day, and increased muscle weakness may result from underdosage, drug resistance, or overdosage. Differentiating between a toxic response and myasthenic crisis may be difficult. When edrophonium is used to distinguish between the two, respiratory support equipment, atropine, and other emergency drugs must be available to counteract cholinergic crisis.

Nursing considerations

✦ Have respiratory support equipment available. Keep suction equipment, oxygen, and a mechanical ventilator on hand if edrophonium is used.
✦ Observe the patient for adverse reactions and interactions and notify the prescriber if they occur.
✦ Monitor the patient's vital signs and respiratory status.

Possible drug interactions

✦ Aminoglycosides
✦ Anesthetics
✦ Antiarrhythmics
✦ Anticholinergics
✦ Carbamazepine
✦ Cholinergic agonists
✦ Corticosteriods
✦ Dexamethasone
✦ Magnesium
✦ Phenobarbital
✦ Phenytoin
✦ Rifampin

Adverse reactions to watch for

✦ Blurred vision, decreased accommodation, miosis
✦ Hypotension
✦ Increased salivation, belching, nausea, vomiting, intestinal cramps, diarrhea
✦ Increased sweating
✦ Irritability, anxiety, fear
✦ Seizures
✦ Shortness of breath, wheezing, tightness in the chest

PATIENT TEACHING

Teaching a patient about anticholinesterases

Whenever an anticholinesterase drug is prescribed, teach the patient and his family the drug's name, dose, frequency, action, and adverse effects and take the following actions.
◆ Help the patient develop a system for keeping track of each dose and its effects.
◆ Suggest ways to manage common adverse reactions. For example, tell the patient to take the drug with food or milk if nausea occurs after oral administration.
◆ Advise the patient to avoid over-the-counter cold or sleep remedies because of the risk of increased anticholinergic effects.
◆ Show the patient how to assess and record changes in muscle strength. Then help the patient practice this assessment.
◆ Advise the patient to report adverse reactions to the prescriber.

Key nursing actions
◆ Keep respiratory support equipment nearby.
◆ Monitor vital signs and respiratory status.
◆ Watch for evidence of a toxic response.
◆ Keep atropine nearby.
◆ Use seizure precautions.
◆ Watch for and document changes in muscle strength.

◆ Monitor the patient closely for signs of a toxic response, such as generalized weakness, fasciculations, dysphagia, and respiratory weakness.
◆ Keep 0.6 mg atropine readily available in a syringe as an antidote.
◆ Take seizure precautions.
◆ Maintain a calm environment.
◆ Encourage the patient to express feelings of anxiety.
◆ Monitor the patient daily for changes in muscle strength during anticholinesterase therapy and record all changes.
◆ Teach the patient and his family about the prescribed drug. (See *Teaching a patient about anticholinesterases.*)

ANTICHOLINERGICS

Anticholinergics interrupt parasympathetic nerve impulses in the central and autonomic nervous systems. These drugs also are called *cholinergic blockers* because they prevent acetylcholine from stimulating cholinergic receptors. Anticholinergics only block muscarinic receptors, which are stimulated by the alkaloid muscarine and blocked by atropine.

Features of anticholinergics
◆ Interrupt parasympathetic nerve impulses in the central and autonomic nervous systems
◆ Also called *cholinergic blockers*
◆ Prevent cholinergic receptor stimulation by acetylcholine

Types of anticholinergics include belladonna alkaloids, quaternary ammonium drugs, and tertiary amines. As the major anticholinergics, belladonna alkaloids include atropine, belladonna, homatropine, hyoscyamine, and scopolamine. Quaternary ammonium drugs, which are synthetic derivatives of belladonna alkaloids, include glycopyrrolate, methscopolamine, and propantheline. Tertiary amines include benztropine, dicyclomine, oxybutynin, tolterodine, and trihexyphenidyl. Because benztropine and trihexyphenidyl are used almost exclusively to treat parkinsonism, they're discussed in chapter 3, Neurologic and neuromuscular drugs.

Pharmacokinetics
The belladonna alkaloids are absorbed from the eyes, GI tract, mucous membranes, and skin. The quaternary ammonium drugs and tertiary amines are absorbed primarily through the GI tract, although not as readily as the belladonna alkaloids.

The belladonna alkaloids are distributed more widely throughout the body than the quaternary ammonium drugs or dicyclomine. Unlike other anticholinergics, the belladonna alkaloids readily cross the blood-brain barrier. The alkaloids exhibit low to moderate binding with serum proteins, are metabolized in the liver, and are excreted by the kidneys as unchanged drug and metabolites.

The quaternary ammonium drugs undergo hydrolysis in the GI tract and liver and are excreted in feces and urine. Dicyclomine's metabolism is unknown, but its excretion appears equal in feces and urine.

Pharmacodynamics

Anticholinergics can have paradoxical effects on the body. For example, they can produce stimulating or depressing effects, depending on the dosage and target organ. In the brain, they cause both — low drug levels stimulate and high drug levels depress.

The effects of anticholinergics also depend on the patient's disorder. Parkinsonism, for example, is characterized by a low dopamine level that intensifies acetylcholine's stimulating effects. Cholinergic blockers, however, depress these effects. In other disorders, the drugs stimulate the CNS.

Pharmacotherapeutics

In many patients, anticholinergics are used to treat GI disorders and complications:
+ Anticholinergics are used to treat spastic or hyperactive conditions of the GI and urinary tracts because they relax muscles and decrease GI secretions. The quaternary ammonium compounds, such as propantheline, are the drugs of choice for these conditions because they cause fewer adverse reactions than the belladonna alkaloids.
+ The belladonna alkaloids are used with morphine to treat biliary colic, which is pain caused by calculi in the bile duct.
+ Anticholinergics are injected before diagnostic tests, such as endoscopy or sigmoidoscopy, to relax GI smooth muscles.
+ Atropine and similar anticholinergics are given before surgery to reduce oral and gastric secretions, reduce respiratory secretions, and prevent a drop in heart rate caused by vagal nerve stimulation during anesthesia.

The belladonna alkaloids can be used to affect the brain in several ways:
+ When given with the analgesics morphine or meperidine, scopolamine is used to cause drowsiness and amnesia in patients having surgery.
+ By itself, scopolamine is used to treat motion sickness.
+ Anticholinergics can be used to treat extrapyramidal symptoms caused by drugs or Parkinson's disease.

The belladonna alkaloids also have important therapeutic effects on the heart. Atropine is the drug of choice to treat symptomatic sinus bradycardia, in which the slow heart rate causes hypotension and dizziness. (See *How atropine speeds the heart rate*, page 38.) It's particularly useful when bradycardia results from anesthetics, choline esters, or succinylcholine.

Anticholinergics also are used as cycloplegics: they paralyze the ciliary muscles and alter the lens shape. In addition, they act as mydriatics to dilate the pupils. This makes it easier to measure refractive errors during an eye examination or to perform eye surgery.

The belladonna alkaloids, particularly atropine and hyoscyamine, are effective antidotes to cholinergics and anticholinesterases. Atropine is the drug of choice to treat organophosphate pesticide poisoning. Atropine and hyoscyamine also counteract the effects of neuromuscular blockers by competing for the same receptor sites. (See *Contraindications and precautions for anticholinergics,* page 39.)

Paradoxical effects
+ Anticholinergics can produce stimulating or depressing effects, depending on the dosage, target organ, and disease being treated.

Uses of anticholinergics
+ To treat spastic or hyperactive conditions of the GI or urinary tract
+ To treat biliary colic
+ To treat motion sickness
+ To treat extrapyramidal symptoms caused by drugs or Parkinson's disease
+ To treat symptomatic sinus bradycardia
+ To paralyze ciliary muscles, alter the shape of the ocular lens, and dilate pupils
+ To relax GI smooth muscles before diagnostic tests
+ To reduce oral, gastric, and respiratory secretions and prevent decreased heart rate during anesthesia
+ To cause perioperative drowsiness and amnesia
+ To provide an antidote to cholinergics and anticholinesterases
+ To treat organophosphate pesticide poisoning
+ To counteract the effects of neuromusclar blockers

EYE ON DRUG ACTION

How atropine speeds the heart rate

To understand how atropine affects the heart, first consider how the heart's electrical conduction system functions.

WITHOUT THE DRUG

When the neurotransmitter acetylcholine is released, the vagus nerve stimulates the sinoatrial (SA) node (the heart's pacemaker) and atrioventricular (AV) node, which controls conduction between the atria and ventricles of the heart. This stimulation inhibits electrical conduction and causes the heart rate to slow down.

WITH THE DRUG

When a patient receives the anticholinergic atropine, the drug competes with acetylcholine for binding with cholinergic receptors on the SA and AV nodes. By blocking acetylcholine, atropine speeds up the heart rate.

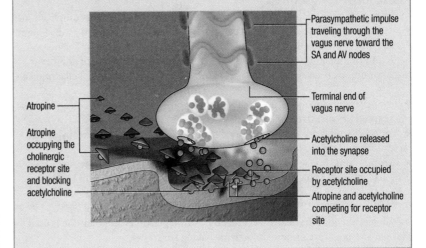

- Parasympathetic impulse traveling through the vagus nerve toward the SA and AV nodes
- Terminal end of vagus nerve
- Acetylcholine released into the synapse
- Receptor site occupied by acetylcholine
- Atropine and acetylcholine competing for receptor site
- Atropine
- Atropine occupying the cholinergic receptor site and blocking acetylcholine

Possible drug interactions

- ✦ Anticholinesterases
- ✦ Antidyskinetics
- ✦ Antiemetics
- ✦ Antipsychotics
- ✦ Antivertigo drugs
- ✦ Cholinergic agonists
- ✦ Cyclobenzaprine
- ✦ Digoxin
- ✦ Disopyramide
- ✦ Orphenadrine
- ✦ Phenothiazines
- ✦ Tetracyclic antidepressants
- ✦ Tricyclic antidepressants

Interactions

Because anticholinergics slow the passage of food and drugs through the stomach, drugs remain in prolonged contact with the GI mucous membranes. This increases the amount of drug absorbed—and the risk of adverse effects.

Drugs that increase the effects of anticholinergics include antidyskinetics (such as amantadine), antiemetics and antivertigo drugs (such as buclizine, cyclizine, diphenhydramine, and meclizine), antipsychotics (such as haloperidol, phenothiazines, and thioxanthenes), cyclobenzaprine, disopyramide, orphenadrine, and tricyclic and tetracyclic antidepressants.

Drugs that decrease the effects of anticholinergics include cholinergic agonists and anticholinesterases.

Besides increased and decreased effects of anticholinergics, other interactions may occur.

✦ When digoxin tablets are taken with an anticholinergic, the risk of digoxin toxicity increases, possibly because the anticholinergic decreases GI motility. For patient safety, monitor the digoxin level and use it to guide dosage adjustments. Or use the elixir or capsule form of digoxin to help prevent toxicity.

✦ Anticholinergics may decrease the therapeutic effects of phenothiazines (such as chlorpromazine, fluphenazine, prochlorperazine, and thioridazine) by antagonizing the CNS pathways involved in cholinergic mechanisms or by accelerating GI metabolism of phenothiazine. This interaction may occur because increasing the metabolism of a drug clears it more quickly from the body, possibly before the therapeutic benefit is achieved.

Adverse reactions

An anticholinergic's widespread actions commonly produce therapeutic benefits as well as undesirable effects. Giving drugs that interact with anticholinergics further increases the risk of adverse reactions.

Adverse reactions are a function of the muscarinic receptor's affinity for specific drugs and of the drug dosage. Dosage is crucial: the difference between a therapeutic and a toxic dose is small with anticholinergics. Some people are much more susceptible than others to the effects of these drugs. These include infants, children with spastic paralysis or brain damage, patients with Down syndrome, and geriatric patients.

As the dosage increases, adverse reactions increase in severity. Small doses may cause decreased salivation, bronchial secretions, and sweating—reducing the patient's ability to cope with heat. With higher doses, the pupils dilate, visual accommodation decreases, and the heart rate increases. Still larger doses inhibit urination and intestinal motility, followed by a decrease in gastric secretions and motility.

With drug overdose, all these effects are exaggerated. At a toxic level, CNS excitation is prominent. The patient becomes restless, irritable, and disoriented, even hallucinatory or delirious. If the process isn't reversed, the excitatory phase leads to CNS depression, unconsciousness, medullary paralysis, and death.

Anticholinergics may precipitate problems in patients with some underlying diseases. The drugs sometimes cause a dangerous rise in intraocular pressure in those with unrecognized narrow-angle glaucoma.

In a patient with coronary artery disease, anticholinergic-induced tachycardia can lead to circulatory failure. This may be compounded by the atrial and ventricular arrhythmias that sometimes occur with these drugs.

Adverse reactions to watch for

✦ Decreased salivation, bronchial secretions, and sweating, which decreases heat tolerance
✦ Dilated pupils, decreased accommodation, increased heart rate
✦ Decreased urination, GI motility, gastric secretions

Evidence of overdose

✦ Prominent CNS excitation
✦ Restlessness, irritability, disorientation, hallucinations or delirium
✦ Eventual CNS depression, unconsciousness, medullary paralysis, death

LIFESPAN

Preventing heatstroke in geriatric patients

For a geriatric patient who takes an anticholinergic and lives in a warm climate or an area with hot summers, discuss heatstroke. Anticholinergics increase the risk of heatstroke, especially in older individuals, especially those with cardiovascular disease. To help prevent heatstroke, instruct the patient to remain indoors during hot weather, use an air conditioner or fan, and drink plenty of cool liquids.

When to use extra caution
+ Narrow-angle glaucoma
+ Coronary artery disease
+ Benign prostatic hyperplasia
+ Advanced age
+ Hot weather
+ Strenuous activity

In a patient with benign prostatic hyperplasia, anticholinergics may cause urine retention. That's why these drugs should be used cautiously in geriatric men.

Heatstroke, another danger for patients taking these drugs because they inhibit such heat-regulating mechanisms as sweating, produces extreme elevation in body temperature, dehydration, flushing, and mental changes. It occurs more commonly with strenuous activity, high environmental temperatures, and advanced age. (See *Preventing heatstroke in geriatric patients*.)

Nursing considerations
+ Teach the patient and his family about the prescribed drug. (See *Teaching a patient about anticholinergics*.)
+ Monitor the patient regularly for adverse reactions and interactions and notify the prescriber if they occur. Adverse reactions increase in severity as the dosage increases.

Key nursing actions
+ Watch for evidence of heatstroke, such as dehydration, flushing, and decreased level of consciousness.
+ Encourage extra fluids, unless contraindicated, during strenuous activity or hot weather.
+ Watch for evidence of urine retention.

PATIENT TEACHING

Teaching a patient about anticholinergics

Whenever an anticholinergic is prescribed, teach the patient and his family its name, dose, frequency, action, and adverse effects and take the following actions.
+ Teach the patient to avoid drug toxicity by taking the drug dose only as ordered. Advise the patient to take a missed dose as soon as possible. If it's almost time for the next dose, tell the patient to wait until then and take a single dose only. Urge the patient not to double the dose without consulting his prescriber.
+ Advise the patient to avoid driving and other hazardous activities if drowsiness, dizziness, or blurred vision occurs.
+ Teach the patient to reduce the risk of heatstroke by moving slowly and staying in the shade in hot weather, avoiding strenuous exercise, and using fans or air conditioners.
+ Advise the patient to limit milk and bedtime snacks because they increase gastric secretions.
+ Teach the patient to consume a high-fiber diet and plenty of fluids to help prevent constipation. If needed, suggest the use of an over-the-counter stool softener.
+ Instruct the patient to notify the prescriber if urine retention or urinary hesitancy occurs.
+ Recommend that the patient wear dark glasses and avoid driving if the drug produces pupil dilation and blurred vision.
+ Teach the patient about the need for thorough oral hygiene to decrease the likelihood of cavities and gum disease caused by decreased salivation.
+ Recommend sugarless gum, hard sugarless candies, or ice to reduce dry mouth.

CLINICAL ALERT An anticholinergic overdose may produce curarelike effects, such as respiratory paralysis. Keep emergency equipment readily available.

✦ Give an anticholinergic 30 to 60 minutes before meals and at bedtime when used to reduce GI motility.

 CLINICAL ALERT Dicyclomine labeling may be misleading. The ampule label reads 10 mg/ml, but doesn't state that the ampule contains 2 ml of solution — or 20 mg of drug.

✦ Monitor the patient for signs of heatstroke, such as dehydration, flushing, and decreased level of consciousness. Anticholinergic-induced heatstroke is more common during strenuous activity, in hot weather, and in geriatric patients.
✦ Keep the patient's room temperature cool.
✦ Encourage the patient to drink additional fluids (if not contraindicated) when engaging in a strenuous activity or when the weather is hot.
✦ Monitor the patient for signs and symptoms of urine retention, such as urinary frequency with voiding of small amounts.

ADRENERGICS

Adrenergics also are called sympathomimetics because they produce effects similar to those produced by the sympathetic nervous system. Based on their chemical structure, adrenergics are classified into two groups: catecholamines (including natural and synthetic) and noncatecholamines.

Adrenergics are divided further by how they act. Direct-acting drugs work directly on the organ or tissue innervated by the sympathetic nervous system. Indirect-acting drugs trigger the release of a neurotransmitter, usually norepinephrine, to produce their actions. Dual-acting drugs have direct and indirect actions. (See *Understanding adrenergics,* page 42.)

The therapeutic use of catecholamines and noncatecholamines alike depends on which receptors they stimulate and to what degree. Adrenergics can affect alpha-adrenergic receptors, beta-adrenergic receptors, and dopaminergic receptors. (See *How drugs affect adrenergic receptor sites,* page 43.)

Most adrenergics produce their effects by stimulating alpha-adrenergic receptors and beta-adrenergic receptors. Basically, these drugs mimic the action of norepinephrine or epinephrine. Dopaminergics act primarily on receptors in the sympathetic nervous system stimulated by dopamine.

CATECHOLAMINES

Because of their common basic chemical structure, catecholamines share certain properties. They stimulate the nervous system, constrict peripheral blood vessels, increase the heart rate, and dilate the bronchi. They can be manufactured in the body or in a laboratory. Common catecholamines include dobutamine, dopamine, epinephrine, isoproterenol, and norepinephrine.

Pharmacokinetics

Catecholamines can't be taken orally because the digestive enzymes MAO and COMT destroy them. When given by the sublingual (S.L.) route, these drugs are absorbed rapidly through the mucous membranes. Any S.L. drug that isn't completely absorbed is metabolized rapidly by swallowed saliva. After giving S.C., ab-

Features of adrenergics

✦ Two types, based on chemical structure: catecholamines (natural and synthetic) and non-catecholamines
✦ May be direct-acting, thus acting directly on organ or tissue innervated by sympathetic nervous system
✦ May be indirect-acting, thus triggering release of a neurotransmitter to produce an action
✦ May be dual-acting and work directly and indirectly

Features of catecholamines

✦ Stimulate the nervous system
✦ Constrict peripheral blood vessels
✦ Increase the heart rate
✦ Dilate the bronchi

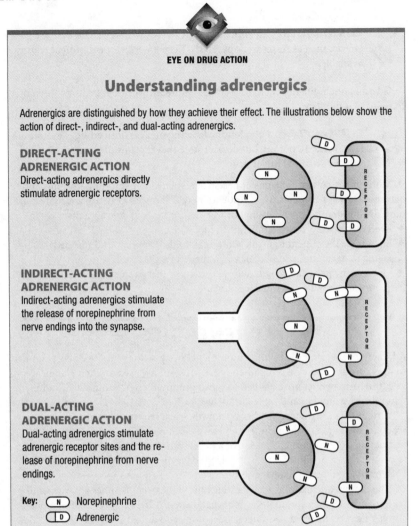

Understanding adrenergics

Adrenergics are distinguished by how they achieve their effect. The illustrations below show the action of direct-, indirect-, and dual-acting adrenergics.

DIRECT-ACTING ADRENERGIC ACTION
Direct-acting adrenergics directly stimulate adrenergic receptors.

INDIRECT-ACTING ADRENERGIC ACTION
Indirect-acting adrenergics stimulate the release of norepinephrine from nerve endings into the synapse.

DUAL-ACTING ADRENERGIC ACTION
Dual-acting adrenergics stimulate adrenergic receptor sites and the release of norepinephrine from nerve endings.

Key: (N) Norepinephrine
(D) Adrenergic

sorption is slowed because these drugs cause vasoconstriction of vessels around the injection site. After giving I.M., absorption is faster because less vasoconstriction occurs.

Catecholamines are widely distributed in the body. They're metabolized and inactivated primarily in the liver, but also in the GI tract, kidneys, lungs, plasma, and other tissues.

Excretion of catecholamines occurs primarily in the urine. However, a small amount of isoproterenol is excreted in feces, and some epinephrine is excreted in breast milk.

Pharmacodynamics

Catecholamines are primarily direct-acting. When they combine with alpha or beta receptors, they can produce an excitatory or inhibitory effect. Typically, activation of alpha receptors generates an excitatory response, except for intestinal relaxation.

How drugs affect adrenergic receptor sites

This table lists receptor types, locations, and effects of adrenergic or dopaminergic drugs on receptors.

RECEPTOR TYPE	LOCATION	EFFECT
Adrenergics		
alpha$_1$	Arterioles	Constriction
	Urinary bladder sphincters	Contraction
	Eye (radial) and skin (pilomotor) muscles	Contraction
	Liver	Glyconeogenesis and glycogenolysis
alpha$_2$	Pancreas	Decreased insulin secretion
	Skeletal blood vessels	Constriction
beta$_1$	Heart	Increased rate, conduction, and contractility
	Adipose tissue	Lipolysis
	Kidneys	Renin release
beta$_2$	Bronchi, GI, and urinary bladder smooth muscles	Relaxation
	Skeletal blood vessels	Dilation
	Uterus	Relaxation
	Liver	Glyconeogenesis and glycogenolysis
Dopaminergics		
dopaminergic	Coronary arteries, renal blood vessels, and mesenteric or visceral blood vessels	Dilation

Activation of beta receptors mostly causes an inhibitory response, except in cardiac cells, where norepinephrine produces excitatory effects.

The effects of catecholamines depend on the dosage and administration route. Catecholamines are potent inotropes, which means that they make the heart contract more forcefully. As a result, the ventricles empty more effectively with each heartbeat, increasing the heart's workload and oxygen demand. Catecholamines also produce a positive chronotropic effect, which means they cause the heart to beat faster. That's because they make pacemaker cells in the sinoatrial node of the heart depolarize at a faster rate. Reflex bradycardia may occur from increased vasoconstriction and blood pressure.

In the heart, catecholamines can cause the Purkinje fibers, a web of fibers that carry electrical impulses into the ventricles, to fire spontaneously, producing arrhythmias, such as premature ventricular contractions and fibrillation. Epinephrine is more likely than norepinephrine to produce this spontaneous firing.

Effects of catecholamines

+ Excitatory response from activation of alpha receptors (except intestinal relaxation)
+ Inhibitory response from activation of beta receptors (except in cardiac cells)
+ More forceful heart contractions (inotropic effect)
+ Faster heart beat (positive chronotropic effect)
+ Spontaneous firing of Purkinje fibers, possibly producing arrhythmias

Pharmacotherapeutics

The therapeutic use of a catecholamine depends on which receptor or receptors it activates. Norepinephrine has the most nearly pure alpha-adrenergic activity. Dobutamine and isoproterenol have only beta-related therapeutic uses. Epinephrine stimulates alpha and beta receptors. Dopamine primarily exhibits dopaminergic activity.

Catecholamines that stimulate alpha receptors are used to treat hypotension. Hypotension may result from many conditions, including sympathectomy, pheochromocytomectomy, spinal anesthesia, myocardial infarction (MI), transfusion reaction, septicemia, drug reactions, or shock. As a rule, catecholamines work best when used to treat hypotension caused by loss of vasomotor tone, which is the relaxation of the muscles of the blood vessels, or loss of adequate circulating blood volume, such as from hemorrhage.

Catecholamines that stimulate $beta_1$ receptors are used to treat bradycardia, heart block, low cardiac output, and paroxysmal atrial or nodal tachycardia. Because they're believed to make the heart more responsive to defibrillation, $beta_1$ adrenergics are used to treat asystole, cardiac arrest, and ventricular fibrillation.

Drugs that exert $beta_2$ activity are used to treat acute hypersensitivity reactions to drugs, bronchial asthma, bronchitis, and emphysema.

Dopamine may be used in doses of 1 to 2 mcg/kg/minute to improve blood flow to the kidneys because it dilates the renal blood vessels. At doses of 2 to 10 mcg/kg/minute, it acts on beta receptors to increase cardiac output. At doses above 10 mcg/kg/minute, it acts on alpha receptors to cause vasoconstriction.

Interactions

When taken with catecholamines, some drugs can cause serious interactions, such as hypotension, hypertension, arrhythmias, seizures, and hyperglycemia in patients with diabetes.

+ Use with alpha-adrenergic blockers, such as phentolamine, can produce hypotension.
+ Use with insulin and oral antidiabetics can increase the glucose level.
+ Use with beta blockers, such as propranolol, can lead to hypertension, bronchial constriction, or asthma.
+ Use with other adrenergics can produce additive effects, such as hypertension and arrhythmias, and enhanced adverse effects.
+ Use with tricyclic antidepressants can inhibit catecholamine reuptake in neurons, increasing or decreasing its effect on receptors, depending on the catecholamine. Direct-acting catecholamines are potentiated, possibly leading to arrhythmias or hypertension. Indirect-acting drugs may have a decreased pressor response.

Adverse reactions

Because of a catecholamine's widespread actions, adverse reactions affect the CNS, cardiovascular system, GI tract, skeletal and smooth muscles, and all other body systems. Although reactions vary from drug to drug, you must be aware of their possibility and must monitor and assess patients carefully during catecholamine therapy.

Many CNS manifestations may be noted, including restlessness, nervousness, anxiety, fear, dizziness, vertigo, headache, insomnia, seizures, and stroke. Adverse cardiovascular reactions include palpitations, arrhythmias, tachycardia, hypotension or hypertension, and angina. Adverse respiratory reactions include dyspnea and asthmatic episodes. Adverse skeletal muscle reactions may include weakness or

Teaching a patient about catecholamines

Whenever a catecholamine is prescribed, teach the patient and his family the drug's name, dose, frequency, action, and adverse effects and take the following actions,

✦ Instruct the patient to report discomfort at the I.V. insertion site.
✦ Teach the patient and family how to take a pulse rate.
✦ Show the patient and family how to use the prescribed inhaler correctly. Emphasize using the lowest number of inhalations possible.
✦ Instruct the patient to rinse his mouth with water after using an inhaler to prevent dry mouth.
✦ Advise the patient using an intranasal drug that rebound congestion and hyperemia commonly occur with too-frequent use of epinephrine.
✦ Advise the patient using an intranasal drug that it will sting, but that the discomfort will be temporary.
✦ Teach the diabetic patient to notify the prescriber if glucose test results change or if signs and symptoms of hyperglycemia occur.
✦ Tell the patient to notify the prescriber if adverse reactions occur.

mild tremors. The most common adverse GI reactions include nausea, vomiting, and diarrhea. Catecholamines can induce hyperglycemia, which may require insulin dosage adjustment in a diabetic patient. They may also cause vasoconstriction, which can lead to hypertensive crisis.

Extravasation of I.V. catecholamines may cause necrosis because of local vasoconstriction. Tissue sloughing may follow. To minimize injury to the area, inject phentolamine, an alpha-adrenergic antagonist.

Nursing considerations

✦ Have oxygen and emergency respiratory equipment readily available.
✦ Correct hypovolemia before therapy begins.
✦ Check the prescription closely, particularly noting the solution concentration, dosage, and rate.
✦ During infusions, monitor the patient's electrocardiogram (ECG) tracing, blood pressure, cardiac output, central venous pressure, pulmonary artery wedge pressure, pulse rate, urine output, and limb color and temperature.
✦ Monitor the patient for adverse reactions and interactions and notify the prescriber if they occur.
✦ Check the glucose level in a diabetic patient.
✦ When giving epinephrine or isoproterenol, monitor the patient's respiratory rate to detect rebound bronchospasm.
✦ Prepare and give the drug carefully.
✦ Monitor the patient's heart rate when giving isoproterenol. If it exceeds 130 beats/minute, notify the prescriber and be alert for ventricular arrhythmias.
✦ Teach the patient about the prescribed drug. (See *Teaching a patient about catecholamines.*)

 CLINICAL ALERT Be careful not to confuse epinephrine with ephedrine or norepinephrine. Also, make sure not to confuse dopamine with dobutamine.

Adverse reactions to watch for

✦ Angina
✦ Dizziness, vertigo
✦ Dyspnea and asthmatic episodes
✦ Headache
✦ Hyperglycemia
✦ Hypotension or hypertension
✦ Insomnia
✦ Nausea, vomiting, and diarrhea
✦ Necrosis and sloughing from extravasation
✦ Palpitations, arrhythmias, tachycardia
✦ Restlessness, nervousness, anxiety, fear
✦ Seizures
✦ Stroke
✦ Vasoconstriction
✦ Weakness or mild tremors

Key nursing actions

✦ Correct hypovolemia.
✦ Monitor ECG, blood pressure, cardiac output, central venous pressure, pulmonary artery wedge pressure, and pulse rate.
✦ Measure urine output.
✦ Assess limb color and temperature.

NONCATECHOLAMINES

Noncatecholamine adrenergics have a wide variety of therapeutic uses because they produce many effects on the body, including local and systemic vasoconstriction (mephentermine and phenylephrine), nasal and eye decongestion and bronchodilation (albuterol, bitolterol, ephedrine, formoterol, isoetharine, isoproterenol, levalbuterol, metaproterenol, pirbuterol, salmeterol, and terbutaline), and smooth-muscle relaxation (terbutaline).

Pharmacokinetics

Absorption of noncatecholamines happens in different ways and depends on the administration route. Inhalants, such as albuterol, are absorbed gradually from the bronchi and result in lower levels in the body. Oral noncatecholamines are absorbed well from the GI tract and distributed widely in the body fluids and tissues. Some noncatecholamines, such as ephedrine, cross the blood-brain barrier and can reach high levels in the brain and cerebrospinal fluid. Metabolism and inactivation of noncatecholamines occur primarily in the liver, but also can take place in the lungs, GI tract, and other tissues. Noncatecholamines and their metabolites are excreted primarily in urine. Some, such as inhaled albuterol, are excreted within 24 hours; others, such as oral albuterol, within 3 days. Acidic urine increases the excretion of many noncatecholamines; alkaline urine slows their excretion.

Pharmacodynamics

Unlike catecholamines, which are primarily direct-acting, noncatecholamines can be direct-acting, indirect-acting, or dual-acting. Direct-acting noncatecholamines achieve their effects by occupying receptor sites on organs and structures innervated by the sympathetic nervous system. For example, phenylephrine exhibits primarily alpha-adrenergic activity; albuterol, isoetharine, metaproterenol, and terbutaline selectively exert $beta_2$ activity.

Indirect-acting noncatecholamines, such as ephedrine, produce their effects by stimulating norepinephrine release from its storage sites. Dual-acting noncatecholamines combine both actions.

Pharmacotherapeutics

Noncatecholamines stimulate the sympathetic nervous system and produce various effects in the body. Because generalized statements about these drugs aren't useful, you need to become familiar with each drug's indications, administration routes, dosages, and administration techniques. You also need to monitor the patient closely for therapeutic effects and drug tolerance.

Interactions

✦ General anesthetics, cyclopropane, and halogenated hydrocarbons can interact to cause arrhythmias.
✦ MAO inhibitors can interact, leading to severe hypertension and possibly death.
✦ When taken with terbutaline, oxytocics (uterine muscle stimulants) can be inhibited. When taken with other noncatecholamines, oxytocics can cause hypertensive crisis or stroke.
✦ Tricyclic antidepressants can interact with noncatecholamines to cause hypertension and arrhythmias.
✦ Urine alkalizers, such as acetazolamide and sodium bicarbonate, can slow the excretion of noncatecholamines, prolonging their action.

Adverse reactions

For any noncatecholamine, adverse reactions depend on the drug's receptor activity. Other factors include the drug's intended therapeutic effects and its ability to cross the blood-brain barrier. For example, if ephedrine is given to produce bronchodilation and then interferes with sleep, the insomnia is considered an adverse reaction. However, if the drug is given to treat narcolepsy, the insomnia is the desired therapeutic effect. Although adverse reactions vary from drug to drug, you must be aware of their potential and must monitor the patient appropriately.

In the CNS, adverse reactions to noncatecholamines include headache, restlessness, nervousness, anxiety or euphoria, irritability, trembling, drowsiness or insomnia, lethargy, dizziness, light-headedness, incoherence, seizures, and cerebral hemorrhage. Adverse cardiovascular reactions include hypertension or hypotension, palpitations, bradycardia or tachycardia, arrhythmias, cardiac arrest, tingling or coldness in the limbs, pallor or flushing, anginal pain, and alterations in maternal and fetal heart rates and blood pressures. Geriatric patients are particularly susceptible to CNS reactions, such as confusion and anxiety, and to cardiovascular reactions, such as increased systolic blood pressure, limb coldness, and anginal pain.

Adverse skeletal muscle reactions may include weakness, mild tremors, or muscle cramps. Other adverse reactions include sweating, urinary urgency or incontinence, urine retention, pilomotor stimulation, stinging and burning of the nasal mucosa or eyes, blurred vision, sneezing, dry mouth, nausea, vomiting, unusual taste, erythema, and transient elevations in glucose level and increased insulin requirements in diabetic patients.

Hypotension can occur after discontinuation of these drugs because of depletion of the intrinsic catecholamines in the storage granules of the nerve endings.

Nursing considerations

+ Monitor the patient's vital signs, mental status, and muscle strength at least every 4 hours.
+ Obtain electrolyte levels in all patients who are beginning therapy; obtain pH, carbon dioxide partial pressure, and bicarbonate level in patients during prolonged therapy.
+ Monitor the patient's potassium level to detect hypokalemia during prolonged infusion of terbutaline.
+ Check the glucose level in a diabetic patient and observe him for signs of hyperglycemia.
+ Monitor the patient for paradoxical bronchospasm. If it occurs, discontinue the drug and begin alternative therapy.
+ Give an oral noncatecholamine with food to reduce GI distress, unless otherwise indicated.
+ Inject S.C. terbutaline in the lateral deltoid area.
+ Although not FDA approved for this use, terbutaline may be given I.V. or S.C. to manage preterm labor. If so, place the patient in a left lateral recumbent position to prevent hypotension during the infusion.
+ Infuse I.V. terbutaline into a large vein to avoid extravasation.
+ Discontinue ephedrine and notify the prescriber if wheezing or bronchospasm occurs after therapy.
+ Notify the prescriber if adverse reactions or interactions occur.

 CLINICAL ALERT Take care not to confuse terbutaline with tolbutamide or terbinafine. Also, make sure you don't confuse epinephrine with ephedrine.

Adverse reactions to watch for

+ Altered maternal and fetal heart rates and blood pressures
+ Drowsiness, insomnia, lethargy
+ Headache, light-headedness, dizziness, incoherence, seizures, cerebral hemorrhage
+ Hypertension or hypotension, palpitations, bradycardia or tachycardia, arrhythmias, cardiac arrest, anginal pain
+ Nausea, vomiting, unusual taste
+ Pilomotor stimulation, stinging and burning of the nasal mucosa or eyes, blurred vision, sneezing, dry mouth
+ Restlessness, nervousness, anxiety, euphoria, irritability, trembling
+ Sweating, urinary urgency or incontinence, urine retention
+ Tingling or coldness in limbs and pallor, erythema, or flushing
+ Transient elevation of glucose level in diabetic patients
+ Weakness, mild tremors, muscle cramps

Key nursing actions

+ Monitor vital signs, mental status, and muscle strength.
+ Assess electrolyte levels, pH, carbon dioxide partial pressure, and bicarbonate level during prolonged therapy.
+ Monitor the potassium level.
+ Watch for paradoxical bronchospasm.

Teaching a patient about noncatecholamines

Whenever a noncatecholamine is prescribed, teach the patient and family its name, dose, frequency, action, and adverse effects, and the following procedures.

◆ Instruct the patient to perform inhalation therapy before meals to improve lung ventilation and to reduce fatigue caused by eating.

◆ Teach the patient self-assessment techniques to determine the need for administration or repeat administration of the drug. For example, instruct the patient to assess for dyspnea, wheezing, and chest discomfort.

◆ Teach the patient to perform oral inhalation correctly by providing these instructions:
 – Shake the inhaler.
 – Clear your nasal passages and throat.
 – Breathe out, expelling as much air from your lungs as possible.
 – Place the mouthpiece well into your mouth, and inhale deeply as you release a dose from the inhaler. Or, hold the inhaler about 1" (2 finger widths) from your open mouth, and inhale while the dose is released.
 – Hold your breath for several seconds, remove the mouthpiece, and exhale slowly.
 – If the prescriber orders more than 1 inhalation, wait at least 2 minutes before repeating the procedure.

◆ Teach the patient to blow his nose gently, with both nostrils open to clear nasal passages before administering a nasal medication.

◆ Instruct the patient to avoid contact between the inhaled drug and his eyes.

◆ Advise the patient to rinse his mouth after inhalation to minimize dryness and irritation.

◆ Teach the patient to take the drug only as prescribed because of possible adverse reactions.

◆ Instruct the patient to protect the drug from light, excessive heat or cold, and moisture and not to use discolored drug.

◆ Teach the patient to notify the prescriber if symptoms aren't relieved or if adverse reactions occur.

Features of adrenergic blockers

◆ Disrupt sympathetic nervous system function by blocking impulse transmission at adrenergic neurons or receptor sites
◆ Interrupt the action of adrenergics, reduce norepinephrine, or prevent the action of cholinergics

Features of alpha blockers

◆ Interrupt the action of epinephrine and norepinephrine at alpha-adrenergic receptors
◆ Relax vascular smooth muscle
◆ Increase vasodilation
◆ Decrease blood pressure
◆ Block stimulation of alpha$_1$ and, possibly, alpha$_2$ receptors

◆ Teach the patient about the prescribed drug. (See *Teaching a patient about noncatecholamines.*)

ADRENERGIC BLOCKERS

Adrenergic blockers, or sympatholytics, are used to disrupt sympathetic nervous system function. These drugs work by blocking impulse transmission (and thus sympathetic nervous system stimulation) at adrenergic neurons or adrenergic receptor sites. Their action at these sites interrupts the action of adrenergics, reduces available norepinephrine, or prevents the action of cholinergics.

Adrenergic blockers are classified by their site of action as alpha-adrenergic blockers or beta blockers.

ALPHA BLOCKERS

Alpha blockers work by interrupting the actions of the catecholamines epinephrine and norepinephrine at alpha-adrenergic receptors. This relaxes smooth muscles in the blood vessels, increases vasodilation, and decreases blood pressure.

Drugs in this class include doxazosin, ergoloid mesylates, ergotamine derivatives, phenoxybenzamine, phentolamine, prazosin, and terazosin. Ergotamine is a mixed alpha-adrenergic agonist and antagonist; at high doses, it acts as an alpha blocker.

Pharmacokinetics

The action of alpha blockers in the body isn't well understood. Most of these drugs are absorbed erratically when given orally and more rapidly and completely when given S.L. They differ considerably in their onset of action, peak level, and duration of action.

Pharmacodynamics

Alpha blockers work in one of two ways. They may interfere with, or block, norepinephrine's synthesis, storage, release, and reuptake by neurons. Or they may antagonize epinephrine, norepinephrine, or adrenergics (sympathomimetics) at alpha-adrenergic receptor sites.

Although alpha-adrenergic receptor sites include alpha $_1$ and alpha$_2$ receptors, alpha blockers include drugs that block stimulation of alpha$_1$ receptors and that may or may not block alpha$_2$ stimulation. Alpha blockers occupy alpha-adrenergic receptor sites on the smooth muscles of blood vessels. (See *How alpha blockers affect peripheral blood vessels,* page 50.) This prevents catecholamines from occupying and stimulating those sites. As a result, blood vessels dilate, increasing local blood flow to the skin and other organs. The decreased peripheral vascular resistance helps decrease blood pressure.

An alpha-adrenergic blocker's therapeutic effects depend on the body's sympathetic tone before drug administration. For instance, if a drug is given with the patient lying down, only a small change in blood pressure occurs. In this position, the sympathetic nerves release very little norepinephrine. However, if the drug is given to a standing patient, the blood pressure may drop dramatically. This happens because norepinephrine is normally released to constrict the veins and push blood back up to a standing patient's heart. In the presence of an alpha-adrenergic blocker, however, the veins can't constrict and blood pools in the legs. Because blood return to the heart is reduced, the blood pressure drops. (See *Minimizing first-dose effect,* page 51.)

Pharmacotherapeutics

Because alpha-adrenergic blockers cause smooth muscles to relax and blood vessels to dilate, they increase local blood flow to the skin and other organs and reduce blood pressure. As a result, they're used to treat hypertension, pheochromocytoma, and peripheral vascular disorders, especially those in which blood vessel spasm causes poor local blood flow, such as Raynaud's disease, acrocyanosis, and frostbite.

Interactions

Many drugs interact with alpha-adrenergic blockers, producing synergistic or exaggerated effects. The most serious include severe hypotension or vascular collapse. The following interactions can occur with ergoloid mesylates and ergotamine derivatives.

✦ Caffeine and macrolide antibiotics can increase ergotamine's effects.
✦ Dopamine can increase the drug's pressor effect.
✦ Nitroglycerin can produce hypotension because of excessive vasodilation.
✦ Adrenergics, including over-the-counter products, can increase cardiac stimulation, leading to hypotension with rebound hypertension.

Conditions that call for alpha blockers

✦ Hypertension
✦ Peripheral vascular disorders, such as Raynaud's disease, acrocyanosis, and frostbite
✦ Pheochromocytoma

Possible drug interactions

✦ Adrenergics
✦ Caffeine
✦ Dopamine
✦ Macrolide antibiotics
✦ Nitroglycerin

How alpha blockers affect peripheral blood vessels

By occupying alpha-adrenergic receptor sites, alpha blockers cause the blood vessel walls to relax. This leads to dilation of blood vessels and reduced peripheral vascular resistance (the pressure that blood must overcome as it flows in a vessel).

ONE RESULT: ORTHOSTATIC HYPOTENSION
These effects can cause orthostatic hypotension, which is a drop in blood pressure that occurs when changing position from lying down to standing. Redistribution of blood to the dilated blood vessels of the legs causes hypotension.

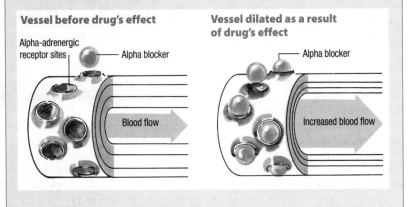

Adverse reactions to watch for
+ Bradycardia, tachycardia
+ Edema, dyspnea, light-headedness
+ Flushing, arrhythmias, angina, MI, cerebrovascular spasm, shock
+ Increased uric acid and blood urea nitrogen levels
+ Nasal stuffiness, blurred vision, increased nasopharyngeal secretions, epistaxis, miosis, conjunctival infection, red sclera, ptosis, tinnitus, dry mouth
+ Orthostatic hypotension, severe hypertension
+ Paresthesia, tingling in limbs, muscle weakness, fatigue, nervousness, depression, insomnia, drowsiness, lethargy, sedation, vertigo, syncope, confusion, headache, CNS stimulation
+ Rash, allergic dermatitis, pruritus, alopecia, lichen planus
+ Shock, diaphoresis, arthralgia
+ Sublingual irritation, nausea, vomiting, heartburn, diarrhea, abdominal pain, worsening of peptic ulcer
+ Urinary frequency, impotence, incontinence, priapism
+ Granulocytopenia, neutropenia, eosinophilia, leukopenia, thrombocytopenia, pancytopenia

Adverse reactions

Adverse reactions caused by alpha-adrenergic receptor blockade are related primarily to vasodilation. However, because the alpha-adrenergic blockers have varied mechanisms of action, they can produce many adverse reactions.

Cardiovascular reactions may include orthostatic hypotension or severe hypertensive episodes, bradycardia or tachycardia, edema, dyspnea, light-headedness, flushing, arrhythmias, angina, MI, cerebrovascular spasm, and a shocklike state. With long-acting noncompetitive alpha-adrenergic blockers, such as phenoxybenzamine, the beta receptors are left unopposed, which can lead to an exaggerated hypotensive response and tachycardia.

In the CNS, manifestations may include paresthesia, tingling in the limbs, muscle weakness, fatigue, nervousness, depression, insomnia, drowsiness, lethargy, sedation, vertigo, syncope, confusion, headache, and CNS stimulation.

Eye, ear, nose, and throat manifestations may occurs, such as nasal stuffiness, blurred vision, increased nasopharyngeal secretions, epistaxis, miosis, conjunctival infection, reddened sclera, ptosis, tinnitus, and dry mouth.

In the GI tract, reactions are common and may consist of sublingual irritation, nausea, vomiting, heartburn, diarrhea, abdominal pain, and exacerbation of peptic ulcer.

Adverse genitourinary reactions may include urinary frequency, impotence, incontinence, or priapism.

WARNING

Minimizing first-dose effect

With the first few doses, alpha-adrenergic blockers may cause significant hypotension (especially orthostatic hypotension) and syncope. To minimize this first-dose effect, make sure the initial doses are low and the dosage is increased gradually. Also, use other antihypertensives or beta blockers with caution.

Hematologic manifestations are rare; however, granulocytopenia, neutropenia, eosinophilia, leukopenia, thrombocytopenia, and pancytopenia have been reported with some drugs.

Various dermatologic effects may occur, including rash, allergic dermatitis, pruritus, alopecia, or lichen planus. Other adverse reactions are allergic phenomena, including shock, diaphoresis, and arthralgia. Increased uric acid and blood urea nitrogen levels may also occur.

Nursing considerations

✦ Teach the patient and his family about the prescribed drug. (See *Teaching a patient about alpha blockers.*)

✦ Monitor the patient for adverse reactions and signs of interactions and notify the prescriber if they occur.

✦ Monitor the patient's vital signs frequently, noting any change in blood pressure when the patient stands.

✦ Take safety measures if the patient develops light-headedness, weakness, or changes in mental status. Raise the side rails and assist with ambulation.

Key nursing actions

✦ Monitor vital signs and blood pressure, especially when patient stands.

✦ Notify the prescriber immediately if patient develops chest pain, obtain ECG, and provide treatment.

✦ If shock develops, place the patient in Trendelenburg position unless contraindicated. Notify the prescriber immediately, and provide treatment.

PATIENT TEACHING

Teaching a patient about alpha blockers

Whenever an alpha blocker is prescribed, teach the patient and his family the drug's name, dose, frequency, action, and adverse effects and take the following actions.

✦ Teach the patient to minimize orthostatic hypotension by rising slowly from a supine position and by dangling his feet for a few minutes before standing.

✦ Instruct the patient to assume a head-low position or to lie down if light-headedness, faintness, or weakness occurs.

✦ Advise the patient not to exceed the prescribed dosage. Explain that adverse reactions can result from higher dosages.

✦ Teach the patient to avoid alcohol use. Explain that alcohol used with alpha-adrenergic blockers may cause hypotension.

✦ Instruct the patient to avoid over-the-counter cough, cold, allergy, or weight-loss drugs that contain alcohol or caffeine unless they have been approved by the prescriber.

✦ Advise the patient to store the drug in a light-resistant, airtight container.

✦ Instruct the patient to notify the prescriber if adverse reactions occur.

✦ Notify the prescriber immediately if the patient develops chest pain. Obtain an ECG tracing and treat the patient.

✦ Place the patient in the Trendelenburg position if shock occurs (and if not contraindicated). Also, notify the prescriber immediately and begin emergency interventions.

✦ Give oral drugs with food or milk to reduce GI distress.

BETA·BLOCKERS

The most widely used adrenergic blockers, beta blockers, prevent stimulation of the sympathetic nervous system by inhibiting the action of catecholamines at beta-adrenergic receptors. These drugs are commonly called beta blockers.

Beta blockers may be selective or nonselective. Selective beta blockers primarily affect $beta_1$ sites, located mainly in the heart. They include acebutolol, atenolol, betaxolol, bisoprolol, esmolol, and metoprolol.

Nonselective beta blockers affect $beta_1$ receptor sites as well as $beta_2$ receptor sites, located in the bronchi, blood vessels, and uterus. These drugs include carteolol, carvedilol, labetalol, levobunolol, nadolol, penbutolol, pindolol, propranolol, sotalol, and timolol.

Some beta blockers, such as acebutolol and pindolol, also have intrinsic sympathetic activity. This means that, instead of attaching to beta receptors and blocking them, these drugs attach to beta receptors and stimulate them. Because of this action, they're sometimes classified as partial agonists.

Pharmacokinetics

Usually, beta blockers are absorbed rapidly and well from the GI tract and are protein-bound to some extent. Food doesn't inhibit their absorption and can enhance absorption for some of them. Some beta blockers are absorbed more completely than others.

Beta blockers are distributed widely in body tissues and reach the highest concentrations in the heart, liver, lungs, and saliva.

With the exception of nadolol and atenolol, beta blockers are metabolized in the liver. They're excreted primarily in urine, as metabolites or in unchanged form, but also can be excreted in feces and bile. They may also appear in breast milk.

The onset of action of beta blockers is primarily dose- and drug-dependent. The time it takes to reach the peak concentration level depends on the administration route. For example, a beta blocker given by I.V. infusion reaches peak level much more rapidly than one given by mouth.

Pharmacodynamics

Beta blockers have widespread effects because they produce their blocking action not only at adrenergic nerve endings but also in the adrenal medulla.

Cardiovascular effects include increased peripheral vascular resistance, decreased blood pressure, decreased force of cardiac contractions, decreased oxygen consumption by the heart, slowed impulse conduction between the atria and ventricles, and decreased cardiac output. (See *How beta blockers work*.)

Some effects of beta blockers depend on whether the drug is selective or nonselective. Selective drugs, which preferentially block $beta_1$-receptor sites, reduce stimulation of the heart. They're often called cardioselective beta blockers.

Nonselective drugs, which block $beta_1$- and $beta_2$-receptor sites, reduce stimulation of the heart and cause bronchoconstriction. For instance, nonselective beta blockers can cause bronchospasm in patients with chronic obstructive pulmonary

Features of beta blockers

✦ Prevent stimulation of sympathetic nervous system.
✦ Selective drugs affect mainly $beta_1$ sites.
✦ Nonselective drugs affect $beta_1$ and $beta_2$ sites.
✦ Some have intrinsic sympathetic activity.

Effects of beta blockers

✦ Increased peripheral vascular resistance
✦ Decreased blood pressure
✦ Decreased force of cardiac contractions
✦ Decreased oxygen consumption by heart
✦ Slowed impulse conduction between atria and ventricles
✦ Decreased cardiac output
✦ Reduced stimulation of heart (selective)
✦ Reduced stimulation of heart and bronchoconstriction (nonselective)

EYE ON DRUG ACTION

How beta blockers work

By occupying beta-receptor sites, beta blockers prevent catecholamines (norepinephrine and epinephrine) from occupying these sites and exerting their stimulating effects. This illustration shows the effects of beta blockers on the heart, lungs, and blood vessels.

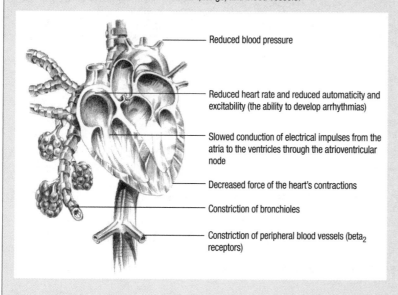

Reduced blood pressure

Reduced heart rate and reduced automaticity and excitability (the ability to develop arrhythmias)

Slowed conduction of electrical impulses from the atria to the ventricles through the atrioventricular node

Decreased force of the heart's contractions

Constriction of bronchioles

Constriction of peripheral blood vessels (beta$_2$ receptors)

Actions of beta blockers

✦ Block norepinephrine and epinephrine receptors
✦ Prevent norepinephrine and epinephrine from stimulating the heart, lungs, and blood vessels

Conditions that call for beta blockers

✦ Angina
✦ Anxiety
✦ Cardiovascular symptoms of thyrotoxicosis
✦ Essential tremor
✦ Heart failure
✦ Hypertension
✦ Hypertrophic cardiomyopathy ·
✦ MI (to prevent another MI)
✦ Migraine headaches
✦ Open-angle glaucoma
✦ Pheochromocytoma
✦ Supraventricular arrhythmias

disease. This adverse reaction doesn't occur when cardioselective drugs are given at low doses.

Pharmacotherapeutics

Beta blockers are used to treat many conditions. Their clinical usefulness is based largely (but not exclusively) on how they affect the heart.

These drugs can be prescribed after an MI to prevent another MI or to treat angina, heart failure, hypertension, hypertrophic cardiomyopathy, and supraventricular arrhythmias.

Other uses for beta blockers include the treatment of anxiety, cardiovascular symptoms of thyrotoxicosis, essential tremor, migraine headaches, open-angle glaucoma, and pheochromocytoma. (See *Contraindications and precautions for beta blockers,* page 54.)

Interactions

Many drugs can interact with beta blockers to cause potentially dangerous effects. The most serious effects include cardiac depression, arrhythmias, respiratory depression, severe bronchospasm, severe hypotension, and vascular collapse.
✦ When digoxin is taken with a beta blocker, digoxin's effects are decreased.
✦ When a calcium channel blocker (primarily verapamil), flecainide, or haloperidol is taken with a beta blocker, the effects of both drugs are increased.

Possible drug interactions

✦ Adrenergics
✦ Ampicillin
✦ Anti-inflammatories
✦ Barbiturates
✦ Calcium channel blockers
✦ Calcium
✦ Cholestyramine

Contraindications and precautions for beta blockers

Beta blockers are contraindicated in patients with bradycardia, heart block greater than first-degree, cardiogenic shock, heart failure (unless caused by tachyarrhythmia treatable with beta blockers), overt heart failure, and hypersensitivity to beta blockers.

Nonselective drugs shouldn't be used in patients with bronchial asthma, including those with severe chronic obstructive pulmonary disease. Sotalol shouldn't be used in patients with congenital or acquired long QT syndromes.

Possible drug interactions
(continued)

+ Cimetidine
+ Clonidine
+ Colestipol
+ Digoxin
+ Flecainide
+ Haloperidol
+ Insulin
+ Lidocaine
+ Oral antidiabetics
+ Rifampin
+ Theophylline

+ Taking cimetidine with a beta blocker may increase the beta blocker's effect and cause toxicity.
+ Taking ampicillin or a calcium salt with atenolol may decrease atenolol's effect.
+ Taking a calcium salt, a barbiturate, an anti-inflammatory (such as indomethacin and salicylates), or rifampin with a beta blocker may decrease the beta blocker's effect.
+ Taking cholestyramine or colestipol with propanolol may decrease the effect of propanolol.
+ When lidocaine is taken with beta blockers, lidocaine toxicity can occur.
+ Beta blockers can interact with insulin and oral antidiabetics altering their requirements in diabetic patients.
+ Nonselective beta blockers can impair theophylline's ability to produce bronchodilation.
+ Use of clonidine with a nonselective beta blocker can lead to life-threatening hypertension when clonidine is stopped.
+ Use of adrenergics with nonselective beta blockers can cause hypertension and reflex bradycardia.

Adverse reactions

Generally, beta blockers cause few adverse reactions, with most being drug- or dose-dependent. Adverse reactions usually occur with I.V. rather than oral administration and in geriatric patients and those with impaired renal or hepatic function.

Primarily, arrhythmias, orthostatic hypotension, CNS disturbances, and GI or respiratory distress signal beta blocker toxicity. Adverse cardiovascular reactions include hypotension, bradycardia, peripheral vascular insufficiency (Raynaud's disease), atrioventricular block, and heart failure. Geriatric patients are especially likely to experience peripheral vascular insufficiency and heart failure.

The most common respiratory reaction is bronchospasm. Although selective drugs are less likely than nonselective ones to cause bronchospasm, you should use caution when giving any beta blocker, particularly to a patient with bronchial asthma, bronchitis, or emphysema. GI manifestations commonly include diarrhea, nausea, vomiting, constipation, abdominal discomfort, anorexia, and flatulence.

Adverse CNS effects may include dizziness, insomnia, fatigue, weakness, lethargy, disorientation, memory loss, vision disturbances, sedation, hallucinations, and behavioral changes. Geriatric patients, in particular, are at increased risk for CNS effects, such as cognitive impairment and depression.

Evidence of beta blocker toxicity

+ Arrhythmias
+ Orthostatic hypotension
+ CNS disturbances
+ GI or respiratory distress

Teaching a patient about beta blockers

Whenever a beta blocker is prescribed, teach the patient and his family the drug's name, dose, frequency, action, and adverse effects and take the following action.

◆ Advise the patient not to stop taking the drug abruptly or alter the prescribed dosage unless ordered. Explain that abrupt withdrawal can cause a myocardial infarction, arrhythmias, or other serious complications.

◆ Teach the patient to take his pulse rate and report slowing or irregularity to the prescriber.

◆ Teach the patient to minimize the effects of orthostatic hypotension by changing position slowly, especially when rising, and to dangle his legs over the bedside for a few minutes before standing.

◆ Instruct the patient to sit or lie down immediately if dizziness or faintness occurs.

◆ Advise the patient not to drive or operate machinery until after adjusting to the drug's central nervous system effects.

◆ Teach the patient with impaired renal function to report a weight gain of 3 to 4 lb per day, cough, difficulty breathing while lying down, fatigue, tachycardia, shortness of breath, anxiety, or swelling of his hands, feet, or lower legs.

◆ Teach the patient to store the drug at room temperature and to protect it from moisture, light, and air.

◆ Tell the patient and his family to notify the prescriber of any adverse drug reactions.

Although rare, adverse hematologic reactions include agranulocytosis, nonthrombocytopenic or thrombocytopenic purpura, thrombocytopenia, eosinophilia, leukopenia, anemia, and leukocytosis. Other adverse reactions include headache, impotence or decreased libido, nasal stuffiness, diaphoresis, tinnitus, and dry mouth, eyes, and skin.

Adverse reactions indicating an allergic response include rash, fever with sore throat, laryngospasm, and possibly respiratory distress. Although most patients tolerate beta blockers fairly well, patients with certain preexisting chronic conditions are at special risk for adverse reactions to beta blocker therapy.

Nursing considerations

◆ Teach the patient about the prescribed drug. (See *Teaching a patient about beta blockers.*)

◆ Monitor the patient periodically for adverse reactions. Adverse reactions are most common when given I.V. and in geriatric patients and those with impaired renal or hepatic function.

◆ Check the glucose level carefully in a diabetic patient because the drug may potentiate hypoglycemia and mask its signs and symptoms.

◆ These drugs may also mask signs and symptoms of shock and hyperthyroidism. Look for secondary signs and symptoms of these disorders.

◆ Give oral drugs before meals or at bedtime to promote absorption. Avoid giving a late-evening dose if insomnia occurs.

◆ When injecting I.V., keep emergency drugs on hand to treat bradycardia, hypotension, and bronchospasm.

Adverse reactions to watch for

◆ Allergic response (rash, fever, sore throat, laryngospasm, respiratory distress)
◆ Atrioventricular block
◆ Bradycardia
◆ Bronchospasm
◆ Diaphoresis
◆ Diarrhea, nausea, vomiting, constipation, abdominal discomfort, anorexia, flatulence
◆ Dizziness, insomnia, fatigue, weakness, lethargy, disorientation, memory loss, vision disturbances, sedation, hallucinations, behavioral changes
◆ Dry mouth, eyes, and skin
◆ Headache, impotence, decreased libido
◆ Heart failure
◆ Hypotension
◆ Nasal stuffiness, tinnitus
◆ Peripheral vascular insufficiency
◆ Agranulocytosis, nonthrombocytopenic or thrombocytopenic purpura, thrombocytopenia, eosinophilia, leukopenia, anemia, leukocytosis

Key nursing actions

◆ Check the glucose level carefully in a diabetic patient.
◆ Look for secondary signs and symptoms of shock and hyperthyroidism.
◆ Check the apical rate before giving the drug.
◆ Notify the prescriber immediately if the patient develops cardiac or respiratory depression, arrhythmias, bronchospasm, or hypotension.
◆ Stop the drug gradually over 2 weeks.

CLINICAL ALERT **Check the patient's apical rate before giving the drug, especially if he takes digoxin. Withhold the drug if the patient has a heart rate below 60 beats/minute or exhibits adverse reactions.**

✦ Notify the prescriber immediately if the patient experiences cardiac or respiratory depression, arrhythmias, bronchospasm, or hypotension.

✦ Give an antacid several hours before or after giving the drug.

✦ Stop the drug gradually over 2 weeks.

Neurologic and neuromuscular drugs

The kind of drugs that qualify as neurologic and neuromuscular drugs is surprising. In this group, you'll find three classes of skeletal muscle relaxants, two classes of neuromuscular blockers, three classes of antiparkinsonians, six classes of anticonvulsants, one class of drugs for Alzheimer's disease, and two classes of antimigraine drugs.

What do these diverse drugs have in common? They all act on the nervous system, although they produce their effects in different ways. To give you a head start on understanding their actions and effects, a brief review of the nervous system can help.

ANATOMY AND PHYSIOLOGY

The nervous system directs all movement, sensation, thought, and emotion. It's composed of the central and peripheral divisions. The central nervous system (CNS) consists of the brain and spinal cord. (See *Exploring central nervous system structures*, page 58.)

The peripheral nervous system consists of cranial and spinal nerves, which carry sensory messages from organs and tissues to the brain and motor instructions from the brain to target organs.

The 12 pairs of cranial nerves primarily address the sensory and motor needs of the head as well as the neck, chest, and abdomen. Cranial nerves I and II originate in the frontal lobe; III through XII originate in the brain stem.

The 31 pairs of spinal nerves originate in the spinal cord. These paired nerves include 8 cervical, 12 thoracic, 5 lumbar, 5 sacral, and 1 coccygeal. Cervical 3 through thoracic 2 innervate the arms; thoracic 9 through 12 innervate the legs.

Anatomy and physiology highlights
+ The nervous system directs movement, sensation, thought, and emotion.
+ The central nervous system includes the brain and spinal cord.
+ The peripheral nervous system includes cranial and spinal nerves that carry sensory and motor messages between the brain and body.

Exploring central nervous system structures

The brain and spinal cord make up the central nervous system and work together to control movement, sensation, thought, and emotion. Their major structures and functions are shown below.

BRAIN STRUCTURES

The brain is composed of the cerebrum, diencephalon, cerebellum, and brain stem. Two hemispheres make up the cerebrum, the largest portion of the brain. Each hemisphere contains four lobes—frontal, parietal, temporal, and occipital. The surface of the cerebrum (cortex) is composed of gray matter made of neuron cell bodies, axon terminals, and dendrites. The interior of the cerebrum is composed of white matter made of basal ganglia. The corpus callosum allows communication between corresponding areas in the two hemispheres.

In front of the brain stem, the diencephalon includes the hypothalamus and thalamus. The cerebellum lies at the base of the brain below the occipital lobes.

The brain stem, composed of the midbrain, pons, and medulla oblongata, relays all messages between the upper and lower levels of the nervous system; cranial nerves III through XII originate there.

SPINAL CORD STRUCTURES

The spinal cord serves as a communication pathway between the brain and the peripheral nervous system, and its gray matter functions as a reflex center for spinal reflexes. It joins the brain stem at the level of the foramen magnum and terminates near the second lumbar vertebra. The spinal cord comprises a central H-shaped mass of gray matter divided into dorsal (or posterior) and ventral (or anterior) horns. Cell bodies in the dorsal horn relay sensory (afferent) impulses. White matter around these horns consists of myelinated axons of sensory and motor nerves grouped in ascending and descending tracts.

CROSS SECTION OF THE BRAIN

Cerebrum — Thalamus — Midbrain — Cerebellum — Pituitary gland — Hypothalamus — Pons — Medulla — Spinal cord

CROSS SECTION OF THE SPINAL CORD

Ventral horn (relays motor impulses) Dorsal horn (relays sensory impulses)

White matter (forms ascending and descending tracts) Gray matter

Functions of neuroglial cells

✦ Supply nutrients to neurons
✦ Assist in producing CSF
✦ Provide electrical insulation for axons of CNS neurons
✦ Perform additional specialized support functions

NEUROGLIAL CELLS AND NEURONS

Two types of cells make up the nervous system: neuroglial cells and neurons. Neuroglial cells perform specialized support functions, such as supplying nutrients to neurons, assisting in cerebrospinal fluid (CSF) production, and providing electrical insulation for the axons of CNS neurons.

The neuron consists of a cell body and two types of appendages—a long one (an axon) and one or more shorter ones (dendrites). Cell bodies form the gray matter in the brain, brain stem, and spinal cord. The axon transmits impulses from the cell body to other neurons. Dendrites receive impulses from nearby cells and guide them toward the cell body for processing.

Neurons perform one of three roles in transmitting impulses: reception of sensory stimuli, transmission of motor responses, or coordination of communication between body parts. Sensory neurons carry stimuli from the peripheral sensory organs, such as the skin, to the spinal cord and brain. Motor neurons carry impulses from the brain and spinal cord to tissues and organs. Interneurons relay impulses within the CNS.

All body functions rely on the electrical and chemical transmission of impulses from neuron to neuron. This transmission occurs across a synapse (the contact point between two neurons). Neurotransmission is facilitated by neurotransmitters, such as acetylcholine and dopamine.

SKELETAL MUSCLE RELAXANTS

Spasticity is a motor disorder characterized by increased muscle tone from hyperexcitability of anterior motor neurons. This hyperexcitability may arise from a lack of inhibition or from excess stimulation by signals transmitted from the brain through the spinal cord's interneurons to the anterior motor neurons. Spasticity is caused by various upper motor neuron disorders, such as multiple sclerosis (MS), cerebral palsy, stroke, and spinal cord injuries.

To varying degrees, skeletal muscle relaxants reduce spasticity, possibly by reducing hyperexcitability. This section discusses the two main classes of skeletal muscle relaxants—centrally acting and direct-acting drugs—as well as three other drugs that are used to relax skeletal muscles.

CENTRALLY ACTING SKELETAL MUSCLE RELAXANTS

Exposure to severe cold, lack of blood flow to a muscle, or overexertion can send sensory impulses from the posterior sensory nerve fibers to the spinal cord and brain. These sensory impulses can cause involuntary muscle contractions or spasms from trauma, epilepsy, hypocalcemia, or muscular disorders. The muscle contraction further stimulates the sensory receptors to cause a more intense contraction, establishing a cycle.

Centrally acting skeletal muscle relaxants may break this cycle by acting as CNS depressants. By acting on the CNS, they can treat acute spasms caused by such conditions as anxiety, inflammation, pain, and trauma.

For acute muscle spasms, a patient may receive one of these centrally acting skeletal muscle relaxants: carisoprodol, chlorphenesin, chlorzoxazone, cyclobenzaprine, metaxalone, methocarbamol, or orphenadrine.

Pharmacokinetics

Little is known about the pharmacokinetics of centrally acting skeletal muscle relaxants. In general, these drugs are absorbed from the GI tract, widely distributed in the body, metabolized in the liver, and excreted by the kidneys.

When given orally, these drugs can take 30 to 60 minutes to achieve their effects. For most of these drugs, the duration of action ranges from 4 to 6 hours; for cyclobenzaprine, it ranges from 12 to 25 hours.

Functions of neurons
+ Receive sensory stimuli (sensory neurons)
+ Transmit motor responses (motor neurons)
+ Coordinate communication in the CNS (interneurons)

Function of a skeletal muscle relaxant
+ To reduce spasticity, possibly by reducing hyperexcitability

Features of centrally acting skeletal muscle relaxants
+ Act as CNS depressants
+ Treat acute spasms from such conditions as anxiety, inflammation, pain, trauma

Uses of centrally acting skeletal muscle relaxants

+ To treat acute, painful musculo-skeletal conditions
+ To supplement rest and physical therapy

Possible drug interactions

+ Anticholinesterases
+ Cholinergic blockers
+ Clonidine
+ CNS depressants
+ Guanethidine
+ MAO inhibitors
+ Phenothiazines
+ Propoxyphene

Adverse reactions to watch for

+ Abdominal distress, heartburn
+ Areflexia, flaccid paralysis, respiratory depression
+ Asthenia, ataxia
+ Blurred vision
+ Bradycardia, tachycardia
+ Constipation, diarrhea
+ Dizziness, syncope, vertigo, lack of coordination
+ Drowsiness. lethargy
+ Dry mouth, urine retention, urinary hesitancy
+ Hypotension, flushing
+ Nausea, vomiting

WARNING

Managing carisoprodol reactions

After the first through the fourth doses of carisoprodol, monitor the patient for idiosyncratic reactions, such as weakness, ataxia, vision and speech difficulties, fever, skin eruptions, and mental changes. Also monitor him for severe reactions, including bronchospasm, hypotension, and anaphylactic shock. If you detect any unusual reaction, withhold the dose and notify the prescriber immediately.

Pharmacodynamics

The centrally acting drugs don't relax skeletal muscles directly or depress neuronal conduction, neuromuscular transmission, or muscle excitability. Although their precise mechanism of action is unknown, these drugs are known to be CNS depressants. Their skeletal muscle relaxant effects may be related to their sedative effects.

Pharmacotherapeutics

Patients receive centrally acting skeletal muscle relaxants to treat acute, painful musculoskeletal conditions. These drugs usually are prescribed along with rest and physical therapy.

Interactions

The centrally acting skeletal muscle relaxants interact with other CNS depressants (including alcohol, opioids, barbiturates, anticonvulsants, tricyclic antidepressants, and anxiolytics), causing increased sedation, impaired motor function, and respiratory depression. In addition, some of these drugs have other interactions.
+ Cyclobenzaprine may interact with monoamine oxidase (MAO) inhibitors, resulting in fever, excitation, and seizures.
+ Cyclobenzaprine also can decrease the antihypertensive effects of guanethidine and clonidine.
+ Cyclobenzaprine and orphenadrine sometimes enhance the effects of cholinergic blockers.
+ Methocarbamol can antagonize the cholinergic effects of anticholinesterases used to treat myasthenia gravis.
+ Orphenadrine can reduce the effects of phenothiazines.
+ When taken together, orphenadrine and propoxyphene can cause additive CNS effects, including confusion, anxiety, and tremors.

Adverse reactions

The most common adverse reactions to centrally acting skeletal muscle relaxants are extensions of their therapeutic effects on the CNS. A few are idiosyncratic. (See *Managing carisoprodol reactions.*)

Drowsiness and dizziness are the most common adverse reactions to these drugs. Occasionally, nausea, vomiting, diarrhea, constipation, heartburn, abdominal distress, or ataxia occurs. Areflexia, flaccid paralysis, respiratory depression, and hypotension are seen occasionally after oral administration of any of these drugs, except methocarbamol. With parenteral administration, reactions may include syn-

PATIENT TEACHING

Teaching a patient about centrally acting skeletal muscle relaxants

Whenever a centrally acting skeletal muscle relaxant is prescribed, teach the patient and his family the drug's name, dose, frequency, action, and adverse effects, and take the following actions.
+ Inform the patient that the drug may impair his alertness or physical coordination, increasing the risk of operating machinery or driving a motor vehicle.
+ Advise the patient to avoid sudden changes in position if dizziness occurs.
+ Instruct the patient to take the oral form with meals or milk to prevent GI distress.
+ Advise the patient to relieve dry mouth with sugarless candy or gum and cool beverages, if permitted.
+ Inform the patient that chlorzoxazone may harmlessly discolor urine orange or purple-red; methocarbamol, green, black, or brown.
+ Teach the patient to notify the prescriber if adverse reactions or urine retention occur.

cope, hypotension, flushing, blurred vision, asthenia, lethargy, vertigo, lack of coordination, and bradycardia.

Because orphenadrine has anticholinergic effects, adverse reactions may include dry mouth, urine retention, urinary hesitancy, blurred vision, and tachycardia. Orphenadrine overdose may cause seizures, shock, respiratory arrest, coma, or death. At high doses, cyclobenzaprine, which is structurally similar to a tricyclic antidepressant, shares its toxic potential. Therefore, additional reactions to cyclobenzaprine may include temporary confusion, disturbed concentration, transient visual hallucinations, agitation, hyperactive reflexes, muscle rigidity, vomiting, and hyperpyrexia. Abrupt cessation of the drug may cause severe withdrawal symptoms.

Rarely, parenteral orphenadrine causes an anaphylactic reaction. Chlorphenesin contains tartrazine dye, which may cause an allergic reaction. Parenteral methocarbamol contains polyethylene glycol that may increase preexisting acidosis and urine retention in patients with renal impairment.

Nursing considerations
+ Teach the patient and his caregiver about the prescribed drug. (See *Teaching a patient about centrally acting skeletal muscle relaxants.*)
+ Monitor the patient periodically for adverse reactions to the centrally acting skeletal muscle relaxant.
+ Avoid abrupt discontinuation of the centrally acting skeletal muscle relaxant and reduce the dosage gradually.
+ Give parenteral orphenadrine over 5 minutes with the patient lying down and keep him this way for 5 to 10 more minutes afterwards. Then help the patient to a sitting position and supervise walking.
+ Monitor the I.V. site in a patient who receives parenteral methocarbamol. Watch for extravasation because thrombophlebitis, sloughing, and pain may result.
+ Give I.V. methocarbamol slowly at no more than 3 ml/minute. Inject I.M. methocarbamol deeply and slowly, only in the upper outer quadrant of the buttocks, with a maximum of 5 ml in each buttock. Avoid subcutaneous (S.C.) administration.

Key nursing actions
+ Avoid stopping the drug abruptly; instead, reduce the dosage gradually.
+ Keep epinephrine, antihistamines, and corticosteroids nearby for persistent syncope.
+ Monitor the patient's respiratory status; keep emergency equipment nearby.

Features of direct-acting skeletal muscle relaxants

✦ Most effective for spasticity of central origin

How dantrolene works

✦ Acts on the muscle itself
✦ Interferes with calcium ion release from the sarcoplasmic reticulum
✦ Weakens the force of muscle contractions
✦ Little effect on cardiac or intestinal smooth muscle

Conditions that call for dantrolene

✦ Cerebral palsy
✦ Malignant hyperthermia (prevention and treatment)
✦ MS
✦ Spinal cord injury
✦ Stroke

EYE ON DRUG ACTION

How dantrolene reduces muscle rigidity

Dantrolene appears to decrease the number of calcium ions released from the sarcoplasmic reticulum (a structure in muscle cells involved in muscle contractions and relaxation by releasing and storing calcium). The lower the calcium level in the muscle plasma or myoplasm, the less energy produced when calcium prompts the muscle's actin and myosin filaments (responsible for muscle contraction) to interact. Less energy means weaker muscle contractions.

By promoting muscle relaxation, dantrolene prevents or reduces the rigidity that contributes to the life-threatening body temperatures of malignant hyperthermia.

✦ Keep epinephrine, antihistamines, and corticosteroids on hand during methocarbamol therapy to correct syncope that doesn't resolve with supportive therapy.
✦ Monitor the respiratory status of a patient receiving a CNS depressant and a centrally acting skeletal muscle relaxant. Keep emergency equipment available.
✦ Notify the prescriber if the centrally acting skeletal muscle relaxant doesn't relieve pain or muscle spasms.

DIRECT-ACTING SKELETAL MUSCLE RELAXANTS

Dantrolene is the most common direct-acting skeletal muscle relaxant. Although dantrolene has a similar therapeutic effect to the centrally acting drugs, it works through a different mechanism of action. Because its major effect is on the muscle, dantrolene poses a lower risk of adverse CNS effects. High therapeutic doses, however, are toxic to the liver.

Dantrolene seems most effective for spasticity of cerebral origin. Because it produces muscle weakness, dantrolene is of questionable benefit in patients with borderline strength.

Pharmacokinetics

Although the peak dantrolene level occurs within about 5 hours after it's ingested, the patient may not notice therapeutic benefits for a week or more.

Dantrolene is absorbed poorly from the GI tract and is highly plasma protein-bound. This means that only a small portion of the drug is available to produce a therapeutic effect.

Dantrolene is metabolized by the liver and excreted in urine. In healthy adults, its elimination half-life is about 9 hours. Because dantrolene is metabolized in the liver, its half-life can be prolonged in patients with impaired liver function.

Pharmacodynamics

Dantrolene is chemically and pharmacologically unrelated to other skeletal muscle relaxants. The drug works by acting on the muscle itself. It interferes with calcium ion release from the sarcoplasmic reticulum and weakens the force of muscle contractions. At therapeutic levels, dantrolene has little effect on cardiac or intestinal smooth muscles.

WARNING

Spotting dantrolene-induced hepatitis

During dantrolene therapy, fatal or nonfatal hepatitis may occur as an idiosyncratic reaction. To help detect such reactions, take these measures.

◆ Monitor the patient for nausea, anorexia, vomiting, and abdominal discomfort, which may precede hepatitis.

◆ Be aware that hepatitis most commonly affects patients who receive more than 300 mg daily for longer than 2 months, but also may occur in patients who take short courses of 800 mg or more daily.

◆ Check for factors that increase the risk of dantrolene hepatotoxicity, which is more likely to affect women, patients older than age 35, patients who also take other drugs (especially estrogens), and patients with baseline liver function test abnormalities.

If signs of hepatitis are detected, expect to withhold dantrolene. The drug-induced liver function test abnormalities may return to normal when the drug is stopped.

Pharmacotherapeutics

Dantrolene helps manage all types of spasticity, but is most effective in patients with cerebral palsy, MS, spinal cord injury, and stroke. Dantrolene also is used to treat and prevent malignant hyperthermia. This rare but potentially fatal complication of anesthesia is characterized by skeletal muscle rigidity and high fever. (See *How dantrolene reduces muscle rigidity.*)

Interactions

◆ CNS depressants (including alcohol) can increase dantrolene's depressant effects; combined use may lead to sedation, lack of coordination, and respiratory depression.

◆ Estrogens combined with dantrolene can increase the risk of liver toxicity.

◆ Together, verapamil and dantrolene may result in cardiovascular collapse. Don't give verapamil to a patient receiving dantrolene.

◆ Sun exposure may cause photosensitivity reactions during dantrolene therapy.

Adverse reactions

Dose-related adverse reactions to dantrolene usually are transient, lasting up to 4 days after therapy begins. The most common is muscle weakness, rarely severe enough to cause slurred speech, drooling, and enuresis. Other common reactions include drowsiness, dizziness, light-headedness, diarrhea, nausea, malaise, and fatigue. If weakness or diarrhea is severe, the dosage may be decreased or the drug discontinued. Other adverse GI reactions that may respond to a dosage decrease include anorexia, vomiting, gastric irritation, abdominal cramps, constipation, difficulty swallowing, and GI bleeding. Constipation sometimes is severe enough to resemble a bowel obstruction. (See *Spotting dantrolene-induced hepatitis.*)

Adverse neurologic reactions include vision and speech disturbances, headache, taste alteration, depression, confusion, hallucinations, nervousness, insomnia, and seizures.

Genitourinary reactions include urinary frequency, incontinence, nocturia, difficult urination, urine retention, hematuria, crystalluria, and difficult erection.

Possible drug interactions

◆ CNS depressants
◆ Estrogens
◆ Verapamil

Adverse reactions to watch for

◆ Abdominal cramps, anorexia, constipation, diarrhea, difficulty swallowing, gastric irritation, GI bleeding, vomiting

◆ Acneiform rash, pruritus, urticaria, excessive tearing, chills, fever, feeling of suffocation.

◆ Dizziness, drowsiness, light-headedness

◆ Fatigue, malaise

◆ Muscle weakness

◆ Urinary frequency, incontinence, nocturia, difficult urination, urine retention, hematuria, crystalluria, difficult erection

◆ Tachycardia, bradycardia, erratic blood pressure, arrhythmias, phlebitis, pleural effusion with pericarditis

◆ Vision and speech disturbances, headache, taste alteration, depression, confusion, hallucinations, nervousness, insomnia, and seizures

Teaching a patient about dantrolene

Whenever dantrolene is prescribed, teach the patient and his family the drug's name, dose, frequency, action, and adverse effects, and take the following actions.
+ Reassure the patient that dantrolene's adverse effects, such as weakness, drowsiness, and dizziness, usually subside in a few days.
+ Instruct the patient to take dantrolene with meals or milk to prevent GI irritation.
+ Advise the patient to expect frequent blood tests of liver function.
+ Tell the patient to notify the prescriber if he develops yellow skin or eyes, itchy skin, or fever.
+ Tell the patient to avoid photosensitivity reactions by using sunblock and wearing protective clothing, to report abdominal discomfort or GI problems immediately, and to follow the prescriber's orders for rest and physical therapy.
+ Tell the patient and his family to notify the prescriber if adverse reactions occur.

Cardiovascular reactions include tachycardia, bradycardia, erratic blood pressure, arrhythmias, phlebitis, and pleural effusion with pericarditis.

Other reactions include acneiform rash, pruritus, urticaria, excessive tearing, chills, fever, and a feeling of suffocation.

Nursing considerations

+ Frequently monitor any patient with severe cardiac or pulmonary disease who receives dantrolene.
+ Monitor the patient's liver function test results before and during dantrolene therapy. If it doesn't produce a benefit in 45 days, stop the drug.

 CLINICAL ALERT Be alert for severe diarrhea, severe weakness, and signs of hepatitis (such as fever and jaundice) or sensitivity reactions (such as fever and skin eruptions). If any of these occur, withhold the dose and notify the prescriber.

+ Prepare oral suspension for a single dose by dissolving capsule contents in juice or another liquid. For multiple doses, dilute in an acidic liquid, refrigerate, and use within several days.
+ Reconstitute dantrolene with 60 ml of sterile, not bacteriostatic, water for I.V. administration. Use the solution within 6 hours. Dantrolene isn't compatible with normal saline solution or dextrose 5% in water.
+ Monitor the patient for sedation, motor skill impairment, and respiratory depression if he receives dantrolene and a CNS depressant.
+ Keep emergency equipment nearby to treat respiratory depression.
+ Monitor the patient's level of spasticity during therapy.
+ Notify the prescriber if the patient's physical mobility doesn't improve during therapy.
+ Teach the patient and his caregiver about the drug. (See *Teaching a patient about dantrolene.*)

Key nursing actions

+ Monitor liver function tests before, during, and after therapy.
+ Watch for severe diarrhea, severe weakness, and evidence of hepatitis or sensitivity reactions.
+ Monitor the patient for sedation, impaired motor skills, respiratory depression.
+ Assess the level of spasticity.

Diazepam as a skeletal muscle relaxant

Diazepam is a benzodiazepine that's used to treat acute muscle spasms as well as spasticity caused by chronic disorders. Other uses of diazepam include treating anxiety, alcohol withdrawal, and seizures. It seems to work by promoting the inhibitory effect of the neurotransmitter gamma-aminobutyric acid, or GABA, on muscle contraction.

Diazepam can be used alone or with other drugs to treat spasticity, especially in patients with spinal cord lesions and, occasionally, in patients with cerebral palsy. It's also helpful in patients with painful, continuous muscle spasms who aren't susceptible to the drug's sedative effects. However, its central nervous system effects, such as sedation, and the tolerance that develops with prolonged therapy limit its use.

OTHER SKELETAL MUSCLE RELAXANTS

Three other drugs are used to relax skeletal muscle, especially in intermittent and chronic spasticity: baclofen, diazepam, and tizanidine. Because diazepam is used primarily an anxiolytic, this section focuses on baclofen and tizanidine. (See *Diazepam as a skeletal muscle relaxant.*)

BACLOFEN

Structurally resembling gamma-aminobutyric acid (GABA), baclofen is typically given orally to treat MS and spinal cord injuries and diseases.

Pharmacokinetics

Baclofen is absorbed rapidly from the GI tract. It's distributed widely (with only small amounts crossing the blood-brain barrier), undergoes minimal liver metabolism, and is excreted primarily unchanged in urine.

The drug can take hours to weeks to produce noticeable beneficial effects. Its elimination half-life ranges from 2½ to 4 hours.

Pharmacodynamics

It isn't known exactly how baclofen works. Because the drug is chemically similar to the neurotransmitter GABA, it probably acts in the spinal cord.

Baclofen reduces nerve impulses from the spinal cord to skeletal muscles, decreasing the number and severity of muscle spasms and reducing pain. The drug produces less sedation than diazepam and less peripheral muscle weakness than dantrolene. Therefore, it's the drug of choice to treat spasticity.

Pharmacotherapeutics

Baclofen's major clinical use is for paraplegic or quadriplegic patients with spinal cord lesions, most commonly caused by MS or trauma. For these patients, the drug significantly reduces the number and severity of painful flexor spasms; however, it doesn't improve stiff gait, manual dexterity, or residual muscle function.

For the patient who doesn't respond to the oral form or who experiences intolerable adverse reactions, baclofen may be administered intrathecally. If the patient shows a positive response to a bolus dose, he may receive an implantable pump for long-term therapy. (See *Using an implantable pump in children,* page 66.)

Features of baclofen
+ Is structurally similar to GABA
+ Probably acts in the spinal cord
+ Reduces nerve impulses from the spinal cord to skeletal muscles
+ Reduces the severity of muscle spasms and pain, but doesn't improve stiff gait, manual dexterity, residual muscle function in paraplegia or quadriplegia

Conditions that call for baclofen
+ Spasticity (drug of choice)
+ Spinal cord injury or disease
+ MS

Possible drug interactions
+ CNS depressants, including alcohol
+ Fentanyl
+ Lithium
+ Tricyclic antidepressants

LIFESPAN

Using an implantable pump in children

In children younger than age 4, the safety of intrathecal baclofen therapy hasn't been established. Before implanting a pump for intrathecal baclofen therapy, the prescriber must determine if the child has sufficient body mass for the pump.

Interactions
✦ When baclofen is given with other CNS depressants, including alcohol, increased CNS depression may occur.
✦ When fentanyl and baclofen are given together, analgesia can be prolonged.
✦ Together, lithium and baclofen can aggravate hyperkinesia.
✦ Tricyclic antidepressants combined with baclofen can increase muscle relaxation.

Adverse reactions
The most common adverse reaction to baclofen is transient drowsiness. Other, less frequent adverse reactions include nausea, fatigue, vertigo, hypotonia, muscle weakness, depression, and headache. These can be avoided by adjusting the dose slowly.

Geriatric patients or patients with psychotic disorders, schizophrenia, or confusion may experience psychiatric disturbances, such as hallucinations, euphoria, depression, confusion, and anxiety. Dosage increases should be made slowly in these patients.

Other rare neuropsychiatric disturbances include insomnia, muscle pain, paresthesia, tinnitus, slurred speech, tremor, rigidity, ataxia, seizures, blurred vision, strabismus, nystagmus, diplopia, and dysarthria. Abrupt discontinuation can cause hallucinations, seizures, and worsening of spasticity. Baclofen rarely causes adverse genitourinary reactions. Cardiovascular reactions include hypotension and, rarely, dyspnea, chest pain, and syncope. Adverse GI reactions include nausea, vomiting, constipation and, rarely, dry mouth, anorexia, taste disorders, and diarrhea.

Rash, allergic skin disorders and pruritus may occur, as may ankle edema, weight gain, and excessive diaphoresis.

Nursing considerations
✦ Teach the patient and his caregiver about the drug. (See *Teaching a patient about baclofen*.)
✦ Monitor the patient periodically for adverse reactions and notify the prescriber if they occur.
✦ Monitor the patient for signs of renal impairment by documenting his fluid intake and output and body weight daily. Impaired renal function may require a dosage reduction because the drug is excreted primarily in urine.

 CLINICAL ALERT Don't discontinue baclofen abruptly, especially when given intrathecally. Abrupt withdrawal can result in high fever, altered mental status, seizures, exaggerated rebound spasticity, and muscle rigidity. Although rare, it can progress to rhabdomyolysis, multiple organ failure, and death.

Adverse reactions to watch for
✦ Ankle edema, weight gain, excessive diaphoresis
✦ Constipation, nausea, vomiting
✦ Depression, headache
✦ Fatigue, vertigo, hypotonia, muscle weakness
✦ Hypotension
✦ Psychiatric disturbances in geriatric patients or patients with psychotic disorders, schizophrenia, or confusion
✦ Rash, allergic skin disorders, pruritus
✦ Transient drowsiness

Key nursing actions
✦ Watch for evidence of renal impairment.
✦ Don't stop the drug abruptly.
✦ Monitor the number and severity of painful flexor spasms.
✦ Assess the patient's bowel and bladder control.

+ Monitor the number and severity of painful flexor spasms.
+ Assess the patient's degree of bowel and bladder control.

 CLINICAL ALERT Don't confuse baclofen with Bactroban (mupirocin), which is a topical anti-infective usually prescribed for impetigo, certain wound infections, or nasal colonization by drug-resistant bacteria.

TIZANIDINE

Tizanidine is a skeletal muscle relaxant that's used to manage acute and intermittent increases in muscle tone related to spasticity.

Pharmacokinetics

Tizanidine is rapidly absorbed and undergoes first pass metabolism. It's metabolized somewhat by the liver and reaches its peak level in 1 to 2 hours and its action endures for 3 to 6 hours. Its terminal half-life is 4 to 8 hours.

Pharmacodynamics

Chemically related to clonidine, tizanidine is an alpha-adrenergic agonist. It's thought to decrease spasticity by decreasing excitatory input and increasing presynaptic inhibition of motor neurons at the spinal cord.

Pharmacotherapeutics

Tizanidine may be used for acute and intermittent spasticity. Its off-label uses include tension headaches, back pain, and trigeminal neuralgia.

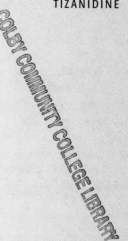

Features of tizanidine
+ Is used for acute, intermittent increases in muscle tone related to spasticity
+ Is an alpha-adrenergic agonist
+ May decrease spasticity by decreasing excitatory input and increasing presynaptic inhibition of motor neurons

Conditions that call for tizanidine
+ Acute and intermittent spasticity
+ Tension headaches, back pain, trigeminal neuralgia (off-label uses)

Possible drug interactions

- Antihypertensives
- CNS depressants
- Diuretics
- Hormonal contraceptives
- Other central alpha-adrenergic agonists

Adverse reactions to watch for

- Drowsiness, sedation, somnolence
- Hypotension
- Xerostomia

Key nursing actions

- Monitor liver function tests at start of therapy; after 1, 3, and 6 months; and periodically thereafter.
- Reduce the dosage if needed in patients with liver or kidney impairment.

Features of neuromuscular blockers

- Relax skeletal muscles by disrupting nerve transmission at motor end plates
- Are used to relax skeletal muscles during surgery, reduce the intensity of muscle spasms in induced seizures, and manage patients fighting mechanical ventilation
- Belong to two classes: nondepolarizing and depolarizing blockers

PATIENT TEACHING

Teaching a patient about tizanidine

Whenever tizanidine is prescribed, teach the patient and his family the drug's name, dose, frequency, action, and adverse effects, and take the following actions.
- Caution the patient to avoid alcohol and activities that require alertness because the drug may cause drowsiness.
- Instruct the patient to minimize orthostatic hypotension by rising slowly and avoiding sudden position changes.

Interactions

♦ When combined with diuretics, other central alpha-adrenergic agonists, or antihypertensives, additive hypotension may occur.
♦ Use with CNS depressants (including baclofen, benzodiazepines, and alcohol) may cause additive CNS depression.
♦ Hormonal contraceptives may reduce tizanidine clearance, requiring a dosage reduction.
♦ Use with herbs, such as gotu kola, kava, St. John's wort, and valerian, may lead to increased CNS depression.

Adverse reactions

Common adverse reactions may include hypotension, sedation, drowsiness, somnolence, and xerostomia. Uncommon adverse reactions include arrhythmia, syncope, fatigue, anxiety, nervousness, skin rash, nausea, vomiting, elevated liver enzyme levels, muscle weakness, and tremor. The patient also may experience palpitations, ventricular extrasystoles, visual hallucination, delusions, and hepatic failure.

Nursing considerations

♦ Use cautiously in a patient taking an antihypertensive because of the increased risk of orthostatic hypotension.
♦ Because of the risk of life-threatening liver impairment, monitor liver function tests results when therapy begins; after 1, 3, and 6 months of therapy; and periodically thereafter.
♦ Reduce the dosage if needed in a patient with kidney or liver impairment because drug clearance may be reduced. (See *Using tizanidine safely in geriatric patients,* page 67.)
♦ Teach the patient and his caregiver about the drug. (See *Teaching a patient about tizanidine.*)

NEUROMUSCULAR BLOCKERS

Neuromuscular blockers relax skeletal muscles by disrupting nerve impulse transmission at motor end plates (branching terminals of a motor nerve axon). (See *How motor end plates work.*)

Neuromuscular blockers have three major clinical indications: to relax skeletal muscles during surgery, to reduce the intensity of muscle spasms in drug or electrically induced seizures, and to manage patients who are fighting a mechanical venti-

How motor end plates work

The motor nerve axon divides to form branching terminals called motor end plates. These plates are enfolded in muscle fibers, but separated from the fibers by the synaptic cleft.

COMPETING WITH CONTRACTION
A stimulus to the nerve causes the release of acetylcholine into the synaptic cleft. There, acetylcholine occupies receptor sites on the muscle cell membrane, depolarizing the membrane and causing muscle contraction. Neuromuscular blockers act at motor end plates by competing with acetylcholine for the receptor sites or by blocking depolarization.

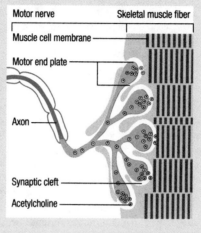

lator. Two main classes of natural and synthetic drugs are used as neuromuscular blockers: nondepolarizing and depolarizing blockers.

NONDEPOLARIZING BLOCKERS

Also called *competitive* or *stabilizing* drugs, nondepolarizing blockers are derived from curare alkaloids and synthetically similar compounds. They include atracurium, cisatracurium, doxacurium, mivacurium, pancuronium, rocuronium, tubocurarine, and vecuronium.

Pharmacokinetics

Because nondepolarizing blockers are absorbed poorly from the GI tract, they're administered parenterally. The I.V. route is preferred because the action is more predictable.

Nondepolarizing blockers are distributed rapidly throughout the body. A variable but large proportion of the drug is excreted unchanged in urine. Some drugs, such as atracurium, pancuronium, and vecuronium, are partially metabolized in the liver.

Pharmacodynamics

Nondepolarizing blockers compete with acetylcholine at cholinergic receptor sites on the skeletal muscle membrane. This action blocks acetylcholine's neurotransmitter action, preventing muscle contraction. Anticholinesterases, such as neostigmine or pyridostigmine, which inhibit the action of acetylcholinesterase, the enzyme that destroys acetylcholine, can counteract it.

Features of nondepolarizing blockers

✦ Compete with acetylcholine at cholinergic receptors on the skeletal muscle membrane
✦ Block acetylcholine's transmitter action, preventing muscle contraction
✦ Don't cross the blood-brain barrier, so the patient remains conscious and aware but can't communicate

Coping with neuromuscular blocker resistance in burn patients

Resistance to neuromuscular blockers in burn patients can be substantial, depending on the extent of the injury and the time elapsed since the burn. Resistance is most likely to happen in a patient with burns over 25% to 30% or more of his body and to occur 1 week or more after the injury, generally peaking 2 or more weeks after the burn and lasting for several months. Resistance will decrease gradually with healing, but these patients may require substantially larger doses of these drugs.

Uses for nondepolarizing blockers

+ Easing passage of an ET tube
+ Decreasing needed anesthetic
+ Assisting in the realignment of broken bones and dislocated joints
+ Paralyzing a patient who needs mechanical ventilation
+ Preventing muscle injury during ECT

Possible drug interactions

+ Aminoglycosides
+ Anticholinesterases
+ Beta blockers
+ Carbamazepine
+ Clindamycin
+ Corticosteroids
+ Drugs that alter calcium, magnesium, and potassium levels
+ Hydantoins
+ Inhaled anesthetics
+ Ketamine
+ Lithium
+ Magnesium salts
+ Nitrates
+ Piperacillin
+ Polymyxin
+ Quinine derivatives
+ Ranitidine
+ Tetracyclines
+ Theophylline
+ Thiazide diuretics
+ Verapamil

The initial muscle weakness produced by these drugs quickly changes to flaccid paralysis that affects the muscles in a specific sequence. The first muscles to exhibit flaccid paralysis are those of the eyes, face, and neck. Next, the limb, abdomen, and trunk muscles become flaccid. Finally, the intercostal muscles and diaphragm are paralyzed. Recovery from the paralysis usually occurs in the reverse order.

Because these drugs don't cross the blood-brain barrier, the patient remains conscious and can feel pain, even though he's paralyzed. The patient is aware of what's happening and may experience extreme anxiety, but can't communicate his feelings. For this reason, an analgesic or anxiolytic should be given with the nondepolarizing blocker.

Pharmacotherapeutics

Nondepolarizing blockers are used for intermediate or prolonged muscle relaxation. They're commonly prescribed to:
+ ease the passage of an endotracheal (ET) tube
+ decrease the amount of anesthetic required during surgery
+ facilitate the realignment of broken bones and dislocated joints
+ paralyze a patient who needs ventilatory support, but who fights the ET tube and ventilation
+ prevent muscle injury during electroconvulsive therapy (ECT) by reducing the intensity of muscle spasms. (See *Coping with neuromuscular blocker resistance in burn patients.*)

Interactions

+ Aminoglycosides, clindamycin, inhalation anesthetics, ketamine, lithium, magnesium salts, nitrates, piperacillin, polymyxin, quinine derivatives, tetracyclines, thiazide diuretics, and verapamil can increase the intensity and duration of paralysis when taken with a nondepolarizing blocker.
+ Anticholinesterases (edrophonium, neostigmine, and pyridostigmine) antagonize nondepolarizing blockers and are used as antidotes to them.
+ Beta blockers may potentiate, counteract, or have no effect on nondepolarizing blockers.
+ Carbamazepine, corticosteroids, hydantoins, ranitidine, and theophylline can decrease neuromuscular blockade when taken with a nondepolarizing blocker.
+ Drugs that alter the calcium, magnesium, or potassium levels also can alter the effects of nondepolarizing blockers.

PATIENT TEACHING

Teaching a patient about nondepolarizing neuromuscular blockers

Whenever a nondepolarizing neuromuscular blocker is prescribed, explain the drug's purpose to the patient and family, and take the following actions.
✦ Encourage the patient and his family to ask questions about the nondepolarizing blocker be-fore administration, if possible.
✦ Inform the patient and his family about all procedures in advance.
✦ Provide reassurance that the patient will be carefully monitored during administration of the nondepolarizing blocker.
✦ Tell the patient that he'll also receive sedation during neuromuscular blocker use.

Adverse reactions

Nondepolarizing blockers most commonly produce adverse reactions when they're given to patients who are debilitated, have fluid and electrolyte imbalances, or have respiratory, hepatic, neuromuscular, cardiac, endocrine, or renal disorders.

The prolonged pharmacologic effects of these drugs are responsible for most adverse reactions. The most serious adverse reaction is apnea. Ganglionic blockade and histamine release may cause a cardiovascular reaction, usually hypotension. Histamine release also may produce skin reactions, bronchospasm, and excessive bronchial and salivary secretions. Antidotes used to restore breathing may accentu-ate the hypotension and bronchospasms. Allergic reactions are rare.

Pancuronium selectively blocks the vagus nerve and may result in tachycardia, arrhythmias, and hypertension.

Nursing considerations

✦ Teach the patient and his caregiver about the drug. (See *Teaching a patient about nondepolarizing neuromuscular blockers.*)
✦ Keep antidotes (such as atropine, edrophonium, and neostigmine) readily avail-able.
✦ Keep endotracheal equipment, oxygen, and suction equipment available for res-piratory support.
✦ Don't combine mivacurium, pancuronium, tubocurarine, or vecuronium with alkaline solutions, such as barbiturates; they're physically incompatible and may produce a precipitate.
✦ Calculate the drug dosage carefully. Always verify the dosage with the prescriber or another health care professional.
✦ Notify the prescriber if adverse reactions or drug interactions occur.
✦ Monitor the patient's respirations frequently until he has fully recovered from neuromuscular blockade, as evidenced by tests of muscle strength (peripheral nerve stimulator, hand grip, head lift, and ability to cough).
✦ Keep the drug refrigerated to maintain potency.
✦ Check the mechanical ventilator's settings and functions frequently to ensure that it's operating properly. Never turn off the ventilator alarm.
✦ Turn the patient every 2 hours and provide chest physiotherapy.
✦ Suction the patient because the nondepolarizing blocker suppresses the cough reflex and may increase respiratory secretions.

Adverse reactions to watch for

✦ Apnea
✦ Arrhythmias, tachycardia
✦ Bronchospasm
✦ Excessive bronchial and salivary secretions
✦ Hypertension, hypotension
✦ Skin reactions

Key nursing actions

✦ Keep antidotes (atropine, edro-phonium, neostigmine) nearby.
✦ Keep endotracheal equipment, oxygen, suction equipment near-by.
✦ Verify the dosage carefully.
✦ Monitor respirations frequently until recovery is complete.
✦ Reassure the patient that breathing will return to normal.

+ Reassure the patient that breathing will return to normal after the drug is stopped.

DEPOLARIZING BLOCKERS

Succinylcholine is the only therapeutic drug in this category. Although it's similar to the nondepolarizing blockers in its therapeutic effect, its mechanism of action differs. Succinylcholine acts like acetylcholine, but isn't inactivated by cholinesterase. It's the drug of choice when short-term muscle relaxation is needed.

Pharmacokinetics

Because succinylcholine is absorbed poorly from the GI tract, the preferred administration route is I.V.; the I.M. route can be used if needed.

Succinylcholine is hydrolyzed in the liver and plasma by the enzyme pseudocholinesterase, producing a metabolite with a nondepolarizing blocking action. Succinylcholine is excreted by the kidneys, with a small amount excreted unchanged.

Pharmacodynamics

After administration, succinylcholine is metabolized rapidly but still more slowly than acetylcholine. As a result, succinylcholine remains attached to receptor sites on skeletal muscle membranes for a longer time. This prevents repolarization of the motor end plate and results in muscle paralysis.

Pharmacotherapeutics

Succinylcholine is the drug of choice for short-term muscle relaxation, such as during intubation and ECT.

Interactions

+ Many drugs may potentiate succinylcholine's action, including amphotericin B, beta blockers, chloroquine, cimetidine, cyclophosphamide, inhalation anesthetics, I.V. procaine, isoflurane, lidocaine, lithium carbonate, magnesium sulfate, narcotic analgesics, nondepolarizing blockers, certain nonpenicillin antibiotics, oxytocin, phenelzine, procainamide, promazine, quinidine, quinine, thiazide diuretics, and trimethaphan.
+ Anticholinesterases increase succinylcholine blockade.
+ The herbal remedy melatonin may potentiate succinylcholine's blocking properties.

Adverse reactions

The primary adverse reactions to succinylcholine are the same as those to nondepolarizing blockers: prolonged apnea and cardiovascular alterations.

Patients commonly experience muscle pain from the fasciculations that occur in phase I. These also may cause myoglobinemia and myoglobinuria, especially in children. The concomitant rise in the potassium level can be dangerous to patients with renal or neuromuscular disorders. The transient elevation of intraocular pressure that occurs during phase I may be harmful to patients with previously elevated intraocular pressure.

Neuromuscular blockade may be potentiated by certain genetic predispositions, such as a low pseudocholinesterase level and the tendency to develop malignant hyperthermia. A low pseudocholinesterase level also is present in liver disorders because pseudocholinesterase is synthesized in the liver. To determine the patient's sensitivity to succinylcholine, an initial test dose of 10 mg may be given.

Phase II blockade may occur with repeated doses of succinylcholine.

Nursing considerations

✦ Monitor the patient periodically for adverse reactions. Keep in mind that genetic factors, such as a low pseudocholinesterase level and a tendency to develop malignant hyperthermia, may potentiate neuromuscular blockade. Also monitor the patient for drug interactions.

✦ Notify the prescriber immediately if adverse reactions or drug interactions occur. Be prepared to give emergency care according to facility guidelines.

✦ Don't use reversing drugs. Unlike nondepolarizing drugs, neostigmine or edrophonium may worsen neuromuscular blockade.

✦ Maintain a patent airway for the patient.

✦ Keep endotracheal equipment, oxygen, suction equipment, and a mechanical ventilator available for respiratory support.

✦ Check the patient's respiratory rate and pattern every 5 to 10 minutes during the infusion.

✦ Notify the prescriber of any change in the patient's respiratory status.

✦ Monitor the patient closely until recovery from neuromuscular blockade is complete. Signs of complete recovery include a renewed ability to cough and a return to previous levels of muscle strength on hand-grip and head-lift tests.

✦ Teach the patient and his caregiver about succinylcholine. (See *Teaching a patient about depolarizing neuromuscular blockers.*)

ANTIPARKINSONIANS

Drug therapy is an important part of treatment for Parkinson's disease, a progressive neurologic disorder characterized by four main features: muscle rigidity, akinesia, tremors at rest, and disturbances of posture and balance. The disease causes movement disorders by affecting the extrapyramidal system, which includes the corpus striatum, globus pallidus, and substantia nigra of the brain.

In Parkinson's disease, a dopamine deficiency occurs in the basal ganglia, the dopamine-releasing pathway that connects the substantia nigra to the corpus striatum. Dopamine reduction in the corpus striatum upsets the normal balance be-

Key nursing actions

✦ Maintain a patent airway.

✦ Keep endotracheal equipment, oxygen, suction equipment nearby.

✦ Check the respiratory rate and pattern every 5 to 10 minutes during infusion.

✦ Monitor the patient closely until recovery is complete.

Facts about Parkinson's disease

✦ Is a progressive neurologic disorder

✦ Has four main features: muscle rigidity, akinesia, tremors at rest, disturbed posture and balance

tween two neurotransmitters, acetylcholine and dopamine. This results in a relative excess of acetylcholine. The excessive excitation caused by cholinergic activity creates the movement disorders of Parkinson's disease. Parkinsonism also can result from drugs, encephalitis, neurotoxins, trauma, arteriosclerosis, or other neurologic disorders and environmental factors.

The goal of drug therapy is to relieve symptoms of Parkinson's disease and maintain the patient's independence and mobility. To achieve these goals, drug therapy aims to correct the neurotransmitter imbalance by inhibiting cholinergic effects (with anticholinergics) and enhancing dopamine's effects (with dopaminergics).

ANTICHOLINERGICS

Sometimes anticholinergics are called parasympatholytics because they inhibit the action of acetylcholine at special receptors in the parasympathetic nervous system. Anticholinergics used to treat parkinsonism are classified in two categories based on chemical structure: synthetic tertiary amines — such as benztropine, biperiden, procyclidine, and trihexyphenidyl — and antihistamines — such as diphenhydramine.

Pharmacokinetics

Typically, anticholinergics are well absorbed from the GI tract and cross the blood-brain barrier to their action site in the brain. Their exact distribution is unknown. Most of these drugs are metabolized in the liver, at least partially, and are excreted by the kidneys as metabolites and unchanged drug.

Benztropine has a duration of action up to 24 hours in some patients but an unknown half-life. Biperiden, procyclidine, and trihexyphenidyl have half-lives of 18 to 24, 12 to 13, and 5 to 10 hours, respectively. In addition to the oral route, some anticholinergics also can be given by the I.M. or I.V. route.

Pharmacodynamics

A high acetylcholine level produces an excitatory effect on the CNS, which can cause parkinsonian tremor. In patients with Parkinson's disease, anticholinergics inhibit the action of acetylcholine at receptor sites in the CNS and autonomic nervous system, which reduces the tremor.

Pharmacotherapeutics

Anticholinergics are used to treat all forms of parkinsonism. They're used most commonly in the early stages of Parkinson's disease when symptoms are mild and don't have a major impact on the patient's lifestyle. These drugs effectively control sialorrhea (excessive flow of saliva) and are about 20% effective in reducing the risk and severity of akinesia and rigidity.

In the early stages of Parkinson's disease, anticholinergics can be used alone or with amantadine. In the later stages, they can be given with levodopa to relieve symptoms further.

Interactions

✦ Amantadine can increase the anticholinergics' adverse effects.
✦ Anticholinergics may decrease levodopa absorption, which may lead to worsening of parkinsonian signs and symptoms.

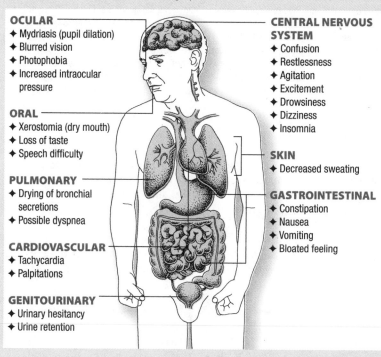

Assessing dose-related adverse reactions to anticholinergics

Common dose-related adverse reactions to anticholinergics are listed below. Use this illustration as a head-to-toe guide when assessing a patient.

OCULAR
+ Mydriasis (pupil dilation)
+ Blurred vision
+ Photophobia
+ Increased intraocular pressure

ORAL
+ Xerostomia (dry mouth)
+ Loss of taste
+ Speech difficulty

PULMONARY
+ Drying of bronchial secretions
+ Possible dyspnea

CARDIOVASCULAR
+ Tachycardia
+ Palpitations

GENITOURINARY
+ Urinary hesitancy
+ Urine retention

CENTRAL NERVOUS SYSTEM
+ Confusion
+ Restlessness
+ Agitation
+ Excitement
+ Drowsiness
+ Dizziness
+ Insomnia

SKIN
+ Decreased sweating

GASTROINTESTINAL
+ Constipation
+ Nausea
+ Vomiting
+ Bloated feeling

+ Antipsychotics (such as phenothiazines, thiothixene, haloperidol, and loxapine) can increase the risk of the anticholinergics' adverse effects. Their interaction can decrease the effectiveness of anticholinergics and antipsychotics.
+ Over-the-counter cough or cold preparations, diet aids, or analeptics (drugs used to stay awake) increase anticholinergic effects.
+ Alcohol increases anticholinergic-induced CNS depression.

Adverse reactions

Most adverse reactions to anticholinergics are an extension of their pharmacologic effects. Mild, dose-related adverse reactions occur in 30% to 50% of patients. Typically, reactions decrease as treatment continues, but they may limit the dosage that the patient can tolerate. One way to review the various dose-related adverse reactions is to start at the head of the body and move down. (See *Assessing dose-related adverse reactions to anticholinergics.*)

Anticholinergics also can produce patient-sensitivity-related adverse reactions, including urticaria and allergic rashes that may lead to exfoliation. Diphenhydramine also can produce a photosensitivity reaction (abnormal reaction of the skin to sunlight), causing burning and redness with minimal exposure.

Possible drug interactions
(continued)

+ Levodopa
+ Over-the-counter cough or cold preparations, diet aids, analeptics

Adverse reactions to watch for

+ About 30% to 50% of patients develop mild, dose-related adverse reactions.
+ Reactions typically decrease as treatment continues, but they may limit dosage.
+ Some patients develop sensitivity reactions that include urticaria, allergic rash, and exfoliation.

Understanding adverse effects of anticholinergics in geriatric patients

Although therapeutically necessary, an anticholinergic can cause serious adverse reactions in a geriatric patient. For example, dry mouth may decrease the desire to eat and increase the risk of oral infections, thus reducing the overall nutrient intake. Mydriasis decreases the ability to accommodate and may increase the patient's risk of falls. Decreased GI motility and constipation may lead to fecal impaction. Tachycardia from anticholinergic use may worsen an existing cardiac condition. Hyperthermia may result from poor thermoregulation. Finally, the central nervous system effects of an anticholinergic may worsen confusion, impaired concentration, and dementia.

Rare adverse effects include blood dyscrasias. Prolonged therapy with some antihistamines may precipitate angle-closure glaucoma. High dosages of an anticholinergic can cause psychiatric disturbances that differ from the confusion usually caused by anticholinergic therapy.

Nursing considerations
✦ Give anticholinergics cautiously to geriatric patients, especially to those over age 60. Their increased sensitivity to anticholinergics may result in confusion, agitation,

Teaching a patient about anticholinergics

Whenever an anticholinergic is prescribed, teach the patient and his family the drug's name, dose, frequency, action, and adverse effects, and take the following actions.
✦ Encourage the patient and his family to ask questions about the prescribed drug.
✦ Teach the patient to relieve dry mouth by drinking cold beverages, sucking on sugarless hard candy, or using a nonprescription saliva substitute. Encourage proper oral hygiene.
✦ Instruct the patient to use caution when performing tasks that require alertness because drowsiness or blurred vision may occur.
✦ Advise the patient to avoid prolonged exposure to high temperatures because an anticholinergic increases the risk of heatstroke by reducing sweating.
✦ Teach the patient not to stop long-term anticholinergic therapy before consulting the prescriber.
✦ Instruct the patient not to take over-the-counter cough or cold preparations, diet aids, or agents used to stay awake without consulting the prescriber because of potential interactions with the prescribed anticholinergic.
✦ Teach the patient that alcohol may increase the drowsiness produced by the anticholinergic.
✦ Advise the patient and his family to inform the prescriber of improving or worsening of parkinsonian signs and symptoms.
✦ Advise the patient to notify the prescriber of adverse reactions.
✦ Instruct family members to inform the prescriber of any signs of confusion or mental changes in the patient, especially a geriatric patient.

hallucinations, and psychotic symptoms. (See *Understanding adverse effects of anticholinergics in geriatric patients,*.)
✦ Give these drugs cautiously to patients with tachycardia, arrhythmias, hypertension, hypotension, liver or kidney disorders, obstructive diseases of the GI or GU tract, prostatic hypertrophy (especially in geriatric patients), or a tendency toward urine retention and to those at risk for heatstroke.
✦ Monitor the patient's vital signs and respiratory status.
✦ Give the drug during or shortly after meals to prevent adverse GI reactions.
✦ Notify the prescriber if the patient experiences adverse reactions.
✦ Record the patient's fluid intake and output during therapy. Observe for decreased urine output.
✦ Teach the patient and his caregiver about the prescribed drug. (See *Teaching a patient about anticholinergics.*)

DOPAMINERGICS

Dopaminergics include these chemically unrelated drugs:
✦ levodopa, the metabolic precursor to dopamine
✦ levodopa-carbidopa, a combination drug composed of levodopa and carbidopa
✦ amantadine, an antiviral with dopaminergic activity
✦ bromocriptine and pergolide, ergot-type dopamine agonists
✦ pramipexole and ropinirole, non–ergot-type dopamine agonists
✦ selegiline, a MAO type B inhibitor.

Pharmacokinetics

Like anticholinergics, dopaminergics are absorbed from the GI tract into the bloodstream and are delivered to their action site in the brain.

Levodopa absorption is slowed and reduced when it's ingested with food. The body absorbs most of a levodopa, levodopa-carbidopa, pramipexole, ropinirole, or amantadine dose from the GI tract after oral administration, but only about 28% of bromocriptine is absorbed. The body can absorb a significant amount of pergolide, although how much is absorbed isn't fully known. About 73% of an oral dose of selegiline is absorbed.

Levodopa is widely distributed in body tissues, including the GI tract, liver, pancreas, kidneys, salivary glands, and skin. Levodopa-carbidopa and pramipexole also are widely distributed. Amantadine is distributed in saliva, nasal secretions, and breast milk. Bromocriptine and pergolide are highly protein-bound. The distribution of selegiline is unknown.

Dopaminergics are metabolized extensively in various areas of the body and eliminated by the liver, the kidneys, or both. Large amounts of levodopa are metabolized in the stomach and during its first pass through the liver. It's metabolized extensively to various compounds that are excreted by the kidneys. Carbidopa isn't metabolized extensively. The kidneys excrete approximately one-third of it as unchanged drug within 24 hours.

Amantadine, pramipexole, and ropinirole are excreted mostly unchanged by the kidneys. Almost all of a bromocriptine dose is metabolized by the liver to pharmacologically inactive compounds and primarily eliminated in feces; only a small amount is excreted in urine. After pergolide is metabolized, the kidneys excrete it. Selegiline is metabolized to amphetamine, methamphetamine, and N-desmethylselegiline (the major metabolite), which are eliminated in urine.

Key nursing actions
✦ Monitor vital signs and respiratory status.
✦ Document fluid intake and output.
✦ Watch for a decrease in urine output.

Features of dopaminergics
✦ Group includes chemically unrelated drugs.
✦ Action takes place in the brain.
✦ Motor function improves through increased dopamine levels or enhanced neurotransmission.
✦ Distribution, metabolism, and excretion vary with each drug.

WARNING

Levodopa toxicity or worsening Parkinson's disease?

Although levodopa is commonly used to treat Parkinson's disease, this use is controversial. Initially, levodopa is effective in controlling symptoms. After several years, however, the drug's effects sometimes don't last as long (the wearing-off effect) or lead to sharp fluctuations in symptoms (the on-off phenomenon).

Some prescribers order levodopa in low doses when the diagnosis is first made. Others start the drug later once symptoms compromise function. Those who advocate starting early feel that fluctuations in response to levodopa stem from the progression of Parkinson's disease and not from the drug's effects. Yet some prescribers are concerned that levodopa accelerates the progression of Parkinson's disease by providing a source of free radicals that contribute to the degeneration of dopaminergic neurons.

Pharmacodynamics

Dopaminergics act in the brain to improve motor function either by increasing dopamine's concentration or by enhancing its neurotransmission.

Levodopa is inactive until it crosses the blood-brain barrier and is converted to dopamine by enzymes in the brain, increasing dopamine concentrations in the basal ganglia. Carbidopa enhances levodopa's effectiveness by blocking the peripheral conversion of levodopa, thus permitting increased amounts of levodopa to be transported to the brain.

Amantadine's mechanism of action isn't clear. It may release dopamine from intact neurons but may also have non-dopaminergic effects. Bromocriptine, pramipexole, and ropinirole stimulate dopamine receptors in the brain, producing effects that are similar to dopamine's. Pergolide directly stimulates postsynaptic dopamine receptors in the CNS. Selegiline can increase dopaminergic activity by inhibiting the activity of MAO type B or by other mechanisms.

Pharmacotherapeutics

The choice of therapy is highly individualized and is determined by the patient's symptoms and level of disability. Patients with mild Parkinson's disease and with tremor as the predominant symptom receive anticholinergics or amantadine. Although selegiline is used to extend levodopa's duration by blocking its breakdown, it also may be used in early Parkinson's disease for its neuroprotective properties and ability to slow disease progression.

Usually, dopaminergics are used to treat patients with severe parkinsonism or those who don't respond to anticholinergics alone. Levodopa is the most effective drug used to treat Parkinson's disease. However, it loses its effectiveness after 3 to 5 years. (See *Levodopa toxicity or worsening Parkinson's disease?*)

When the patient's response to levodopa fluctuates, the drug dose and frequency of administration may be adjusted. Alternatively, another dopaminergic, such as selegiline or amantadine, or a COMT inhibitor may be added to the regimen.

Controlled-release formulations of levodopa-carbidopa may help manage the wearing-off effect, or delayed-onset motor fluctuations. When carbidopa is given with levodopa, the levodopa dosage can be reduced, decreasing the risk of adverse

---

When to use dopaminergics

- In severe parkinsonism
- When anticholinergics alone don't produce desired response
- For mild disease with tremor as main symptom (amantadine)
- In early disease for neuroprotective and disease-slowing properties (selegiline)

Facts about levodopa-carbidopa

- This drug combination is standard therapy for Parkinson's disease.
- Controlled-release forms help manage the wearing-off effect and delayed-onset motor fluctuations.

Contraindications and precautions for levodopa-carbidopa

Levodopa-carbidopa is contraindicated in patients with angle-closure glaucoma, melanoma, or undiagnosed skin lesions. It's also contraindicated within 14 days of therapy with a monoamine oxidase inhibitor.

Levodopa-carbidopa may be used cautiously in patients with severe cardiovascular, renal, hepatic, endocrine, or pulmonary disorders; a history of peptic ulcer; psychiatric illness; myocardial infarction with residual arrhythmias; bronchial asthma; emphysema; and well-controlled, chronic open-angle glaucoma.

GI and cardiovascular effects. Levodopa-carbidopa is the standard therapy for Parkinson's disease. Nevertheless, it isn't appropraite for all patients. (See *Contraindications and precautions for levodopa-carbidopa.*)

Before discontinuation, some dopaminergics, such as amantadine, pramipexole, and bromocriptine, must be tapered gradually to avoid causing a parkinsonian crisis (sudden, marked deterioration) and possible life-threatening complications.

Interactions

✦ Pyridoxine (vitamin B_6), phenytoin, benzodiazepines, reserpine, and papaverine can reduce levodopa's effectiveness.
✦ Use of dopaminergics with an MAO type A inhibitor increases the risk of hypertensive crisis.
✦ Antipsychotics, such as phenothiazines, thiothixene, haloperidol, and loxapine, can reduce the effectiveness of levodopa and pergolide.
✦ Anticholinergics can increase the anticholinergic effects of amantadine and reduce levodopa absorption.
✦ When taken with selegiline, opiate agonists can cause a fatal reaction.
✦ The herbal products 5-hydroxytryptophan, jimsonweed, kava, and octacosanol may cause worsening parkinsonian symptoms or increased adverse reactions to dopaminergics.
✦ High-tyramine foods may cause hypertensive crisis in a patient taking selegiline.
✦ Dietary amino acids can decrease levodopa's effectiveness by competing with it for intestinal absorption and slowing its transport to the brain.

Adverse reactions

Among the dopaminergics, amantadine produces the fewest adverse reactions. Adverse reactions to bromocriptine, pergolide, and levodopa are mainly dose-related and can occur peripherally or in the CNS. With daily-recommended dosages, selegiline produces few adverse reactions.

Levodopa and levodopa-carbidopa

Adverse reactions to levodopa or levodopa-carbidopa usually are dose-related and reversible. Levodopa commonly produces adverse GI reactions, such as nausea, vomiting, and anorexia. It also can cause orthostatic hypotension as well as other, less common adverse cardiovascular reactions, such as palpitations, tachycardia, ar-

Facts about levodopa-carbidopa
(continued)

✦ Because the levodopa dosage can be reduced, the risk of adverse GI and cardiovascular effects is lessened.

Possible drug interactions

✦ Anticholinergics
✦ Antipsychotics
✦ Benzodiazepines
✦ MAO type A inhibitors
✦ Opiate agonists
✦ Papaverine
✦ Phenytoin
✦ Pyridoxine (vitamin B_6)
✦ Reserpine

Adverse reactions to watch for

Levodopa and levodopa-carbidopa

✦ Anorexia, nausea, vomiting
✦ Arrhythmias, flushing, hypertension, palpitations, tachycardia
✦ CNS disturbances, such as irritability, confusion, hallucinations
✦ Dark-colored urine and sweat, urinary frequency, urine retention
✦ Orthostatic hypotension
✦ Vision changes

Levodopa withdrawal

✦ Decreased hemoglobin and hematocrit
✦ Granulocytopenia, hemolytic anemia, leukopenia, thrombocytopenia
✦ Hyperpyrexia
✦ Neuroleptic malignant syndrome

Loss of levodopa effect

✦ Sharp fluctuations between mobility and immobility

Adverse reactions to watch for
(continued)

♦ Progressive decrease in beneficial effects from each dose

Adverse reactions to amantadine

♦ Anorexia, constipation, nausea
♦ Anxiety, confusion, dizziness, hallucinations, inability to concentrate, insomnia, irritability, light-headedness
♦ Livedo reticularis
♦ Orthostatic hypotension
♦ Urine retention

Adverse reactions to bromocriptine

♦ Confusion, hallucinations, delusions, nightmares
♦ Edema of the ankles and feet, palpitations, ventricular tachycardia, bradycardia, worsening angina, persistent orthostatic hypotension, syncope
♦ Erythromelalgia
♦ GI reactions, such as nausea
♦ Incontinence, urinary frequency, urine retention
♦ Initial reactions: orthostatic hypotension, vomiting, acute anxiety, dizziness, and sedation
♦ Numbness and tingling of the arms and legs, cold feet, muscle cramps in the legs and feet
♦ Pulmonary infiltrates, pleural effusions, thickening of pleura

rhythmias, flushing, and hypertension. Additional adverse reactions include dark-colored urine and sweat, urinary frequency or urine retention, CNS disturbances (irritability, confusion, and hallucinations), and vision difficulties.

After levodopa withdrawal, some patients experience hyperpyrexia and neuroleptic malignant syndrome (characterized by hyperthermia, akinesia, altered consciousness, muscular rigidity, and profuse sweating). Both reactions can be fatal. Hematologic effects — such as leukopenia, granulocytopenia, thrombocytopenia, hemolytic anemia, and decreased hemoglobin and hematocrit — also may occur. When used alone, levodopa can cause a transient increase in liver enzyme, bilirubin, and blood urea nitrogen (BUN) levels. When combined with carbidopa, levodopa may produce lower BUN, creatinine, and uric acid levels.

The most distressing problem with levodopa is the drug's loss of effectiveness after 3 to 5 years. The problem takes one of two forms: the on-off phenomenon, characterized by sharp fluctuations between mobility and immobility, or the end-of-dose deterioration (also known as the wearing-off effect), a progressive decrease in the duration of beneficial effects from each levodopa dose. The use of smaller, more frequent doses of levodopa and adjunctive therapy (such as with selegiline or pergolide) can reduce both problems.

Amantadine

At usual dosages, amantadine produces relatively few adverse reactions. However, long-term therapy may produce livedo reticularis (diffuse, mottled reddening of the skin usually confined to the leg), which commonly is accompanied by mild ankle edema. Other relatively common adverse reactions include urine retention, orthostatic hypotension, anorexia, nausea, and constipation. Adverse CNS reactions may include inability to concentrate, confusion, light-headedness, anxiety, insomnia, irritability, dizziness, and hallucinations. Rare reactions include rash, leukopenia, eczematoid dermatitis, seizures, oculogyric episodes, and lingual and facial dyskinesias.

Bromocriptine

Besides cost, adverse reactions are the most important factor limiting the use of bromocriptine. Adverse reactions are more common at the start of therapy and when the dosage exceeds 20 mg/day. Adverse GI reactions, such as nausea, occur commonly. Other common initial adverse reactions include orthostatic hypotension, vomiting, acute anxiety, dizziness, and sedation. Erythromelalgia also may occur. This drug can cause adverse cardiovascular reactions by producing edema in the ankles and feet, palpitations, ventricular tachycardia, bradycardia, exacerbation of angina, and persistent orthostatic hypotension, which may result in syncope. Confusion, hallucinations, delusions, nightmares, and erythromelalgia are notable especially during long-term therapy or dosages of 100 mg or more daily bromocriptine therapy, but they usually are reversible. The presence of adverse CNS reactions usually limits the dosage and is the main reason for stopping therapy.

Bromocriptine therapy has been linked to pleuropulmonary reactions, such as pulmonary infiltrates, pleural effusions, and thickening of the pleura. It also has been linked to bladder dysfunction with incontinence, urinary frequency, and urine retention. Signs and symptoms of ergotism, including numbness and tingling of the arms and legs, cold feet, and muscle cramps in the legs and feet, also may occur.

Other dopaminergics

The most common adverse reactions to pergolide include confusion, dyskinesia, hallucinations, somnolence, orthostatic hypotension, nausea, and constipation.

Teaching a patient about dopaminergics

Whenever a dopaminergic is prescribed, teach the patient and his family the drug's name, dose, frequency, action, and adverse effects, and take the following actions.

✦ Advise the patient not to exceed the prescribed daily dosage because serious adverse reactions could result.

✦ Explain the importance of frequent blood pressure measurements and teach the patient to recognize the symptoms of hypotension (such as dizziness and light-headedness) as well as hypertension (such as headache and vision changes).

✦ Advise the patient that somnolence may occur and to avoid activities that require alertness until the drug's effects are known.

✦ Inform the patient that hallucinations can occur, especially if the patient is elderly.

✦ Teach the family how to maintain a safe environment to prevent patient injury during periods of confusion.

✦ Inform the patient that levodopa may cause harmless discoloration of urine and sweat.

✦ Teach the patient who is taking levodopa about the on-off phenomenon.

✦ Instruct the patient to notify her prescriber if she becomes pregnant or is breast-feeding during therapy.

✦ Inform the patient that the levodopa-carbidopa dosage may be decreased after adjunct therapy begins with another dopaminergic.

✦ Tell the patient not to chew or crush extended-release forms.

✦ Inform the patient who is beginning levodopa therapy that the drug may take several weeks or months to reach its maximum effectiveness.

✦ Teach the patient not to discontinue long-term drug therapy before consulting the prescriber.

✦ Instruct the patient to notify the prescriber if adverse reactions occur.

✦ Instruct family members to inform the prescriber if the patient experiences confusion or mental changes.

Other adverse reactions may include abdominal pain, dizziness, drowsiness, flulike symptoms, lower back pain, rhinitis, and weakness; they may require medical attention if they continue or are bothersome. Rarely, pergolide has caused cerebrovascular hemorrhage, myocardial infarction (MI), chills, diarrhea, xerostomia, facial edema, appetite loss, and vomiting.

Common adverse reactions to pramipexole and ropinirole include nausea, dizziness, somnolence, dyspepsia, constipation, asthenia, and hallucinations. When used with levodopa, these drugs commonly produce dyskinesia, dizziness, extrapyramidal syndrome or aggravated parkinsonism, somnolence, insomnia, injury, hallucinations, confusion, urinary frequency and infection, constipation, and dry mouth.

Selegiline usually doesn't cause serious adverse reactions. However, it may produce nausea, dry mouth, dizziness, light-headedness, fainting, confusion, and hallucinations. Additional adverse reactions include vivid dreams, dyskinesia, headache, generalized achiness, anxiety, tension, diarrhea, insomnia, lethargy, leg pain, low back pain, palpitations, urine retention, and weight loss.

Nursing considerations

✦ Teach the patient and his caregiver about the prescribed drug. (See *Teaching a patient about dopaminergics.*)

Key nursing actions
+ Consider combination therapy.
+ Assess the patient for orthostatic hypotension by monitoring his blood pressure
+ Monitor the patient's degree of mobility.
+ Report decreased mobility to the prescriber,.

+ Consider combination therapy. Levodopa-carbidopa typically decreases the amount of levodopa needed by 75%, reducing the risk of adverse reactions. If the patient takes levodopa, discontinue it at least 8 hours before starting levodopa-carbidopa.
+ Adjust your technique for using urine glucose test strips during levodopa or levodopa-carbidopa therapy. These drugs may produce false-positive results on cupric sulfate strips or false-negative results on glucose oxidase strips. To measure urine glucose accurately, immerse the paper strip only partially in the urine sample. Allow urine to migrates up the strip, as with an ascending chromatographic system. Then read only the top of the strip.
+ Avoid giving levodopa with meals to prevent drug-food interactions that may decrease the rate and extent of drug absorption.
+ Give the second daily dose of amantadine earlier in the evening if the patient experiences insomnia.

 CLINICAL ALERT Don't confuse Eldepryl (selegiline) with enalapril, which is an angiotensin-converting enzyme inhibitor typically prescribed to treat hypertension or heart failure.

+ Monitor the patient's blood pressure for orthostatic hypotension.
+ Monitor the patient's degree of physical mobility.
+ Report decreased mobility to the prescriber.

COMT INHIBITORS

Catechol-*O*-methyltransferase (COMT) inhibitors are used with levodopa-carbidopa to manage Parkinson's disease in patients who experience a wearing-off effect at the end of the dosing interval. These drugs include entacapone and tolcapone.

Pharmacokinetics

Entacapone and tolcapone are absorbed rapidly from the GI tract and offer absolute bioavailability of 35% and 65%, respectively. Because both drugs are highly bound to albumin, they have limited distribution to tissues. They're almost completely metabolized in the liver to inactive metabolites and are excreted in urine.

Pharmacodynamics

Entacapone and tolcapone are selective and reversible COMT inhibitors. COMT is the major enzyme that metabolizes levodopa in the presence of carbidopa. Inhibition of COMT alters the pharmacokinetics of levodopa, leading to a sustained levodopa level. This results in more constant dopaminergic stimulation in the brain and improves signs and symptoms of Parkinson's disease.

Pharmacotherapeutics

Entacapone or tolcapone may be added to levodopa-carbidopa in patients who experience the wearing-off effect at the end of a dosing interval or random on-off fluctuations in response to levodopa-carbidopa. When used alone, COMT inhibitors have no antiparkinsonian effects; they should always be combined with levodopa-carbidopa. The addition of a COMT inhibitor usually requires a decrease in the levodopa-carbidopa dosage, particularly in patients who receive more than 800 mg of levodopa per dose.

Rapid withdrawal of a COMT inhibitor may lead to emergence of parkinsonian symptoms and may cause a syndrome of high fever and confusion similar to neu-

Features of COMT inhibitors
+ Are used with levodopa-carbidopa when that drug begins wearing off too early or causing random on-off fluctuations
+ Have no antiparkinsonian effects when used alone

roleptic malignant syndrome. Although tapering schedules haven't been evaluated, gradual tapering of COMT inhibitors is suggested.

Interactions

✦ COMT inhibitors shouldn't be used with nonselective MAO-type inhibitors, such as phenelzine and tranylcypromine, since COMT and MAO are two major enzyme systems involved in catecholamine metabolism. They may be used with a selective MAO-B inhibitor such as selegiline.

✦ COMT inhibitors combined with catecholamines (such as dopamine, dobutamine, epinephrine, methyldopa, norepinephrine, and isoproterenol) can cause significant cardiac effects or arrhythmias.

✦ Use of COMT inhibitors with CNS depressants (such as alcohol, antipsychotics, benzodiazepines, opioid analgesics, other sedative-hypnotics, and tricyclic antidepressants) may cause additive CNS effects.

✦ Use of entacapone with iron may cause chelation and decreased absorption of iron.

✦ Use of entacapone with bromocriptine or pergolide has caused fibrotic complications.

✦ Drugs that interfere with glucuronidation (such as ampicillin, chloramphenicol, cholestyramine, erythromycin, probenecid, and rifampin) may decrease entacapone elimination.

✦ Entacapone or tolcapone may increase the warfarin level.

Adverse reactions

Common adverse reactions to COMT inhibitors include dyskinesia, sleep disorders, dystonia, excessive dreaming, somnolence, confusion, headache, hallucinations, orthostatic hypotension, anorexia, nausea, vomiting, diarrhea, and hyperkinesias or hypokinesia. Entacapone also may cause brown-orange urine discoloration.

   Less common adverse reactions include syncope, dizziness, fatigue, abdominal pain, constipation, dry mouth, back pain, and diaphoresis. Tolcapone may cause life-threatening liver failure.

Nursing considerations

✦ Don't begin tolcapone therapy in a patient with evidence of liver disease or with liver enzyme levels that exceed the normal range.

✦ Because of the risk of acute, fatal liver failure, use tolcapone only when a patient with Parkinson's disease starts responding differently to levodopa and doesn't respond to or isn't appropriate for other adjunctive drugs. Advise the patient of the risk of liver injury and provide written informed consent before starting tolcapone therapy.

✦ Obtain liver function test results at baseline and every 2 weeks for the first year of tolcapone therapy. Then obtain them every 4 weeks for the next 6 months and every 8 weeks thereafter.

✦ Give entacapone or tolcapone with the levodopa-carbidopa dose. Discontinue tolcapone if the patient shows no improvement within 3 weeks.

✦ When using a COMT inhibitor with a dopaminergic, monitor the patient for orthostatic hypotension because of the increased risk of this adverse reaction.

✦ Ask the patient about diarrhea, which commonly occurs 2 to 12 weeks or more after therapy begins. Reassure the patient that diarrhea usually resolves when therapy is discontinued and rarely requires hospitalization.

Possible drug interactions

✦ Bromocriptine
✦ Catecholamines
✦ CNS depressants
✦ Drugs that interfere with glucuronidation
✦ Iron
✦ Nonselective MAO-type inhibitors
✦ Pergolide
✦ Warfarin

Adverse reactions to watch for

✦ Anorexia, nausea, vomiting, diarrhea
✦ Brown-orange urine discoloration
✦ Confusion, dyskinesia, dystonia, excessive dreaming, hallucinations, headache, sleep disorders, somnolence
✦ Hyperkinesias, hypokinesia
✦ Less common: abdominal pain, back pain, constipation, diaphoresis, dizziness, dry mouth, fatigue, syncope
✦ Life-threatening liver failure
✦ Orthostatic hypotension

Key nursing actions

✦ Monitor liver function tests if the patient receives tolcapone.
✦ Don't give tolcapone if the patient has liver impairment.
✦ Assess the patient for the onset of diarrhea.

Teaching a patient about COMT inhibitors

Whenever a COMT inhibitor is prescribed, teach the patient and his family the drug's name, dose, frequency, action, and adverse effects, and take the following actions.
+ Encourage the patient and his family to ask questions about the prescribed drug.
+ Advise the patient to take the drug as prescribed without regard to meals.
+ Teach the patient to recognize the signs and symptoms of liver injury, such as jaundice, fatigue, loss of appetite, persistent nausea, pruritus, dark urine, or right upper quadrant tenderness. Tell him to report these effects immediately.
+ Advise the patient to avoid hazardous activities until the drug's central nervous system effects are known.
+ Tell the patient that dyskinesia or dystonia may increase.
+ Inform the patient that entacapone may turn his urine brownish orange.
+ Advise the patient to report adverse reactions, such as nausea, diarrhea, dizziness, and lightheadedness, to the prescriber.
+ Advise the patient to report suspected or planned pregnancy. Also, instruct her to notify the prescriber if she wants to breast-feed.

+ Teach the patient and his family about the prescribed drug.(See *Teaching a patient about COMT inhibitors.*)

ANTICONVULSANTS

Accurate diagnosis of a seizure requires a reliable patient history, careful patient observations, and an electroencephalogram. It also may require computerized tomography or magnetic resonance imaging.

Proper diagnosis is important because treatment varies with the type of seizure. The goal of anticonvulsant therapy is to control or prevent seizures. For many patients, anticonvulsant therapy is lifelong. For others, drug therapy may be tapered and eventually discontinued if they don't experience seizures for a year.

Anticonvulsants inhibit neuromuscular transmission. They may be used for:
+ long-term management of chronic epilepsy (recurrent seizures)
+ short-term management of acute isolated seizures not caused by epilepsy, such as after trauma or brain surgery
+ emergency treatment of status epilepticus (a continuous seizure state).

Treatment of epilepsy should begin with a single drug and increase in dosage until seizures are controlled or adverse reactions become problematic. Generally, an alternative drug should be tried as monotherapy before it's used in combination therapy. The choice of drug depends on its characteristics and cost as well as the patient's medical history, seizure type, age, gender, occupation, fatigue and stress levels, and personal preferences and habit.

Anticonvulsants fall into several major classes, including hydantoins, barbiturates, benzodiazepines, succinimides, sulfonamides, and other anticonvulsants.

Features of anticonvulsants

+ Can control or prevent seizures
+ Are used for long-term management of chronic epilepsy, short-term management of seizures not caused by epilepsy, and emergency treatment of status epilepticus
+ Belong to several major classes, including hydantoins, barbiturates, benzodiazepines, succinimides, sulfonamides, other anticonvulsants

HYDANTOINS

The most commonly prescribed anticonvulsant—phenytoin—belongs to a class called hydantoins. Less commonly used hydantoins include ethotoin, fosphenytoin, and mephenytoin.

Pharmacokinetics

The pharmacokinetics of hydantoins vary from drug to drug.

Phenytoin is absorbed slowly after oral and I.M. administration. It's distributed rapidly to all tissues and is 90% protein-bound. Phenytoin is metabolized in the liver. Inactive metabolites are excreted in bile and then reabsorbed from the GI tract. Eventually they're excreted in urine. The enzyme system responsible for phenytoin metabolism is saturable. When it becomes saturated, a change in the dose can result in a disproportionate change in drug level.

The liver metabolizes ethotoin. Extensively protein-bound, ethotoin is excreted in urine, primarily as metabolites.

After I.M. or I.V. administration, fosphenytoin is widely distributed throughout the body and 90% protein-bound. The drug is metabolized by the liver and excreted in urine.

Mephenytoin is absorbed rapidly after oral administration and is only 60% protein-bound. The liver metabolizes it to an active metabolite believed to produce the drug's therapeutic and toxic effects. Excretion occurs in urine.

Pharmacodynamics

In most cases, hydantoins stabilize nerve cells to keep them from getting overexcited. Phenytoin appears to work in the motor cortex of the brain, where it stops the spread of seizure activity. The pharmacodynamics of ethotoin, fosphenytoin, and mephenytoin are thought to mimic those of phenytoin. Phenytoin also exerts antiarrhythmic properties similar to those of quinidine or procainamide.

Pharmacotherapeutics

Because of its effectiveness and relatively low toxicity, phenytoin is the most commonly prescribed anticonvulsant. It's one of the drugs of choice to treat complex partial seizures (also called psychomotor or temporal lobe seizures) and tonic-clonic seizures.

Hydantoins are the long-acting anticonvulsants of choice for status epilepticus after initial treatment with I.V. benzodiazepines. Prescribers sometimes order ethotoin and mephenytoin with other anticonvulsants to treat partial and tonic-clonic seizures in patients who are resistant to or intolerant of other anticonvulsants.

Interactions

Hydantoins interact with a number of other drugs. Some interactions have major to moderate significance.

✦ Antacids, carbamazepine, diazoxide, phenobarbital, rifampin, sucralfate, and theophylline reduce phenytoin's effects.

✦ Allopurinol, amiodarone, benzodiazepines, chloramphenicol, cimetidine, disulfiram, fluconazole, isoniazid, metronidazole, omeprazole, oral anticoagulants, succinimides, sulfonamides, and valproic acid increase phenytoin's effects and risk of toxicity.

✦ A hydantoin can reduce the effects of amiodarone, carbamazepine, corticosteroids, cyclosporine, dicumarol, doxycycline, hormonal contraceptives, levodopa,

Features of hydantoins

✦ Are the most commonly prescribed anticonvulsants

✦ Stabilize nerve cells to keep them from getting overexcited

✦ May work in the motor cortex of the brain

✦ Are the drugs of choice for complex partial and tonic-clonic seizures and status epilepticus

Possible drug interactions

✦ Allopurinol
✦ Amiodarone
✦ Antacids
✦ Benzodiazepines
✦ Carbamazepine
✦ Chloramphenicol
✦ Cimetidine
✦ Corticosteroids
✦ Cyclosporine
✦ Diazoxide
✦ Dicumarol
✦ Disulfiram
✦ Doxycycline
✦ Fluconazole
✦ Hormonal contraceptives
✦ Isoniazid
✦ Levodopa
✦ Lithium
✦ Meperidine
✦ Methadone
✦ Metronidazole
✦ Metyrapone
✦ Omeprazole
✦ Oral anticoagulants
✦ Phenobarbital
✦ Primidone
✦ Quinidine
✦ Rifampin
✦ Succinimides

Possible drug interactions
(continued)

- Sucralfate
- Sulfonamides
- Theophylline
- Thyroid hormone
- Valproic acid
- Warfarin

Adverse reactions to watch for

- Agranulocytosis, anemias, eosinophilia, leukocytosis, leukopenia, macrocytic anemia from folic acid deficiency, pancytopenia, macrocytosis, thrombocytopenia
- Anorexia, epigastric pain, nausea, vomiting
- Ataxia, dizziness, drowsiness, dysarthria, headache, irritability, nystagmus, restlessness, vertigo
- Depressed atrial and ventricular conduction, ventricular fibrillation (in toxic states)
- Gingival hyperplasia, facial skin coarsening, hirsutism
- Glycosuria, hyperglycemia, osteomalacia
- Hypersensitivity reactions: arthralgia, fever, measleslike rash, pruritus; exfoliative, purpuric, or bullous dermatitis; Stevens-Johnson syndrome; lymphadenopathy; acute renal failure; hepatitis; liver necrosis

Key nursing actions

- Monitor the phenytoin level.
- Keep oxygen, suction, and resuscitation equipment nearby.
- Stop the drug and notify the prescriber if a rash develops.

methadone, metyrapone, quinidine, theophylline, thyroid hormone, and valproic acid.

✦ A hydantoin can increase the adverse effects of lithium, meperidine, primidone, and warfarin.

✦ Enteral tube feedings may interfere with oral phenytoin absorption, requiring feeding to stop for 2 hours before and after phenytoin administration.

Adverse reactions

The adverse effects of hydantoins involve the central nervous, cardiovascular, GI, and hematopoietic systems, as well as cosmetic effects. The adverse reactions presented here relate directly to phenytoin. As a prodrug of phenytoin, fosphenytoin shares many of its predecessor's precautions. Ethotoin produces similar reactions; mephenytoin may produce more serious blood dyscrasias, including aplastic anemia.

In the CNS, adverse reactions to hydantoins include drowsiness, ataxia, irritability, headache, restlessness, nystagmus, dizziness, vertigo, and dysarthria. Adverse CNS reactions to phenytoin correspond to the drug level. Most patients tolerate a drug level of less than 25 mcg/ml; in others, nystagmus, diplopia, and ataxia may occur. A drug level that exceeds 30 mcg/ml can produce drowsiness, lethargy, and asterixis. A level that exceeds 50 mcg/ml may lead to coma. Phenytoin also may cause toxic amblyopia and mental dullness.

The major adverse GI reactions include nausea, vomiting, epigastric pain, and anorexia. The adverse cardiovascular reactions are depressed atrial and ventricular conduction and, in toxic states, ventricular fibrillation. With I.V. administration, the adverse cardiovascular reactions include bradycardia, hypotension, and potential cardiac arrest. The primary adverse reaction of the hematopoietic system is a folic acid deficiency that can cause macrocytic anemia.

Cosmetic toxicity includes gingival hyperplasia, hirsutism, and facial skin coarsening. Other adverse reactions include hyperglycemia, glycosuria, and osteomalacia. Toxic doses of phenytoin paradoxically may induce seizures.

Hypersensitivity reactions to hydantoins typically are manifested as pruritus, fever, arthralgia, and a measleslike rash; exfoliative, purpuric, or bullous dermatitis; Stevens-Johnson syndrome; lymphadenopathy; acute renal failure; hepatitis; and liver necrosis. Several adverse reactions also relate to the hematopoietic system, including thrombocytopenia, leukopenia, leukocytosis, agranulocytosis, pancytopenia, eosinophilia, macrocytosis, and various anemias.

Nursing considerations

✦ Monitor the patient's phenytoin level because many adverse reactions are dose-related.

✦ Keep oxygen, suction, and resuscitation equipment available when giving I.V. phenytoin.

✦ Monitor the patient regularly for adverse reactions to the prescribed hydantoin.

✦ Give I.V. phenytoin at no more than 50 mg/minute (or 50 mg/3 minute in a geriatric patient with heart disease) because of its cardiotoxicity. Also monitor the patient's blood pressure, pulse, and respirations every 5 minutes during administration and every 15 minutes thereafter until the patient becomes stable. If his blood pressure decreases during administration, reduce the infusion rate.

✦ Give I.V. fosphenytoin at no more than 150 phenytoin sodium equivalents (PEs)/minute.

✦ Stop the drug and notify the prescriber if rash appears. If rash is exfoliative, purpuric, or bullous, or if lupus erythematosus, Stevens-Johnson syndrome, or toxic

Teaching a patient about hydantoins

Whenever a hydantoin is prescribed, teach the patient and his family the drug's name, dose, frequency, action, and adverse effects, and take the following actions.
+ Warn the patient not to stop taking the drug abruptly.
+ Advise the patient to avoid driving and other potentially hazardous activities that require alertness until the drug's central nervous system effects are known.
+ For a patient who takes a hormonal contraceptive with a hydantoin, suggest that she use an additional or different contraceptive method.
+ Encourage the patient with gingival hyperplasia to practice good oral hygiene.
+ Remind the patient to notify his dentist about hydantoin therapy.
+ Inform the patient that phenytoin may cause harmless pink, red, or red-brown discoloration of urine.
+ Advise the patient to report adverse reactions — especially rash — to the prescriber.
+ Advise the patient with diabetes to monitor his glucose level closely because a hydantoin may increase it.

epidermal necrolysis is suspected, stop the drug and consider alternative therapy. If rash is mild (measleslike or scarlatiniform), resume therapy after rash disappears. If rash recurs when therapy is resumed, further fosphenytoin or phenytoin administration is contraindicated. Document that the patient is allergic to the drug.

 CLINICAL ALERT Fosphenytoin should always be prescribed and dispensed in PEs. Don't adjust the recommended doses when substituting fosphenytoin for phenytoin or vice versa.

+ Minimize vein irritation by infusing normal saline solution after I.V. phenytoin administration.
+ Don't mix I.V. phenytoin with any other drug to avoid phenytoin precipitation.
+ Avoid I.M. injections (except for fosphenytoin) because phenytoin precipitates in muscle tissue, which decreases drug bioavailability.
+ Give an oral hydantoin with meals to minimize GI distress.
+ Shake a suspension preparation vigorously before pouring to ensure uniform distribution and exact measurement of the drug.
+ Don't stop the drug abruptly.

 CLINICAL ALERT Don't confuse Cerebyx (fosphenytoin) with Cerezyme (imiglucerase, an enzyme), Celexa (citalopram, an antidepressant), or Celebrex (celecoxib, a nonsteroidal anti-inflammatory drug).

+ Teach the patient and his caregiver about the drug. (See *Teaching a patient about hydantoins*.)

BARBITURATES

In the past, the long-acting barbiturate phenobarbital was one of the most widely used anticonvulsants. Now it's used less frequently because of its sedative effects. Phenobarbital may be prescribed for long-term treatment of epilepsy or for treatment of status epilepticus when hydantoins and I.V. diazepam aren't effective.

Features of barbiturates
+ May be used for long-term treatment of epilepsy or for status epilepticus
+ May have sedative effects

Mephobarbital, also a long-acting barbiturate, sometimes is used as an anticonvulsant. Primidone, which is closely related chemically to the barbiturates, is also used in the long-term treatment of epilepsy.

Pharmacokinetics
Each barbiturate has slightly different pharmacokinetic properties. Phenobarbital is absorbed slowly but well from the GI tract. Peak plasma levels occur 8 to 12 hours after a single dose. The drug is 20% to 45% bound to proteins and to a similar extent to other tissues, including the brain. The liver metabolizes about 75% of a phenobarbital dose, and 25% is excreted unchanged in urine.

Almost half of a mephobarbital dose is absorbed from the GI tract and well distributed in body tissues. The drug is bound to tissue and plasma proteins. Mephobarbital undergoes extensive metabolism by the liver; only 1% to 2% is excreted unchanged in urine.

About 60% to 80% of a primidone dose is absorbed from the GI tract and distributed evenly among body tissues. The drug is protein-bound to a small extent in the plasma. Primidone is metabolized by the liver to two active metabolites: phenobarbital and phenylethylmalonamide (PEMA). From 15% to 25% of primidone is excreted unchanged in urine, 15% to 25% is metabolized to phenobarbital, and 50% to 70% is excreted in urine as PEMA. Primidone also appears in breast milk.

Pharmacodynamics
Barbiturates exhibit anticonvulsant action at doses below those that produce hypnotic effects. For this reason, these drugs usually don't produce addiction when used to treat epilepsy. Barbiturates raise the seizure threshold by decreasing postsynaptic excitation.

Pharmacotherapeutics
The barbiturate anticonvulsants are effective alternative therapy for partial seizures, tonic-clonic seizures, and febrile seizures. They can be used alone or with other anticonvulsants. I.V. phenobarbital also is used to treat status epilepticus. The major disadvantage of using phenobarbital for status epilepticus is that it has a delayed onset of action when an immediate response is needed. Barbiturate anticonvulsants are ineffective in treating absence seizures.

Mephobarbital has no advantage over phenobarbital and is used when the patient can't tolerate phenobarbital's adverse effects. In general, phenobarbital is tried before primidone because primidone requires higher monitoring costs and more frequent dosing. Primidone may be effective in patients who don't respond to phenobarbital therapy.

Interactions
+ When taken with rifampin, barbiturates can exhibit reduced effects.
+ The risk of toxicity increases when phenobarbital is taken with chloramphenicol, cimetidine, CNS depressants, felbamate, phenytoin, or valproic acid.
+ When taken with a barbiturate, many drugs, such as beta blockers, carbamazepine, corticosteroids, cyclosporine, digoxin, doxycycline, estrogens, felodipine, hormonal contraceptives, metronidazole, oral anticoagulants, phenothiazine, quinidine, theophylline, tricyclic antidepressants, and verapamil, exhibit reduced effects.
+ Barbiturates may increase the adverse effects of tricyclic antidepressants.
+ Evening primrose oil and herbs or dietary supplements that contain thujones or vitamin B_6 may decrease the seizure threshold, requiring an increase in the barbiturate dosage.

Conditions that call for barbiturates
+ Partial, tonic-clonic, or febrile seizures (alternate therapy)
+ Status epilepticus
+ Lack of response to phenobarbital (primidone)

Possible drug interactions
+ Beta blockers
+ Carbamazepine
+ Chloramphenicol
+ Cimetidine
+ CNS depressants
+ Corticosteroids
+ Cyclosporine
+ Digoxin
+ Doxycycline
+ Estrogens
+ Felbamate
+ Felodipine
+ Hormonal contraceptives
+ Metronidazole
+ Oral anticoagulants
+ Phenothiazine
+ Phenytoin
+ Quinidine
+ Rifampin
+ Theophylline
+ Tricyclic antidepressants
+ Valproic acid
+ Verapamil

✦ The appetite stimulant wormwood may increase phenobarbital's effects.

Adverse reactions

The toxicity of barbiturate anticonvulsants results primarily in adverse CNS reactions. Significant GI reactions, blood dyscrasias, and emotional or psychiatric reactions also occur.

The most common dose-related CNS effects of phenobarbital include drowsiness, lethargy, and dizziness; nystagmus; confusion; and ataxia with large doses.

Adverse GI reactions include nausea and vomiting. These reactions are most common when primidone therapy begins, which explains why the primidone dosage is increased gradually.

Folate deficiencies and osteomalacia caused by the induced metabolism of vitamin D also may occur. When administered I.V., phenobarbital can cause laryngospasm, respiratory depression, and hypotension related to decreased cardiac output. Signs of overdose include respiratory depression, pupillary constriction, oliguria, hypothermia, circulatory collapse, and pulmonary edema.

Mephobarbital produces adverse reactions similar to phenobarbital. Primidone evokes the same CNS and GI adverse reactions as phenobarbital. Primidone also has been linked to acute psychoses in patients with complex partial seizures. In addition, it may cause alopecia, impotence, and osteomalacia.

Rare hematologic adverse effects of barbiturates include agranulocytosis, thrombocytopenia, leukopenia, eosinophilia, decreased folate level, and megaloblastic anemia. All three barbiturate anticonvulsants can produce a hypersensitivity rash. These drugs also may produce a morbilliform rash, lupus-like syndrome, and lymphadenopathy. Paradoxical excitement in geriatric patients and children and hyperkinetic behavior in children may occur.

Nursing considerations

✦ Teach the patient and his caregiver about the prescribed drug. (See *Teaching a patient about barbiturates*.)
✦ When giving an I.V. barbiturate, keep resuscitative drugs and equipment nearby and don't exceed 60 mg/minute.

Adverse reactions fo watch for
✦ Ataxia with large doses
✦ Confusion, dizziness, nystagmus
✦ Drowsiness, lethargy
✦ Folate deficiency
✦ Hypersensitivity rash, morbilliform rash
✦ Lupus-like syndrome
✦ Lymphadenopathy
✦ Nausea, vomiting
✦ Osteomalacia
✦ Paradoxical excitement in geriatric and pediatric patients
✦ Phenobarbital I.V.: laryngospasm, respiratory depression, hypotension
✦ Primidone: acute psychoses in patients with complex partial seizures, alopecia, impotence, osteomalacia

Key nursing actions
✦ Monitor vital signs often, especially respirations and blood pressure.
✦ Monitor the phenobarbital level.
✦ Watch for evidence of toxicity.
✦ Monitor the patient's level of mobility. Notify the prescriber if the drug reduces it.

CLINICAL ALERT Don't confuse phenobarbital with pentobarbital (Nembutal), which is a sedative-hypnotic (controlled substance schedule II, III for suppositories) prescribed for insomnia or sedation.

✦ When giving an I.V. barbiturate, don't use a cloudy solution. Give a reconstituted solution within 30 minutes of preparation.
✦ Monitor the patient's vital signs frequently—especially respirations and blood pressure—when administering an I.V. barbiturate.
✦ Monitor the patient's phenobarbital level. The therapeutic level is 15 to 40 mcg/ml.
✦ Watch for signs of toxicity, including coma, cyanosis, asthmatic breathing, clammy skin, and hypotension. Overdose can be fatal.
✦ Notify the prescriber of fever, sore throat, mouth sores, easy bruising or bleeding, or tiny broken blood vessels under the skin.
✦ Monitor the patient's physical mobility during therapy.
✦ If sedative effects interfere with mobility, notify the prescriber.

BENZODIAZEPINES

Four benzodiazepines provide anticonvulsant effects: clonazepam, clorazepate, diazepam, and lorazepam. Only clonazepam is recommended for long-term treatment of epilepsy. Clorazepate is prescribed as an adjunct in treating partial seizures. Parenteral diazepam is restricted to acute treatment of status epilepticus; rectal diazepam, to repetitive seizures. I.V. lorazepam and I.V. diazepam are considered drugs of choice for acute management of status epilepticus.

Pharmacokinetics

The patient can receive benzodiazepines orally, parenterally, or in certain situations, rectally. These drugs are absorbed rapidly and almost completely from the GI tract, but are distributed at different rates. Protein binding of benzodiazepines ranges from 85% to 90%.

Benzodiazepines are metabolized in the liver to multiple metabolites and are then excreted in urine. They readily cross the placenta and appear in breast milk.

Pharmacodynamics

Benzodiazepines act as anticonvulsants, anxiolytics, sedative-hypnotics, and muscle relaxants. Their mechanism of action is poorly understood.

Pharmacotherapeutics

Each benzodiazepine is used in slightly different ways. Clonazepam is used to treat absence (petit mal), atypical absence (Lennox-Gastaut syndrome), atonic, and myoclonic seizures.

Clorazepate is used with other drugs to treat partial seizures.

Diazepam isn't recommended for long-term treatment because of the risk of addiction and the high level needed to control seizures. I.V. diazepam is used to control status epilepticus. Because the drug provides only short-term effects of less than 1 hour, the patient also must receive a long-acting anticonvulsant, such as phenytoin or phenobarbital, during therapy. Diazepam rectal gel is approved for treatment of repetitive seizures.

I.V. lorazepam also is used to treat status epilepticus.

Actions of benzodiazepines
✦ Anticonvulsant
✦ Anxiolytic
✦ Muscle relaxant
✦ Sedative-hypnotic

Conditions that call for benzodiazepines
✦ Clonazepam: absence, atypical absence, atonic, and myoclonic seizures
✦ Clorazepate: adjunct for partial seizures
✦ Diazepam: status epilepticus (I.V.), repetitive seizures (rectal gel)
✦ Lorazepam: status epilepticus (I.V.)

WARNING

Giving rectal diazepam safely

To give diazepam rectal gel (Diastat) safely, it should be given only by caregivers who:
+ can distinguish the distinct cluster of increased seizure activity from the patient's ordinary seizure activity
+ have been instructed in and can give the treatment competently
+ understand which seizures may be treated with Diastat
+ can monitor the patient's response and recognize when immediate professional medical evaluation is needed.

Interactions
+ When benzodiazepines are taken with CNS depressants, the interaction enhances sedative and other depressant effects, which can cause motor skill impairment, respiratory depression, and even death at high doses.
+ When combined with benzodiazepines, cimetidine and hormonal contraceptives can cause excessive sedation and CNS depression.
+ The combination of clonazepam and phenytoin may decrease the phenytoin level.
+ The herbal product kava may increase the adverse CNS effects of benzodiazepines.
+ St. John's wort may reduce the level of certain benzodiazepines by stimulating the production of the hepatic and intestinal enzymes responsible for their metabolism.

Adverse reactions
Dose-related adverse reactions to benzodiazepines are primarily neurologic and include drowsiness, confusion, ataxia, weakness, dizziness, nystagmus, vertigo, syncope, dysarthria, headache, tremor, and a glassy-eyed appearance. Geriatric or debilitated patients, children, patients with liver disease or a low serum albumin level are most likely to experience adverse CNS reactions and generally should receive reduced initial doses of the drugs. These dose-related reactions diminish as therapy continues. Cardiorespiratory depression may occur with high doses and with I.V. diazepam. Geriatric patients are particularly susceptible to confusion, ataxia, and paradoxical excitement.

Idiosyncratic reactions to benzodiazepines include rash and acute hypersensitivity reactions. Hepatomegaly, leukopenia, thrombocytopenia, agranulocytosis, aplastic anemia, hemolytic anemia, leukocytosis, and eosinophilia rarely occur.

Nursing considerations
+ Monitor the patient for adverse reactions.
+ Be familiar with the different forms and how to give them. (See *Giving rectal diazepam safely*.)
+ While giving I.V. diazepam, monitor the patient's vital signs and keep resuscitation equipment readily available.
+ Give I.V. diazepam no faster than 5 mg/minute in an adult and at least 2 to 5 minutes in a child. Avoid starting an I.V. line in a small vein. Use care to prevent extravasation.

Possible drug interactions
+ Cimetidine
+ CNS depressants
+ Hormonal contraceptives
+ Phenytoin

Adverse reactions to watch for
+ Acute hypersensitivity reactions, rash
+ Ataxia, confusion, dizziness, drowsiness, dysarthria, glassy-eyed appearance, headache, nystagmus, vertigo, weakness, syncope, tremor
+ Cardiorespiratory depression
+ Agranulocytosis, aplastic anemia, eosinophilia, hemolytic anemia, hepatomegaly, leukocytosis, leukopenia, thrombocytopenia

Key nursing actions
+ With I.V. diazepam, monitor vital signs and keep resuscitation equipment nearby.
+ Monitor hepatic, renal, and hematopoietic function.
+ Watch for evidence of abuse or addiction.

+ Don't mix I.V. diazepam with other drugs in the same syringe.
+ Monitor the results of hepatic, renal, and hematopoietic function studies in a patient receiving repeated or prolonged therapy.
+ Be alert for signs of abuse or addiction. Don't withdraw the drug abruptly after long-term use; withdrawal symptoms may occur.
+ Store an oral benzodiazepine in a light-resistant container at room temperature, unless otherwise specified by the manufacturer.
+ Teach the patient and his caregiver about the prescribed drug. (See *Teaching a patient about benzodiazepines.*)

SUCCINIMIDES

The succinimides, ethosuximide and methsuximide, are used to manage absence seizures. Because ethosuximide is the drug of choice for absence seizures, this section focuses on that drug.

Pharmacokinetics

The succinimides are readily absorbed from the GI tract. Ethosuximide reaches its peak level in 3 to 7 hours. The succinimides are metabolized in the liver and excreted in urine. Metabolites are probably inactive. The elimination half-life of ethosuximide is about 60 hours in adults and 30 hours in children. At a high blood level, ethosuximide may exhibit nonlinear metabolism similar to phenytoin.

Pharmacodynamics

Ethosuximide's exact mechanism of action is unknown. The drug inhibits an enzyme needed to form gamma-hydroxybutyrate, which has been linked to the induction of absence seizures.

Succinimides suppress the paroxysmal, three cycle/second, spike-and-wave activity that occurs on the EEG in absence seizures. These drugs elevate the seizure threshold in the cortex and basal ganglia and reduce synaptic response to low-frequency repetitive stimulation.

Features of succinimides

+ Inhibit an enzyme needed to form gamma-hydroxybutyrate, linked to absence seizures
+ Suppress paroxysmal, three cycle/second, spike-and-wave activity in absence seizures
+ Elevate the seizure threshold in cortex and basal ganglia
+ Reduce synaptic response to low-frequency repetitive stimulation

Teaching a patient about succinimides

Whenever a succinimide is prescribed, teach the patient and his family the drug's name, dose, frequency, action, and adverse effects, and take the following actions.

✦ Instruct the patient to take the drug with food or milk to prevent GI distress.

✦ Advise the patient not to discontinue the drug abruptly or change the dosage unless directed by the prescriber.

✦ Tell the patient to avoid alcohol.

✦ Warn the patient to use caution while driving or performing other tasks requiring alertness, coordination, or physical dexterity.

✦ Advise the patient to notify the prescriber if he notices skin rash, joint pain, unexplained fever, sore throat, unusual bleeding or bruising, drowsiness, dizziness, or blurred vision.

✦ Tell the patient to notify the prescriber if she becomes—or plans to become—pregnant.

✦ Advise the patient to carry identification indicating that he takes a drug to treat epilepsy.

Pharmacotherapeutics

The only indication for ethosuximide is the treatment of absence seizures. Although it's the treatment of choice for these seizures, it also may be used with valproic acid for absence seizures that are difficult to control.

Interactions

Ethosuximide isn't protein bound, so it can't participate in interactions involving displacement from plasma proteins.

✦ Carbamazepine may aid ethosuximide metabolism.

✦ Valproic acid may inhibit ethosuximide metabolism that's near saturation.

✦ Ethosuximide may increase the level of hydantoins.

✦ Primidone and phenobarbital levels may decrease when the patient is taking ethosuximide.

Adverse reactions

Ethosuximide is well tolerated. The most common adverse reactions include nausea, vomiting, epigastric and abdominal pain, anorexia, and constipation. Other common adverse reactions include drowsiness, fatigue, lethargy, dizziness, diplopia, hiccups, headaches, and mood changes. Rarely, the drug can cause blood dyscrasias, rashes (including Steven-Johnson syndrome and erythema multiforme), lupus-like syndrome, and psychotic behaviors.

Nursing considerations

✦ Teach the patient and his caregiver about the drug. (See *Teaching a patient about succinimides.*)

✦ Monitor blood counts periodically. Fatal blood dyscrasias may occur.

✦ Monitor the patient for signs of blood dyscrasias, such as sore throat, fever, and unusual bleeding or bruising.

✦ Monitor the level of a succinimide and the level of a concomitant anticonvulsant; these drugs may interact and affect the drug levels. The therapeutic range of ethosuximide is 40 to 100 mcg/ml.

✦ Monitor the patient for signs of toxicity, including nausea, vomiting, and profound CNS depression.

Possible drug interactions

✦ Carbamazepine
✦ Hydantoins
✦ Phenobarbital
✦ Primidone
✦ Valproic acid

Adverse reactions to watch for

✦ Abdominal pain, anorexia, constipation, epigastric pain, nausea, vomiting

✦ Diplopia, headaches, hiccups, mood changes

✦ Dizziness, drowsiness, fatigue, lethargy

✦ Blood dyscrasias, lupus-like syndrome, psychosis, rash (including Steven-Johnson syndrome and erythema multiforme)

Key nursing actions

✦ Monitor blood counts.
✦ Watch for evidence of blood dyscrasias.
✦ Watch for evidence of toxicity.

SULFONAMIDES

The sulfonamide zonisamide is approved as an adjunct treatment for partial seizures in adults and children older than age 16. It's also the most commonly prescribed sulfonamide.

Pharmacokinetics

After zonisamide is absorbed, it achieves a peak level within 2 to 6 hours. The drug is widely distributed and extensively bound to erythrocytes. It's metabolized by cytochrome P450 (CYP) 3A4 enzymes in the liver and is excreted in urine, primarily as unchanged drug and the glucuronide of a metabolite.

Pharmacodynamics

Zonisamide's precise mechanism of action is unknown, but it may stabilize neuronal membranes and suppress neuronal hypersynchronization.

Pharmacotherapeutics

Zonisamide is approved only as adjunctive therapy for partial seizures in adults and children older than 16 years. Despite this single indication, the drug appears to be effective in other types of seizures (infantile spasms and myoclonic, generalized, and atypical absence seizures) and has been used in other countries as monotherapy for these and other seizure types in children and adults.

Interactions

+ Drugs that induce liver enzymes, such as carbamazepine, phenobarbital, and phenytoin, increase the metabolism and decrease the half-life of zonisamide.
+ Use of zonisamide with drugs that inhibit or induce CYP 3A4 may increase or decrease the serum zonisamide level. (Because zonisamide doesn't induce CYP 3A4 enzymes, it isn't likely to affect other drugs metabolized by this system.)

Adverse reactions

Common adverse reactions include somnolence, dizziness, confusion, headache, irritability, agitation, anorexia, nausea, diarrhea, weight loss, and rash. Slowly adjust dosage and give with meals to decrease the risk of these reactions. More serious reactions to zonisamide include fatal Stevens-Johnson syndrome, toxic epidermal necrolysis, psychosis, aplastic anemia, and agranulocytosis. Although not approved for use in children in the United States, the drug may cause decreased sweating, hyperthermia, and heatstroke in children. Renal calculi composed of calcium or urate salts have formed in patients who take zonisamide.

WARNING

Giving sulfonamides cautiously

In patients receiving sulfonamides, rare fatalities have occurred because of severe adverse reactions, such as Stevens-Johnson syndrome, fulminant hepatic necrosis, aplastic anemia, otherwise unexplained rashes, and agranulocytosis.

If signs and symptoms of hypersensitivity or other serious reactions occur, discontinue the drug immediately and notify the prescriber.

Teaching a patient about sulfonamides

Whenever a sulfonamide is prescribed, teach the patient and his family the drug's name, dose, frequency, action, and adverse effects, and take the following actions.
✦ Tell the patient to take the drug with or without food and not to bite or break the capsule.
✦ Advise the patient to call the prescriber immediately if a rash appears or if seizures worsen.
✦ Tell the patient to contact the prescriber immediately if he develops sudden back pain, abdominal pain, pain when urinating, bloody or dark urine, fever, sore throat, mouth sores, easy bruising, decreased sweating, fever, depression, or speech or language problems.
✦ Tell the patient to drink 6 to 8 glasses of water per day.
✦ Caution the patient that the drug may cause drowsiness and not to drive or operate dangerous machinery until the drug's effects are known.
✦ Advise the patient not to stop taking the drug without the prescriber's approval.
✦ Instruct the patient to call the prescriber if she is pregnant or breast-feeding or if she plans to become pregnant or breast-feed.
✦ Advise a woman of childbearing age to use a contraceptive while taking the drug.

Nursing considerations

✦ Zonisamide is contraindicated in patients with an allergy to sulfonamides. Use of zonisamide in patients with a renal clearance below 50 ml/minute isn't recommended.
✦ Begin therapy with low doses in geriatric patients because they're more likely than younger patients to have renal impairment.
✦ Monitor the patient closely during sulfonamide therapy. (See *Giving sulfonamides cautiously*.)
✦ Because of the drug's long half-life, it may take 2 weeks to achieve a steady state level.
✦ Monitor the patient's temperature, especially in the summer, because decreased sweating can occur, resulting in heatstroke and dehydration.
✦ When reducing the dosage or stopping zonisamide, do so gradually. Abrupt withdrawal of the drug may increase the frequency of seizures or cause status epilepticus.
✦ Increase the fluid intake and urine output to help prevent renal calculi, especially in patients with predisposing factors.
✦ Monitor the patient's renal function periodically.
✦ Teach the patient and his caregiver about the prescribed drug. (See *Teaching a patient about sulfonamides*.)

Key nursing actions

✦ Monitor the patient's temperature, especially in hot weather.
✦ Don't stop the drug abruptly.
✦ Increase fluid intake and urine output to help prevent renal calculi.
✦ Monitor renal function.

OTHER ANTICONVULSANTS

Because they belong to many different classes, several other anticonvulsants must be discussed separately. These drugs include carbamazepine, felbamate, gabapentin, lamotrigine, levetiracetam, oxcarbazepine, tiagabine, topiramate, and valproic acid.

Features of carbamazepine

+ Has an anticonvulsant effect similar to that of phenytoin
+ Inhibits the spread of seizure activity and neuromuscular transmission
+ Is the drug of choice for generalized tonnic-clonic, simple, and complex seizures
+ Relieves the pain of trigeminal neuralgia
+ May help certain psychiatric disorders
+ May worsen absence or generalized convulsive seizures

Possible drug interactions

+ Barbiturates
+ Bupropion
+ Cimetidine
+ Danazol
+ Diltiazem
+ Doxycycline
+ Erythromycin
+ Felbamate
+ Haloperidol
+ Hormonal contraceptives
+ Isoniazid
+ Ketoconazole
+ Lamotrigine
+ Lithium
+ Oral anticoagulants
+ Phenytoin
+ Propoxyphene
+ Selective serotonin reuptake inhibitors
+ Theophylline
+ Tricyclic antidepressants
+ Troleandomycin
+ Valproic acid
+ Verapamil
+ Warfarin

WARNING

Contraindications and precautions for carbamazepine

Carbamazepine is contraindicated in patients who are hypersensitive to it or to tricyclic antidepressants and in those with a history of bone marrow suppression. The drug also is contraindicated in patients who have taken a monoamine oxidase inhibitor in the last 14 days. The drug falls within pregnancy risk category D and isn't recommended during breast-feeding.

CARBAMAZEPINE

Carbamazepine is the most commonly used iminostilbene anticonvulsant. It effectively treats partial and generalized tonic-clonic seizures and mixed seizure types. It's the first choice anticonvulsant for complex partial seizures.

Pharmacokinetics

Carbamazepine is absorbed slowly and erratically from the GI tract. It's distributed rapidly to all tissues; 75% to 90% is bound to plasma proteins. Metabolism occurs in the liver, and carbamazepine is excreted in urine. A small amount crosses the placenta, and some appears in breast milk. The half-life varies greatly. The drug aids its own metabolism; the level typically falls after 3 to 5 weeks of treatment.

Pharmacodynamics

Carbamazepine's anticonvulsant effect is similar to that of phenytoin. Its anticonvulsant action can occur because of its ability to inhibit the spread of seizure activity or neuromuscular transmission in general.

Pharmacotherapeutics

In adults and children, carbamazepine is the drug of choice for treating generalized tonic-clonic seizures and simple and complex partial seizures. The drug also relieves pain when used to treat trigeminal neuralgia (tic douloureux, characterized by excruciating facial pain along the trigeminal nerve) and may be useful in selected psychiatric disorders. The drug may worsen absence or generalized convulsive seizures.

Interactions

+ Carbamazepine can reduce the effects of bupropion, doxycycline, felbamate, haloperidol, hormonal contraceptives, lamotrigine, oral anticoagulants, theophylline, tricyclic antidepressants, and valproic acid.
+ Cimetidine, danazol, diltiazem, erythromycin, isoniazid, ketoconazole, propoxyphene, selective serotonin reuptake inhibitors, troleandomycin, valproic acid, and verapamil can increase the carbamazepine level and lead to toxicity.
+ Together, lithium and carbamazepine increase the risk of toxic neurologic effects.
+ Barbiturates, felbamate, phenytoin, and warfarin can decrease the carbamazepine level.
+ Grapefruit juice can increase the carbamazepine level, increasing the drug's pharmacologic and adverse effects.

Teaching a patient about carbamazepine

Whenever carbamazepine is prescribed, teach the patient and his family the drug's name, dose, frequency, action, and adverse effects, and take the following actions.
✦ Advise the patient to take the drug with meals to decrease GI distress and enhance absorption.
✦ Tell the patient not to crush or chew extended-release forms and not to take broken or chipped tablets.
✦ Tell the patient that the drug may cause mild to moderate dizziness when first taken. Advise him to avoid hazardous activities until these effects disappear, usually within 3 or 4 days.
✦ For a patient who uses a hormonal contraceptive, recommend that she use an additional or different contraceptive method. Discuss the advantages and disadvantages of various contraceptive methods, if requested.
✦ Instruct the patient and his family to notify the prescriber immediately if the patient displays early signs of hematologic problems, such as fever, sore throat, malaise, unusual fatigue, or a tendency to bruise or bleed.

Adverse reactions

Most adverse reactions are tolerable and relatively minor if drug therapy begins slowly at a low dosage and advances gradually to tolerance. Occasionally serious hematologic toxicity may occur.

Dose-related adverse reactions include drowsiness, diplopia, ataxia, vertigo, nystagmus, headaches, tremor, and dry mouth. Because carbamazepine is related to tricyclic antidepressants, it can produce many of the same adverse reactions, including heart failure, hypertension or hypotension, syncope, arrhythmias, and MI. Its action as a mild anticholinergic may result in urine retention, constipation, and increased intraocular pressure. With long-term use, the drug also can cause syndrome of inappropriate antidiuretic hormone secretion and water intoxication.

Urticaria and Stevens-Johnson syndrome may occur. The occasional but significant hematologic reactions include aplastic anemia (rare), agranulocytosis, thrombocytopenia, and leukopenia. Rare instances of cholestatic and hepatocellular jaundice also have been noted. Rare psychiatric reactions have been noted, including activation of latent psychosis, mental depression with agitation, and talkativeness.

Nursing considerations

✦ Assess the patient for conditions that may contraindicate or require cautious use. (See *Contraindications and precautions for carbamazepine.*)
✦ Teach the patient and his caregiver about the drug. (See *Teaching a patient about carbamazepine.*)
✦ Monitor the patient for worsening of seizures, especially in mixed seizure disorders, including atypical absence seizures.
✦ Sprinkle the contents of extended-release capsules over applesauce if the patient has trouble swallowing capsules. Capsules or tablets shouldn't be crushed or chewed unless labeled as chewable form.
✦ If the patient develops thrombocytopenia or leukopenia, take bleeding and infection precautions.
✦ If the patient exhibits drowsiness, diplopia, ataxia, vertigo, or syncope, take safety precautions.

Adverse reactions to watch for

✦ Arrhythmias, heart failure, hypertension, hypotension, MI, syncope
✦ Ataxia, diplopia, drowsiness, vertigo, dry mouth, headache, nystagmus, tremor
✦ Constipation, increased intraocular pressure, urine retention
✦ Agranulocytosis, aplastic anemia, cholestatic and hepatocellular jaundice, leukopenia, psychiatric reactions, thrombocytopenia
✦ Stevens-Johnson syndrome, urticaria
✦ Syndrome of inappropriate antidiuretic hormone secretion, water intoxication.

Key nursing actions

✦ Watch for worsening seizures.
✦ Monitor the patient for evidence of fluid retention.
✦ Document intake and output and changes in vital signs.
✦ Limit fluid and salt intake.
✦ Monitor the drug level.
✦ Watch for anorexia or appetite changes.

Features of felbamate

✦ Is structurally similar to meprobamate, without tolerance or dependence
✦ May work by antagonizing N-methyl-D-aspartate receptors
✦ Is a second-line drug and usually limited to patients with severe refractory epilepsy

Possible drug interactions

✦ Carbamazepine
✦ Phenobarbital
✦ Phenytoin
✦ Valproic acid

Adverse reactions to watch for

✦ Acute liver failure
✦ Anorexia, diarrhea, nausea, taste disturbance, vomiting, weight loss
✦ Aplastic anemia
✦ Ataxia
✦ Diplopia
✦ Headache
✦ Insomnia, somnolence
✦ Rash
✦ Rhinitis

✦ If the patient develops adverse reactions to carbamazepine, notify the prescriber.
✦ Assess the patient for signs of fluid retention, such as crackles, dependent edema, and weight gain.
✦ Document fluid intake and output and note changes in vital signs, such as increased blood pressure, pulse, and respirations, at least daily.
✦ Limit the patient's fluid and salt intake.
✦ Monitor drug level; the therapeutic level is 4 to 12 mcg/ml.
✦ Watch for anorexia or appetite changes, which may indicate an abnormally high drug level.

 CLINICAL ALERT Don't confuse Tegretol with Toradol (ketorolac, a nonsteroidal anti-inflammatory drug) or Tegopen (cloxacillin, an antibiotic). Don't confuse Carbatrol with carvedilol (Coreg, an antihypertensive).

FELBAMATE

Felbamate is structurally similar to meprobamate but doesn't cause tolerance or dependence.

Pharmacokinetics

Felbamate is rapidly and well absorbed. It's partially metabolized in the liver by hydroxylation and conjugation and excreted in urine as metabolites and unchanged drug. The drug displays dose-related linear pharmacokinetics.

Pharmacodynamics

Felbamate appears to act as an antagonist on N-methyl-D-aspartate receptors. This inhibits the initiation and propagation of seizure activity.

Pharmacotherapeutics

Felbamate is approved for use alone or as an adjunct to other drugs in adults with partial and secondarily generalized seizures and as an adjunct in children with Lennox-Gastaut syndrome. However, the drug should be used only as second-line therapy. Because of serious hematologic and hepatic reactions, its use generally is limited to patients with severe refractory epilepsy.

Interactions

✦ Felbamate inhibits the clearance of phenobarbital, phenytoin, valproic acid, and a metabolite of carbamazepine, requiring a dosage reduction of these drugs.
✦ Carbamazepine, phenobarbital, and phenytoin can increase the clearance of felbamate.

Adverse reactions

Adverse reactions are more likely with polytherapy than monotherapy. Common reactions include anorexia, weight loss, insomnia, somnolence, nausea, vomiting, and headache. Less common ones include diarrhea, rash, diplopia, ataxia, rhinitis, and taste disturbances

Serious adverse reactions may be aplastic anemia and acute liver failure. Aplastic anemia is more likely to affect patients with a history of low cell counts, anticonvulsant allergy, viral infection, or other immunologic problems.

Nursing considerations

✦ Obtain informed consent in writing before beginning therapy.

Teaching a patient about felbamate

Whenever felbamate is prescribed, teach the patient and his family the drug's name, dose, frequency, action, and adverse effects, and take the following actions.
+ Advise the patient to discuss his informed consent with the prescriber before therapy.
+ Instruct the patient to alert the prescriber if he notices fever, sore throat, increased bleeding or bruising, fatigue, rash, abdominal pain, anorexia, dark urine, light stools, or jaundice.
+ Advise the patient to schedule laboratory tests as prescribed.
+ Tell the patient to avoid prolonged exposure to sunlight or sunlamps.

+ Use only in patients whose response to alternative treatments is inadequate and whose epilepsy is so severe that the benefits of the drug outweigh the risk of severe hepatic failure or aplastic anemia.
+ Obtain liver function test results before therapy begins and then every 1 to 2 weeks. Discontinue felbamate if the patient's liver enzyme levels are elevated.
+ Obtain complete blood, platelet, and reticulocyte counts before therapy begins. Be alert for signs of aplastic anemia, which may occur from 5 to 30 weeks after treatment starts.
+ Monitor hematologic test results for signs of bone marrow depression. Also monitor the patient for signs of infection, bleeding, or anemia.
+ Advise the patient not to stop taking felbamate abruptly or change the dosage unless directed by the prescriber.
+ Teach the patient and his caregiver about the drug. (See *Teaching a patient about felbamate*.)

GABAPENTIN

Gabapentin was designed to be a GABA agonist, but its exact mechanism is unknown.

Pharmacokinetics

Gabapentin is absorbed in the stomach by an active process that's subject to saturation. Because of this active-transport process, bioavailability may decrease as the dose increases. Gabapentin isn't metabolized; it's excreted exclusively by the kidneys.

Pharmacodynamics

The exact mechanism of gabapentin's action isn't known. Originally designed as a GABA agonist, it doesn't appear to act at GABA receptors, affect GABA uptake, or interfere with GABA transaminase. Instead, the drug seems to bind with a carrier protein and act at unique receptors, elevating the GABA level in the brain.

Pharmacotherapeutics

Gabapentin is used for adjunct therapy in adults and children older than age 12 with partial seizures (with and without secondary generalization) and in children ages 3 to 12 with partial seizures. Like carbamazepine, gabapentin may worsen myoclonic seizures.

Key nursing actions
+ Give only to patients unresponsive to other drugs and when benefits outweigh risks.
+ Monitor liver function tests.
+ Monitor complete blood, platelet, and reticulocyte counts.
+ Evaluate hematologic test results for evidence for bone marrow depression.
+ Assess the patient for evidence of infection, bleeding, anemia.

Features of gabapentin
+ Acts by unknown mechanism
+ May bind with carrier protein and act at unique receptors to elevate GABA levels in the brain
+ Is used as an adjunct for partial seizures with and without secondary generalization
+ Is used for partial seizures in children ages 3 to 12
+ May worsen myoclonic seizures
+ Is used to prevent migraines and to treat pain and tremor in MS, bipolar disorder, Parkinson's disease

The drug also may be used to prevent migraines and to treat pain, tremor in MS, bipolar disorder, and Parkinson's disease.

Interactions
Gabapentin doesn't induce or inhibit liver enzymes or affect the metabolism of other anticonvulsants. That's why it's involved in few drug interactions.
- ✦ Antacids may decrease gabapentin level.
- ✦ Cimetidine may increase gabapentin level.

Adverse reactions
In adults and children older than age 12, common adverse reactions include fatigue, somnolence, dizziness, ataxia, leukopenia, and nystagmus. In children ages 3 to 12, common reactions are viral infection, fever, nausea, vomiting, somnolence, and hostility.

Nursing considerations
- ✦ Reduce the dosage in a patient with a creatinine clearance of less than 60 ml/minute.
- ✦ Give the first dose at bedtime to minimize drowsiness, dizziness, fatigue, and ataxia.
- ✦ Discontinue gabapentin gradually over at least 1 week to minimize the risk of precipitating seizures. Do this even if another anticonvulsant is being substituted for gabapentin.
- ✦ Don't suddenly withdraw other anticonvulsants in a patient starting gabapentin therapy.
- ✦ Routine monitoring of the gabapentin level isn't necessary. The drug doesn't alter the levels of other anticonvulsants.
- ✦ Teach the patient and his caregiver about the drug. (See *Teaching a patient about gabapentin*.)

LAMOTRIGINE
Lamotrigine is chemically unrelated to other anticonvulsants. Lamotrigine is FDA-approved for adjunctive therapy in adults with partial seizures and in children older than age 2 with generalized seizures of Lennox-Gastaut syndrome. It's also ap-

Possible drug interactions
- ✦ Antacids
- ✦ Cimetidine

Adverse reactions to watch for
- ✦ Ataxia, dizziness, nystagmus
- ✦ Fatigue, somnolence
- ✦ Leukopenia
- ✦ Children ages 3 to 12: fever, hostility, nausea, somnolence, viral infection, vomiting

Key nursing actions
- ✦ Give the first dose at bedtime.
- ✦ Stop the drug gradually over at least a week.
- ✦ Don't withdraw other anticonvulsants abruptly when the patient starts gabapentin.

proved for conversion to monotherapy in adults with partial seizures who are receiving treatment with a single anticonvulsant that induces enzymes.

Pharmacokinetics

Lamotrigine is rapidly and well absorbed, but isn't significantly bound to plasma proteins. The drug is metabolized by the liver and excreted by the kidneys. Its clearance is increased in the presence of other enzyme-inducing anticonvulsants.

Pharmacodynamics

Although lamotrigine's precise mechanism of action is unknown, it's thought to involve a use-dependent blocking effect on sodium channels, which inhibits the release of the excitatory neurotransmitters, glutamate and aspartate.

Pharmacotherapeutics

Lamotrigine appears effective for many types of generalized seizures, but can worsen myoclonic seizures. The drug may be used as an adjunct in adults with partial seizures and in children younger than age 2 with Lennox-Gastaut syndrome. In adults, it also may be used for conversion to monotherapy.

Specific dosing guidelines are available for the addition of lamotrigine to regimens with an anticonvulsant that induces enzymes (such as carbamazepine, phenobarbital, phenytoin, or primidone) with or without valproic acid.

Interactions

✦ Acetaminophen, carbamazepine, phenobarbital, phenytoin, and primidone may decrease lamotrigine's effects.
✦ Valproic acid may decrease lamotrigine's clearance and increase its effects.
✦ Lamotrigine may produce additive effects when combined with folate inhibitors.
✦ Lamotrigine may increase the carbamazepine metabolite level and decrease the valproic acid level.

Adverse reactions

Common reactions to lamotrigine include dizziness, ataxia, somnolence, headache, blurred vision, diplopia, nausea, vomiting, and rash.

Several types of rash may occur with this drug, including Stevens-Johnson syndrome. The generalized, erythematous, morbilliform rash usually appears in the first 3 to 4 weeks of therapy and usually is mild to moderate, but may be severe. Stop lamotrigine at the first sign of rash. Starting at high doses, rapidly increasing doses, or using the drug with valproic acid may increase the risk of rash.

Nursing considerations

✦ Don't discontinue lamotrigine abruptly because of the risk of increased seizure frequency. Instead, taper the drug dosage over at least 2 weeks.

 CLINICAL ALERT Withhold lamotrigine at the first sign of rash unless the rash isn't drug related. Rash is more severe in children. Safety and efficacy in children younger than age 16 (other than those with Lennox-Gastaut syndrome) haven't been established.

✦ Reduce the dose when lamotrigine is added to a multidrug regimen that includes valproic acid.
✦ Monitor the patient for changes in seizure activity and check the serum level of all adjunct anticonvulsants.

Teaching a patient about lamotrigine

Whenever lamotrigine is prescribed, teach the patient and his family the drug's name, dose, frequency, action, and adverse effects, and take the following actions.

✦ Inform the patient that he may develop a rash. If he's also taking valproic acid, a serious rash may develop. Tell the patient to report a rash or signs and symptoms of hypersensitivity promptly to the prescriber because the drug may need to be stopped.

✦ Warn the patient not to engage in hazardous activities until the drug's central nervous system effects are known.

✦ Warn the patient that photosensitivity reactions may occur. Suggest that he avoid prolonged or unprotected exposure to sunlight until his tolerance is known.

✦ Advise the patient not to stop taking the drug abruptly.

✦ Advise the patient to discuss drug therapy with the prescriber if she plans to become pregnant.

✦ Advise the patient that she shouldn't breast-feed during therapy.

✦ Teach the patient and his caregiver about lamotrigine. (See *Teaching a patient about lamotrigine*.)

LEVETIRACETAM

A pyrrolidone derivative, levetiracetam is chemically unrelated to other anticonvulsants. It's approved for use as adjunctive therapy for partial seizures in adults.

Pharmacokinetics
Levetiracetam is rapidly absorbed and reaches almost complete bioavailability. Metabolism of levetiracetam isn't extensive and involves hydrolysis, not liver CYP isoenzymes. The drug is excreted through the kidneys as unchanged drug.

Pharmacodynamics
The mechanism of action of levetiracetam is unknown; it doesn't appear to involve known mechanisms relating to inhibitory and excitatory neurotransmission.

Pharmacotherapeutics
Levetiracetam is approved as an adjunct to treat partial seizures in adults. It also may be effective, alone or with other anticonvulsants, for generalized seizures or myoclonus in adults, but hasn't been approved for these indications. Some patients have rapidly developed tolerance to levetiracetam's anticonvulsant effects.

Interactions
Levetiracetam doesn't seem to be affected by the use of other anticonvulsants, and vice versa.

Adverse reactions
Common adverse reactions to levetiracetam include dizziness, asthenia, somnolence, weakness, irritability, coordination difficulties, infection, headache, depres-

---

Features of levetiracetam

✦ Is chemically unrelated to other anticonvulsants
✦ Acts by an unknown mechanism
✦ Is adjunct therapy for partial seizures in adults
✦ May be effective for generalized seizures or myoclonus in adults
✦ May produce tolerance quickly in some patients

Adverse reactions to watch for

✦ Asthenia, coordination difficulties, weakness
✦ Depression, headache, irritability, nervousness
✦ Dizziness, somnolence
✦ Infection
✦ Pharyngitis, rhinitis
✦ Mild decreases in hemoglobin, hematocrit, and RBC count

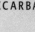

PATIENT TEACHING

Teaching a patient about levetiracetam

Whenever levetiracetam is prescribed, teach the patient and his family the drug's name, dose, frequency, action, and adverse effects, and take the following actions.
✦ Caution the patient to use extra care when sitting or standing to avoid falling.
✦ Advise the patient to call the prescriber and not to stop taking the drug abruptly if adverse reactions occur.
✦ Tell the patient to take the drug with other prescribed seizure drugs.
✦ Inform the patient that the drug can be taken with or without food.

---

sion, rhinitis, nervousness, and pharyngitis. Asthenia, somnolence, and dizziness are most common during the first 4 weeks of treatment.

Less common reactions are mild decreases in hemoglobin, hematocrit, and red blood cell count.

Nursing considerations

✦ Reduce the dosage in a patient with renal impairment or a geriatric patient at risk for renal impairment.
✦ Use the drug cautiously in immunocompromised patients, such as those with cancer or human immunodeficiency virus infection, because it may cause leukopenia and neutropenia.
✦ Give the drug with or without food.
✦ Use the drug only with other anticonvulsants; it isn't recommended for monotherapy.
✦ Don't stop the drug abruptly because seizures can result. Instead, gradually taper the drug dosage.
✦ Monitor the patient closely for such adverse reactions as dizziness, which may lead to falls.
✦ Teach the patient and his caregiver about the drug. (See *Teaching a patient about levetiracetam.*)

OXCARBAZEPINE

The prodrug oxcarbazepine is chemically similar to carbamazepine but causes less induction of liver enzymes. It may be used alone or with other anticonvulsants to treat adults with partial seizures, and with other anticonvulsants to treat children with partial seizures.

Pharmacokinetics

Oxcarbazepine is completely absorbed and extensively metabolized via liver enzymes to the 10-monohydroxy (MHD) metabolite, which is responsible for its pharmacologic activity. MHD is further metabolized by conjugation and excreted primarily by the kidneys. The half-life of MHD is about 9 hours. Unlike carbamazepine, oxcarbazepine doesn't induce its own metabolism.

Key nursing actions
✦ Give the drug only with other anticonvulsants.
✦ Don't stop the drug abruptly.
✦ Assess the patient for adverse reactions that could lead to falls.

Features of oxcarbazepine
✦ Is chemically similar to carbamazepine but doesn't induce liver enzymes as much
✦ May stabilize excitatory neuronal membranes
✦ May inhibit repetitive neuronal firing
✦ May decrease propagation of synaptic impulses by blocking sodium-sensitive channels
✦ Is an adjunct for partial seizures in adults and children over age 4; also as monotherapy in adults
✦ Is also effective for generalized seizures
✦ May worsen myoclonic and absence seizures

Teaching a patient about oxcarbazepine

Whenever oxcarbazepine is prescribed, teach the patient and his family the drug's name, dose, frequency, action, and adverse effects, and take the following actions.

✦ Inform the patient that the drug can be taken with or without food.

✦ Tell the patient to contact the prescriber before interrupting or stopping the drug.

✦ Advise the patient to report signs and symptoms of hyponatremia, such as nausea, malaise, headache, lethargy, confusion, and decreased sensation.

✦ Caution the patient to avoid driving and operating heavy machinery until the drug's central nervous system effects are known.

✦ Advise a woman using hormonal contraception to use an additional method while taking oxcarbazepine.

✦ Tell the patient to avoid alcohol while taking the drug.

✦ Advise the patient to inform the prescriber if he has ever experienced a hypersensitivity reaction to carbamazepine.

Possible drug interactions

✦ Carbamazepine
✦ Felodipine
✦ Hormonal contraceptives
✦ Phenobarbital
✦ Phenytoin
✦ Valproic acid
✦ Verapamil

Adverse reactions to watch for

✦ Abdominal pain, dyspepsia, nausea, rectal bleeding, vomiting
✦ Abnormal gait, ataxia, dizziness, fatigue, somnolence
✦ Abnormal vision, diplopia
✦ Aggravated seizures, tremor
✦ Less common: agitation, back pain, confusion, hyponatremia, hypotension, rhinitis, speech disorder, upper respiratory tract infection

Key nursing actions

✦ Stop the drug gradually.
✦ Watch for evidence of hyponatremia.
✦ Monitor the sodium level.
✦ Watch for psychomotor slowing, trouble concentrating, problems with language, fatigue, abnormal coordination.

Pharmacodynamics

The exact mechanism of oxcarbazepine and its metabolite is unknown. However, the drug may stabilize excitatory neuronal membranes, inhibit repetitive neuronal firing, and decrease propagation of synaptic impulses by blocking sodium-sensitive channels, which prevents seizure spread in the brain.

Pharmacotherapeutics

Oxcarbazepine is FDA-approved as an adjunct to treat partial seizures in adults and children older than age 4, and as monotherapy in adults. Like carbamazepine, it's also effective for generalized seizures, but may worsen myoclonus and absence seizures.

Interactions

✦ Carbamazepine, phenobarbital, phenytoin, valproic acid, and verapamil may decrease the level of the active metabolite MHD.

✦ Oxcarbazepine may decrease the effectiveness of hormonal contraceptives and felodipine.

Adverse reactions

With oxcarbazepine therapy, common reactions include somnolence, dizziness, fatigue, abnormal vision, diplopia, ataxia, nausea, vomiting, abdominal pain, dyspepsia, abnormal gait, tremor, aggravated seizures, and rectal bleeding.

Less common reactions include agitation, confusion, hypotension, hyponatremia, rhinitis, speech disorder, back pain, and upper respiratory tract infection.

Nursing considerations

✦ Reduce the dosage in a patient with a creatinine clearance below 30 ml/minute.

✦ Shake the oral suspension well. The suspension can be mixed with water or swallowed directly from a syringe.

✦ Interchange the oral suspension and tablets at equal doses if needed.

CLINICAL ALERT Ask the patient if he has had carbamazepine hypersensitivity because cross-sensitivity with carbamazepine allergy occurs in 20% to 30% of patients. Stop the drug immediately if signs or symptoms of hypersensitivity occur.

◆ Withdraw the drug gradually to minimize the risk of increased frequency of seizures.
◆ Watch for signs and symptoms of hyponatremia, including nausea, malaise, headache, lethargy, confusion, and decreased sensation.
◆ Monitor the sodium level, especially in a patient receiving other therapies that may decrease the sodium level.
◆ Oxcarbazepine has been linked to adverse CNS reactions. Monitor the patient for psychomotor slowing, difficulty with concentration, speech or language problems, somnolence, fatigue, and coordination abnormalities. Notify the prescriber if any adverse reactions occur.
◆ Teach the patient and his caregiver about the drug. (See *Teaching a patient about oxcarbazepine*.)

TIAGABINE

A structurally unique anticonvulsant, tiagabine is a potent and specific inhibitor of GABA uptake into glial cells and other neuronal elements.

Pharmacokinetics

After oral administration, tiagabine is rapidly and completely absorbed. It is 96% bound to plasma proteins, and it's unknown if drug appears in breast milk. It undergoes metabolism in the liver, primarily by cytochrome P450 3A4 enzymes, and is excreted in urine and feces. Enzyme inducers, such as carbamazepine, phenobarbital, phenytoin, and primidone, increase tiagabine's clearance. Children may metabolize the drug faster than adults.

Pharmacodynamics

Tiagabine is believed to block GABA reuptake into nerve cells, thus enhancing this neurotransmitter's action and decreasing the propagation of impulses that cause seizures.

Pharmacotherapeutics

Tiagabine is approved for use as an adjunct to treat partial seizures in patients age 12 and older.

Interactions

◆ Carbamazepine, phenobarbital, and phenytoin may increase tiagabine's clearance and reduce its level though the implications are unknown.
◆ Use of tiagabine with CNS depressants may enhance CNS effects.
◆ Tiagabine may decrease valproic acid's bioavailability though the implications are unknown.

Adverse reactions

Common adverse reactions to tiagabine include dizziness, asthenia, somnolence, nervousness, tremor, and nausea. Less common ones are cognitive problems, speech disturbances, vomiting, diarrhea, rash, and pharyngitis.

Features of tiagabine
◆ Is a structurally unique anticonvulsant
◆ Is a potent and specific inhibitor of GABA uptake
◆ May metabolize faster in children than adults
◆ Is an adjunct for partial seizures

Possible drug interactions
◆ Carbamazepine
◆ CNS depressants
◆ Phenobarbital
◆ Phenytoin
◆ Valproic acid

Adverse reactions to watch for
◆ Asthenia, dizziness, somnolence
◆ Nausea
◆ Nervousness, tremor
◆ Less common: cognitive problems, diarrhea, pharyngitis, rash, speech disturbances, vomiting

Key nursing actions

+ Don't stop the drug abruptly.
+ Assess the patient for generalized weakness.
+ Explain that weakness resolves when drug is reduced or stopped.

Features of topiramate

+ May potentiate GABA activity by blocking sodium channels
+ May antagonize kainate's ability to activate glutamate (excitatory amino acid) receptors
+ Is an adjunct for partial and primary generalized tonic-clonic seizures in adults and children over age 2
+ Is used for Lennox-Gastaut syndrome in children and adults
+ May be useful for other seizure types and as monotherapy

Nursing considerations

+ In a patient with hepatic impairment, reduce the initial and maintenance doses.
+ Don't withdraw the drug abruptly because seizure frequency may increase. Discontinue the drug gradually unless safety concerns require a more rapid withdrawal.
+ When starting therapy, a patient who doesn't already receive at least one enzyme-inducing anticonvulsant may need lower doses or more gradual dosage adjustment of tiagabine.
+ In breast-feeding women, use the drug cautiously and only if the benefits to the mother outweigh the risks to the infant.
+ Monitor the patient for generalized weakness, which may be moderately severe to incapacitating. Reassure him that weakness resolves after dosage reduction or drug discontinuation.
+ Teach the patient and his caregiver about the drug. (See *Teaching a patient about tiagabine.*)

TOPIRAMATE

Topiramate is a sulfamate-substituted monosaccharide that's used to treat partial, tonic-clonic, and other seizures. Topiramate also may be used off-label for cluster headaches and infantile spasms.

Pharmacokinetics

Topiramate is rapidly absorbed and partially metabolized in the liver. The drug is excreted mostly unchanged in urine.

Pharmacodynamics

This anticonvulsant may act by blocking sodium channels, potentiating GABA activity, or antagonizing kainate's ability to activate particular excitatory amino acid (glutamate) receptors.

Pharmacotherapeutics

Topiramate is approved as an adjunct to treat partial seizures and primary generalized tonic-clonic seizures in adults and children ages 2 and older, and to treat

Lennox-Gastaut syndrome in children and adults. It also may prove beneficial for other types of seizures and as monotherapy.

Interactions
✦ Carbamazepine, phenytoin, and valproic acid may decrease the topiramate level.
✦ Topiramate may decrease the effectiveness of hormonal contraceptives.
✦ Topiramate may decrease the valproic acid level.
✦ Together, topiramate and CNS depressants may cause additive CNS effects.

Adverse reactions
Common reactions include drowsiness, fatigue, somnolence, dizziness, headache, ataxia, nervousness, confusion, paresthesias, weight loss, and diplopia. Psychomotor slowing, difficulty finding words, impaired concentration, and memory impairment also are common and may require stopping the drug. Low starting doses and slow titration may minimize these effects.

Serious, but infrequent, adverse reactions include secondary angle-closure glaucoma, liver failure, heatstroke, and renal calculi.

Nursing considerations
✦ Reduce the dosage by 50% for a patient with a creatinine clearance less than 70 ml/minute.
✦ Withdraw drug gradually to minimize the risk of increased seizures.
✦ Monitoring of the drug level isn't necessary.
✦ Teach the patient and his caregiver about the drug. (See *Teaching a patient about topiramate.*)

VALPROIC ACID
Valproic acid is structurally unrelated to other anticonvulsants. Valproic acid is also available as valproate and divalproex.

Pharmacokinetics
Valproate is converted rapidly to valproic acid in the stomach. Divalproex is a precursor of valproic acid and separates into valproic acid in the GI tract. Valproic acid is absorbed well, is strongly protein-bound, and is metabolized in the liver. Metab-

Possible drug interactions
✦ Carbamazepine
✦ CNS depressants
✦ Hormonal contraceptives
✦ Phenytoin
✦ Valproic acid

Adverse reactions to watch for
✦ Ataxia, dizziness, drowsiness, fatigue, somnolence
✦ Confusion, headache, nervousness
✦ Diplopia
✦ Impaired concentration and memory, psychomotor slowing, trouble finding words
✦ Paresthesias
✦ Weight loss
✦ Infrequent: heatstroke, liver failure, renal calculi, angle-closure glaucoma

Key nursing actions
✦ Reduce the dosage by one-half if the creatinine clearance is below 70 ml/minute.
✦ Don't stop the drug abruptly.

Features of valproic acid
✦ Acts by an unknown mechanism
✦ May increase GABA level by increasing potassium conductance
✦ Isn't used routinely because of the risk of serious liver toxicity
✦ Is used for long-term treatment of absence, partial, myoclonic, and tonic-clonic seizures

**Features of
valproic acid**
(continued)
+ Is used with caution in children under age 2, especiialy those most susceptible to liver toxicity

**Possible drug
interactions**
+ Aspirin
+ Benzodiazepines
+ Carbamazepine
+ Cimetidine
+ CNS depressants
+ Erythromycin
+ Ethosuximide
+ Felbamate
+ Lamotrigine
+ Phenobarbital
+ Phenytoin
+ Primidone
+ Rifampin
+ Tricyclic antidepressants
+ Warfarin
+ Zidovudine

**Adverse reactions to
watch for**
+ Appetite changes, constipation, diarrhea, nausea, vomiting
+ Ataxia, decreased alertness, dizziness, drowsiness, headache, muscle weakness, sedation
+ Blood dyscrasias, such as anemia, aplastic anemia, bone marrow suppression, hemorrhage, leukopenia, pancytopenia, thrombocytopenia
+ Hyperammonemia
+ Inhibited platelet aggregation, prolonged bleeding time
+ Depression, hallucinations, behavioral disorders in children

olites and unchanged drug are excreted in urine. Valproic acid is a liver enzyme inhibitor. It readily crosses the placenta and appears in breast milk.

Pharmacodynamics

The mechanism of action for valproic acid remains unknown. It's thought to increase the level of the inhibitory neurotransmitter GABA, which directly stabilizes membranes and inhibits neuronal activity by increasing potassium conductance.

Pharmacotherapeutics

Valproic acid is prescribed for long-term treatment of absence seizures, partial seizures, myoclonic seizures, and tonic-clonic seizures. The drug must be used cautiously in children younger than age 2, particularly those receiving multiple anticonvulsants, those with congenital metabolic disorders, those with severe seizures and mental retardation, and those with organic brain disease. In these patients, valproic acid carries a risk of potentially fatal liver toxicity. This toxicity usually occurs within the first 6 months of treatment. This risk limits the use of valproic acid as a drug of choice for seizure disorders.

Interactions

+ Aspirin, cimetidine, erythromycin, and felbamate may increase the drug level.
+ Carbamazepine, lamotrigine, phenobarbital, phenytoin, primidone, and rifampin may decrease the drug level.
+ Valproic acid may increase the effects of benzodiazepines, CNS depressants, ethosuximide, lamotrigine, phenobarbital, primidone, tricyclic antidepressants, warfarin, and zidovudine.

Adverse reactions

Most adverse reactions are tolerable and dose related; however, rare fatal hepatotoxicity may occur. The drug isn't prescribed routinely because of the risk of hepatotoxicity.

Dose-related adverse reactions affect the GI tract and CNS. Adverse GI reactions include nausea, vomiting, appetite changes, diarrhea, and constipation. Divalproex produces fewer adverse GI reactions than valproic acid. Adverse CNS reactions include sedation, drowsiness, dizziness, ataxia, headache, decreased alertness, and muscle weakness.

Adverse hematologic reactions include inhibited platelet aggregation and prolonged bleeding time. Rare adverse psychiatric reactions include depression, hallucinations, and behavioral disorders in children.

The rare, fatal hepatotoxicity that has been reported usually is preceded by nonspecific symptoms, such as loss of seizure control, malaise, jaundice, weakness, lethargy, facial edema, anorexia, and vomiting. The reaction may develop at any time from 3 days to 6 months after therapy begins. At the greatest risk are children and patients who receive other anticonvulsants with valproic acid.

A drug rash may occur, as may hyperammonemia with normal liver function. The use of valproic acid also may produce blood dyscrasias, such as anemia, leukopenia, thrombocytopenia, hemorrhage, bone marrow suppression, pancytopenia, and aplastic anemia.

Nursing considerations

+ Obtain liver function test results, platelet count, and prothrombin time, or PT, and International Normalized Ratio, or INR, before therapy begins. The drug is contraindicated in patients with hepatic disease or dysfunction.

Teaching a patient about valproic acid

Whenever valproic acid is prescribed, teach the patient and his family the drug's name, dose, frequency, action, and adverse effects, and take the following actions.

✦ Instruct the patient to swallow each capsule whole because the free drug can irritate the GI mucosa.

✦ Advise the patient not to mix valproate sodium oral solution in carbonated drinks; local irritation to the mouth and throat and unpleasant taste will occur.

✦ Tell the patient and parents to keep the drug out of children's reach.

✦ Alert the diabetic patient that the drug may produce a false-positive result on a urine ketone test.

✦ Teach the patient to recognize the signs and symptoms of hepatotoxicity (such as fever, malaise, abdominal pain, dark urine, light stools, and jaundice) and to contact the prescriber immediately if any occur.

✦ Remind the patient to report immediately signs of bleeding (such as dark stool, increased bleeding or bruising, and pallor) so that platelet function can be assessed.

✦ Instruct the patient to inform the surgeon of valproic acid therapy before surgery, including dental surgery.

✦ Use a lower starting dosage and more gradual dosage adjustment for a geriatric patient.

✦ Monitor the patient for adverse reactions.

✦ Use caution when converting a patient from a brand to a generic product because breakthrough seizures can occur.

✦ If decreased alertness occurs, take safety measures. For example, keep the bedside rails up at all times, maintain the bed in a low position, and supervise all patient activity.

✦ Administer valproic acid with meals to decrease adverse GI reactions. Keep the flavorful red syrup out of the reach of children.

 CLINICAL ALERT Watch for early, nonspecific signs of severe or fatal hepatotoxicity, such as loss of seizure control, malaise, weakness, lethargy, anorexia, and vomiting.

✦ Monitor the valproic acid level regularly. The therapeutic level is 50 to 100 mcg/ml.

✦ Monitor the patient's seizure activity.

✦ Notify the prescriber of any change in seizure activity and serum drug level.

✦ Teach the patient and his caregiver about the drug. (See *Teaching a patient about valproic acid.*)

DRUGS FOR ALZHEIMER'S DISEASE

Alzheimer's disease, a gradually progressive and eventually fatal dementia, is the most common form of dementia. The disease affects cognitive function and behavior. Personality, memory, and functional abilities decline until the patient becomes totally dependent on a caregiver for all his basic needs.

Although the precise pathophysiology of the disorder remains unclear, the brains of patients with Alzheimer's disease display structural changes, such as neurofibrillary tangles, neuritic plaques, and beta-amyloid proteins. These changes

Adverse reactions to watch for
(continued)

✦ Fatal hepatotoxicity, usually preceded by nonspecific symptoms, such as loss of seizure control, malaise, jaundice, weakness, lethargy, facial edema, anorexia, vomiting

✦ Rash

Key nursing actions

✦ Obtain liver function tests, platelet count, PT, and INR before therapy starts.

✦ Take safety precautions if the patient's level of alertness declines.

✦ Watch for early, nonspecific evidence of liver toxicity.

✦ Monitor the drug level regularly.

Reviewing Alzheimer's disease

✦ Affects cognition and behavior

✦ Has unclear pathology, but affected brains show neurofibrillary tangles, neuritic plaques, and beta-amyloid proteins

Reviewing Alzheimer's disease
(continued)

♦ May cause memory and cognitive impairment through loss of cholinergic cells
♦ May occur through immune system involvement
♦ May also involve neurotransmitters, estrogen, head trauma, environmental factors

Features of drugs for Alzheimer's disease

♦ Act by competitive, reversible inhibition of central acetylcholinesterase
♦ Increase the acetylcholine level in brain
♦ Treat mild to moderate dementia; don't alter disease progression but may improve cognition

Possible drug interactions

♦ Amiodarone
♦ Anticholinergics
♦ Beta blockers
♦ Calcium channel blockers
♦ Carbamazepine
♦ Cholinergic agonists, such as bethanechol
♦ Dexamethasone
♦ Digoxin
♦ Drugs that inhibit CYP 450
♦ Phenobarbital
♦ Phenytoin
♦ Rifampin
♦ Succinylcholine

have led to theories about the causes of Alzheimer's disease. Genetic research has linked early-onset and late-onset Alzheimer's disease to changes in chromosomes that affect the production of beta-amyloid proteins and apolipoprotein-E. The presence of inflammatory mediators and other immune system components near the plaques suggests that the immune system plays a role in the development of Alzheimer's disease. Cholinergic cell loss has been implicated as the cause of memory and cognitive impairments in Alzheimer's disease. (Today's cognition-enhancing drugs may work by increasing cholinergic function.) Other theories involve neurotransmitters (such as MAO type B, serotonin, and glutamate), estrogen, head trauma, and environmental exposure.

For assessment and treatment, Alzheimer's disease symptoms are divided into two groups:
♦ cognitive symptoms, including memory loss, dysphasia, disorientation, and impaired calculation and problem-solving skills
♦ behavioral symptoms, including depression, psychotic symptoms, nonpsychotic disruptive behaviors (such as aggression, uncooperativeness, combativeness, and repetitive activities).

Cognitive symptoms affect all patients in the final stages of Alzheimer's disease; behavioral symptoms are less predictable. Usually, behavioral symptoms are managed with antidepressants, antipsychotics, and anxiolytics. Cognitive symptoms may be treated with four drugs: donepezil, galantamine, rivastigmine, and tacrine—the first drug introduced in this class, but rarely used today.

Pharmacokinetics

All drugs in this class are rapidly absorbed and metabolized in the liver. Donepezil, galantamine, and tacrine are metabolized by the CYP enzyme system. Rivastigmine is metabolized primarily by hydrolysis mediated by cholinesterase.

The elimination half-life is about 2 hours for rivastigmine and tacrine, 6 to 8 hours for galantamine, and up to 70 hours for donepezil.

Pharmacodynamics

The drugs for Alzheimer's disease are competitive and reversible inhibitors of central acetylcholinesterase. They increase the acetylcholine level in the brain by decreasing acetylcholine degradation. Donepezil, galantamine, and rivastigmine are specific inhibitors of acetylcholinesterase; tacrine is a nonspecific inhibitor that causes more peripheral adverse effects.

Pharmacotherapeutics

All four cholinesterase inhibitors are approved to treat mild to moderate dementia. These drugs don't alter the progression of Alzheimer's disease, but may improve cognitive function in some patients. Improvement is typically subtle, but noticeable by caregivers. Because tacrine may produce significant adverse effects and requires monitoring, it isn't commonly prescribed for Alzheimer's disease.

Interactions

♦ Cholinesterase inhibitors can reduce the activity of anticholinergics.
♦ When combined with cholinesterase inhibitors, succinylcholine and other cholinergic agonists, such as bethanechol, may show increased effects.
♦ Together, cholinesterase inhibitors and amiodarone, beta blockers, calcium channels blockers, or digoxin may cause additive bradycardia.
♦ Drugs that inhibit CYP may increase the effects of donepezil, galantamine, or tacrine.

Teaching a patient about drugs for Alzheimer's disease

Whenever a drug is prescribed for Alzheimer's disease, teach the patient and his family the drug's name, dose, frequency, action, and adverse effects, and take the following actions.

✦ Advise the patient that memory improvement may be subtle and that a more likely result is a slower decline in memory loss. These drugs may enhance cognitive function but not alter the disease process.

✦ Advise the patient and caregiver that abrupt discontinuation or dosage reduction may cause reduced cognitive function and behavioral disturbances.

✦ Instruct the patient to report adverse reactions promptly.

✦ Tell the patient to alert other health care providers about this drug therapy before receiving anesthesia.

✦ Instruct the patient or his caregiver to report nausea, vomiting, and diarrhea.

✦ Advise the patient to take the drug with food and fluid to minimize adverse GI effects.

✦ Urge the patient to consult the prescriber before taking any over-the-counter preparations.

✦ Carbamazepine, dexamethasone, phenobarbital, phenytoin, and rifampin may decrease donepezil's effects.

✦ Smoking increases the clearance of rivastigmine.

Adverse reactions

Common adverse reactions include nausea, vomiting, diarrhea, dizziness, and headache. Less common ones are bradycardia, insomnia, confusion, and weakness. Tacrine may elevate the transaminase level.

Nursing considerations

✦ Teach the patient and his caregiver about the drug. (See *Teaching a patient about drugs for Alzheimer's disease.*)

✦ Use these drugs cautiously in patients who take NSAIDs or have cardiovascular disease, asthma, obstructive pulmonary disease, impaired urine outflow, renal disease, or a history of ulcer disease.

✦ Use tacrine cautiously in patients with hepatic disease.

✦ Monitor the patient for signs of GI bleeding because of increased gastric acid secretion.

✦ Monitor the patient for severe nausea, vomiting, and diarrhea, which may lead to dehydration and weight loss.

✦ Use proper technique when dispensing an oral galantamine solution with a pipette. Dispense the measured amount in a nonalcoholic beverage and administer it right away.

✦ Monitor the patient's ALT level weekly during the first 18 weeks of tacrine therapy. After 18 weeks, if the ALT level is elevated up to twice the upper limit of normal, continue weekly monitoring. If no problems are detected, monitor the ALT level every 3 months. Whenever the dosage is increased, resume weekly monitoring for at least 6 weeks.

✦ Advise the patient and family that dramatic memory improvement is unlikely. As the disease progresses, the benefits of drug therapy may decline.

Adverse reactions to watch for

✦ Bradycardia
✦ Confusion
✦ Diarrhea, nausea, vomiting
✦ Dizziness, headache
✦ Insomnia
✦ Weakness

Key nursing actions

✦ Watch for evidence of GI bleeding.
✦ Monitor the patient for severe nausea, vomiting, and diarrhea.
✦ Monitor the ALT level weekly for first 18 weeks of tacrine therapy.
✦ Explain that dramatic memory improvement isn't likely and that the drug's benefits may decline over time.

CLINICAL ALERT Don't confuse Aricept (donepezil) with Ascriptin, which is a nonopioid analgesic that contains aspirin, magnesium hydroxide, aluminum hydroxide, and calcium carbonate.

ANTIMIGRAINE DRUGS

An episodic headache disorder, migraine is one of the most common primary headache disorders, affecting about 24 million people in the United States. Typically, migraine produces unilateral headaches, with pounding, pulsating, or throbbing pain, that may be preceded by an aura. Other common symptoms of migraine are sensitivity to light or sound, nausea, vomiting, and constipation or diarrhea.

Migraine symptoms may result from cranial vasodilation or the release of vasoactive and proinflammatory substances from nerves in an activated trigeminal system. One class of antimigraine drugs, the 5-hydroxytriptamine (5-HT$_1$ or serotonin) agonists, constricts cranial vessels, inhibits neuropeptide release, and reduces transmission in the trigeminal pathway. These actions may abort a migraine or relieve its symptoms.

Migraine treatment may aim to alter attacks with abortive or symptomatic therapy or to prevent them with prophylactic therapy. The choice of therapy depends on the headache's severity, duration, frequency, and resulting degree of disability as well as the patient's characteristics. Abortive treatments may include analgesics (such as aspirin and acetaminophen), nonsteroidal anti-inflammatory drugs (NSAIDs), ergotamine, 5-HT$_1$ agonists, and such miscellaneous drugs as corticosteroids, intranasal butorphanol, isometheptene combinations, and metoclopramide. Prophylactic treatments include beta blockers, methysergide, NSAIDs, tricyclic antidepressants, and valproic acid.

5-HT$_1$ AGONISTS

Also known as *triptans*, 5-HT$_1$ agonists are the treatment of choice for moderate to severe migraine. This drug class includes almotriptan, eletriptan, frovatriptan, naratriptan, rizatriptan, sumatriptan, and zolmitriptan.

Pharmacokinetics

When comparing the 5-HT$_1$ agonists, key pharmacokinetic features are onset and duration of action. Most of these drugs have a half-life of about 2 hours. However, the half-life of almotriptan and eletriptan is 3 to 4 hours, of naratriptan is about 6 hours, and of frovatriptan is 25 hours. Frovatriptan's long half-life accounts for its delayed onset of action.

All of these drugs are available in standard oral forms. In addition, rizatriptan is available in disintegrating tablets; sumatriptan is available in injectable and intranasal forms. The injectable form of sumatriptan offers the fastest onset of action.

Pharmacodynamics

These drugs constrict cranial vessels, inhibit neuropeptide release, and reduce transmission in the trigeminal pain pathway. These actions may abort or provide symptomatic relief for a migraine. These drugs are effective in controlling the pain, nausea, and vomiting caused by migraine.

Contraindications for 5-HT₁ agonists

The 5-HT₁ agonists are contraindicated for patients with ischemic heart disease (such as angina pectoris, a history of myocardial infarction, or documented silent ischemia) and those with symptoms or findings consistent with ischemic heart disease, coronary artery vasospasm (including Prinzmetal's variant angina), or other significant underlying cardiovascular conditions. These drugs also shouldn't be prescribed for patients with cerebrovascular syndromes, such as stroke and transient ischemic attacks, or those with peripheral vascular disease, including ischemic bowel disease. In addition, they shouldn't be used in patients with uncontrolled hypertension or hemiplegic or basilar migraine.

Pharmacotherapeutics

These drugs are used to treat migraine headaches, not to prevent them. The choice of drug depends on patient preference for dosage form, presence of recurrent migraine, and use restrictions. A patient with nausea and vomiting may prefer to take injectable or intranasal sumatriptan. Recurrent migraine may respond better to a drug with a longer half-life, such as frovatriptan and naratriptan. Because a drug with a long half-life also has a delayed onset of action, the prescriber may compromise by ordering almotriptan or eletriptan, which have a rapid onset and an intermediate half-life.

The 5-HT₁ agonists aren't recommended for patients who have risk factors for unrecognized coronary artery disease (CAD) — such as hypertension, hypercholesterolemia, smoking, obesity, diabetes, strong family history of CAD, surgical or physiologic menopause in a woman, and age over 40 in a man — unless a cardiovascular evaluation demonstrates that the patient is reasonably free of underlying cardiovascular disease. If a 5-HT₁ agonist is used in such a patient, the first dose should be given in the prescriber's office or other medically staffed and equipped facility. Also, patients who use 5-HT₁ agonists intermittently for a long time and those who have or acquire risk factors should undergo periodic cardiovascular evaluation. Many conditions contraindicate the use of these drugs. (See *Contraindications for 5-HT₁ agonists.*)

Interactions

✦ Giving 5-HT₁ agonists within 24 hours of each other is contraindicated because of the increased risk of vasospastic reactions.
✦ Use of drugs containing ergotamine or ergot-type drugs (such as dihydroergotamine or methysergide) within 24 hours of 5-HT₁ agonist use may cause prolonged vasospastic reactions; combined use should be avoided.
✦ Eletriptan shouldn't be used within 72 hours of treatment with a CYP 3A4 inhibitor, such as clarithromycin, itraconazole, ketoconazole, nefazodone, nelfinavir, ritonavir, and troleandomycin because of the decreased eletriptan metabolism.
✦ Ketoconazole increases the almotriptan level.
✦ Almotriptan, rizatriptan, sumatriptan, and zolmitriptan shouldn't be used within 2 weeks of an MAO inhibitor because of the risk of a vasospastic reaction.
✦ Together, 5-HT₁ agonists and selective serotonin reuptake inhibitors (SSRIs), such as citalopram, fluoxetine, fluvoxamine, paroxetine, and sertraline, or sibu-

When not to use a 5-HT₁ agonist

✦ Patient has risk factors for coronary artery disease (unless examination shows little or no underlying cardiac disease).

Possible drug interactions

✦ Citalopram
✦ Clarithromycin
✦ Ergotamine or ergot-type drugs
✦ Fluoxetine
✦ Fluvoxamine
✦ Hormonal contraceptives
✦ Itraconazole
✦ Ketoconazole
✦ MAO inhibitors
✦ Nefazodone
✦ Nelfinavir
✦ Paroxetine
✦ Propranolol
✦ Ritonavir
✦ Sertraline
✦ Sibutramine
✦ Troleandomycin

Adverse reactions to watch for

✦ Acute MI, arrhythmias (may be fatal)
✦ Chest pain or pressure; neck, throat, or jaw pain or pressure
✦ Dizziness, fatigue, somnolence, weakness
✦ Dry mouth, dyspepsia, nausea
✦ Flushing, paresthesias, sweating, tingling, warm or hot sensations
✦ Injection site reactions (S.C. sumatriptan)
✦ Nose or throat discomfort, taste disturbance (intranasal sumatriptan)
✦ Vision disturbances

Key nursing actions

✦ Ask about risk factors for CAD.
✦ Give the drug only if the patient has a definitve diagnosis of migraine.
✦ Give the drug as soon as migraine symptoms appear.
✦ Keep in mind that safety information isn't available for treating more than four migraines in 30 days

tramine may cause weakness, hyperreflexia, and incoordination, requiring close patient monitoring if combined treatment is required.
✦ Hormonal contraceptives may increase frovatriptan's bioavailability.
✦ Propranolol may increase the bioavailability of eletriptan, frovatriptan, rizatriptan, and zolmitriptan.

Adverse reactions

The 5-HT₁ agonists may cause a wide range of adverse reactions. These include tingling; warm or hot sensations; flushing; nasal discomfort; vision disturbances; paresthesias; dizziness; fatigue; somnolence; chest pain or pressure; neck, throat, or jaw pain or pressure; weakness; dry mouth; dyspepsia; nausea; sweating; injection site reactions (with S.C. sumatriptan); and nasal or throat discomfort and taste disturbances (with intranasal sumatriptan).

Serious cardiac reactions, including acute MI, arrhythmias, and death have occurred a few hours after use. However, the risk of such reactions is extremely low.

Nursing considerations

✦ Assess the patient for conditions that contraindicate or require cautious drug use.
✦ Ask the patient about risk factors for CAD, such as hypertension, hypercholesterolemia, smoking, obesity, diabetes, strong family history of CAD, surgical or physiological menopause in a woman, and age over 40 in a man.
✦ Use these drugs only in a patient with a definitive diagnosis of migraine.
✦ Administer the drug as soon as migraine symptoms appear; 5-HT₁ agonists aren't for prophylactic use.
✦ Reduce the dose in a patient with renal or hepatic impairment.
✦ The safety of treating an average of more than three or four migraine attacks in a 30-day period hasn't been established.

CLINICAL ALERT When giving a 5-HT$_1$ agonist to a patient with risk factors for CAD, such as obesity, smoking, hypertension, and diabetes, but not a diagnosis, give the first dose in a facility or physician's office with medical personnel and emergency equipment present. Serious adverse cardiac reactions can occur.

◆ Teach the patient and his caregiver about the prescribed drug. (See *Teaching a patient about 5-HT$_1$-receptor agonists.*)

ERGOTAMINE PREPARATIONS

Ergotamine and its derivatives may be used as abortive or symptomatic therapy for migraine. Commonly used drugs in this class include: ergotamine, which is available as a sublingual or oral tablet or a rectal suppository combined with caffeine, and dihydroergotamine, which is available in injectable or intranasal forms.

Methysergide is a semisynthetic ergot derivative approved for the prophylaxis of vascular headaches, such as migraine. The drug has no vasoconstrictive properties, but acts as a potent 5-HT$_2$-receptor antagonist, possibly stabilizing neurotransmission in the trigeminal area and preventing neurogenic inflammation. Despite its effectiveness as a preventative, methysergide is rarely used because it can cause severe fibrotic changes in the retroperitoneal area, lungs, and cardiac valves.

Pharmacokinetics

In the GI tract, ergotamine absorption is incomplete and erratic. However, caffeine increases the absorption rate. After inhalation or I.M. injection, drug absorption is more complete. The liver metabolizes ergotamine; 90% of the metabolites are excreted in bile. The drug's half-life is about 2 hours, but the drug has lasting effects, possibly because of tissue storage.

Pharmacodynamics

For ergotamine preparations, antimigraine effects may result from blockade of neurogenic inflammation. These drugs also may act as partial agonists or antagonists at serotonin, dopaminergic, and alpha-adrenergic receptors. Ergotamine preparations usually need to be prescribed with antiemetics when used for migraine.

Dihydroergotamine, a hydrogenated form of ergotamine, differs mainly in its degree of activity. It's less vasoconstrictive than ergotamine and has a much lower chance of emesis.

Pharmacotherapeutics

Ergotamine preparations are used to prevent or treat vascular headaches, such as migraine, migraine variant, and cluster headache. Dihydroergotamine is used when rapid control of migraine is desired or when other oral or rectal routes are undesirable. However, these drugs must be avoided during pregnancy and breast-feeding. (See *Safety of ergotamine preparations for pregnant and breast-feeding patients*, page 116.)

Interactions

◆ Propranolol and other beta blockers block the vasodilation pathway in patients receiving these drugs, resulting in excessive vasoconstriction and cold arms and legs.

Features of ergotamine preparations

◆ May block neurogenic inflammation
◆ May act as partial agonists or antagonists at serotonin, dopaminergic, and alpha-adrenergic receptors
◆ Prevent or treat vascular headaches (migraine, migraine variant, cluster headaches)
◆ Ergotamine usually used with an antiemetic
◆ Dihydroergotamine is used for rapid control or when oral or rectal routes are undesirable and is less vasoconstrictive and emetic than ergotamine.

Possible drug interactions

- Beta blockers such as propranolol
- Drugs that inhibit CYP 3A4
- SSRIs
- Sumatriptan
- Vasoconstrictors

Adverse reactions to watch for

- Abdominal pain, diarrhea, heartburn, nausea, vomiting
- Bradycardia, localized edema, precordial pain, tachycardia
- Itching, leg weakness, muscle pain, numbness and tingling of fingers and toes
- Ergotism, gangrene, rebound headaches (with prolonged use)

✦ Use with SSRIs may increase the risk of weakness, hyperflexion, and incoordination.

✦ Sumatriptan and ergotamine preparations may cause additive effects, increasing the risk of coronary vasospasm and prohibiting the use of these drugs within 24 hours of each other.

✦ Vasoconstrictors and ergotamine preparations may cause additive effects, increasing the risk of high blood pressure.

✦ CYP 3A4 enzyme inhibitors, such as azole-derivative antifungals, clarithromycin, erythromycin, indinavir, nelfinavir, ritonavir, and troleandomycin, may alter ergotamine metabolism, increasing the serum ergotamine level and the risk of vasospasm and cerebral or peripheral ischemia. These drugs shouldn't be used together.

Adverse reactions

Adverse GI reactions include nausea, vomiting, diarrhea, heartburn, and abdominal pain. A gradual dosage increase and administration with food may help minimize these reactions. More serious adverse reactions include numbness and tingling of the fingers and toes, precordial pain, localized edema, tachycardia, bradycardia, muscle pain, leg weakness, and itching.

Smoking or other nicotine use can contribute to peripheral vasoconstriction, increasing the risk of peripheral ischemia, especially in patients who take methysergide. (See *Recognizing methysergide-induced ischemia*.) That's why these patients should avoid smoking.

PATIENT TEACHING

Teaching a patient about ergotamine preparations

Whenever an ergotamine preparation is prescribed, teach the patient and his family the drug's name, dose, frequency, action, and adverse effects, and take the following actions.
◆ Tell the patient to begin therapy at the first sign of an attack and not to exceed the recommended dosage.
◆ Instruct the patient to lie down and relax in a quiet, low-light environment after taking the drug.
◆ Tell the patient to notify the prescriber if he experiences irregular heart beat, nausea, vomiting, numbness or tingling in the fingers or toes, or pain or weakness in the arms or legs.
◆ Advise the patient to notify the prescriber if she becomes pregnant or plans to become pregnant.

Prolonged administration of ergotamine preparations may result in ergotism, gangrene, and rebound headaches.

Nursing considerations

◆ Assess the patient for contraindications, including coronary, cerebral, or peripheral vascular disease; hypertension; sepsis; malnutrition; severe pruritus; and liver or kidney disease.
◆ For maximum effectiveness, give the drug at the first sign of a migraine headache or soon after it begins.
◆ Avoid prolonged use and don't exceed the recommended dosage.
◆ Patients who take the drug over an extended period of time may become dependent on it and require progressively increasing doses to relieve migraine headaches and prevent the dysphoric effects that follow withdrawal.
◆ Teach the patient and his caregiver about the prescribed drug. (See *Teaching a patient about ergotamine preparations*.)

Key nursing actions
◆ Give the drug as soon as possible after the first sign of migraine headache.
◆ Avoid prolonged use; don't exceed the recommended dosage.
◆ Give increased doses over time if needed to relieve migraines and prevent dysphoric effects that follow withdrawal.

Analgesics

A nalgesics are drugs that relieve pain. These drugs range from mild, over-the-counter (OTC) preparations, such as acetaminophen, to potent general anesthetics. Types of analgesics include non-opioid analgesics, antipyretics, and non-steroidal anti-inflammatory drugs (NSAIDs), opioid agonist and antagonist drugs, and anesthetics.

To understand how these drugs achieve their effects, you need to be familiar with nervous system anatomy and the physiology of pain.

ANATOMY AND PHYSIOLOGY

A basic protective mechanism, pain is a symptom of an underlying physiologic or psychological problem. Pain usually indicates that something is wrong and that medical care is needed.

Because pain is subjective, only the patient can describe it. Pain is whatever sensation the patient perceives it to be; one person's pain perception may vary widely from another's. Emotional states and ethnic, cultural, and religious factors all contribute to the patient's pain perception.

PAIN DETECTION AND TRANSMISSION

Pain sensation begins in the nociceptors, which are part of afferent neurons. Nociceptors are free nerve endings located primarily in the skin, periosteum, joint surfaces, and arterial walls. They may be activated by mechanical, chemical, or thermal stimuli. They also may be activated by chemical mediators, such as prostaglandins, histamine, bradykinin, and serotonin, which are released or synthesized in response to tissue damage. Even minor tissue damage can trigger the synthesis of chemical mediators—and stimulation of nociceptors. Once the pain process is initiated, the impulse is communicated from the nociceptors' peripheral terminals to the spinal cord. (See *Understanding pain pathways*.)

ANATOMY & PHYSIOLOGY

Understanding pain pathways

When stimulated, A-delta fiber and C fiber nociceptors transmit an afferent impulse through the dorsal root ganglia to the dorsal horn. Peripheral nerves also transmit information to the dorsal horn. The dorsal horn then controls this information and may transmit an impulse via the spinothalamic tract to the cerebral cortex. Descending pathways carry inhibitory information from the brain to the dorsal horn to be used by the peripheral nervous system.

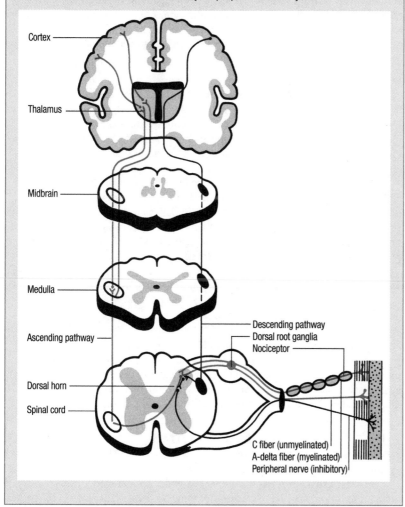

Somatostatin, cholecystokinin, and substance P may act as neurotransmitters in the afferent neurons. Analgesics may block the effects of any of those neurotransmitters. The two types of nociceptors are the myelinated A-delta fibers and the smaller, unmyelinated, more numerous C fibers. The faster-conducting A-delta fibers signal sharp, well-localized pain; the slower-conducting C fibers signal dull, poorly localized pain.

All nociceptors terminate in the dorsal horn of the spinal cord. The dorsal horn is the control center for incoming information from the afferent neurons, pain impulse regulation, and descending influences from higher centers in the central nervous system (CNS), such as emotion, attention, and memory.

PAIN THEORY

The Melzack-Wall gate-control theory, the most widely accepted pain theory, states that neural mechanisms in the dorsal horn act as regulators between the peripheral fibers and the higher processing centers in the CNS. The dorsal horn receives pain and other signals from various peripheral nerves; pain messages depend on the total information. This process, called the gating effect, regulates afferent input before an impulse is sent to the CNS and pain is perceived. Therefore, pain perception may be inhibited by the simultaneous activation of sensory neurons carrying non-pain information.

INFLAMMATION AND FEVER

Pain may occur alone or with inflammation. Both are reactions to tissue irritation. Inflammation is a process mediated by the immune system and characterized by redness, heat, swelling, loss of function, and pain at the site. Some chemical mediators of pain, including prostaglandins, bradykinin, and histamine, also mediate the inflammatory response.

The hypothalamus regulates body temperature by balancing heat production and loss. Pyrogens, secreted by toxic bacteria or released from protein breakdown, can cause the hypothalamic thermostat to rise. This in turn increases body temperature. Pyrogens may also increase body temperature by causing production of prostaglandin E_1 in the hypothalamus. Some drugs used to control pain inhibit prostaglandins and produce an antipyretic effect.

NON-OPIOID ANALGESICS, ANTIPYRETICS, AND NSAIDS

Non-opioid analgesics, antipyretics, and NSAIDs represent a broad group of analgesics. They're discussed together because, in addition to pain control, they also produce antipyretic and anti-inflammatory effects. The drug classes in this group include salicylates (especially aspirin), the para-aminophenol derivative acetaminophen, NSAIDs, and cyclooxygenase-2 (COX-2) inhibitors.

SALICYLATES

Salicylates are among the most commonly used analgesics. They're used regularly to control pain and reduce fever and inflammation.

Salicylates usually cost less than other analgesics and are readily available without a prescription. Aspirin, the most commonly used salicylate, remains the cornerstone of anti-inflammatory drug therapy. Other common salicylates include choline magnesium trisalicylate, choline salicylate, diflunisal, salsalate, and sodium salicylate.

Pharmacokinetics

When given orally, salicylates are absorbed partly in the stomach, but primarily in the upper part of the small intestine. The pure and buffered forms of aspirin are

---

Evidence of inflammation

+ Redness
+ Heat
+ Swelling
+ Loss of function
+ Localized pain

Features of salicylates

+ Are commonly used, especially aspirin
+ Are usually inexpensive
+ Are available over the counter
+ Reduce pain, fever, inflammation
+ Inhibit prostaglandin synthesis to reduce pain and inflammation
+ Stimulate the hypothalamus to reduce fever
+ Don't relieve visceral pain or severe pain from trauma
+ Reduce the risk and severity of MI via effects on platelets

Contraindications and precautions for salicylates

Salicylates are contraindicated in patients who are hypersensitive to nonsteroidal anti-inflammatory drugs and those with glucose-6-phosphate dehydrogenase deficiency or bleeding disorders, such as hemophilia, von Willebrand's disease, telangiectasia, bleeding ulcers, and hemorrhagic states. In addition, magnesium salicylate is contraindicated in patients with advanced chronic renal insufficiency.

All salicylates should be used cautiously in patients with GI lesions, impaired renal function, hypoprothrombinemia, vitamin-K deficiency, thrombocytopenia, severe hepatic impairment, or thrombotic thrombocytopenic purpura (TTP).

absorbed readily; sustained-release and enteric-coated salicylate preparations or food or antacids in the stomach delay absorption. When given rectally, salicylates have a slower, more erratic absorption.

Salicylates are distributed widely throughout body tissues and fluids, including breast milk. In addition, they easily cross the placenta.

The liver metabolizes salicylates extensively into several metabolites. The kidneys excrete the metabolites and some unchanged drug.

Pharmacodynamics

The different effects of salicylates stem from their separate mechanisms of action. They relieve pain primarily by inhibiting the synthesis of prostaglandin (a chemical mediator that sensitizes nerve cells to pain). They also may reduce inflammation by inhibiting prostaglandin synthesis and release during inflammation.

Salicylates reduce fever by stimulating the hypothalamus, dilating the peripheral blood vessels and increased sweating. This promotes heat loss through the skin and cooling by evaporation. Also, because prostaglandin E increases body temperature, inhibiting its production lowers a fever.

One salicylate, aspirin, inhibits platelet aggregation by interfering with the production of thromboxane A_2, a substance needed for platelet aggregation. Aspirin interferes with platelet aggregation for the entire 7 to 10 days of the platelet's life. NSAIDs' effect on platelet aggregation is reversible.

Pharmacotherapeutics

Salicylates are used primarily to relieve pain. However, they don't effectively relieve visceral pain or severe pain from trauma. (See *Contraindications and precautions for salicylates,* page 122.)

These drugs won't reduce a normal body temperature, but they can reduce a fever and can relieve headache and muscle ache at the same time.

When used to reduce inflammation in rheumatic fever, rheumatoid arthritis, or osteoarthritis, salicylates can provide considerable relief in 24 hours.

Because of its effects on platelets, aspirin can be used to enhance blood flow during a myocardial infarction (MI). It's also used to reduce the risk of death or nonfatal MI in patients with previous infarction or unstable angina and to reduce the risk of recurrent transient ischemic attacks or strokes in men.

Avoiding Reye's syndrome

In a child with varicella or flulike symptoms, salicylates may lead to Reye's syndrome, a life-threatening disorder that causes encephalopathy and fatty infiltration of internal organs. Although a direct causal relationship hasn't been established, discourage salicylate use in children and adolescents with varicella or influenza to avoid Reye's syndrome.

No matter what the indication, the main guideline of salicylate therapy is to use the lowest dose that provides relief. This reduces the likelihood of adverse reactions. Even so, salicylates should be used with caution.

Interactions

Because salicylates are highly protein bound, they can interact with many other protein-bound drugs, displacing them from sites to which they normally bind. This raises the level of the unbound drug, increasing its pharmacologic effects.

♦ When taken with a salicylate, heparin, insulin, methotrexate, oral anticoagulants, and oral antidiabetics may have increased effects or risks of toxicity.

♦ When taken with a salicylate, probenecid, spironolactone, and sulfinpyrazone may have decreased effects.

♦ Corticosteroids may decrease the serum salicylate level and increase the risk of ulcers.

♦ Alkalinizing drugs and antacids may reduce the salicylate level.

♦ When combined with a salicylate, angiotensin-converting enzyme (ACE) inhibitors and beta blockers may display reduced antihypertensive effects.

♦ When taken with a salicylate, NSAIDs may have reduced therapeutic effects and an increased risk of adverse GI effects.

♦ Herbal products that contain dong quai, feverfew, ginkgo, horse chestnut, kelpware, or red clover may increase the risk of bleeding related to salicylate use.

♦ White willow may increase the salicylate's adverse effects.

♦ Caffeine may increase aspirin absorption.

♦ Alcohol may increase the risk of GI bleeding related to salicylate use.

Possible drug interactions

♦ ACE inhibitors
♦ Alkalinizing drugs
♦ Antacids
♦ Beta blockers
♦ Corticosteroids
♦ Heparin
♦ Insulin
♦ Methotrexate
♦ NSAIDs
♦ Oral anticoagulants
♦ Oral antidiabetics
♦ Probenecid
♦ Spironolactone
♦ Sulfinpyrazone

Using salicylates effectively with antacids

Many patients take salicylates with an antacid to reduce the risk of GI distress. Although a single antacid dose probably won't affect the salicylate significantly, long-term use of an antacid may reduce the salicylate's effectiveness. Because antacids can increase urine pH, they can reduce renal reabsorption of a salicylate and increase its clearance.

For a patient who has been stabilized on a high dose of salicylate, monitor salicylate level and adjust salicylate dosage when antacid therapy begins or ends.

LIFESPAN

Using salicylates during pregnancy

Because salicylates may be teratogens, they shouldn't be used during pregnancy, especially in the third trimester. In the mother, aspirin may produce such adverse reactions as anemia, hemorrhage, and prolonged gestation and labor. In the infant, maternal aspirin use in the third trimester may cause low birth weight, increased risk of intracranial hemorrhage in a premature infant, stillbirth, or neonatal death. All salicylates cross the placenta; by inhibiting prostaglandin synthesis, they may constrict the ductus arteriosis and lead to other adverse fetal effects.

Adverse reactions

The most common adverse reactions to salicylates involve the GI tract. Other reactions may include respiratory alkalosis, metabolic acidosis, hearing problems, salicylate toxicity, hypersensitivity reactions, and Reye's syndrome. (See *Avoiding Reye's syndrome.*)

Gastric distress, nausea, and vomiting commonly result from the central action of the salicylates on the emetic center of the medulla and their local action on gastric secretions that protect the stomach from gastric acid. GI irritation may be minimized if the patient takes the drug with food, an antacid, or 8 ounces (240 ml) of water or milk, or if the preparation is enteric-coated, extended-release, or an oral solution. (See *Using salicylates effectively with antacids.*)

Large or toxic salicylate doses can cause respiratory alkalosis and increase the rate and depth of respiration. If the respiratory problem isn't corrected, metabolic acidosis can occur as the body tries to compensate for the respiratory alkalosis.

In some patients, prolonged use of salicylates causes bilateral hearing loss of 20 to 40 decibels that usually resolves within 24 to 72 hours after therapy is discontinued. Tinnitus may occur with dosages needed to treat inflammatory conditions and when the salicylate level is 200 to 300 mcg/ml. A geriatric patient or a patient with impaired hearing (who may not notice tinnitus until it's severe) should be monitored closely.

Adverse hematologic reactions include prolonged bleeding time, leukopenia, thrombocytopenia, purpura, decreased iron concentration, and shortened erythrocyte survival time.

Mild salicylate toxicity, or salicylism, characteristically causes nausea, vomiting, diarrhea, diaphoresis, difficulty hearing, tinnitus, confusion, dizziness, CNS depression, headache, lethargy, and hyperventilation. Indications of severe toxicity include respiratory alkalosis, metabolic acidosis and related acid-base imbalances, nausea, vomiting, hypokalemia, hemorrhagic tendencies, hypoglycemia, restlessness, irritability, incoherent speech, apprehension, delirium, hallucinations, seizures, dehydration, and hyperthermia.

Common hypersensitivity reactions to salicylates include rash and, in asthmatics with nasal polyps, bronchospasm and asthma. Anaphylaxis rarely occurs.

Nursing considerations

✦ Don't give aspirin to a patient in her third trimester of pregnancy. If she ingests aspirin or an aspirin-containing product up to 2 weeks before delivery, observe neonate for bleeding. (See *Using salicylates during pregnancy.*)

Adverse reactions to watch for

✦ Decreased iron level, shortened erythrocyte lifespan
✦ Gastric distress, nausea, vomiting
✦ Hearing loss, tinnitus
✦ Prolonged bleeding time, leukopenia, thrombocytopenia, purpura
✦ Respiratory alkalosis, increased rate and depth of respiration, metabolic acidosis

Evidence of salicylate toxicity

Mild toxicity
✦ CNS depression, confusion, dizziness
✦ Diaphoresis
✦ Diarrhea, nausea, vomiting
✦ Difficulty hearing, tinnitus
✦ Headache
✦ Hyperventilation
✦ Lethargy

Severe toxicity
✦ Acid-base imbalances (respiratory alkalosis, metabolic acidosis, others)
✦ Dehydration
✦ Nausea, vomiting
✦ Hemorrhagic tendency
✦ Hyperthermia
✦ Hypoglycemia
✦ Hypokalemia
✦ Restlessness, irritability, incoherent speech, apprehension, delirium, hallucinations
✦ Seizures

Teaching a patient about salicylates

Whenever a salicylate is prescribed, teach the patient and his family the drug's name, dose, frequency, action, and adverse effects, and take the following actions.

✦ Discourage the use of salicylates — even children's aspirin — in a child younger than age 18.

✦ Advise an aspirin-sensitive patient to read labels carefully on over-the-counter drugs because many contain aspirin or another salicylate.

✦ Teach the patient to watch for such signs as gum bleeding, prolonged bleeding from a cut, black or tarry stools, dark urine (which may indicate blood in the urine), petechiae, and bruises. Advise the patient to report these signs to the prescriber immediately.

✦ Instruct the patient to keep the salicylate in a cool, dry place because exposure to heat and moisture will weaken its potency.

✦ Advise the patient to discard tablets with a vinegary odor — a sign of salicylate deterioration.

✦ Suggest that the patient take aspirin with food or milk to prevent GI distress.

✦ Advise the patient not to crush or chew sodium salicylate tablets or take them within 1 hour of ingesting milk or antacids, which may disrupt the enteric coating.

✦ Advise the patient not to crush or chew diflunisal tablets. Expect to give a smaller diflunisal dosage to a patient with renal failure.

✦ Inform the patient that use of alcohol with a salicylate increases the risk of bleeding.

✦ Caution a pregnant woman to consult her prescriber before considering salicylate use.

✦ Advise the asthmatic patient with nasal polyps to avoid using salicylates when self-medicating for minor aches and pains because these drugs may induce an acute asthma attack.

✦ Advise a patient with hypertension or on a sodium-restricted diet not to use effervescent aspirin products, which have a lot of sodium.

✦ Instruct the patient to notify the prescriber of hearing changes or other adverse reactions to the salicylate.

Key nursing actions

✦ Closely monitor a patient who has asthma and nasal polyps.

✦ Don't give aspirin to a patient in her third trimester of pregnancy.

✦ Monitor the salicylate level.

✦ Stop aspirin 1 week before major surgery.

✦ Assess for pain relief.

 CLINICAL ALERT Closely monitor a patient who has asthma and nasal polyps. Such a patient is particularly vulnerable to acute asthmatic attack and bronchospasm, usually 15 to 30 minutes after salicylate ingestion.

✦ Teach the patient and his caregiver about the prescribed drug. (See *Teaching a patient about salicylates.*)

✦ Don't give diflunisal to reduce fever.

✦ Question any prescription for sodium salicylate in a patient with hypertension or sodium restriction.

✦ Observe the patient frequently for adverse reactions. Dehydrated children and febrile or geriatric patients may be more susceptible to these reactions.

✦ Monitor the patient's salicylate level. With long-term therapy, severe toxic effects may occur if the level exceeds 400 mcg/ml.

✦ Check the diflunisal dose carefully before administration. Small dosage changes may cause large changes in the drug level, leading to toxicity.

✦ Give with at least 8 ounces (240 ml) of liquid, unless contraindicated.

✦ Don't check the diabetic patient's urine for glucose with Diastix, Chemstrip uG, Clinitest, and Benedict's solution. These tests may provide incorrect results during salicylate therapy.

✦ Discontinue aspirin 1 week before major surgery to reduce the risk of bleeding.

✦ Monitor the patient for pain relief during therapy. If pain relief doesn't occur, notify the prescriber. Concomitant use of certain drugs, such as corticosteroids and antacids, may decrease the salicylate's analgesic effects.

ACETAMINOPHEN

Although the class of para-aminophenol derivatives includes two drugs—acetaminophen and phenacetin—only acetaminophen is available in the United States. Acetaminophen is an OTC drug that produces analgesic and antipyretic effects. It appears in many products designed to relieve pain and symptoms of colds and influenza.

Pharmacokinetics

Acetaminophen is absorbed rapidly and completely from the GI tract. It's also absorbed well from the mucous membranes of the rectum.

The drug is distributed widely in body fluids and readily crosses the placenta. After the liver metabolizes acetaminophen, the kidneys excrete it. Small amounts also appear in breast milk.

Pharmacodynamics

Acetaminophen reduces pain and fever, but unlike salicylates, it doesn't affect inflammation or platelet function.

The pain-control effects of acetaminophen aren't well understood. It may work in the CNS by inhibiting prostaglandin synthesis and in the peripheral nervous system in some unknown way. It reduces fever by acting directly on the heat-regulating center in the hypothalamus.

Pharmacotherapeutics

Acetaminophen is used to reduce fever and relieve headache, muscle ache, and general pain. It's the drug of choice to treat fever and flulike symptoms in children. Acetaminophen also is an effective pain reliever for some types of arthritis.

Interactions

✦ Acetaminophen may slightly increase the effects of oral anticoagulants and thrombolytics.
✦ When acetaminophen is combined with long-term alcohol use or with barbiturates, carbamazepine, isoniazid, or phenytoin, the risk of liver toxicity increases.
✦ Acetaminophen may reduce the effects of lamotrigine, loop diuretics, and zidovudine.
✦ Watercress may inhibit oxidative metabolism of acetaminophen.
✦ Caffeine may enhance acetaminophen's analgesic effects. Products may combine caffeine and acetaminophen for therapeutic advantage.

Adverse reactions

Most patients tolerate acetaminophen well. Unlike the salicylates, acetaminophen rarely causes gastric irritation or hemorrhagic tendencies.

Similar to an overdose, long-term use of high doses of acetaminophen can cause hypoglycemia, methemoglobinemia, leukopenia, neutropenia, pancytopenia, thrombocytopenia, hemolytic anemia, kidney damage, renal failure, hepatotoxicity leading to coagulation defects, cyanosis, and vascular collapse.

Hypersensitivity reactions to acetaminophen usually take the form of rashes, but rarely may include fever and angioedema. Such reactions are much less common with acetaminophen than with aspirin.

Features of acetaminophen

✦ Appears in many pain, cold, and flu relievers
✦ Reduces pain and fever, but has no effect on inflammation or platelet function
✦ May control pain by reducing peripheral prostaglandin synthesis
✦ Reduces fever by acting directly on the heat-regulating center in the hypothalamus
✦ Is used for fever, headache, muscle aches, general pain, some types of arthritis
✦ Is the drug of choice for fever and flulike symptoms in children

Possible drug interactions

✦ Barbiturates
✦ Carbamazepine
✦ Isoniazid
✦ Lamotrigine
✦ Long-term alcohol use
✦ Loop diuretics
✦ Oral anticoagulants
✦ Phenytoin
✦ Thrombolytics
✦ Zidovudine

Adverse reactions to watch for

✦ Cyanosis, vascular collapse
✦ Hemolytic anemia, leukopenia, methemoglobinemia, neutropenia, pancytopenia, thrombocytopenia
✦ Hepatotoxicity leading to coagulation defects
✦ Hypersensitivity reactions (usually rash, rarely fever and angioedema
✦ Hypoglycemia
✦ Kidney damage, renal failure

Teaching a patient about acetaminophen

Whenever acetaminophen is prescribed, teach the patient and his family the drug's name, dose, frequency, action, and adverse effects, and take the following actions.
+ Tell the parents to consult the prescriber before giving acetaminophen to a child younger than age 2.
+ Advise the patient that acetaminophen is for short-term use and that he should consult the prescriber before using the drug for more than 10 days in an adult or for more than 5 days in a child.
+ Tell the patient not to use acetaminophen to control a fever above 103.1° F (39.5° C), a fever persisting longer than 3 days, or a recurrent fever unless directed by the prescriber.
+ Warn the patient that high doses or unsupervised long-term use of acetaminophen can cause liver damage. Excessive alcohol use may increase the risk of liver damage. Caution an alcoholic patient to limit his acetaminophen intake to no more than 2 grams per day.
+ Tell a breast-feeding patient that less than 1% of a dose of acetaminophen appears in breast milk. If drug therapy is short and doesn't exceed the recommended dose, she may use acetaminophen safely while breast-feeding.

Key nursing actions

+ Check for acetaminophen in all OTC products the patient takes; include all sources when calculating the patient's total consumption.
+ Don't exceed five doses in 24 hours for a child.

Features of nonsteroidal anti-inflammatory drugs

+ Reduce prostaglandin synthesis by inhibiting COX enzyme
+ Relieves pain and inflammation via COX-2 inhibition; may cause adverse GI effects via COX-1 inhibition
+ Are used mainly for inflammation, secondarily to reduce pain
+ Are used to reduce fever in children (ibuprofen only)
+ Treat ankylosing spondylitis, rheumatoid arthritis, osteoarthritis, acute gouty arthritis, mild to moderate pain, dysmenorrhea, tendinitis, bursitis, migraine

Nursing considerations

+ Use the drug cautiously in patients with a history of long-term alcohol use because hepatotoxicity can occur even with therapeutic doses.
+ Many OTC products contain acetaminophen. Be sure to include their acetaminophen content when calculating the patient's total daily dose.
+ Use a liquid form of acetaminophen for a child or another patient who has difficulty swallowing.
+ Don't exceed five doses in 24 hours for a child.
+ Teach the patient and his caregiver about the drug. (See *Teaching a patient about acetaminophen.*)

NONSTEROIDAL ANTI-INFLAMMATORY DRUGS

With an anti-inflammatory action equal to that of aspirin, NSAIDs typically are used to combat inflammation. They also have analgesic and antipyretic effects. However, they're seldom prescribed for fever, except for ibuprofen, which is used in children.

Drugs in this class include diclofenac, etodolac, indomethacin, ibuprofen, ketoprofen, ketorolac, meloxicam, nabumetone, naproxen, oxaprozin, piroxicam, and sulindac.

Pharmacokinetics

All NSAIDs are absorbed in the GI tract. They're mostly metabolized in the liver and excreted primarily by the kidneys.

Pharmacodynamics

Researchers believe that NSAIDs produce their effects by inhibiting prostaglandin synthesis. NSAIDs inhibit cyclooxygenase (COX), the enzyme that catalyzes the conversion of arachidonic acid to prostaglandins. Two COX isoenzymes have been identified. COX-1 is needed for homeostatic maintenance, such as platelet aggregation, regulation of blood flow in the kidneys and stomach, and regulation of gastric acid secretion. COX-2 is induced by pain and inflammatory stimuli. NSAIDs inhibit both isoenzymes. COX-1 inhibition may be responsible for the drugs' GI toxicity. COX-2 inhibition alleviates pain and inflammation.

Pharmacotherapeutics

Primarily, NSAIDs are used to decrease inflammation. Secondarily, they're used to relieve pain. Although they're seldom prescribed to reduce fever, ibuprofen is used for this purpose in children. Many conditions respond favorably to NSAIDs, including ankylosing spondylitis, moderate to severe rheumatoid arthritis, osteoarthritis accompanied by inflammation; acute gouty arthritis, mild to moderate pain, dysmenorrhea, tendinitis, bursitis, migraines, and osteoarthritis in the hip, shoulder, or other large joints.

Interactions

Because they're highly protein bound, NSAIDs are likely to interact with other protein-bound drugs, such as oral anticoagulants, prednisolone, salicylates, and tolbutamide.

✦ Cholestyramine and salicylates may decrease an NSAID's therapeutic effects.
✦ Salicylates may increase the risk of serious adverse reactions to ketorolac; they shouldn't be used together.
✦ Colestipol and sucralfate may decrease diclofenac's effects.
✦ Diflunisal may significantly increase the indomethacin level.
✦ Phenobarbital may decrease fenoprofen's half-life.
✦ Probenecid may increase NSAID toxicity; it shouldn't be used with ketorolac.
✦ Ritonavir may increase the risk of piroxicam toxicity.
✦ NSAIDs may decrease the therapeutic effects of ACE inhibitors, beta blockers, and diuretics.
✦ When used with anticoagulants, NSAIDs may increase the prothrombin time (PT) and international normalization ratio (INR).
✦ Use of cyclosporine with an NSAID may increase the nephrotoxicity of both drugs.
✦ Use of ibuprofen or indomethacin with digoxin may increase digoxin level.
✦ Combined use with an NSAID may lead to hydantoin, lithium, or methotrexate toxicity.
✦ Use of an NSAID with dong quai, feverfew, garlic, ginger, ginkgo biloba, horse chestnut, or red clover may increase the risk of bleeding.
✦ An NSAID's interactions with white willow are similar to its interactions with aspirin because the body converts the salicin in the herb to salicylic acid.
✦ Alcohol use during NSAID therapy may increase the risk of adverse GI reactions.

Adverse reactions

All NSAIDs produce similar adverse reactions that rarely require discontinuation of therapy. In general, NSAIDs are better tolerated than salicylates or corticosteroids.

GI disturbances are the most common adverse reactions to NSAIDs. Common GI reactions include nausea, vomiting, diarrhea, abdominal pain, dyspepsia, flatulence, ulcer, and GI bleeding. Elevated liver enzyme levels and hepatotoxicity may occur. (See *Detecting NSAID-induced GI toxicity*, page 128.)

Other reactions affect the CNS, renal system, and eyes. Adverse CNS and renal reactions are particularly common in geriatric patients. In the CNS, NSAID use may result in dizziness, headache, somnolence, nervousness, asthenia, malaise, and

Possible drug interactions

✦ ACE inhibitors
✦ Anticoagulants
✦ Beta blockers
✦ Cholestyramine
✦ Colestipol
✦ Cyclosporine
✦ Diflunisal
✦ Digoxin
✦ Diuretics
✦ Hydantoin
✦ Lithium
✦ Methotrexate
✦ Oral anticoagulants
✦ Phenobarbital
✦ Prednisolone
✦ Probenecid
✦ Ritonavir
✦ Salicylates
✦ Sucralfate
✦ Tolbutamide

Detecting NSAID-induced GI toxicity

In any patient taking a nonsteroidal anti-inflammatory drug (NSAID), be alert for signs and symptoms of GI toxicity, which can cause inflammation, bleeding, ulceration, and perforation of the stomach or intestines. This adverse reaction can occur at any time—with or without warning—during long-term NSAID therapy.

To detect it, assess the patient for minor upper GI problems, such as dyspepsia, which are common and usually occur early in NSAID therapy. Also, stay alert for signs and symptoms of ulceration and bleeding, such as pain or dark, tarry stools, even in patients who didn't display early, minor problems. Often, a patient who experiences a serious adverse GI reaction won't exhibit earlier symptoms.

Adverse reactions to watch for

✦ Abdominal pain, diarrhea, dyspepsia, flatulence, GI bleeding, nausea, ulcer, vomiting
✦ Anemia, decreased hemoglobin and hematocrit, ecchymosis, hemolysis, leukopenia, thrombocytopenia
✦ Asthenia, dizziness, headache, malaise, nervousness, seizures, somnolence
✦ Asthma, bronchospasm, dyspnea, pharyngitis, rhinitis
✦ Blurred or reduced vision, change in color vision, corneal deposits, retinal disturbances
✦ Bullous eruption, erythema multiforme, exfoliative dermatitis, Stevens-Johnson syndrome
✦ Dysuria, hyperkalemia, hyponatremia, increased BUN and creatinine levels, renal insufficiency, renal failure, urinary frequency, UTI
✦ Elevated liver enzyme levels, hepatotoxicity
✦ Fluid retention, hypertension, pedal edema
✦ Hypersensitivity reactions with rash, urticaria, angioedema, hypotension, dyspnea, asthmalike syndrome

seizures. In the renal system, hyperkalemia, hyponatremia, urinary tract infection (UTI), increased blood urea nitrogen (BUN) and creatinine levels, dysuria, urinary frequency, renal insufficiency, and renal failure may occur. In the eyes, vision may be blurred or diminished. The patient may experience a change in color vision, corneal deposits, and retinal disturbances. That's why routine ophthalmologic examinations are needed.

Adverse cardiovascular effects include hypertension, fluid retention, and pedal edema. Dyspnea, pharyngitis, rhinitis, asthma, and bronchospasm may occur. Asthmatics who are hypersensitive to aspirin shouldn't take NSAIDs.

Decreased hemoglobin and hematocrit, hemolysis, ecchymosis, anemia, leukopenia, and thrombocytopenia may occur with NSAID use and require hematologic monitoring during long-term therapy.

NSAIDs can cause hypersensitivity reactions, evidenced by rashes, urticaria, angioedema, hypotension, dyspnea, and asthmalike syndrome. Photosensitivity may occur, requiring patients to take protective measures. Stevens-Johnson syndrome, bullous eruption, erythema multiforme, and exfoliative dermatitis have occurred with NSAID use. With any NSAID, therapy should be stopped at the first sign of a hypersensitivity reaction.

Nursing considerations
✦ Ask the patient if he has had a hypersensitivity reaction, such as asthma, urticaria, or other allergic-type reactions, after taking aspirin or another NSAID.
✦ Stop therapy and notify the prescriber at the first sign of a hypersensitivity reaction to the drug.
✦ Monitor the patient's vision. If an alteration or problem develops, withhold the drug until an ophthalmic examination rules out drug therapy as the cause.
✦ Give NSAIDs with food or milk to decrease GI irritation.
✦ Monitor the patient with a history of peptic ulcer for ulcer reactivation and gastric bleeding during NSAID therapy.
✦ Monitor the patient for signs of GI irritation, such as nausea, vomiting, abdominal pain, and black, tarry stools. Notify the prescriber immediately if the patient displays signs of GI irritation.
✦ Monitor the patient's hepatic, hematologic, and renal function studies.
✦ Monitor the patient for signs of infection. Keep in mind that NSAIDs may mask infection.

Teaching a patient about NSAIDs

Whenever a nonsteroidal anti-inflammatory drug (NSAID) is prescribed, teach the patient and his family the drug's name, dose, frequency, action, and adverse effects, and take the following actions.

✦ Stress the importance of returning periodically for blood tests.
✦ Advise the patient to avoid driving or operating machinery until the effects are known because drowsiness and dizziness commonly occur at the beginning of therapy.
✦ Advise the patient that some NSAIDs, such as ibuprofen, fenoprofen, and naproxen, may take several weeks to produce their maximum therapeutic effect.
✦ Instruct the patient to take the drug with milk or food to decrease GI irritation, unless directed otherwise.
✦ Advise the patient with aspirin hypersensitivity to avoid NSAIDs.
✦ Instruct the patient who self-medicates to discontinue the drug and consult his prescriber if pain lasts longer than 72 hours.
✦ Advise the patient to avoid alcohol, aspirin, and other drugs that may cause GI irritation and bleeding.
✦ Instruct the patient taking an oral anticoagulant and the prescribed NSAID to be alert for bleeding tendencies, such as easy bruising, nosebleeds, and black, tarry stools. Also, advise the patient to take bleeding precautions, such as using an electric razor when shaving and avoiding forceful nose blowing and bumps and trauma to the skin.
✦ Teach the patient to recognize the signs and symptoms of liver damage, including nausea, fatigue, lethargy, itching, yellowed skin or eyes, right upper quadrant tenderness, and flulike symptoms. Advise the patient to contact the prescriber if any of these findings occur.
✦ Advise the patient to use sunblock, wear protective clothing, and avoid prolonged exposure to sunlight because photosensitivity may occur.
✦ Advise the patient not to take ketorolac at the same time as a salicylate.
✦ Inform the patient that fluid retention can occur; advise him to ask his prescriber about related dietary restrictions, such as avoiding high-sodium food and limiting fluids.
✦ Instruct the patient to notify the prescriber if adverse reactions occur.

Key nursing actions

✦ Stop the drug and notify the prescriber if the patient has evidence of a hypersensitivity reaction.
✦ Monitor the patient's vision.
✦ Watch for evidence of GI irritation.
✦ Monitor hepatic, hematologic, and renal function tests.
✦ Watch for evidence of infection.
✦ Evaluate pain relief.
✦ Check vital signs at least every 8 hours.
✦ Weigh the patient daily and report rapid, unexpected gain.

✦ Evaluate the degree of pain relief during NSAID therapy. Note that 2 to 4 weeks may elapse before the prescribed NSAID provides relief.
✦ Monitor the patient's vital signs at least every 8 hours. Note a significant increase in blood pressure, fluid retention, or signs of heart failure.
✦ Weigh the patient daily and report sudden, unexplained weight gain. Fluid retention and edema may occur during NSAID therapy.
✦ Teach the patient and his caregiver about the prescribed drug. (See *Teaching a patient about NSAIDs.*)

COX-2 INHIBITORS

Although COX-2 inhibitors are considered NSAIDs, they act only on the isoenzyme COX-2, selectively relieving pain and inflammation. These drugs are as effective as NSAIDs for providing analgesia and anti-inflammatory effects. Unlike NSAIDs, they also can be used perioperatively because they don't affect platelet function and have a longer duration of action. Drugs in this class include celecoxib, rofecoxib, and valdecoxib.

Features of COX-2 inhibitors

✦ Act only on COX-2 to inhibit prostaglandin synthesis
✦ Relieve pain and inflammation with fewer adverse GI effects than other NSAIDs
✦ Don't affect platelets, so can be used perioperatively
✦ Treat osteoarthritis, rheumatoid arthritis, acute pain, primary dysmenorrhea, familial adenomatous polyposis

Pharmacokinetics

After oral administration, COX-2 inhibitors are well absorbed through the GI tract and provide relief within 1 to 2 hours. They're widely distributed throughout the body and metabolized by the liver. Celecoxib is metabolized principally by CYP 2C9; rofecoxib is minimally metabolized by the CYP enzyme system; and valdecoxib is metabolized by CYP 3A4 and CYP 2C9 isoenzymes and by glucuronidation.

The kidneys excrete all three drugs. Celecoxib is excreted in urine and feces; rofecoxib and valdecoxib are excreted in urine only.

Pharmacodynamics

COX-2 inhibitors produce their effects by blocking COX-2 enzymes, thereby inhibiting prostaglandin synthesis. This selective action produces analgesic and anti-inflammatory effects without the adverse GI effects caused by COX-1 inhibitors.

Pharmacotherapeutics

The primary use of COX-2 inhibitors is to provide analgesia and decrease inflammation. These drugs are particularly effective in treating osteoarthritis, rheumatoid arthritis, acute pain, and primary dysmenorrhea. Celecoxib also is effective in managing familial adenomatous polyposis.

Interactions

◆ A COX-2 inhibitor can reduce the antihypertensive effects of ACE inhibitors.
◆ Antacids that contain aluminum or magnesium can reduce the celecoxib level.
◆ When used with a COX-2 inhibitor, aspirin may increase the risk of ulcers.
◆ Fluconazole and ketoconazole may increase the celecoxib or valdecoxib level.
◆ Lithium toxicity may occur when lithium is taken with a COX-2 inhibitor.
◆ Rofecoxib may increase the serum methotrexate or theophylline level.
◆ When used with warfarin, a COX-2 inhibitor may increase PT and INR and the risk of bleeding complications.
◆ Rifampin may reduce the rofecoxib level by 50%.
◆ Valdecoxib may increase the dextromethorphan level.
◆ Use of a COX-2 inhibitor with dong quai, feverfew, garlic, ginger, ginkgo biloba, horse chestnut, and red clover may increase the risk of bleeding.
◆ A COX-2 inhibitor's interactions with white willow are similar to its interactions with aspirin because the body converts the salicin in the herb into salicylic acid.
◆ Long-term alcohol use and smoking during COX-2 inhibitor therapy may cause GI irritation or bleeding.

Adverse reactions

Common adverse reactions to COX-2 inhibitors include dyspepsia, abdominal pain, nausea, diarrhea, flatulence, abdominal fullness, upper respiratory tract infection, sinusitis, headache, dizziness, accidental injury, peripheral edema, back pain, flulike symptoms, rash, hypertension, and myalgia.

Valdecoxib may raise liver enzyme levels by at least three times the upper limit of normal. Rarely, COX-2 inhibitors may cause erythema multiforme, exfoliative dermatitis, Stevens-Johnson syndrome, and toxic epidermal necrolysis. Severe anaphylactic reactions have occurred, especially in patients with asthma, bronchospastic aspirin sensitivity, or aspirin triad. That's why COX-2 inhibitors shouldn't be used in these patients.

Possible drug interactions

◆ ACE inhibitors
◆ Antacids
◆ Aspirin
◆ Dextromethorphan
◆ Fluconazole
◆ Ketoconazole
◆ Lithium
◆ Methotrexate
◆ Rifampin
◆ Theophylline
◆ Warfarin

Adverse reactions to watch for

◆ Abdominal fullness or pain, diarrhea, dyspepsia, flatulence, nausea
◆ Accidental injury
◆ Back pain, flulike symptoms, myalgia, peripheral edema
◆ Dizziness, headache
◆ Hypertension
◆ Increased liver enzyme levels
◆ Rash
◆ Sinusitis, upper respiratory tract infection
◆ Erythema multiforme, exfoliative dermatitis, Stevens-Johnson syndrome, toxic epidermal necrolysis

PATIENT TEACHING

Teaching a patient about COX-2 inhibitors

Whenever a COX-2 inhibitor is prescribed, teach the patient and his family the drug's name, action, frequency, and adverse effects, and take the following actions.
✦ Instruct the patient to promptly report signs of GI bleeding, such as blood in vomit, urine, or stool; or black, tarry stools.
✦ Advise the patient to immediately report rash, unexplained weight gain, or swelling.
✦ Tell the patient to notify the prescriber if she becomes pregnant or plans to become pregnant during therapy.
✦ Instruct the patient to take the drug with food if GI distress occurs.
✦ Teach the patient that COX-2 inhibitors may harm the liver. Signs and symptoms of liver toxicity include nausea, fatigue, lethargy, itching, yellowing of the skin or eyes, right upper quadrant tenderness, and flulike syndrome. Advise the patient to stop therapy and alert the prescriber if any of these effects occur.
✦ Inform the patient that the drug may take several days to produce consistent pain relief.

Nursing considerations
✦ Use COX-2 inhibitors cautiously in patients with a history of ulcers or GI bleeding, advanced renal disease, dehydration, anemia, symptomatic liver disease, hypertension, edema, heart failure, or asthma. Also use these drugs cautiously in geriatric or debilitated patients.

 CLINICAL ALERT Don't administer celecoxib or valdecoxib to any patient who reports being allergic to sulfonamides or to products that contain sulfa.

✦ Use COX-2 inhibitors cautiously in patients with ischemic heart disease. Because these drugs don't inhibit platelet aggregation or prolong bleeding time, they aren't substitutes for aspirin in preventing MI or other cardiovascular events.
✦ Give COX-2 inhibitors with meals, if needed to minimize GI distress.
✦ Monitor the patient for signs and symptoms of hepatotoxicity, including nausea, fatigue, lethargy, yellowed skin or eyes, right upper quadrant tenderness, and flulike symptoms.

 CLINICAL ALERT Don't confuse Celebrex (celecoxib) with Cerebyx (fosphenytoin, an anticonvulsant prescribed for status epilepticus or seizures) or Celexa (citalopram, an antidepressant).

✦ Teach the patient and his caregiver about the prescribed drug. (See *Teaching a patient about COX-2 inhibitors.*)

Key nursing actions
✦ Give COX-2 inhibitors with food, if needed to reduce GI distress.
✦ Watch for evidence of hepatotoxicity.

OPIOID AGONISTS AND ANTAGONISTS

Also called *opioid analgesics,* opioid agonists include opium derivatives and synthetic drugs with similar properties. They're used to relieve or decrease pain without causing unconsciousness. Some opioid agonists also have antitussive effects that suppress coughing and antidiarrheal actions that can control diarrhea.

Features of opioid agonists and antagonists

Agonists
+ Are known as *opioid analgesics*
+ Include opium derivatives and synthetics with similar properties
+ Reduce pain without causing unconsciousness
+ May help control coughing and diarrhea

Antagonists
+ Block the effects of opioid agonists
+ Reverse adverse effects of opioids, such as respiratory and CNS depression
+ Cause pain to recur

Mixed agonist-antagonists
+ Relieve pain
+ Reduce the risk of toxicity and dependence
+ Are used for moderate to severe pain, preoperative anxiety and pain, and analgesia during childbirth

How opioid agonists work
+ Bind to opiate receptors in the peripheral nervous system and CNS
+ Mimic the effects of endorphins
+ Relieve pain and suppress cough
+ Affect GI and genitourinary smooth muscles
+ Cause blood vessels to dilate

Opioid antagonists aren't analgesics. Instead, they block the effects of opioid agonists and are used to reverse their adverse reactions, such as respiratory and CNS depression. By reversing the analgesic's effects, however, opioid antagonists also cause the pain to recur.

Some opioid analgesics, called mixed opioid agonist-antagonists, have agonist and antagonist properties. The agonist component relieves pain, and the antagonist component decreases the risk of toxicity and drug dependence. These mixed opioid agonist-antagonists reduce the risk of respiratory depression and drug abuse.

OPIOID AGONISTS

Opioid agonists include codeine, fentanyl, hydrocodone, hydromorphone, levorphanol, meperidine, methadone, morphine (including sustained-release tablets and intensified oral solution), oxycodone, oxymorphone, propoxyphene, remifentanil, and sufentanil. Tramadol has characteristics similar to those of other opioid analgesics. Although it isn't classified as an opioid, it may become habit-forming, causing mental or physical dependence.

Morphine sulfate is the standard against which the effectiveness and adverse reactions of other analgesics are measured.

Pharmacokinetics

A patient may receive opioid agonists by any administration route, although the inhalation route is rarely used. After oral administration, these drugs are absorbed readily from the GI tract.

After I.V. administration, opioid agonists provide the most rapid and reliable pain relief. Opioid agonists given by the transmucosal or intrathecal routes also provide very fast action. Administration by the S.C. or I.M. route may result in delayed absorption, especially in patients with poor circulation.

Opioid agonists are distributed widely throughout body tissues. They have plasma protein-binding capacity of 30% to 35%.

The drugs are metabolized extensively in the liver. For example, meperidine is metabolized to normeperidine, a toxic metabolite with a longer half-life than meperidine. The metabolite accumulates in patients with renal dysfunction and may lead to CNS excitation. Propoxyphene is metabolized to norpropoxyphene, a metabolite that may prolong cardiac conduction intervals.

The kidneys excrete the metabolites. A small amount is excreted in stool through the biliary tract.

Pharmacodynamics

Opioid agonists reduce pain by binding to opiate receptor sites in the peripheral nervous system and the CNS. When these drugs stimulate opiate receptors, they mimic the effects of endorphins (naturally occurring opiates that are part of the body's own pain relief system). This receptor-site binding produces the therapeutic effects of analgesia and cough suppression as well as adverse reactions, such as respiratory depression and constipation. (See *How opioid agonists control pain*.)

Opioid agonists, especially morphine, affect the smooth muscle of the GI and genitourinary tracts. This causes contraction of the bladder and ureters and slows intestinal peristalsis. This explains why constipation is one of the most common adverse effects of opiates.

These drugs also cause blood vessels to dilate, especially in the face, head, and neck. In addition, they suppress the cough center in the brain, producing antitussive effects and causing constriction of the bronchial muscles. Any of these effects

EYE ON DRUG ACTION

How opioid agonists control pain

Opioid agonists, such as meperidine, inhibit pain transmission by mimicking the body's natural pain control mechanisms.

NEURONS RELEASE SUBSTANCE P

In the dorsal horn of the spinal cord, peripheral pain neurons meet central nervous system (CNS) neurons. At the synapse, the pain neuron releases substance P (a pain neurotransmitter). This substance helps transfer pain impulses to the CNS neurons that carry the impulses to the brain.

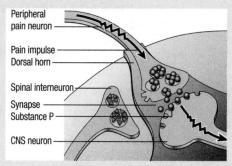

ENDOGENOUS OPIATES BLOCK PAIN IMPULSES

In theory, the spinal interneurons respond to stimulation from the descending neurons of the CNS by releasing endogenous opiates. These opiates bind to the peripheral pain neuron to inhibit the release of substance P and to retard the transmission of pain impulses.

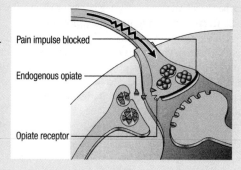

OPIOID AGONISTS HELP BLOCK PAIN

Synthetic opioid agonists supplement this pain-blocking effect by binding with free opiate receptors to inhibit the release of substance P. These drugs also alter consciousness of pain, but how this mechanism works remains unknown.

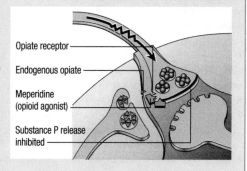

can become adverse reactions if they occur in excess. For example, if the blood vessels dilate too much, hypotension can result.

Pharmacotherapeutics

Opioid agonists are prescribed to relieve severe pain in acute, chronic, and terminal illnesses. They also reduce anxiety before a patient receives anesthesia and are sometimes prescribed to control diarrhea and suppress coughing. Methadone is

WARNING

Contraindications and precautions for propoxyphene

Use of propoxyphene is contraindicated in patients who are suicidal or addiction-prone. Also, use of the drug requires extreme caution in patients who take tranquilizers or antidepressants or who consume excessive alcohol. High doses of propoxyphene with other CNS depressants may result in death.

When to use an opioid agonist

✦ To relieve severe pain in acute, chronic, and terminal illness
✦ To reduce anxiety before anesthesia
✦ To control coughing or diarrhea
✦ To temporarily maintain drug addiction (methadone)
✦ To induce and maintain general anesthesia
✦ To relieve shortness of breath in pulmonary edema and heart failure

Possible drug interactions

✦ Anticholinergics
✦ Beta blockers
✦ Calcium channel blockers
✦ Carbamazepine
✦ Diuretics
✦ Hydantoins
✦ MAO inhibitors
✦ Phenothiazine
✦ Protease inhibitors
✦ Respiratory depressants
✦ Rifampin
✦ Tricyclic antidepressants
✦ Warfarin

used for temporary maintenance of drug addiction. Other opioids, such as remifentanil, are used to induce and maintain general anesthesia. However, some of these drugs pose special contraindications and precautions. (See *Contraindications and precautions for propoxyphene.*)

Patients can take opioids for long-term therapy. Pure opioids have no maximum daily dose, or ceiling, for their analgesic effects. This means that opioids can be prescribed at whatever dose is needed to provide pain relief. They can be combined with acetaminophen to limit the opioid dose.

Opioid agonists cause blood to pool in the arms and legs because they decrease peripheral resistance. They also can decrease venous return, cardiac workload, and pulmonary venous pressure. As blood shifts from the central to the peripheral circulation, cardiac preload decreases. These cardiovascular actions help morphine to relieve shortness of breath in patients with pulmonary edema and left-sided heart failure.

Interactions

✦ Use of an opioid agonist with another drug that decreases respirations (such as alcohol, sedatives, hypnotics, and anesthetics) increases the risk of severe respiratory depression.
✦ Use of a tricyclic antidepressant, phenothiazine, or anticholinergic with an opioid agonist may cause severe constipation and urine retention.
✦ An opioid agonist may potentiate the effects of a tricyclic antidepressant or MAO inhibitor, possibly requiring a dosage reduction and contraindicating the use of meperidine or fentanyl with an MAO inhibitor.
✦ An opioid agonist may decrease the effects of a diuretic.
✦ Use of an opioid agonist with a protease inhibitor may increase CNS and respiratory depression, contraindicating the combination of meperidine or propoxyphene with a protease inhibitor.
✦ Use of sufentanil with a beta blocker or calcium channel blocker may increase bradycardia and hypotension.
✦ Propoxyphene may increase the carbamazepine level.
✦ Propoxyphene and morphine may enhance warfarin's anticoagulant effects.
✦ Rifampin may decrease methadone level, reducing that drug's effect.
✦ A hydantoin may decrease the effects of meperidine or methadone.

Adverse reactions

Opioid agonists produce numerous adverse reactions that affect most body systems. Adverse CNS reactions, the most common, usually affect the respiratory and GI tracts.

CNS, respiratory, and GI reactions

One of the most common adverse reactions to opioid agonists is decreased respiratory rate and depth that worsens as the dosage increases. This may cause periodic, irregular breathing or precipitate asthmatic attacks in susceptible patients. The cough-suppressant effect of opioid agonists usually is considered therapeutic; however, as these adverse reactions indicate, it sometimes may be undesirable.

Adverse GI reactions include nausea, vomiting, biliary colic or spasm, and constipation. Nausea and vomiting are more likely to occur in ambulatory patients; however, these reactions differ with the drug used, even in the same patient. Opioid agonist-induced biliary colic is linked to elevated amylase and lipase levels. Because of this effect, these levels shouldn't be determined for 24 hours or more after an opioid agonist is given so a true value can be obtained. Opioid agonists may cause constipation through sedation that reduces the response to the defecation impulse, through significant reduction in peristalsis, and through increased water absorption from intestinal contents.

Other reactions

Dilation of peripheral arteries and veins from opioid agonists leads to flushing and orthostatic hypotension. The patient may feel drowsy or light-headed, and his arms and legs may feel warm and heavy. (Little change in blood pressure or pulse rate occurs when the patient is lying down.)

Some patients receiving these drugs, especially men with prostatic hypertrophy, may experience urine retention. Opioid agonists also may prolong labor and produce respiratory depression in neonates.

All opioid agonists may cause pupil constriction that persists throughout long-term therapy. Meperidine frequently produces tremors, palpitations, tachycardia, and delirium.

The patient may develop tolerance to the effects of opioid agonists. When an opioid-tolerant patient suddenly stops receiving the drug, withdrawal symptoms may occur, including increased sensory perceptions (especially those of pain and touch), tactile hallucinations, increased GI secretions, nasopharyngeal secretions, diarrhea, dilated pupils, and photophobia.

Severe hypersensitivity reactions to opioid agonists are rare and usually occur as urticaria or a rash. Even I.V. administration rarely causes anaphylaxis. Some patients may experience itching or wheal formation at the injection site, but this is usually a local, histamine-mediated response.

Nursing considerations

+ Observe the patient periodically for adverse reactions.
+ Obtain the patient's baseline blood pressure, pulse, and respirations before giving the initial dose. Continue to monitor these vital signs throughout therapy.
+ Note the patient's respiratory rate, depth, and rhythm before giving each dose. Withhold the dose and notify the prescriber if the patient's respiratory rate is 8 to 10 breaths/minute or less. An infant or a patient with compromised respiratory function may be particularly sensitive to the respiratory effects of the drug.

 CLINICAL ALERT Prolonged administration or high doses may increase the risk of neurotoxicity and seizures from the build-up of normeperidine in patients with sickle cell anemia, burns, or cancer.

+ Notify the prescriber of adverse reactions. Be aware that drug may interfere with CNS evaluation related to level of consciousness, pupillary changes, and respiratory depression. This is especially important in a patient with a head injury.

Teaching a patient about opioid agonists

Whenever an opioid agonist is prescribed, teach the patient and his family the drug's name, dose, frequency, action, and adverse effects, and take the following actions.

✦ Advise the patient to take the drug with food if GI distress occurs.

✦ Instruct the patient not to smoke or walk immediately after receiving an opioid agonist because of its sedative effects. Also caution the patient against driving or performing any other activity that requires alertness.

✦ Advise the patient to avoid alcohol or other central nervous system depressants, which may cause excessive sedation and respiratory depression.

✦ Instruct the patient to lie down if drowsiness, nausea, or light-headedness occurs.

✦ Teach the patient ways to prevent constipation, such as increasing fluid and fiber intake.

✦ Advise the patient to note any change in voiding patterns because urine retention may occur.

✦ Caution the patient to take the drug exactly as prescribed because misuse can lead to dependence.

✦ Teach the patient pain management techniques, such as guided imagery, distraction, and meditation, to minimize the need for prolonged use or large doses.

✦ Instruct the patient to take the drug before the pain becomes severe for greatest effectiveness.

✦ Instruct the patient not to crush or break morphine sulfate sustained- or extended-release tablets because this will negate their sustained-release effect.

✦ Advise the patient and his family to notify the prescriber if adverse reactions occur.

✦ Provide written instructions about the drug.

Key nursing actions
(continued)

✦ Don't stop the drug abruptly.
✦ Assess pain level before and after each dose.

✦ Observe for signs of patient tolerance to the drug's effects, such as inadequate pain relief and requests for increased drug administration.

✦ Don't stop the drug suddenly in a drug-dependent patient. This may cause withdrawal symptoms, such as restlessness, lacrimation, rhinorrhea, yawning, diaphoresis, piloerection, restless sleep, and mydriasis during the first 24 hours. After that, the symptoms may progress and include twitching and muscle spasm; severe aches in the back, abdomen and legs; abdominal and muscle cramps; hot and cold flashes; nausea; vomiting; diarrhea; coryza and severe sneezing; hyperthermia; tachypnea; hypertension; and tachycardia.

✦ Assess the patient's pain before and after each dose. The drug is most effective when given before pain becomes severe.

✦ Don't crush or break morphine sulfate sustained-release tablets; this will negate their sustained-release effect.

✦ Don't abbreviate morphine sulfate, MSO_4; this can be confused with $MgSO_4$ (magnesium sulfate).

✦ Teach the patient and his caregiver about the prescribed drug. (See *Teaching a patient about opioid agonists.*)

TRAMADOL

Although structurally different from opioid agonists, tramadol acts like an opioid agonist. It's used to treat moderate to severe pain after surgery, including oral surgery.

WARNING

Precautions for tramadol

Use tramadol cautiously in patients who are at risk for seizures or respiratory depression and in those with increased intracranial pressure or head injury, acute abdominal conditions, renal or hepatic impairment, or physical dependence on opioids.

Pharmacokinetics

After oral administration, tramadol is rapidly and completely absorbed, exhibits low protein binding, and is extensively metabolized by the liver. About 30% is excreted in urine as unchanged drug and 60% is excreted as metabolites.

Pharmacodynamics

Tramadol is a centrally acting analgesic. Its exact mechanism isn't understood, but the drug may bind to mu-opioid receptors and inhibit the reuptake of norepinephrine and serotonin.

Pharmacotherapeutics

Tramadol is used for the treatment of moderate to severe pain. However, it should be used cautiously in certain patients. (See *Precautions for tramadol.*)

Interactions

✦ Carbamazepine increases tramadol metabolism.
✦ Together, tramadol and CNS depressants cause additive effects.
✦ When used with tramadol, cyclobenzaprine, monoamine oxidase (MAO) inhibitors, neuroleptics, selective serotonin reuptake inhibitors, and tricyclic antidepressants may increase the risk of seizures.
✦ Quinidine increases the tramadol level.
✦ Use of tramadol with paroxetine or sertraline increases risk of serotonin syndrome.

Adverse reactions

Common adverse reactions to tramadol include dizziness, vertigo, headache, somnolence, nausea, vomiting, and constipation.

Other adverse CNS reactions include CNS stimulation, asthenia, anxiety, confusion, coordination disturbance, euphoria, nervousness, sleep disorder, seizures, and malaise.

Vasodilation, vision disturbances, dry mouth, diarrhea, abdominal pain, urine retention or urinary frequency, hypertonia, respiratory depression, and rash also may occur during tramadol therapy.

Nursing considerations

✦ For more effective analgesia, give tramadol before the pain becomes intense.
✦ Reassess the patient's level of pain at least 30 minutes after administration.
✦ Monitor the patient's cardiovascular and respiratory status. Withhold the dose and notify the prescriber if the respirations become shallow or the respiratory rate falls below 12 breaths/minute.

Features of tramadol

✦ Is a centrally acting analgesic
✦ May bind to mu-opioid receptors and inhibit reuptake of norepinephrine and serotonin
✦ Is used for moderate to severe pain

Possible drug interactions

✦ Carbamazepine
✦ CNS depressants
✦ Cyclobenzaprine
✦ MAO inhibitors
✦ Neuroleptics
✦ Paroxetine
✦ Quinidine
✦ Sertraline
✦ SSRIs
✦ Tricyclic antidepressants

Adverse reactions to watch for

✦ Abdominal pain, constipation, diarrhea, nausea, vomiting
✦ Asthenia, anxiety, confusion, coordination disturbance, CNS stimulation, euphoria, malaise, nervousness, seizures, sleep disorder
✦ Dizziness, headache, somnolence, vertigo
✦ Dry mouth, urine retention, urinary frequency
✦ Hypertonia
✦ Rash
✦ Respiratory depression
✦ Vasodilation
✦ Vision disturbances

Key nursing actions

✦ Give the drug before the pain becomes intense.
✦ Assess the pain level at least 30 minutes after giving a dose.

Key nursing actions
(continued)
◆ Monitor cardiovascular and respiratory status.
◆ Monitor bowel function.
◆ Watch for seizures.
◆ Assess the patient for evidence of drug dependence.

Features of mixed opioid agonist-antagonists
◆ Relieve pain while minimizing opioid toxicity and dependence
◆ May act as agonists at some receptors and as antagonists at others
◆ Alter perceptions of and motional response to pain (buprenorphine)
◆ May act on opiate receptors in the limbic system (butorphanol)
◆ Increase pulmonary vascular resistance, blood pressure, and cardiac workload (butorphabol and pentazocine)

◆ Monitor the patient's bowel function. If the patient is constipated, give him a laxative.
◆ Monitor the patient for seizures because tramadol may reduce the seizure threshold.
◆ Assess the patient for signs of drug dependence. Tramadol may produce dependence similar to that of codeine or dextropropoxyphene and has a similar abuse potential.

 CLINICAL ALERT Don't confuse tramadol, a centrally acting analgesic, with trazodone (Desyrel), which is an antidepressant that inhibits serotonin uptake in the brain.

◆ Teach the patient and his caregiver about the drug. (See *Teaching a patient about tramadol.*)

MIXED OPIOID AGONIST-ANTAGONISTS

Mixed opioid agonist-antagonists attempt to relieve pain while reducing the opioid's toxic effects and dependency. This drug class includes buprenorphine, butorphanol, nalbuphine, and pentazocine hydrochloride (combined with pentazocine lactate, naloxone, aspirin, or acetaminophen).

Originally, mixed opioid agonist-antagonists appeared to have less abuse potential than opioid agonists. However, butorphanol and pentazocine have reportedly caused dependence.

Pharmacokinetics
Absorption of mixed opioid agonist-antagonists occurs rapidly from parenteral sites. These drugs are distributed to most body tissues and cross the placenta. They're metabolized in the liver and excreted primarily by the kidneys, although more than 10% of butorphanol and a small amount of pentazocine are excreted in stool.

Pharmacodynamics
The exact mechanism of action of the mixed opioid agonist-antagonists isn't known. Nalbuphine, pentazocine, and the partial agonists buprenorphine and butorphanol may have agonist activity at some receptors and antagonist activity at

other receptors. Partial agonists bind to the receptors but don't always stimulate a response.

Buprenorphine binds with receptors in the CNS, altering the perception of and emotional response to pain through an unknown mechanism. It seems to release slowly from binding sites, producing a longer duration of action than other drugs in this class.

Butorphanol's site of action may be opiate receptors in the limbic system, which is the part of the brain involved in emotion. Like pentazocine, butorphanol also acts on pulmonary circulation, increasing pulmonary vascular resistance (the resistance in the blood vessels of the lungs that the right ventricle must pump against). Both drugs also increase blood pressure and the cardiac workload.

Pharmacotherapeutics

Mixed opioid agonist-antagonists are prescribed primarily to relieve moderate to severe pain and to reduce preoperative anxiety and pain. They're also used for analgesia during childbirth. They shouldn't be used in patients with chronic pain who take opioid agonists.

Sometimes these drugs are prescribed instead of opioid agonists because they have a lower risk of drug dependence. Mixed opioid agonist-antagonists also are less likely to cause respiratory depression and constipation, although they can produce some adverse reactions.

Interactions

✦ Use of a mixed opioid agonist-antagonist with another CNS depressant (such as a barbiturate or alcohol) may result in increased CNS depression and an additive decrease in respiratory rate and depth.
✦ Use of a mixed opioid agonist-antagonist with an opioid agonist can cause withdrawal symptoms, especially in a patient with a history of opioid abuse.

Adverse reactions

Adverse reactions to mixed opioid agonist-antagonists are less common than reactions to opioid agonists and usually affect the CNS and the GI tract.

The most common adverse reactions to these drugs include nausea, vomiting, light-headedness, sedation, and euphoria. Dysphoria, visual hallucinations, confusion, and disorientation also may occur, especially in geriatric patients. These effects limit the long-term use of these drugs in patients with severe pain. Respiratory depression may occur with initial doses, but doesn't worsen as the dosage increases. Insomnia, disturbed dreams, blood pressure changes, and anticholinergic effects (dry mouth, blurred vision, constipation, and urine retention) also may occur. The mixed opioid agonist-antagonists also can cause hypersensitivity reactions. When abused, pentazocine can produce additional serious reactions. (See *Effects of "Ts and Blues,"* page 140.)

Nursing considerations

✦ Rate the patient's pain before and after each dose; determine and record the pain's onset, duration, location, intensity, and quality as well as the degree of pain relief after drug administration.
✦ Observe the patient frequently and take safety precautions if the patient develops mental status changes. For example, keep the bed rails up and place the bed in the low position.
✦ Notify the prescriber if adverse reactions occur or if pain isn't relieved.

Uses for mixed opioid agonist-antagonists
✦ To relieve moderate to severe pain
✦ To reduce anxiety and pain before surgery
✦ To provide analgesia in childbirth

Possible drug interactions
✦ CNS depressants
✦ Opioid agonists

Adverse reactions to watch for
✦ Anticholinergic effects: blurred vision, constipation, dry mouth, urine retention
✦ Blood pressure changes
✦ Confusion, disorientation, dysphoria, visual hallucinations
✦ Disturbed dreams, euphoria, insomnia, light-headedness, sedation
✦ Hypersensitivity reactions
✦ Nausea, vomiting
✦ Respiratory depression

Key nursing actions

✦ Rate the patient's pain before and after each dose.
✦ Assess the patient frequently, and take safety precautions if you note mental status changes.
✦ Monitor respiratory status.

✦ Teach the patient and his caregiver about the prescribed drug. (See *Teaching a patient about mixed opioid agonist-antagonists*.)
✦ Monitor the patient's respiratory status during therapy. Have emergency equipment readily available.

 CLINICAL ALERT Don't administer a mixed opioid agonist-antagonist to a patient who is dependent on opioids; it may precipitate withdrawal symptoms.

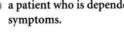

✦ Take safety precautions and provide psychological support if the drug is given inadvertently to an opioid-dependent patient.
✦ Don't mix pentazocine in the same syringe as a barbiturate; a precipitate will form.
✦ To help prevent severe tissue damage, don't give subcutaneous (S.C.) pentazocine. If the patient must receive S.C. pentazocine, record, inspect, and rotate injection sites.
✦ If an overdose occurs, provide emergency care, symptomatic treatment, and mechanical ventilation if needed. Plan to use naloxone to reverse the effects of opioids, butorphanol, methadone, nalbuphine, pentazocine, or propoxyphene.

OPIOID ANTAGONISTS

Opioid antagonists attach to opiate receptors but don't stimulate them. In fact, they have a greater attraction for opiate receptors than opioids do. As a result, they prevent opioid agonists, enkephalins, and endorphins from producing their effects. Opioid antagonists include naloxone and naltrexone.

Pharmacokinetics

Naloxone is given I.M., S.C., or I.V. Naltrexone is given orally in tablet or liquid form. Both drugs are metabolized by the liver and excreted by the kidneys.

Pharmacodynamics

Opioid antagonists block the effects of opioid agonists by occupying the opiate receptor sites. They displace opioids that were attached to opiate receptors and block further opioid binding at these sites. This process is known as competitive inhibition.

Pharmacotherapeutics

Naloxone is the drug of choice for managing opioid agonist overdose. Within seconds after administration, it reverses respiratory depression and sedation and helps stabilize the patient's vital signs. Because naloxone also reverses the opioid's analgesic effects, a patient who received an opioid drug for pain relief may report pain or experience withdrawal symptoms.

Naltrexone is used with psychotherapy or counseling to treat drug abuse. However, it's only given to patients who have gone through a detoxification program to remove all opioids from the body. That's because a patient who still has opioids in the body may experience acute withdrawal symptoms if he receives naltrexone. (See *Managing naltrexone therapy for drug addiction,* page 142.)

Interactions

Naloxone produces no significant drug interactions. Naltrexone may cause a few.
✦ When given to a patient who is receiving or is addicted to an opioid agonist, naltrexone will cause withdrawal symptoms.
✦ Naltrexone may reduce the therapeutic effects of opioid-containing products, such as analgesics and cough, cold, and antidiarrheal preparations.

Adverse reactions

Naloxone may cause nausea, vomiting, and, occasionally, hypertension and tachycardia. An unconscious patient returned to consciousness abruptly after naloxone administration may hyperventilate and experience tremors.

Features of opioid antagonists
✦ Attach to opiate receptors but don't stimulate them
✦ Block the effects of opioid agonists
✦ Displace opioids that were attached to opiate receptors and block further binding at those sites (competitive inhibition)

Uses for opioid antagonists
✦ To manage opioid agonist overdose (naloxone)
✦ To treat drug abuse as adjunct to psychotherapy (naltrexone)

Managing naltrexone therapy for drug addiction

To prevent acute withdrawal during treatment for opioid addiction, plan to use naltrexone as part of a comprehensive rehabilitation program. Also, follow these guidelines.
✦ Don't give naltrexone until a negative naloxone challenge test is obtained.
✦ Don't give naltrexone to a patient receiving an opioid agonist, addicted to an opioid agonist, or in the acute phase of opioid withdrawal because acute withdrawal may occur or worsen.
✦ For a patient who is addicted to a short-acting opioid, such as heroin or meperidine, wait at least 7 days after the last opioid dose before starting naltrexone.
✦ For a patient who is addicted to a longer-acting opioid, such as methadone, wait at least 10 days after the last opioid dose before starting naltrexone.
✦ During naltrexone therapy, be alert for signs of opioid withdrawal, such as drug craving, confusion, drowsiness, visual hallucinations, abdominal pain, vomiting, diarrhea, fever, chills, tachypnea, diaphoresis, salivation, lacrimation, runny nose, and mydriasis.

Adverse reactions to watch for

naloxone
✦ Hypertension
✦ Nausea, vomiting
✦ Tachycardia

naltrexone
✦ Abdominal pain or cramps, nausea, vomiting
✦ Anorexia, constipation, diarrhea
✦ Anxiety, dizziness, headache, difficulty sleeping, increased energy, irritability, nervousness
✦ Chills
✦ Elevated liver enzyme levels
✦ Hypertension
✦ Increased thirst
✦ Joint and muscle pain
✦ Lassitude, low energy, mental depression, suicidal ideation, somnolence
✦ Rash
✦ Tachycardia

Key nursing actions
✦ Give more than one dose of naloxone if the patient has respiratory depression.
✦ In an emergency, the patient taking naltrexone may receive an opioid analgesic, but the dose must be adjusted. Watch for respiratory depression.

Naltrexone produces many adverse reactions in various body systems. In more than 10% of patients taking naltrexone for alcohol or narcotic addiction, adverse reactions include nausea, vomiting, abdominal pain or cramps, headache, lassitude, low energy level, difficulty sleeping, anxiety, nervousness, and joint and muscle pain. Other common adverse reactions include anorexia, constipation, diarrhea, elevated liver enzyme levels, increased energy level, mental depression, suicidal ideation, irritability, somnolence, dizziness, rash, chills, and increased thirst.

The variety and number of adverse reactions to naltrexone have delayed its full acceptance as a treatment for opioid addiction. Because of the drug's adverse reactions, patients who receive it even as outpatients should be monitored frequently.

Nursing considerations
✦ Observe the patient for adverse reactions throughout therapy.
✦ Give more than one dose of naloxone if respiratory depression occurs. The drug's duration of action may exceed naloxone's duration. Naloxone doesn't reverse respiratory depression caused by diazepam.

 CLINICAL ALERT Don't confuse naltrexone with naloxone. Naltrexone is used for maintaining freedom from opioid addiction, and naloxone is used to reverse the adverse effects of opioids.

✦ In an emergency, a patient receiving naltrexone may receive an opioid analgesic. However, the opioid dose must be higher than usual to overcome naltrexone's effects. Watch for respiratory depression from the opioid analgesic; it may be longer and deeper than usual.
✦ Teach the patient and his caregiver about the prescribed drug. (See *Teaching a patient about opioid antagonists.*)

ANESTHETICS

Anesthetics can be divided into three main groups: general, local, and topical anesthetics. General anesthetics can be subdivided into two main types: inhalation anesthetics (volatile liquids or gases vaporized in oxygen and given by inhalation) and injection anesthetics (nonvolatile solutions given by injection).

The practice of general anesthesia includes more than proper administration of anesthetic drugs. Other vital components of anesthesia practice include monitoring and maintaining the patient's vital signs, fluid and electrolyte levels, acid-base balance, body temperature, and positioning as well as ensuring the patient's well-being from the preoperative period through recovery.

Local and topical anesthetics are used to interrupt pain impulse transmission from peripheral nerves by causing a temporary loss of sensation in a limited body area. Local anesthetics must be injected to produce anesthesia; topical anesthetics are applied directly to the skin or mucous membranes. Some local anesthetics can be used topically.

INHALATION ANESTHETICS

General anesthetics that are commonly given by inhalation include desflurane, enflurane, halothane, isoflurane, nitrous oxide, and sevoflurane.

Components of anesthesia practice
+ Properly administering anesthetic drugs
+ Monitoring and maintaining vital signs, fluid and electrolyte levels, acid-base balance, and body temperature and position
+ Ensuring the patient's well-being from the preoperative period through recovery

Using inhalation anesthetics cautiously in geriatric patients

Inhalation anesthetics require cautious use in geriatric patients, especially ones with multiple, coexisting conditions that have caused debilitation. That's because debilitated surgical patients are predisposed to an exaggerated response to inhalation anesthetics. In these patients, even smaller-than-normal drug doses may lead to hypotension, prolonged respiratory depression, and longer recovery. In addition, geriatric patients may experience prolonged recovery from inhalation anesthetics, resulting in confusion, agitation, and memory loss that may be mistaken for signs of dementia.

Features of inhalation anesthetics

- ✦ Depend on solubility in blood for absorption and elimination
- ✦ Distribute most rapidly to organs with high blood flow (brain, liver, kidneys, heart)
- ✦ Work mainly by depressing the CNS
- ✦ Produce muscle relaxation, loss of consciousness, loss of responsiveness

Using inhalation anesthetics

- ✦ They're used for surgery because the depth of anesthesia can be controlled better than with injected drugs.
- ✦ Choice of drug varies with the patient's physiology, medical history, planned surgery, and expected postoperative course.
- ✦ Because drugs are gaseous, doses aren't expressed as weights.

Pharmacokinetics

An anesthetic's absorption and elimination rates depend on its solubility in blood. Inhalation anesthetics enter the blood from the lungs and are distributed to other tissues. Distribution is most rapid to organs with high blood flow, such as the brain, liver, kidneys, and heart. Inhalation anesthetics are eliminated primarily by the lungs; enflurane, halothane, and sevoflurane also are eliminated by the liver. Metabolites are excreted in urine.

Pharmacodynamics

Inhalation anesthetics work primarily by depressing the CNS, producing loss of consciousness, loss of responsiveness to sensory stimulation (including pain), and muscle relaxation. They also affect other organ systems.

Pharmacotherapeutics

Inhalation anesthetics are used for surgery because they offer more precise and rapid control of the depth of anesthesia than injection anesthetics do. Because inhalation anesthetics are liquids at room temperature, they require a vaporizer and special delivery system for safe use.

Of the inhalation anesthetics, desflurane, isoflurane, and nitrous oxide are the most commonly used. The choice of a particular general anesthetic for a patient involves several considerations, including the patient's physiologic state and medical history, the type of surgery, and the expected postoperative course. (See *Using inhalation anesthetics cautiously in geriatric patients*.)

Inhalation anesthetics are given as gases, so dosages aren't expressed in weight, as with other drugs. Because the amount of anesthetic in the lungs is proportional to the amount in the brain at equilibrium, the quantity of anesthetic needed can be determined by the minimum alveolar concentration (MAC). MAC is the alveolar anesthetic concentration at which 50% of patients don't move during a surgical incision.

Inhalation anesthetics are contraindicated in patients who are hypersensitive to the drug and in those with a liver disorder or malignant hyperthermia, which is a life-threatening complication of anesthesia. (See *Controlling malignant hyperthermia*.) These drugs require cautious use in pregnant and breast-feeding patients.

WARNING

Controlling malignant hyperthermia

For a patient who receives an inhalation anesthetic, monitor for malignant hyperthermia, a serious adverse reaction that's characterized by a sudden, potentially fatal increase in body temperature. Malignant hyperthermia only affects genetically susceptible patients and may result from a failure of calcium uptake by muscle cells. To treat this condition, be prepared to give the skeletal muscle relaxant dantrolene.

Interactions

Because inhalation anesthetics can cause serious interactions, be sure the patient's list of current medications is up to date before his preoperative meeting with the anesthesiologist or nurse anesthetist.

✦ When used with labetalol, an inhalation anesthetic (especially enflurane, halothane, and isoflurane) can cause excessive hypotension.

✦ Inhalation anesthetics potentiate the effects of nondepolarizing muscle relaxants and prolong the action of the muscle relaxants.

Adverse reactions

The most common adverse reaction to inhalation anesthetics is an exaggerated response to a normal dose. Postoperative reactions resemble those of other CNS depressants: cardiopulmonary depression, confusion, sedation, nausea, vomiting, ataxia, and hypothermia.

Enflurane may cause renal damage or failure because of fluoride ion release. Desflurane isn't recommended to induce anesthesia in children because of its high risk of moderate to severe upper airway adverse events (including laryngospasm, coughing, breath holding, and secretions). After induction and intubation, desflurane may be used for maintenance of anesthesia.

Halothane administration may be linked to two types of hepatic dysfunction. One type is characterized by increased liver enzyme levels. The other type occurs in about 1 in 7,000 to 1 in 30,000 patients, producing liver necrosis several days after halothane use. Although it isn't infective, the necrosis clinically resembles hepatitis. (See *Identifying halothane hepatitis,* page 146.)

Nursing considerations

✦ Observe the patient for adverse reactions to the drug during administration and recovery.

✦ Monitor the patient's vital signs frequently to detect potential problems. Assess the adequacy, rate, and depth of the patient's respirations. Maintain a patent airway. Assess the patient's level of consciousness, arousal, and orientation.

✦ Keep atropine available to reverse bradycardia.

✦ Monitor the patient's temperature frequently. Be aware that hypothermia is a common reaction and that shivering is normal during recovery. If shivering occurs, give the patient oxygen to compensate for the increased oxygen demand.

✦ Keep the patient warm if hypothermia occurs.

Possible drug interactions
✦ Labetalol
✦ Muscle relaxants
✦ Nondepolarizing muscle relaxants

Adverse reactions to watch for
✦ Ataxia, confusion, sedation
✦ Cardiopulmonary depression
✦ Exaggerated response to a normal dose
✦ Hepatic dysfunction (halothane)
✦ Hypothermia
✦ Nausea, vomiting
✦ Renal damage or failure (enflurane)

Key nursing actions
✦ Monitor vital signs frequently.
✦ Keep atropine readily available.
✦ Monitor the patient's temperature to detect hypothermia.
✦ Keep the patient warm if hypothermia occurs.

Identifying halothane hepatitis

A patient who receives halothane may be at risk for halothane hepatitis, a potentially fatal syndrome that may stem from an immunologic or chemical response to a toxic metabolite. To identify this reaction promptly, first determine if the patient has received halothane before because this form of hepatitis is most common in obese, middle-aged women who have undergone multiple, closely spaced administrations of halothane. Then, monitor the patient closely for the disorder's signs and symptoms, including rash, fever, jaundice, nausea, vomiting, eosinophilia, and altered results on liver function tests. If the patient displays any of these findings, expect to treat symptoms of the syndrome.

CLINICAL ALERT Notify the anesthesiologist immediately if the patient's temperature increases suddenly. This may signal malignant hyperthermia.

✦ Teach the patient and his caregiver about the drug. (See *Teaching a patient about inhalation anesthetics.*)

INJECTION ANESTHETICS

Injection anesthetics are general anesthetics that usually are used when anesthesia is needed for only a short period, such as with outpatient surgery. They're also used to promote rapid induction of anesthesia or to supplement inhalation anesthetics.

Three drugs in this class — etomidate, ketamine, and propofol — are used solely as injection anesthetics. The rest are drawn from other chemical classes, such as barbiturates (methohexital and thiopental) and benzodiazepines (diazepam, lorazepam, and midazolam), and are used secondarily as anesthetics. In addition, various opioids and opiate-like drugs may be used as injection anesthetics, such as alfentanil, fentanyl, meperidine, morphine, and sufentanil.

Pharmacokinetics

All injection anesthetics bypass the mechanisms that reduce bioavailability, distributing rapidly into the CNS. Opioids given by I.M. injection have a more delayed absorption and reduced peak effect than when given by the I.V. route. Barbiturates depend on liver transformation for elimination, as do benzodiazepines, opioids, and the hypnotic etomidate.

Pharmacodynamics

Opioids work by occupying sites on specialized receptors scattered throughout the CNS and modifying the release of neurotransmitters from sensory nerves entering the CNS. Ketamine appears to induce a profound sense of dissociation from the environment by acting directly on the cortex and limbic system in the brain.

Barbiturates, benzodiazepines, and etomidate seem to enhance responses to the CNS neurotransmitter gamma-aminobutyric acid (GABA). This inhibits the brain's response to stimulation of the reticular activating system, the area of the brain stem that controls alertness. Barbiturates also depress the excitability of CNS neurons.

Features of injection anesthetics

✦ Are used for short-term anesthesia, as for outpatient surgery
✦ Are used to promote rapid induction of anesthesia or to supplement inhaled anesthetics
✦ May include anesthetics, barbiturates, benzodiazepines, opioids, opiate-like drugs
✦ Occupy receptor sites throughout the CNS to modify neurotransmitter release from sensory nerves entering the CNS

Teaching a patient about inhalation anesthetics

Whenever an inhalation anesthetic is prescribed, teach the patient and his family the drug's name, dose, frequency, action, and adverse effects, and take the following actions.
+ Advise the patient not to eat for at least 8 hours before surgery to prevent aspiration of stomach contents into the lungs during anesthesia.
+ Inform the patient that psychomotor functions may be impaired for 24 hours or more after administration.
+ Advise the patient not to drink alcohol or use any other central nervous system depressants for at least 24 hours after anesthesia.
+ Instruct the patient to report adverse reactions or unusual symptoms to the prescriber immediately.

Pharmacotherapeutics

Because of the injection anesthetics' short duration of action, they're used in short surgical procedures, including outpatient surgery. Barbiturates are used alone in surgery that isn't expected to be painful and as adjuncts to other drugs in more extensive procedures. Benzodiazepines produce sedation and amnesia, but not pain relief.

Etomidate is used to induce anesthesia and to supplement low-potency inhalation anesthetics, such as nitrous oxide. The opioids provide pain relief and supplement other anesthetic drugs.

Interactions

The injection anesthetics, particularly ketamine, produce a variety of drug interactions. These interactions range from mild to life-threatening.
+ Verapamil enhances the anesthetic effects of etomidate, producing respiratory depression and apnea.
+ Together, ketamine and halothane increase the risk of hypotension and reduce cardiac output (the amount of blood pumped by the heart each minute).
+ Ketamine can increase the neuromuscular effects of a nondepolarizing blocker, resulting in prolonged respiratory depression.
+ Use of a barbiturate or opioid with ketamine may prolong the patient's recovery after anesthesia.
+ Together, ketamine and theophylline may promote seizures.
+ When use with a thyroid hormone, ketamine may cause hypertension and tachycardia.
+ Thiopental can potentiate the effects of another CNS depressant (including sedatives, hypnotics, nitrous oxide, and alcohol) or vice versa.
+ An antipsychotic can potentiate the hypnotic effects of thiopental.
+ Thiopental may displace from binding sites — or be displaced by — another highly protein bound drug, such as aspirin, meprobamate, probenecid, or sulfisoxazole.
+ An opioid, inhalation anesthetic, hypnotic, or sedative can increase propofol's effects.
+ A CNS depressant, inhalation anesthetic, or opioid analgesic can increase the CNS depression cause by propofol or thiopental, possibly requiring dosage reductions when used together.

Using injection anesthetics

+ Barbiturates may be used alone if a procedure isn't painful or as adjunct in extensive procedures.
+ Benzodiazepines produce sedation and amnesia but no pain relief.
+ Etomidate is used to induce anesthesia and as an adjunct to inhalation anesthetics.

Possible drug interactions

+ Alcohol
+ Antipsychotics
+ Aspirin
+ Azole antifungals
+ Barbiturates
+ Cimetidine
+ CNS depressants
+ Fluvoxamine
+ Halothane
+ Hormonal contraceptives
+ Hypnotics
+ Indinavir
+ Inhalation anesthetics
+ Meprobamate
+ Nondepolarizing blockers
+ Opioids
+ Probenecid
+ Rifamycin
+ Ritonavir
+ Sedatives
+ Sulfisoxazole
+ Theophylline
+ Thyroid hormones
+ Valproic acid
+ Verapamil

Adverse reactions to watch for

+ Airway reflex hyperactivity with hiccups, coughing, and muscle twitching and jerking
+ Arrhythmias
+ Delirium, disorientation, excitement, hallucinations, irrational behavior, prolonged recovery, unpleasant dreams
+ Excess salivation, tearing
+ Hypersensitivity reaction, rash
+ Increased CSF and intraocular pressure
+ Increased heart rate, cardiac output, and blood pressure
+ Muscle rigidity and spasms
+ Nausea, vomiting
+ Pain on administraion
+ Peripheral vasodilation
+ Respiratory depression
+ Seizures
+ Shivering

Key nursing actions

+ Keep resuscitation equipment and emergency drugs readily available.
+ Watch for muscle rigidity and spasms after giving ketamine or an opioid.
+ Watch for emergence reaction if patient received ketamine.

◆ Alcohol, azole antifungals, cimetidine, fluvoxamine, hormonal contraceptive, indinavir, ritonavir, valproic acid, or verapamil can increase the CNS depression caused by midazolam.
◆ Rifamycin or theophylline may decrease midazolam's effects.

Adverse reactions

Adverse reactions to injection anesthetics frequently are extensions of their therapeutic effects.

Adverse CNS reactions are most common after ketamine administration; they include prolonged recovery, unpleasant dreams, irrational behavior, excitement, disorientation, delirium, and hallucinations. Barbiturates and propofol cause respiratory depression. Thiopental, etomidate, and propofol can produce airway reflex hyperactivity with hiccups, coughing, and muscle twitching and jerking. Thiopental also depresses cardiac function and causes peripheral vasodilation; ketamine increases the heart rate, cardiac output, and blood pressure in patients who aren't severely ill. Opioids sometimes cause changes in the heart rate, including arrhythmias. The rare circulatory failure and respiratory arrest seen with benzodiazepines may be related to too-rapid drug administration or concomitant opioid administration. Phlebitis may occur with benzodiazepine administration.

Muscle rigidity and spasms follow administration of ketamine and opioids; the reaction seems to be directly proportional to the infusion rate. Fentanyl and ketamine may cause seizures.

Etomidate, ketamine, and propofol can cause nausea and vomiting. Ketamine also may produce excess salivation, tearing, shivering, and increased cerebrospinal fluid (CSF) and intraocular pressure. In a patient under stress, etomidate may reduce the cortisol level. The only other major adverse reaction to etomidate is pain on administration, which can be avoided by rapid administration into a large vein or with use of a preoperative analgesic.

Rash and hypersensitivity reactions are uncommon with etomidate, opioids, and barbiturates; anaphylaxis has been reported with barbiturates only. Extravasation of barbiturates may cause neuritis and vasospasm.

Nursing considerations

◆ Monitor the patient for adverse reactions during administration and recovery.
◆ Keep resuscitation equipment and emergency drugs readily available.
◆ Don't mix barbiturates and ketamine in the same syringe; they're chemically incompatible.
◆ Shake propofol well before use to distribute the emulsion evenly. Because propofol is an I.V. fat emulsion, use sterile technique during preparation.
◆ Notify the prescriber immediately if adverse reactions occur.
◆ Watch for muscle rigidity and spasms after administration of ketamine or an opioid; these signs are directly proportional to the infusion rate.
◆ Watch for emergence reactions, such as pleasant dream-like states, vivid imagery, hallucinations, and emergence delirium sometimes accompanied by confusion, excitement, and irrational behavior, in a patient who has received ketamine. Reactions may last up to 24 hours, and may be reduced by using low dosages of I.V. diazepam and by not overstimulating the patient during recovery.

 CLINICAL ALERT If a patient develops a severe emergence reaction, you may treat it by administering a hypnotic dose of a short-acting barbiturate.

✦ Monitor the patient's I.V. site closely; barbiturate extravasation may cause painful neuritis and vasospasm.
✦ Teach the patient and his caregiver about the drug. (See *Teaching a patient about injection anesthetics*.)

LOCAL ANESTHETICS

Many situations require local anesthetics to prevent or relieve pain. These drugs also offer a safe alternative to general anesthesia for geriatric or debilitated patients. Local anesthetics may be amide drugs (ones with nitrogen in the molecular chain) or ester drugs (ones with oxygen in the molecular chain). Amide anesthetics include bupivacaine, ropivacaine, lidocaine, mepivacaine, and prilocaine. Ester anesthetics include chloroprocaine, procaine, and tetracaine.

Local anesthetics can be given in various places to block different groups of nerves and used for local effects as well as central, peripheral, I.V. regional, retrobulbar, or transtracheal nerve blocks. (See *Blocking the pain pathways*, page 150.)

Local infiltration involves injecting a local anesthetic into an area that has been injured or that will undergo surgery. One particularly useful type of local infiltration is the field block, which uses several injections to produce a wall of anesthetic around a lesion or an incision.

A central nerve block can be given in the spinal, perineal, epidural, caudal, or lumbar area to produce anesthesia in the CNS. A spinal (or subarachnoid) block requires penetrating the second layer of the spinal cord (the arachnoid membrane at the base of the spine) and injecting a local anesthetic into the CSF. In a saddle block, the anesthetic is administered near the lower end of the spinal column, where it's confined to the perineal or saddle area. An epidural block places the local anesthetic next to the outermost covering of the spinal cord, the dura mater. A caudal block, a special type of epidural block, is given near the sacrum. A lumbar block is a type of epidural block given low in the spinal column, near the lumbar vertebrae.

A peripheral nerve block places a local anesthetic next to nerve fibers in the peripheral nervous system. Paracervical and pudendal blocks are peripheral nerve blocks used in obstetric procedures. A sympathetic block is a peripheral nerve block of sympathetic nerve trunks that is used to relieve pain from injury to the arms or legs and injury or disease of the internal organs. An intercostal block is pe-

Features of local anesthetics

✦ Prevent or relieve severe pain that topical anesthetics or analgesics can't relieve
✦ Offer a safe alternative to general anesthesia for geriatric or debilitated patients or those with respiratory disease
✦ May be given with a drug, such as epinephrine that constricts blood vessels
✦ Can be given in different locations to block different sets of nerves
✦ Are used for local effects and in central, peripheral, I.V. regional, retrobulbar, or transtracheal nerve blocks

Reviewing nerve blocks

✦ Central: Given in spinal, perineal, epidural, caudal, or lumbar area to produce anesthesia in CNS
✦ Field: Given around a lesion or incision
✦ Peripheral: Given next to nerve fibers in the peripheral nervous system

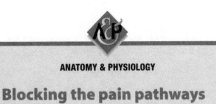

ANATOMY & PHYSIOLOGY

Blocking the pain pathways

Nerve endings transmit pain signals through the peripheral and central nervous systems to the brain. Giving a central nerve block can block the signal transmission and relieve pain. The illustration below shows two key points where an anesthetic may be administered to produce a central nerve block

LATERAL VIEW

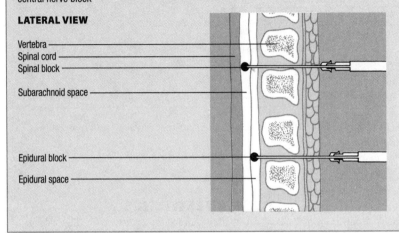

ripheral nerve block produced by injection of an anesthetic near the intercostal nerves.

An I.V. regional nerve block is reserved for specific surgical procedures, such as hand or foot surgery. A tourniquet is applied to the proximal end of the patient's arm or leg, and then a pressure bandage is applied to force blood away from the area to be anesthetized. A local anesthetic solution is infused into the limb to provide regional anesthesia during the procedure.

A retrobulbar nerve block involves injecting a local anesthetic into nerves behind the eyeball in preparation for ocular surgery.

A transtracheal nerve block eliminates reflex activity that occurs from contact with mucous membranes during upper airway surgery. It requires inserting a needle through the cricoid cartilage into the larynx so that an anesthetic solution can be sprayed on the laryngeal mucosa.

Pharmacokinetics

Absorption of local anesthetics varies widely, but distribution occurs throughout the body. Esters and amides undergo different types of metabolism, but both yield metabolites that are excreted in urine.

Pharmacodynamics

Local anesthetics block nerve impulses at the point of contact in all kinds of nerves. They accumulate and cause the nerve cell membrane to expand. As the membrane expands, the cell loses its ability to depolarize, which is necessary for impulse transmission.

Reviewing nerve blocks
(continued)

✦ I.V. regional: Used for specific surgical procedures, such as hand or foot surgery
✦ Retrobulbar: Given into nerves behind the eyeball for ocular surgery
✦ Transtracheal: Given through cricoid cartilage to eliminate reflex activity during upper airway surgery

Pharmacotherapeutics

Local anesthetics are used to prevent and relieve pain from medical procedures, disease, or injury. These drugs are used for severe pain that topical anesthetics or analgesics can't relieve.

Usually, local anesthetics are preferred to general anesthetics for surgery in a geriatric or debilitated patient or a patient with a disorder that affects respiratory function, such as chronic obstructive pulmonary disease or myasthenia gravis.

For some procedures, a local anesthetic is combined with a drug such as epinephrine that constricts blood vessels. Vasoconstriction helps control local bleeding and reduces anesthetic absorption. Reduced absorption prolongs the anesthetic's action at the site and limits its distribution and CNS effects.

Interactions

✦ A local anesthetic that contains a vasoconstrictor, especially norepinephrine, can cause prolonged hypertension in a patient taking an MAO inhibitor, tricyclic antidepressant, or ergot oxytocic and should be used with extreme caution, if at all.
✦ A local anesthetic that contains a vasoconstrictor increases the risk of arrhythmias when used with a halogen general anesthetic; this combination shouldn't be used.
✦ When a local anesthetic is used with a CNS depressant, additive effects may occur.
✦ Procaine, chloroprocaine, and tetracaine inhibit the action of sulfonamides.

Adverse reactions

Adverse reactions to local anesthetics usually result from three main causes: overdose, hypersensitivity, and improper injection technique.

A high anesthetic level can cause CNS and cardiovascular reactions. In the stimulatory phase, dose-related CNS reactions include anxiety, apprehension, restlessness, nervousness, disorientation, confusion, dizziness, blurred vision, tremors, twitching, shivering, and seizures. CNS depression follows, with drowsiness, unconsciousness, and respiratory arrest. The stimulatory phase may not occur, however, if the patient has received lidocaine or another amide anesthetic. Other CNS reactions may include nausea, vomiting, chills, pupil contraction, and tinnitus. Cardiovascular reactions usually are dose-related and may include myocardial depression, bradycardia, arrhythmias, hypotension, cardiovascular collapse, and cardiac arrest.

Local anesthetic solutions that contain vasoconstrictors, such as epinephrine, also can produce CNS and cardiovascular reactions, including anxiety, dizziness, headache, restlessness, tremors, palpitations, tachycardia, anginal pain, and hypertension. Extreme reactions include pulmonary edema and ventricular fibrillation. Norepinephrine may be less likely to cause arrhythmias, but may cause reflex bradycardia. A burning sensation at the injection site also occurs commonly with these drugs. In rare cases, this reaction may be severe, producing pain, skin discoloration, tissue irritation, swelling, neuritis, neurolysis, and tissue necrosis and sloughing.

Ester anesthetics and preservatives in amide anesthetics can cause hypersensitivity reactions, with dermatologic symptoms, edema, status asthmaticus, or anaphylaxis. A patient who is hypersensitive to an ester drug probably won't be sensitive to an amide drug, although he may be hypersensitive to other ester drugs. A local anesthetic solution with a preservative, such as paraben, phenol, or bisulfite, may produce chronic inflammation of the arachnoid membrane if it's used for subarachnoid or epidural anesthesia.

Possible drug interactions

✦ CNS depressants
✦ Ergot oxytocics
✦ Halogen general anesthetics
✦ MAO inhibitors
✦ Sulfonamindes
✦ Tricyclic antidepressants

Adverse reactions to watch for

✦ Anginal pain, arrhythmias, bradycardia, cardiac arrest, cardiovascular collapse, hypertension, hypotension, myocardial depression, palpitations, pulmonary edema, tachycardia, ventricular fibrillation
✦ Anxiety, apprehension, confusion, disorientation, dizziness, headache, nervousness, restlessness, tremors
✦ Blurred vision, chills, pupil contraction, seizures, shivering, tinnitus, tremors, twitching
✦ Burning at injection site
✦ CNS depression drowsiness, unconsciousness, respiratory arrest
✦ Hypersensitivity reactions: dermatologic symptoms, edema, status asthmaticus, anaphylaxis
✦ Methemoglobinemia
✦ Nausea, vomiting

Teaching a patient about local anesthetics

Whenever a local anesthetic is prescribed, teach the patient and his family the drug's name, dose, frequency, action, and adverse effects, and take the following actions.
+ Stress the importance of bedrest for several hours after receiving a spinal anesthetic.
+ Teach the patient to protect numbed areas until sensation returns.
+ Instruct the patient to alert the nurse or prescriber immediately if adverse reactions occur.

Local anesthetics may produce methemoglobinemia (oxidized hemoglobin in the blood, preventing it from efficiently carrying oxygen to tissues). Although this reaction is rare, it occurs most commonly with prilocaine. Cyanosis may be the only symptom, but if it's severe, oxygen and methylene blue may be needed.

Because local anesthetics rapidly cross the placenta, they may produce adverse reactions in the fetus, such as bradycardia and acidosis.

Nursing considerations

+ Monitor the patient's cardiovascular and respiratory status and level of consciousness after each injection.
+ Be alert for signs of CNS toxicity, such as restlessness, anxiety, incoherent speech, light-headedness, numbness and tingling of the mouth and lips, metallic taste, tinnitus, dizziness, blurred vision, tremors, twitching, depression, or drowsiness.
+ Observe the patient for adverse reactions. The higher the dose is, the higher the risk of adverse reactions.
+ Keep emergency drugs and resuscitation equipment on hand when the patient must receive the parenteral form.
+ Don't give with a vasoconstrictor if a halogen inhalation anesthetic may be used later.

 CLINICAL ALERT Don't use the 0.75% concentration of bupivacaine for obstetric anesthesia. It may cause cardiac arrest when used for epidural anesthesia in obstetric patients.

+ Don't use a preparation containing a preservative for caudal epidural anesthesia.
+ Observe the arm or leg that has undergone regional anesthesia. Check its peripheral pulse, color, and temperature, and compare it to the unaffected arm or leg.
+ Don't administer a local anesthetic containing a vasoconstrictor in the fingers, toes, ears, nose, or penis.
+ Ensure that the gag reflex has returned before feeding a patient whose throat has been anesthetized.
+ Discard partially used vials of drug that contains no preservatives.
+ Monitor the patient with angina for anginal pain when giving a local anesthetic that contains a vasoconstrictor. Ensure that his nitroglycerin is nearby.
+ Reassure the patient that a burning sensation at the injection site is normal with the use of a local anesthetic that contains a vasoconstrictor.
+ Teach the patient and his caregiver about the drug. (See *Teaching a patient about local anesthetics.*)

Key nursing actions

+ Monitor cardiovascular and respiratory status.
+ Watch for evidence of CNS toxicity.
+ Keep resuscitation equipment and emergency drugs readily available.
+ Monitor the affected limb in regional anesthesia.
+ Make sure the gag reflex has returned before feeding the patient.
+ Keep nitroglycerin nearby and monitor the patient for angina when giving a local anesthetic with a vasoconstrictor.

TOPICAL ANESTHETICS

Applied directly to the skin or mucous membranes, topical anesthetics include benzocaine, benzyl alcohol, butacaine, butamben picrate, clove oil, cocaine, dibucaine, dyclonine, ethyl chloride, lidocaine, menthol, pramoxine, and tetracaine. Some injectable local anesthetics, such as lidocaine and tetracaine, also are effective topically.

All these drugs may be used alone to prevent or relieve minor pain. Some also are used in combination products for topical anesthesia. Tetracaine also is used as a topical ophthalmic anesthetic. Benzocaine is used with other drugs in several otic preparations.

Pharmacokinetics

Topical anesthetics produce little systemic absorption, except for cocaine when it's applied to mucous membranes. However, systemic absorption may occur if the patient receives frequent or high-dose applications to the eyes or large areas of burned or injured skin.

Tetracaine and other esters are metabolized extensively in the blood and to a lesser extent in the liver. Lidocaine and other amides are metabolized primarily in the liver. Both types of topical anesthetics are excreted in urine.

Pharmacodynamics

Benzocaine, butacaine, butamben, cocaine, dyclonine, and pramoxine produce topical anesthesia by blocking nerve impulse transmission. They accumulate in the nerve cell membrane, causing it to expand and lose its ability to depolarize, thus blocking impulse transmission. Dibucaine, lidocaine, and tetracaine may block impulse transmission across the nerve cell membranes.

The aromatic compounds, such as benzyl alcohol and clove oil, appear to stimulate nerve endings. This stimulation causes counterirritation that interferes with pain perception.

Ethyl chloride superficially freezes the tissue, stimulating the cold sensation receptors and blocking the nerve endings in the frozen area. Menthol selectively stimulates the sensory nerve endings for cold, causing a cool sensation and some local pain relief.

Pharmacotherapeutics

Topical anesthetics are used to relieve or prevent pain, especially minor burn pain; relieve itching and irritation; anesthetize an area before an injection is given; numb mucosal surfaces before a tube, such as a urinary catheter, is inserted; and relieve sore throat or mouth pain when used in a spray or solution.

Tetracaine also is used as a topical anesthetic for the eye. Benzocaine is used with other drugs in several ear preparations.

Interactions

Few drug interactions occur with topical anesthetics because they aren't absorbed well into the systemic circulation. However, these drugs should be used cautiously with class I antiarrhythmics, such as mexiletine and tocainide, because their interaction may produce additive—and possibly synergistic—toxic effects.

Adverse reactions

Adverse reactions to topical anesthetics vary with the chemical class. Drugs that also are used as local anesthetics may produce CNS and cardiovascular reactions.

Features of topical anesthetics

+ Are applied to the skin or mucous membranes
+ Are used to prevent or relieve minor pain, especially burn pain, itching, irritation
+ Are used to anesthetize an area before injection, numb mucous membrane before a tube is inserted, relieve throat or mouth pain (spray form)
+ May be used alone or in combination products
+ May block nerve impulse transmission (benzocaine, butacaine, butamben, cocaine, dyclonine, pramoxine)
+ May interfere with pain perception by irritating nerve endings (benzyl alcohol, clove oil)
+ May freeze tissue (ethyl chloride)

Teaching a patient about topical anesthetics

Whenever a topical anesthetic is prescribed, teach the patient and his family the drug's name, dose, frequency, action, and adverse effects, and take the following actions.
✦ Show the patient and his family how to apply a topical anesthetic if prescribed for home use. Instruct them to use it only as directed.
✦ Advise the patient to protect treated skin against inadvertent trauma from scratching, rubbing, or exposure to extreme temperatures.
✦ Discourage prolonged use without medical supervision.
✦ Advise the patient to keep the drug out of the reach of children to prevent ingestion and accidental poisoning.
✦ Advise the patient whose oropharyngeal mucosa has been anesthetized to delay eating for at least 1 hour or until sensation returns.
✦ Instruct the patient to notify the prescriber if adverse reactions occur.

Adverse reactions to watch for

✦ Burning
✦ Hypersensitivity reactions: rash, pruritus, urticaria, swelling of the mouth and throat, difficulty breathing
✦ Sloughing
✦ Stinging
✦ Tenderness

Key nursing actions

✦ If the patient has severe hepatic impairment, watch for a toxic lidocaine or prilocaine level.
✦ Use the lowest dose needed to relieve symptoms.
✦ Don't let the patient eat for 1 hour after anesthetic use in the mouth or throat.
✦ Stop the drug if a rash develops.

Benzyl alcohol can cause topical reactions such as skin irritation. Refrigerants, such as ethyl chloride, may produce frostbite in the application area.

Any topical anesthetic can cause burning, stinging, tenderness, or sloughing as well as a hypersensitivity reaction that may include a rash, pruritus, urticaria, swelling of the mouth and throat, and breathing difficulty.

Nursing considerations

✦ Don't use lidocaine or prilocaine on mucous membranes because this application increases absorption and the risk of adverse reactions.
✦ Don't use benzocaine, lidocaine, or prilocaine in a patient with congenital or idiopathic methemoglobinemia or in an infant younger than age 12 months who is receiving a drug that induces methemoglobin.
✦ Monitor the patient with severe hepatic impairment for a toxic lidocaine or prilocaine level because this disorder increases the risk of toxicity.
✦ Observe the patient regularly for adverse reactions.
✦ In a patient receiving a refrigerant, such as ethyl chloride, monitor for signs of localized frostbite; in a patient receiving another topical anesthetic, monitor for skin irritation and other topical reactions.
✦ Use the lowest dose necessary to relieve symptoms.
✦ Don't allow the patient to eat for 1 hour after anesthetic use in the mouth or throat because the drug may impair swallowing and increase the risk of aspiration.
✦ Discontinue use if a rash develops.
✦ Notify the prescriber if adverse reactions occur.
✦ Teach the patient and his caregiver about the prescribed drug. (See *Teaching a patient about topical anesthetics*.)

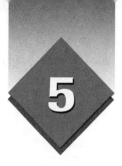

Cardiovascular drugs

Because cardiovascular disorders run the gamut from arrhythmias to hypertension, prescribers need a wide range of drugs to treat them. Cardiovascular drugs include inotropics, antiarrhythmics, antianginals, antihypertensives, and antilipemics. Each of these therapeutic categories consists of drugs from several classes. An understanding of the uses and functions of each drug class requires a working knowledge of the cardiovascular system.

ANATOMY AND PHYSIOLOGY

The heart, arteries, veins, and lymphatics make up the cardiovascular system. These structures transport life-supporting oxygen and nutrients to cells, remove metabolic waste products, and carry hormones from one part of the body to another. Because this system performs such vital functions, any problem with the heart or blood vessels can seriously affect a person's health.

Cardiac function depends on electrical impulse conduction throughout the myocardium. This electrical activity results in contraction of the heart and ejection of blood. (See *Structures of the heart*, page 156.)

Coronary arteries, which arise from the aorta and fill during diastole, supply blood to the myocardium. Coronary veins carry away the waste products of metabolism.

The kidneys dispose of these waste products and regulate the body's fluid and electrolyte balance. Blood enters the kidneys through the renal arteries and is filtered at the glomerulus. The filtrate enters the renal tubular system, where it's altered and concentrated or diluted. Then the concentrated or diluted urine leaves the kidneys through the renal pelvis and ureters to the bladder for excretion. Blood leaves the kidneys through the renal veins.

The kidneys also help regulate blood pressure through the renin-angiotensin-aldosterone system. They release the hormone renin in response to decreased renal blood flow or, more specifically, to a decreased glomerular filtration rate. Renin acts on the plasma protein angiotensinogen to form angiotensin I. Angiotensin I is con-

Anatomy and physiology highlights

♦ The cardiovascular system includes the heart, arteries, veins, and lymphatics.

♦ These structures transport nutrients, oxygen, and hormones to the tissues, and they remove metabolic waste products.

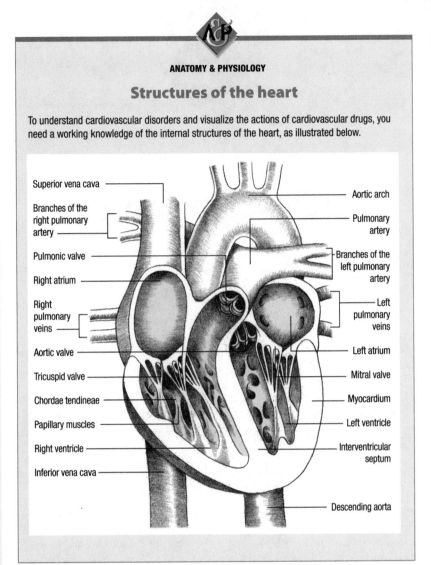

ANATOMY & PHYSIOLOGY

Structures of the heart

To understand cardiovascular disorders and visualize the actions of cardiovascular drugs, you need a working knowledge of the internal structures of the heart, as illustrated below.

Circulatory facts

+ Blood pressure is the force exerted by blood against vessel walls.
+ Blood ejected from the left side of the heart goes to peripheral circulation.
+ Blood ejected from the right side of the heart goes to pulmonary circulation.

verted to angiotensin II as it circulates through the lungs. Angiotensin II, a potent vasoconstrictor, increases peripheral resistance and promotes aldosterone excretion. Aldosterone, in turn, promotes the retention of sodium and water, increasing the volume of blood the heart needs to pump and raising the blood pressure.

Blood flow results from pressure differences in the circulatory system, which are caused by the force of the blood flow through the vessels and the force or resistance to that blood flow.

Blood pressure refers to the force exerted by the blood against the vessel walls. Cardiac output and peripheral resistance determine arterial blood pressure. Usually, an increase or decrease in cardiac output or peripheral resistance will increase or decrease blood pressure correspondingly. Similarly, increases or decreases in blood flow and tissue perfusion will accompany blood pressure changes. Cardiac output is a function of the heart rate and stroke volume.

Peripheral circulation refers to blood ejected from the left side of the heart. Pulmonary circulation refers to blood ejected from the right side.

In peripheral circulation, the heart pumps blood to all body tissues and organs except the lungs. Arteries and arterioles carry the blood away from the heart; capillaries allow the exchange of nutrients for cellular waste products; then the venules and veins return the blood to the right side of the heart.

In pulmonary circulation, the heart pumps blood to the lungs via the pulmonary arteries, and the pulmonary veins return the blood to the left side of the heart. Unlike peripheral circulation, pulmonary circulation uses the veins to carry oxygen-rich blood and the arteries to carry unoxygenated blood and waste products.

INOTROPICS

Inotropics increase the force of cardiac contraction; that is, they exert a positive inotropic effect. They also slow the heart rate, a negative chronotropic effect, and electrical impulse conduction through the atrioventricular (AV) node, a negative dromotropic effect. These actions make inotropics useful in treating heart failure and certain supraventricular arrhythmias.

Heart failure results from decreased cardiac output. It typically decreases myocardial contractility and increases preload (the amount of blood in the ventricles at the end of diastole, when the ventricles are full) and afterload (the resistance against which the left ventricle must eject blood during contraction). To try to maintain vital organ perfusion, the body compensates in other ways: It increases sympathetic tone and renin-angiotensin-aldosterone system activity and it causes ventricular dilation and hypertrophy. Although these compensations help maintain adequate blood flow, they increase the work of the myocardium. Eventually, the patient's condition worsens and requires drug treatment. When this occurs, the prescriber may use inotropics to improve myocardial contractility.

In supraventricular arrhythmias, such as atrial fibrillation or atrial flutter, inotropics are used to slow electrical impulse conduction through the AV node. By doing so, they slow the ventricular rate.

Inotropic drugs include the digitalis glycoside digoxin and the bipyridine derivatives inamrinone and milrinone.

DIGOXIN

The inotropic drug digoxin is used to treat heart failure and supraventricular arrhythmias.

Pharmacokinetics

Intestinal absorption of digoxin varies greatly with the drug form. Capsules are about 90% to 100% absorbed; elixir and tablets are about 60% to 85% absorbed. Capsules produce a higher peak concentration than elixir and tablets do. Patients commonly show variations in digoxin level, therapeutic effects, and toxic effects. The drug is distributed widely throughout the body, reaching its highest level in the heart muscle, liver, and kidneys. It's poorly bound to plasma proteins. A small amount of digoxin is metabolized by the liver and GI flora. Most of the drug is excreted unchanged by the kidneys.

Pharmacodynamics

Digoxin is used to treat heart failure by boosting intracellular calcium at the cell membrane, which strengthens ventricular contractions. It may also enhance calci-

Features of inotropics
+ Increase the force of cardiac contraction (positive inotropic effect)
+ Slow the heart rate (negative chronotropic effect)
+ Slow conduction through the AV node (negative dromotropic effect)
+ Are used for heart failure and certain supraventricular arrhythmias, such as atrial fibrillation and atrial flutter

Features of digoxin
+ Strengthens ventricular contractions by increasing intracellular calcium at the cell membrane, increasing movement of calcium into myocardial cells, and possibly increasing norepinephrine at adrenergic nerve terminals
+ Produces variable drug levels and effects based on patient response
+ Is typically used for heart failure, supraventricular arrhythmias, and paroxysmal atrial tachycardia

Contraindications and precautions for digoxin

Digoxin is contraindicated in patients with ventricular fibrillation or multifocal atrial tachycardia.

The drug requires cautious use in patients with severe pulmonary disease, hypoxia, myxedema, acute myocardial infarction, severe heart failure, acute myocarditis, chronic constrictive pericarditis, acute glomerulonephritis and heart failure, idiopathic hypertrophic subaortic stenosis, incomplete atrioventricular block, increased carotid sinus sensitivity, or frequent premature ventricular contractions or ventricular tachycardia.

I.V. digoxin requires cautious use in patients with hypertension.

Possible drug interactions

- Amiodarone
- Amphotericin B
- Antacids
- Barbiturates
- Beta blockers
- Calcium channel blockers
- Calcium preparations
- Cholestyramine resin
- Clarithromycin
- Cyclosporine
- Erythromycin
- Hydroxychloroquine
- Itraconazole
- Kaolin and pectin
- Metoclopramide
- Neomycin
- Omeprazole
- Potassium-wasting diuretics
- Propafenone
- Quinidine
- Rifampin
- Spironolactone
- Steroids
- Succinylcholine
- Sulfasalazine
- Tetracycline
- Thyroid preparations
- Verapamil

um movement into the myocardial cells and may stimulate the release — or block the reuptake — of norepinephrine at adrenergic nerve terminals.

Digoxin acts on the central nervous system (CNS) to slow the heart rate, thus making it useful for treating supraventricular arrhythmias, such as atrial fibrillation and atrial flutter. It also increases the refractory period.

Pharmacotherapeutics

Digoxin is mainly used to treat heart failure and supraventricular arrhythmias, but also paroxysmal atrial tachycardia. However, the drug can't be used in some patients and requires cautious use in others. (See *Contraindications and precautions for digoxin.*)

Interactions

- Rifampin, barbiturates, cholestyramine resin, antacids, kaolin and pectin, sulfasalazine, neomycin, and metoclopramide can reduce digoxin's therapeutic effects.
- Calcium preparations, quinidine, verapamil, cyclosporine, tetracycline, clarithromycin, propafenone, amiodarone, spironolactone, hydroxychloroquine, erythromycin, itraconazole, and omeprazole increase the risk of digoxin toxicity.
- When taken with digoxin, amphotericin B, potassium-wasting diuretics, or steroids may cause hypokalemia and increase the risk of digoxin toxicity.
- Together, digoxin and a beta blocker or calcium channel blocker may cause an excessively slow heart rate and arrhythmias.
- When given with digoxin, succinylcholine and thyroid preparations increase the risk of arrhythmias.
- St. John's wort may increase digoxin's metabolism and decrease its therapeutic effects.
- Siberian ginseng may falsely elevate digoxin assays or increase the plasma drug level; it shouldn't be used with the drug.

Adverse reactions

Because digoxin has a narrow therapeutic index, the drug may produce digoxin toxicity. To prevent this toxicity, individualize the dosage based on the patient's digoxin level. The therapeutic digoxin level typically ranges from 0.5 to 2 ng/ml. However, patients vary greatly in their response to digoxin. A level that's therapeutic in one patient may cause toxicity in another.

WARNING

Recognizing signs and symptoms of digoxin toxicity

Digoxin toxicity usually produces cardiac, gastrointestinal, and neurologic signs and symptoms. To prevent severe or even life-threatening effects, be prepared to recognize the signs and symptoms listed below. Also assess the patient for the most common early indicators of toxicity: anorexia, nausea, vomiting, and diarrhea.

CARDIAC
- Accelerated junctional rhythms
- Atrial tachycardia with atrioventricular (AV) block
- Second-degree AV block (Wenckebach)
- Sinoatrial arrest or block
- Third-degree AV block (complete)
- Ventricular arrhythmias

GASTROINTESTINAL
- Abdominal pain
- Anorexia
- Diarrhea
- Nausea
- Vomiting

NEUROLOGIC
- Blue-yellow color blindness
- Blurred vision
- Colored dots in vision
- Coma
- Confusion
- Depression
- Disorientation
- Flickering lights
- Headache
- Insomnia
- Irritability
- Lethargy
- Personality change
- Psychosis
- Restlessness
- Seizures
- White halos on dark objects

The following conditions may predispose a patient to digoxin toxicity: hypokalemia, hypomagnesemia, hypothyroidism, hypoxemia, hypercalcemia, advanced myocardial disease, active myocardial ischemia, and altered autonomic (increased vagal) tone. Elevated sympathetic tone and hyperthyroidism may cause resistance to the drug's effect.

The signs and symptoms of digoxin toxicity fall primarily into three categories: GI, neurologic, and cardiac. (See *Recognizing signs and symptoms of digoxin toxicity.*) The GI and neurologic symptoms may precede or follow the potentially life-threatening cardiac symptoms.

Less common and less severe adverse reactions to digoxin include gynecomastia and hypersensitivity reactions, such as rash, fever, and eosinophilia.

Nursing considerations

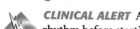 **CLINICAL ALERT** Assess the patient's baseline apical heart rate and rhythm before starting digoxin therapy. Then, take the apical rate before giving each dose. Stop the drug and notify the prescriber if the pulse rate falls below 60 beats/minute or the minimum specified by the prescriber.

- Monitor the patient's digoxin level. To avoid a falsely elevated level, draw blood at least 8 hours after the last oral dose or preferably immediately before giving the daily maintenance dosage (about 24 hours after the last dose).

The importance of the digoxin level
- Digoxin has a narrow therapeutic range, typically 0.5 to 2 ng/ml.
- A level that's therapeutic in one patient may be toxic in another.
- Dosage must be individualized.
- To obtain an accurate drug level, draw blood just before giving the daily maintenance dose or at least 8 hours after last oral dose.
- Some conditions predispose a patient to toxic effects: active myocardial ischemia, advanced myocardial disease, hypercalcemia, hypokalemia, hypomagnesemia, hypothyroidism, hypoxemia, increased vagal tone.

Key nursing actions

+ Assess the baseline apical heart rate before starting digoxin and before giving each dose.
+ Give lower doses of capsules and elixir because they have higher bioavailability.
+ Don't give digoxin I.M.
+ Give the I.V. form over 5 minutes.
+ Notify the prescriber about evidence of toxicity, adverse reactions, and new arrhythmias.

PATIENT TEACHING

Teaching a patient about digoxin

Whenever digoxin is prescribed, teach the patient and his family the drug's name, dose, frequency, action, and adverse effects. Also take the following actions.
+ Show the patient how to take his pulse. Advise him to report a pulse rate below 60 beats/minute, a change in pulse regularity, or signs and symptoms of digoxin toxicity.
+ Instruct the patient to recognize and report the following signs of heart failure: persistent cough; shortness of breath; weight gain of 1 to 2 pounds in 1 day or 5 pounds in a week; swelling of the ankles, legs, or hands; loss of appetite; nausea; and the sensation of abdominal fullness.
+ Teach the patient treated for supraventricular arrhythmias to recognize and report signs of recurrence, such as a rapid heart rate, light-headedness, fluttering in the chest, excessive fatigue, or chest pain.
+ Encourage the patient to eat high-potassium foods, such as orange juice, bananas, spinach, cantaloupe, watermelon, dates, raisins, soybeans, apples, prunes, beans, potatoes, molasses, and squash.
+ Instruct the patient to store digoxin in a tightly covered, light-resistant container and to consult his prescriber before taking herbal remedies, dietary supplements, or over-the-counter medications.
+ Instruct the patient not to substitute one brand of digoxin for another.
+ Tell the patient to avoid using St. John's wort, Siberian ginseng, and other herbal remedies. If he has been using an herbal preparation and has been stabilized on digoxin, advise him not to suddenly discontinue the herbal remedy without alerting his prescriber. His digoxin level may need to be monitored closely.

Giving digoxin to a child

+ To avoid a high peak level in a pediatric patient, give digoxin for maintenance in two divided doses each day.
+ Adjust the loading dose appropriately.

+ Adjust the loading dose in a child, geriatric patient, or a patient with renal failure, heart failure, or hypoalbuminemia, because these conditions affect the volume of drug distribution.
+ Give lower dosages of digoxin capsules and elixir because they have a higher bioavailability than tablets do.
+ Don't give intramuscular (I.M.) digoxin because it causes severe pain at the injection site and increases the creatine phosphokinase level; these effects can complicate interpretation of enzyme levels.
+ Give digoxin in two divided doses for maintenance in a child to avoid a high peak level.
+ Give the intravenous (I.V.) form over 5 minutes, taking care to avoid extravasation, which can cause irritation, necrosis, and sloughing.
+ Monitor the patient for adverse reactions, including signs and symptoms of digoxin toxicity.
+ Stop the drug, notify the prescriber, and obtain the drug level if digoxin toxicity is suspected.
+ Notify the prescriber if new arrhythmias occur during therapy. Also notify him when normal sinus rhythm returns.
+ Teach the patient and his caregiver about the prescribed drug. (See *Teaching a patient about digoxin.*)

INAMRINONE AND MILRINONE

These inotropics typically are used for short-term heart failure management or long-term heart failure management in patients awaiting heart transplantation. Be-

WARNING

Contraindications and precautions for inamrinone and milrinone

Both drugs are contraindicated in patients who are hypersensitive to them. Inamrinone also is contraindicated in those who are hypersensitive to sulfites.

Both drugs should be used cautiously in patients with hypertrophic subaortic stenosis. Inamrinone also requires cautious use in patients with acute myocardial infarction.

cause thrombocytopenia is more common in patients taking inamrinone, this drug is the less desirable choice.

Pharmacokinetics

After I.V. administration, inamrinone produces its onset of action in 2 to 5 minutes and peak effects in about 10 minutes. Its action lasts 30 minutes to 2 hours. The drug is distributed rapidly and is 10% to 49% bound to plasma proteins. Inamrinone is metabolized by the liver and excreted by the kidneys.

After I.V. administration, milrinone produces its onset of action in 5 to 15 minutes and peak effects in 1 to 2 hours. The drug's duration of action is 3 to 6 hours. It's distributed rapidly and is about 70% bound to plasma proteins. The kidneys excrete milrinone, primarily as unchanged drug.

Pharmacodynamics

Inamrinone and milrinone improve cardiac output by strengthening contractions. These drugs may help move calcium into the cardiac cell or may increase calcium storage in the sarcoplasmic reticulum. By directly relaxing vascular smooth muscle, they also decrease preload and afterload.

Pharmacotherapeutics

Both inotropics are used for short-term management of heart failure in patients who haven't responded adequately to treatment with digoxin, diuretics, or vasodilators. For safe therapy, however, the prescriber must observe certain limitations. (See *Contraindications and precautions for inamrinone and milrinone*.)

Interactions

✦ Inamrinone may interact with disopyramide and cause hypotension.
✦ Because inamrinone and milrinone reduce the potassium level, taking them with a potassium-wasting diuretic may lead to hypokalemia.

Adverse reactions

Adverse reactions are uncommon and usually occur only during prolonged therapy. Inamrinone and milrinone can produce arrhythmias and should be stopped if they occur. Other adverse reactions may include nausea, vomiting, headache, fever, chest pain, hypokalemia, thrombocytopenia (more common with inamrinone), and a mild increase in heart rate. Inamrinone may also increase liver enzyme levels and cause burning at the injection site. These effects, however, are uncommon. Ex-

Features of inamrinone and milrinone

✦ Improve cardiac output by strengthening contractions
✦ May help move calcium into cardiac cells or may increase calcium storage in the sarcoplasmic reticulum
✦ Are used for short-term management of heart failure
✦ Are also used for long-term management of heart failure in patients awaiting heart transplantation

Possible drug interactions

✦ Disopyramide
✦ Potassium-wasting diuretics

Adverse reactions to watch for

✦ Arrhythmias
✦ Burning at injection site
✦ Chest pain
✦ Fever
✦ Headache
✦ Hypersensitivity reactions: ascites, pericarditis, pleurisy
✦ Hypokalemia
✦ Hypotension
✦ Increased heart rate
✦ Increased liver enzyme levels
✦ Nausea, vomiting
✦ Thrombocytopenia

cessive vasodilation may lead to hypotension, which may require dosage reduction or drug discontinuation.

Patients on prolonged therapy with inamrinone and milrinone may experience hypersensitivity reactions with such signs and symptoms as pericarditis, pleurisy, and ascites.

Key nursing actions
✦ Correct hypokalemia.
✦ Monitor the heart rate and rhythm, blood pressure, and ECG often.
✦ Watch for petechiae, ecchymosis, and changes in the platelet count.

Nursing considerations
✦ Obtain a platelet count and liver enzyme, electrolyte, blood urea nitrogen (BUN), and creatinine levels before therapy begins. Monitor these test results throughout therapy.
✦ Correct hypokalemia before or during therapy.
✦ Frequently monitor the patient's heart rate, heart rhythm, and blood pressure to detect arrhythmias or hypotension. Also monitor the patient's electrocardiogram (ECG) tracings to detect arrhythmias. Notify the prescriber if the patient develops hypotension or arrhythmias. The dosage may need to be decreased or stopped.
✦ Monitor the patient for therapeutic responses: increased blood pressure; decreased pulmonary venous congestion, pulmonary artery pressure, and pulmonary artery wedge pressure; decreased systemic venous congestion and central venous pressure; increased urine output; decreased weight, peripheral edema, and dyspnea; and elimination of S_3 and basilar crackles.
✦ Assess the patient for petechiae or ecchymosis. Note changes in the patient's platelet count. A platelet count below 150,000/mm³ usually requires the dosage to be reduced, below 100,000/mm³ usually requires the drug to be stopped.
✦ Teach the patient and his caregiver about the prescribed drug. (See *Teaching a patient about inamrinone and milrinone.*)

Facts about arrhythmias
✦ High degree of morbidity and mortality
✦ May be supraventricular (originating in atria, SA node, or AV node) or ventricular
✦ Supraventricular have less effect on cardiac function and output than ventricular

ANTIARRHYTHMICS

Arrhythmias have a high degree of morbidity and mortality. They may be classified as tachyarrhythmias, in which the heart rate is increased, or bradyarrhythmias, in which the heart rate is decreased.

Supraventricular arrhythmias originate in the atria, sinoatrial (SA) node, or AV node. They include supraventricular tachycardia, atrial flutter, and atrial fibrillation. Ventricular arrhythmias include sustained ventricular tachycardia, premature ventricular contractions, and ventricular fibrillation. Supraventricular arrhythmias don't affect cardiac function and output as much as ventricular arrhythmias do. Also, they aren't as likely to be life-threatening.

Although ischemia is the most common cause of arrhythmias, other causes include congenital cardiac conditions, cardiac trauma or surgery, cardiomyopathy, electrolyte or acid-base imbalances, adverse drug reactions, emboli, invasive cardiac diagnostic tests, cardiac valvular diseases, alcoholism, respiratory diseases, and viral infections.

Antiarrhythmics are used to treat abnormal electrical activity of the heart. Specifically, they're used to treat, suppress, or prevent three major mechanisms of arrhythmias: increased automaticity, decreased conductivity, and reentry. They limit cardiac electrical activity to normal conduction pathways and decrease abnormally fast heart rates. Although mainly prescribed for adults, these drugs may be prescribed for children.

Although these drugs can correct an arrhythmia, the underlying condition also must be treated to eliminate the need for continued therapy. Because most antiarrhythmics also can cause new arrhythmias or worsen existing ones, the prescriber must weigh the benefits against the risks.

Antiarrhythmics are categorized into four classes—I (which includes class IA, IB, and IC), II, III, and IV—and adenosine, an AV nodal drug. A few drugs exhibit properties common to more than one class.

CLASS IA ANTIARRHYTHMICS

Class IA antiarrhythmics are used to treat a wide variety of atrial and ventricular arrhythmias. These antiarrhythmics include disopyramide, procainamide, and quinidine.

Pharmacokinetics

When given orally, class IA drugs are rapidly absorbed and metabolized. Their onset of action occurs within 30 minutes. The duration of action ranges from 3 hours for procainamide to 6 to 8 hours for quinidine and disopyramide. Disopyramide and procainamide are 90% absorbed. Quinidine is almost completely absorbed, but the absorption rate depends on the salt with which it's combined.

These drugs are distributed through all body tissues, except for quinidine, which doesn't cross the blood-brain barrier. Protein binding for disopyramide is 20% to 60%, for procainamide is 20%, and for quinidine is 90%.

All class IA antiarrhythmics are metabolized in the liver and excreted unchanged by the kidneys.

Pharmacodynamics

Class IA antiarrhythmics control arrhythmias by altering the myocardial cell membrane and interfering with autonomic nervous system control of pacemaker cells. These antiarrhythmics also block parasympathetic stimulation of the SA and AV nodes. Because stimulation of the parasympathetic nervous system causes the heart rate to slow, drugs that block the parasympathetic nervous system increase the conduction rate of the AV node.

Pharmacotherapeutics

Antiarrhythmics in class IA are prescribed to treat such arrhythmias as premature atrial and ventricular contractions, ventricular tachycardia, atrial fibrillation, atrial flutter, and paroxysmal supraventricular tachycardia. Disopyramide and procainamide are used primarily to treat life-threatening, sustained ventricular tachycardia.

What causes arrhythmias?

+ Ischemia (most common)
+ Adverse drug reactions
+ Alcoholism
+ Cardiac trauma or surgery
+ Cardiac valvular diseases
+ Cardiomyopathy
+ Congenital cardiac conditions
+ Electrolyte or acid-base imbalances
+ Emboli
+ Invasive cardiac diagnostic tests
+ Respiratory diseases
+ Viral infections

Features of class IA antiarrhythmics

+ Alter the myocardial cell membrane, interfere with autonomic nervous system control of pacemaker cells, and block parasympathetic stimulation of SA and AV nodes
+ Are used for many atrial and ventricular arrhythmias, including premature contractions, atrial fibrillation and flutter, paroxysmal supraventricular tachycardia, and life-threatening ventricular tachycardia

Spotting cinchonism

Cinchonism is a reaction to cinchona alkaloids, such as the antiarrhythmic quinidine. To spot these quinidine-related reactions, assess the patient for:
+ Fever
+ Headache
+ Light-headedness
+ Tinnitus
+ Vertigo
+ Vision disturbances.
   These signs of cinchonism are most likely to appear after the first dose or with quinidine toxicity. Syncope also may occur, probably from transient ventricular tachycardia or ectopy.

Possible drug interactions
+ Anticholinergics
+ Digoxin
+ Macrolide antibiotics
+ Neuromuscular blockers
+ Phenobarbital
+ Phenytoin
+ Rifampin
+ Verapamil

Interactions
+ Disopyramide taken with an anticholinergic may increase anticholinergic effects.
+ The combination of disopyramide and verapamil may produce additive myocardial depression and should be avoided.
+ When taken with a macrolide antibiotic, disopyramide may prolong the QT interval.
+ Together with a neuromuscular blocker, quinidine may increase skeletal muscle relaxation.
+ Quinidine increases the risk of digoxin toxicity.
+ Rifampin, phenytoin, or phenobarbital can reduce the effects of quinidine and disopyramide.
+ Grapefruit juice may delay quinidine's onset of action.

Adverse reactions to watch for
+ Anticholinergic effects
+ Arrhythmias
+ Cinchonism
+ GI changes: anorexia, bitter taste, cramping, diarrhea, nausea, vomiting
+ Hypotension
+ Prolonged QT interval

Adverse reactions
Reactions to class IA antiarrhythmics include anticholinergic effects, GI changes, and reactions unique to quinidine's source, cinchona. (See *Spotting cinchonism.*)

   The anticholinergic effect of disopyramide commonly produces dry mouth, blurred vision, constipation, urinary hesitancy, and urine retention. The drug's negative inotropic effect combined with increased peripheral vasoconstriction sometimes result in heart failure, hypotension, chest pain, edema, and dyspnea.

   The class IA antiarrhythmics, especially quinidine, may produce GI symptoms, such as diarrhea, cramping, nausea, vomiting, anorexia, and bitter taste.

   Procainamide, especially the I.V. form, can produce hypotension. The drug's negative inotropic effect less commonly leads to heart failure. Because I.V. quinidine may lead to severe hypotension and cardiovascular collapse, the drug rarely is given this way.

   All class IA antiarrhythmics can induce arrhythmias, especially conduction delays that may compound existing heart blocks. Apparent conduction through the AV node may be increased. This increase may precipitate a dangerously high ventricular rate. As the effective refractory period and the action potential duration increase, the ECG reflects a prolonged QT interval. This is a precursor to a type of ventricular tachycardia known as torsades de pointes.

   Up to 30% of patients using procainamide experience an adverse reaction that mimics systemic lupus erythematosus (SLE). Signs and symptoms include pain in

Systemic lupus erthematous-like adverse effects of procainamide
+ Blood dyscrasias
+ Dyspnea
+ Fever
+ Headache
+ Pain in small joints
+ Pericardial effusion
+ Pleuritic pain
+ Positive antinuclear antibody titer

Teaching a patient about class IA antiarrhythmics

Whenever a class IA antiarrhythmic is prescribed, teach the patient and his family the drug's name, dose, frequency, action, and adverse effects. Also take the following actions.

◆ Demonstrate how to take a pulse. Tell the patient to measure his pulse before taking the prescribed antiarrhythmic. Advise him to notify the prescriber if his pulse is irregular or slower than 60 beats/minute or the rate selected by the prescriber.

◆ Instruct the patient to weigh himself daily, at the same time every day and in similar clothes, to detect fluid retention. Advise him to notify the prescriber of a sudden weight gain of 2 pounds or more in 1 day, shortness of breath, or peripheral edema.

◆ Stress the importance of regularly testing the drug level and obtaining an electrocardiogram to detect abnormalities.

◆ Instruct the patient to take the prescribed drug around-the-clock rather than just during the day to maintain a therapeutic drug level.

◆ Advise the family that the drug may cause confusion in a geriatric patient. Instruct them to take safety measures, such as increased supervision, and to notify the prescriber if the patient becomes confused.

◆ Teach the patient how to manage the anticholinergic effects, such as dry mouth and constipation. Also advise him to report signs of urine retention, such as urinary frequency and a sensation of bladder fullness after voiding.

◆ Teach the patient to recognize and report any signs of drug-induced systemic lupus erythematosus before taking the next dose of procainamide.

◆ Teach the patient to recognize signs of infection and bleeding, especially during procainamide therapy.

◆ Teach the patient to recognize and report signs of cinchonism before taking the next dose of quinidine.

◆ Instruct the patient not to take the drug with food.

◆ Advise the patient receiving sustained-release tablets or capsules that the wax matrix may be excreted intact in the stool. Tell him that this is normal and that the body has absorbed the entire drug.

◆ Instruct a woman of childbearing age to notify the prescriber if she is pregnant or plans to become pregnant.

◆ Tell the patient not to take quinidine with grapefruit juice.

---

small joints, pleuritic pain, dyspnea, fever, headache, pericardial effusion, blood dyscrasias, and positive antinuclear antibody titers. This reaction, called drug-induced lupus erythematosuslike syndrome, is not dose-dependent and resolves when procainamide is stopped. Rarely, quinidine also causes lupuslike symptoms and hypersensitivity reactions manifested by fever, blood dyscrasias, skin eruptions, liver disorders, and anaphylaxis. Class IA antiarrhythmics can precipitate heart failure and can produce confusion in geriatric patients.

Nursing considerations

◆ Teach the patient and his caregiver about the prescribed drug. (See *Teaching a patient about class IA antiarrhythmics.*)

◆ Assess the patient for early signs of heart failure, such as hypotension, edema, and irregular heartbeat.

Key nursing actions

◆ Watch for evidence of heart failure.

◆ Monitor ECG tracings for an increased ventricular rate, prolonged QT interval, and conduction disturbances.

◆ Assess electrolyte levels.

◆ Monitor the drug level.

◆ Check patient for SLE-like syndrome (with procainamide therapy).

◆ Watch for evidence of cinchonism.

✦ Monitor the patient's ECG tracing for an increased ventricular rate, a QT interval 50% longer than normal, and conduction disturbances.

✦ Monitor the patient's electrolyte levels closely when therapy begins and if a diuretic is given. Electrolyte abnormalities, especially hypokalemia, can bring about arrhythmias.

✦ Closely monitor the patient's drug level to detect early signs of toxicity. Notify the prescriber if the level falls outside the therapeutic range.

✦ Observe the patients for signs of drug-induced lupus erythematosuslike syndrome during procainamide therapy.

✦ Monitor the patient for signs of cinchonism during quinidine therapy.

✦ Don't give the drug with food because food may affect absorption.

CLASS IB ANTIARRHYTHMICS

These antiarrhythmics are used to treat ventricular arrhythmias. They include lidocaine, mexiletine, and tocainide.

Pharmacokinetics

After oral administration, most class IB antiarrhythmics are absorbed well from the GI tract. Because lidocaine undergoes significant first-pass metabolism in the liver, it's only given parenterally. Lidocaine's onset of action is 45 to 90 seconds; its duration of action is 10 to 20 minutes. Tocainide's peak level occurs in 30 minutes to 2 hours if the drug is taken on an empty stomach; 2 to 4 hours if it's taken with food. Mexiletine's peak level occurs in 2 to 3 hours.

Lidocaine is distributed widely throughout the body, especially to highly perfused tissues such as the kidneys, lungs, liver, and heart. It readily crosses the blood-brain barrier. Lidocaine and mexiletine are moderately bound to plasma proteins. Tocainide, on the other hand, is mostly unbound.

Class IB antiarrhythmics are metabolized in the liver and excreted in urine.

Pharmacodynamics

Class IB drugs work by blocking the rapid influx of sodium ions during the depolarization phase of the heart's depolarization-repolarization cycle. This results in a shorter refractory period, which reduces the risk of arrhythmias. (See *How lidocaine works.*)

Pharmacotherapeutics

These antiarrhythmics are used to treat ectopic ventricular beats, ventricular tachycardia, and ventricular fibrillation.

Interactions

✦ A class IB antiarrhythmic may exhibit additive or antagonistic effects when given with another antiarrhythmic, such as phenytoin, procainamide, propranolol, or quinidine.

✦ Rifampin may reduce the effects of mexiletine or tocainide.

✦ When given with mexiletine, theophylline's level may increase.

✦ Use of a beta blocker or disopyramide with mexiletine may reduce cardiac contractility.

Adverse reactions

All class IB antiarrhythmics pose a relatively high risk of CNS disturbances, especially drowsiness, confusion, light-headedness, paresthesia, slurred speech, vision and hearing disturbances, tremor, seizures, and coma. Reducing the dosage or stop-

---

Features of class IB antiarrhythmics

✦ Block the rapid influx of sodium ions during depolarization, shortening the refractory period

✦ Are used for ectopic ventricular beats, ventricular tachycardia, ventricular fibrillation

Possible drug interactions

✦ Antiarrhythmics
✦ Beta blockers
✦ Disopyramide
✦ Rifampin
✦ Theophylline

Adverse reactions to watch for

✦ Allergic skin reactions
✦ AV block
✦ Ataxia
✦ Bradycardia
✦ Coma
✦ Confusion
✦ Drowsiness
✦ GI distress
✦ Hearing disturbances
✦ Hypotension
✦ Light-headedness
✦ Paresthesia
✦ Respiratory arrest
✦ Seizures
✦ Slurred speech
✦ Tremor
✦ Vision disturbances

How lidocaine works

Lidocaine works in injured or ischemic myocardial cells to retard sodium influx and restore cardiac rhythm. Normally, the ventricles contract in response to impulses from the sinoatrial (SA) node. But when tissue damage occurs in the ventricles, ischemic cells can create an ectopic pacemaker, which can trigger ventricular arrhythmias. The illustrations below show how these arrhythmias develop at the cellular level — and how lidocaine suppresses them.

ISCHEMIC MYOCARDIAL CELL

Normal myocardial cells permit a limited amount of sodium ions to enter, which leads to controlled depolarization. Ischemic myocardial cells allow a rapid infusion of sodium ions. This causes the cells to depolarize much more quickly than normal and then begin firing spontaneously. The result: a ventricular arrhythmia.

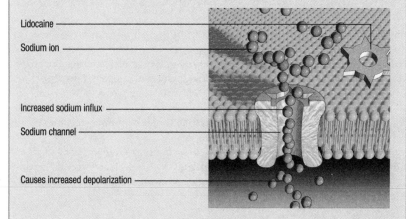

Lidocaine

Sodium ion

Increased sodium influx

Sodium channel

Causes increased depolarization

ISCHEMIC MYOCARDIAL CELL WITH LIDOCAINE

By slowing sodium's influx, lidocaine raises the cells' electrical stimulation threshold (EST). The increased EST prolongs depolarization in the ischemic cells and returns control to the SA node, the heart's main pacemaker.

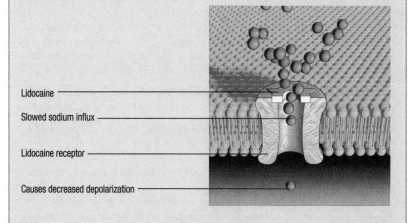

Lidocaine

Slowed sodium influx

Lidocaine receptor

Causes decreased depolarization

Teaching a patient about class IB antiarrhythmics

Whenever a class IB antiarrhythmic is prescribed, teach the patient and his family the drug's name, dose, frequency, action, and adverse effects. Also take the following actions.

✦ Advise the patient not to perform activities that require alertness if adverse CNS reactions occur.

✦ Inform the family or caregiver that the antiarrhythmic may cause confusion.

✦ Teach the patient and his family to recognize and report signs of toxicity, such as decreased level of consciousness, seizures, and vision or hearing disturbances. Reassure them that these reactions will disappear when the dosage is reduced or the drug is stopped.

✦ Instruct the patient to take mexiletine or tocainide with food or an antacid.

ping the drug reverses these reactions. Hypotension and bradycardia sometimes occur.

Lidocaine toxicity can cause seizures and respiratory arrest, requiring the use of resuscitation equipment. Mexiletine or tocainide can cause upper GI distress, which usually is relieved by taking the drug with food or antacids. Adverse reactions to mexiletine commonly include hypotension, AV block, bradycardia, confusion, ataxia, and diplopia. Adverse reactions to tocainide commonly include GI distress and CNS and cerebellar effects.

Tocainide can lead to two rare but serious reactions: blood dyscrasias and pulmonary fibrosis. These disappear when the drug is stopped. Drug fever and hepatitis may occur after tocainide therapy. Tocainide or mexiletine may produce allergic skin reactions.

Nursing considerations

✦ Closely monitor the patient for CNS disturbances, sensory or perceptual alterations (such as vision or hearing disturbances or paresthesias), and other adverse reactions.

✦ Monitor the patient's potassium level because hypokalemia exacerbates arrhythmias.

✦ Give lidocaine I.V. to avoid interfering with the cardiac enzyme measurements used to help diagnose an acute myocardial infarction (MI). If the drug must be given I.M., use the deltoid muscle rather than the gluteus or vastus lateralis muscles because the drug reaches a higher level more rapidly with deltoid administration.

 CLINICAL ALERT Don't use a lidocaine solution that contains epinephrine when lidocaine is prescribed to treat arrhythmias; such solutions are for local anesthesia only.

✦ Give a continuous I.V. infusion using an infusion pump, and monitor the patient's ECG constantly.

✦ Reduce the dosage for a patient with heart failure, cardiogenic shock, liver disease, or severe renal or hepatic impairment.

✦ Give mexiletine or tocainide with food or antacids to reduce GI distress.

✦ Reassure the patient with sensory and perceptual hallucinations that these reactions should disappear with dosage reduction or drug discontinuation.

Key nursing actions

✦ Watch for CNS disturbances and other adverse reactions.

✦ Monitor the potassium level.

✦ Give a continuous I.V. infusion using a pump, and monitor the ECG continuously.

✦ Give lidocaine I.V. to avoid interfering with cardiac enzyme assessments.

✦ Teach the patient and his caregiver about the prescribed drug. (See *Teaching a patient about class IB antiarrhythmics*.)

CLASS IC ANTIARRHYTHMICS

To treat certain severe, refractory ventricular arrhythmias, prescribers may choose from the class IC antiarrhythmics. They include flecainide, moricizine, and propafenone. Moricizine has properties of all three subclasses (A, B, and C).

Pharmacokinetics

After oral administration, class IC antiarrhythmics are absorbed well, distributed in varying degrees, and probably metabolized by the liver. They're excreted primarily in urine, except for propafenone, which is excreted primarily in feces.

After oral administration, about 38% of moricizine is absorbed. It undergoes extensive metabolism, with less than 1% of a dose excreted unchanged in urine. The drug is highly protein-bound, leaving only a small portion free to produce its antiarrhythmic effect.

Pharmacodynamics

Class IC antiarrhythmics primarily slow conduction along the heart's conduction system. Moricizine decreases the fast inward current of sodium ions of the action potential, depressing the depolarization rate and effective refractory period.

Pharmacotherapeutics

Like class IB antiarrhythmics, class IC antiarrhythmics are used to treat life-threatening ventricular arrhythmias. For example, moricizine is used to manage sustained ventricular tachycardia. These drugs also are used to treat supraventricular arrhythmias. In addition, flecainide may be used to prevent paroxysmal supraventricular tachycardia (PSVT) in patients without structural heart disease. However, some patients shouldn't receive these drugs. (See *Precautions for class IC antiarrhythmics*.)

Interactions

✦ A class IC antiarrhythmic may exhibit additive effects when given with another antiarrhythmic.
✦ When used with digoxin, flecainide and propafenone increase the risk of digoxin toxicity.
✦ Quinidine increases the effects of propafenone.
✦ Cimetidine may increase the moricizine level and the risk of moricizine toxicity.

Features of class IC antiarrhythmics

✦ Slow conduction
✦ Are used for life-threatening ventricular arrhythmias, supraventricular arrhythmias, prevention of paroxysmal supraventricular tachycardia (in patients without structural disease)

Possible drug interactions

✦ Antiarrhythmics
✦ Cimetidine
✦ Digoxin
✦ Metoprolol
✦ Propranolol
✦ Quinidine
✦ Theophylline

Teaching a patient about class IC antiarrhythmics

Whenever a class IC antiarrhythmic is prescribed, teach the patient and his family the drug's name, dose, frequency, action, and adverse effects. Also take the following actions.

✦ Demonstrate how to take a pulse and tell the patient to do this before taking each dose of the prescribed antiarrhythmic. Advise him to notify the prescriber if his pulse is irregular or slower than 60 beats/minute.

✦ Stress the importance of taking the drug exactly as prescribed. Instruct the patient to notify the prescriber if he forgets a dose.

✦ Teach the patient who takes digoxin with flecainide or propafenone to watch for and report signs of digoxin toxicity.

✦ Instruct the patient taking propafenone and an oral anticoagulant to have regular prothrombin time testing to detect bleeding problems.

✦ Reassure the patient that adverse central nervous system (CNS) reactions, such as altered taste, may disappear if the propafenone dosage is reduced.

✦ Instruct the patient to avoid activities that require mental alertness if dizziness, blurred vision, or other CNS reactions occur.

✦ Instruct the patient to notify the prescriber if nausea, vomiting, or diarrhea occurs. Suggest ways to relieve or prevent constipation, if needed.

✦ Inform the patient that the drug can cause or worsen heart failure. Review the signs and symptoms of this disorder, and advise the patient to report fluid retention. Instruct him to limit his fluid and salt intake to minimize this reaction.

✦ Combined with moricizine, propranolol or digoxin may prolong the PR interval on ECG tracings.

✦ A patient receiving moricizine and theophylline may have a reduced theophylline level.

✦ Propafenone increases the levels and effects of metoprolol and propranolol.

Adverse reactions

Class IC antiarrhythmics can produce serious adverse reactions, including the development of new arrhythmias.

All class IC agents cause adverse CNS reactions, which may include dizziness, headache, paresthesia, fatigue, and blurred vision. They may also produce adverse GI reactions, such as nausea, vomiting, and constipation or diarrhea. A metallic or bitter taste may result from propafenone and flecainide use. The CNS and GI reactions may be dose-related in some patients and may subside with dosage reduction.

Adverse cardiovascular reactions to these drugs include conduction abnormalities, exacerbation of heart failure, new arrhythmias, and hypotension. Paradoxically, class IC agents can aggravate existing arrhythmias.

Class IC drugs have some negative inotropic potential and may cause or worsen heart failure. This effect is most pronounced with flecainide.

Because propafenone possesses beta-blocking properties, it may cause bronchospasm, although only a few cases have been reported. Rarely, flecainide and propafenone have been linked to hematologic disturbances. More commonly, flecainide causes fever, rash, and allergic reactions.

Adverse reactions to watch for

✦ Allergic reaction, fever, rash
✦ Blurred vision, dizziness, fatigue, headache, paresthesia
✦ Bronchospasm
✦ Conduction abnormalities
✦ Constipation, diarrhea, nausea, vomiting
✦ Hypotension
✦ New arrhythmias
✦ Worsening of heart failure

Nursing considerations

✦ Closely monitor the patient for adverse reactions, especially CNS, cardiovascular, or GI disturbances. Reassure the patient that a dosage reduction may relieve adverse CNS reactions.

✦ Monitor the ECG tracing continuously for a critical care patient when beginning or adjusting drug therapy. If the original arrhythmia worsens, a new arrhythmia occurs, or the PR interval, QRS complex, or QT interval becomes excessively prolonged, notify the prescriber. The drug's arrhythmogenic effects may be misinterpreted as recurrence or spontaneous worsening of the original arrhythmia.

✦ Monitor the patient's vital signs regularly, noting an irregular heartbeat or hypotension.

✦ Observe the patient receiving digoxin with flecainide or propafenone for signs of digoxin toxicity.

✦ When giving a class IC antiarrhythmic, separate dosage adjustments by several days. Give a patient with renal or hepatic impairment a lower dose of flecainide.

✦ Monitor the patient closely for signs of heart failure, such as increased shortness of breath, crackles, jugular vein distension, and peripheral edema.

✦ Limit the patient's fluid and salt intake to decrease fluid retention, as prescribed.

✦ Teach the patient and his caregiver about the prescribed drug. (See *Teaching a patient about class IC antiarrhythmics*.)

CLASS II ANTIARRHYTHMICS

Class II antiarrhythmics are beta blockers with antiarrhythmic activity. They include atenolol, esmolol, metoprolol, and propranolol.

Pharmacokinetics

After oral administration, metoprolol and propranolol are absorbed almost entirely from the GI tract. Atenolol absorption is rapid but incomplete. Esmolol, which can only be given I.V., is immediately available throughout the body.

Atenolol and esmolol have low lipid solubility and don't cross the blood-brain barrier. Metoprolol has moderate lipid solubility, which means it can distribute more rapidly and effectively to underperfused tissue, such as ischemic myocardium, compared to atenolol and esmolol. Propranolol has high lipid solubility and readily crosses the blood-brain barrier. Metoprolol and propranolol undergo significant first-pass metabolism, leaving only a small portion of these drugs available to reach the circulation to be distributed to the body.

About 50% of atenolol is excreted in stool. Esmolol is metabolized exclusively by red blood cells (RBCs) with only 1% excreted in urine. About 3% of a metoprolol dose is excreted in urine. Propranolol's metabolites are excreted in urine.

Pharmacodynamics

Class II antiarrhythmics block beta-adrenergic receptor sites in the cardiac conduction system. As a result, the SA node's ability to fire spontaneously is slowed. The AV node's and other cells' ability to receive and conduct an electrical impulse to nearby cells also is reduced.

These antiarrhythmics also reduce the strength of the heart's contractions. When the heart beats less forcefully, it doesn't require as much oxygen to do its work.

Key nursing actions
✦ Monitor the ECG continuously.
✦ Check vital signs regularly.
✦ Watch closely for evidence of heart failure.

Features of class II antiarrhythmics
✦ Block beta-adrenergic receptors in the cardiac conduction system, slowing spontaneous firing of the SA node
✦ Reduce the strength of the heart's contractions

Teaching a patient about class II antiarrhythmics

Whenever a class II antiarrhythmic is prescribed, teach the patient and his family the drug's name, dose, frequency, action, and adverse effects. Also take the following actions.
- ✦ Demonstrate how to take a pulse. Tell the patient to check his pulse before each dose of the prescribed antiarrhythmic. If his pulse is slower than 60 beats/minute or a rate selected by the prescriber, advise him to withhold the dose and notify the prescriber.
- ✦ Instruct the patient not to perform activities that require alertness if dizziness, fatigue, lethargy, or confusion occurs.
- ✦ Instruct the patient to report nausea, vomiting, diarrhea, or constipation to his prescriber.
- ✦ Stress the importance of limiting fluid and salt intake to minimize fluid retention.

Possible drug interactions
- ✦ Antihypertensives
- ✦ Digoxin
- ✦ NSAIDs
- ✦ Phenothiazines
- ✦ Sulfonylureas
- ✦ Sympathomimetics
- ✦ Verapamil

Adverse reactions to watch for
- ✦ Angina
- ✦ Arrhythmias
- ✦ Blood dyscrasias, depression, rash, vivid dreams
- ✦ Bradycardia
- ✦ Bronchoconstriction
- ✦ Confusion, decreased libido, dizziness, fatigue, lethargy
- ✦ Fluid retention
- ✦ Hypotension with peripheral vascular insufficiency
- ✦ Peripheral edema
- ✦ Shock
- ✦ Syncope
- ✦ Worsening heart failure

Pharmacotherapeutics

Class II antiarrhythmics slow ventricular rates in patients with atrial flutter, atrial fibrillation, and paroxysmal atrial tachycardia.

Interactions

- ✦ Giving a class II antiarrhythmic with another antihypertensive or a phenothiazine increases the antihypertensive effect.
- ✦ A class II antiarrhythmic may reduce the effects of a sympathomimetic.
- ✦ Combined with verapamil, a beta blocker can depress the heart, causing hypotension, bradycardia, AV block, and asystole.
- ✦ A beta blocker can reduce the effects of a sulfonylurea.
- ✦ When digoxin is taken with esmolol, the risk of digoxin toxicity increases.
- ✦ A nonsteroidal anti-inflammatory drug (NSAID) may inhibit the activity of a beta blocker, decreasing its antihypertensive effects.

Adverse reactions

The most common adverse reactions to class II antiarrhythmics involve the cardiovascular system and usually occur when the drugs are first given. Because they inhibit sinus node stimulation, class II antiarrhythmics may produce bradycardia. Hypotension with peripheral vascular insufficiency may also occur, especially with esmolol. Syncope, angina, and shock may accompany these reactions. Occasionally, fluid retention and peripheral edema occur. Because class II antiarrhythmics reduce the force of myocardial contraction and increase preload, they may exacerbate or precipitate heart failure. Arrhythmias, especially AV block, may also occur.

Adverse CNS reactions include dizziness, confusion, fatigue, lethargy, and decreased libido. Typical GI reactions, such as nausea, vomiting, and mild diarrhea or constipation, usually are transient.

Propranolol, a nonselective beta blocker, blocks bronchial beta receptors that otherwise dilate bronchioles; this action can lead to significant bronchoconstriction. I.V. infusions of esmolol cause inflammation and induration at the injection site in about 80% of patients.

Other reactions to class II antiarrhythmics include rashes, blood dyscrasias, depression, and vivid dreams. These reactions, however, are rare.

Nursing considerations

+ Closely monitor the patient for cardiovascular and other adverse reactions, especially when therapy begins. Throughout therapy, closely monitor the patient for signs of fluid retention, such as peripheral edema, crackles, weight gain, shortness of breath, wheezing, and bronchospasm.
+ Monitor the patient's ECG tracings to detect arrhythmias, especially AV block and bradycardia.
+ If the patient's pulse is less than 60 beats/minute or if his systolic blood pressure is less than 90 mm Hg, withhold the dose and notify the prescriber.
+ Observe the esmolol infusion site for signs of inflammation and induration. Use an infusion pump for added control of the dosage when giving esmolol. Monitor the patient's heart rate and blood pressure continuously during esmolol infusion.
+ Observe the patient receiving esmolol with digoxin for signs of digoxin toxicity.
+ Teach the patient and his caregiver about the prescribed drug. (See *Teaching a patient about class II antiarrhythmics*.)

CLASS III ANTIARRHYTHMICS

Class III antiarrhythmics include amiodarone, dofetilide, ibutilide, and sotalol. These drugs are used to treat atrial fibrillation, atrial flutter, and ventricular arrhythmias, such as ventricular tachycardia and ventricular fibrillation. Some also are used to delay the recurrence of atrial fibrillation or atrial flutter.

Pharmacokinetics

Absorption of class III antiarrhythmics varies widely. After oral administration, amiodarone is absorbed slowly at widely varying rates. The drug is distributed extensively and accumulates in many sites, especially in organs with a rich blood supply and fatty tissue. It's highly protein-bound in plasma, mainly to albumin. Sotalol also is absorbed slowly, and is minimally protein-bound. Dofetilide is well absorbed from the GI tract. It's about 70% bound to plasma proteins. Ibutilide's pharmacokinetics vary widely among individuals. The drug is about 40% bound to plasma proteins.

Pharmacodynamics

Although the exact mechanism of action isn't known, class III antiarrhythmics may suppress arrhythmias by converting a unidirectional block to a bidirectional block. They have little or no effect on depolarization.

Pharmacotherapeutics

Class III antiarrhythmics are used to treat various arrhythmias. Amiodarone and sotalol are prescribed for life-threatening ventricular arrhythmias. Dofetilide and sotalol are used to maintain normal sinus rhythm in patients with corrected atrial fibrillation and atrial flutter. Dofetilide may also be used to convert atrial fibrillation or atrial flutter to sinus rhythm; I.V. ibutilide is used to rapidly convert these arrhythmias to sinus rhythm.

Interactions

+ Amiodarone may increase the quinidine, procainamide, or phenytoin level.
+ Amiodarone increases the risk of digoxin toxicity.
+ Combined with ibutilide, a class IA or other class III antiarrhythmic can increase the risk of prolonged refractoriness. These drugs shouldn't be given within 4 hours of each other.

Key nursing actions

+ Watch closely for evidence of fluid retention.
+ Monitor ECG tracings.
+ Withhold the drug and notify the prescriber if the heart rate is below 60 beats/minute or the systolic blood pressure is below 90 mm Hg.

Features of class III antiarrhythmics

+ May suppress arrhythmias by converting a unidirectional block to bidirectional block
+ Are used for various arrhythmias, including life-threatening ventricular arrhythmias
+ Are also used to convert atrial flutter or fibrillation to sinus rhythm or to maintain rhythm after conversion

Possible drug interactions

+ Anticoagulants
+ Class IA or III antiarrhythmics
+ Digoxin
+ Dolasetron
+ Drugs that prolong the QT interval
+ H_1-receptor agonists
+ Ketoconazole
+ Megestrol
+ Phenothiazine
+ Procainamide
+ Prochloperazine
+ Quinidine
+ Sulfamethoxazole
+ Tricyclic or tetracyclic antidepressants
+ Trimethoprim
+ Verapamil

WARNING

Preventing drug-induced arrhythmias

A patient who is starting or restarting therapy with sotalol at a maintenance dosage or dofetilide is at risk for developing drug-induced arrhythmias. To reduce this risk, place the patient in a facility capable of continuous ECG monitoring, cardiac resuscitation, and creatinine clearance calculation. Arrange for him to remain in this facility for at least 3 days.

✦ When given with ibutilide, a phenothiazine, tricyclic and tetracyclic antidepressant, histamine (H_1)-receptor antagonist, or other drug that can prolong the QT interval may increase the risk of arrhythmias.

 CLINICAL ALERT Amiodarone increases the effects of anticoagulants and may cause serious or fatal bleeding. A 30% to 50% reduction in the anticoagulant dose may be required.

✦ Use of dofetilide with cimetidine, ketoconazole, megestrol, prochlorperazine, sulfamethoxazole, trimethoprim, or verapamil may induce life-threatening arrhythmias and should be avoided.
✦ Use of sotalol with dolasetron or droperidol increases the risk of life-threatening arrhythmias and should be avoided.

Adverse reactions

Like most other antiarrhythmics, class III antiarrhythmics can aggravate arrhythmias, and may prolong the QT interval. For some patients, this requires special monitoring. (See *Preventing drug-induced arrhythmias*.) Amiodarone may cause bradycardia in up to 5% of patients.

Other adverse reactions to class III antiarrhythmics may lead to drug discontinuation. Amiodarone may produce hypotension, nausea, and anorexia. In 20% to 40% of patients, it causes adverse CNS reactions, such as malaise, fatigue, tremor, involuntary movements, lack of coordination, abnormal gait, ataxia, dizziness, and paresthesia. Rarely, peripheral neuropathy and proximal myopathy occur. Sotalol may commonly cause fatigue, dizziness, light-headedness, asthenia, weakness, headache, and sleep disturbance. Headache, chest pain, and dizziness are the most common adverse reactions to dofetilide.

Amiodarone causes several reactions that are not dose-related. Pulmonary toxicity consisting of interstitial pneumonia and alveolitis occurs in 10% to 17% of patients and can be fatal; signs and symptoms include dyspnea, cough, and changes in X-ray findings. Dyspnea may occur in up to 21% of patients receiving sotalol. Corneal microdeposits occur in almost all patients being treated with amiodarone for more than 6 months, but only 10% experience vision disturbances. The deposits disappear with dosage reduction or drug discontinuation. Skin photosensitivity occurs with amiodarone, sometimes producing a blue-gray discoloration of exposed skin. The metabolic effects of amiodarone can produce hypothyroidism or hyperthyroidism.

Nursing considerations

✦ Monitor the patient's ECG tracings. Be especially alert for bradycardia, increased ventricular ectopic beats, and prolonged PR intervals, QRS complexes, and QT intervals.

Adverse reactions to watch for

✦ Abnormal gait, asthenia, ataxia, dizziness, fatigue, headache, light-headedness, malaise, tremor, involuntary movements, lack of coordination, paresthesia, sleep disturbance, weakness
✦ Anorexia, nausea
✦ Bradycardia
✦ Chest pain
✦ Corneal microdeposits
✦ Dyspnea
✦ Hypotension
✦ Photosensitivity
✦ Prolonged QT interval
✦ Pulmonary toxicity
✦ Worsened arrhythmia

Teaching a patient about class III antiarrhythmics

Whenever a class III antiarrhythmic is prescribed, teach the patient and his family the drug's name, dose, frequency, action, and adverse effects. Also take the following actions.

◆ Demonstrate how to take a pulse. Tell the patient to check his pulse before each dose and to notify the prescriber if the pulse falls below 60 beats/minute (or the rate selected by the prescriber) or becomes irregular.

◆ Instruct the patient to avoid activities that require alertness or coordination, if adverse CNS reactions occur.

◆ Advise the patient to report nausea or vomiting. An antiemetic may be needed.

◆ Inform the patient that the prescribed amiodarone dosage will be high for the first several weeks and then decreased gradually to a maintenance dosage.

◆ Instruct the patient taking amiodarone to notify the prescriber if signs of pulmonary toxicity occur, such as dyspnea or persistent cough.

◆ Teach the patient taking amiodarone to use protective clothing and sunscreen or to avoid sunlight to protect against photosensitivity.

◆ Reassure the patient that corneal microdeposits produce vision disturbances in only 10% of all patients receiving amiodarone. However, tell the patient to notify the prescriber if vision changes occur.

CLINICAL ALERT During amiodarone therapy, closely monitor the patient for signs of pulmonary toxicity, such as dyspnea, cough, and X-ray findings that show interstitial pneumonia or alveolitis. If the patient shows these signs, notify the prescriber immediately because the drug should be stopped. Continue to monitor the patient for several months after stopping amiodarone; the drug's effects may persist for weeks or months.

◆ Measure the patient's vital signs frequently, noting a slow or irregular pulse or hypotension.

◆ Observe for additive effects in a patient receiving a class III antiarrhythmic and another antiarrhythmic. Monitor the patient closely during therapy with a class III antiarrhythmic and another cardiovascular drug, such as digoxin or an antihypertensive.

◆ Teach the patient and his caregiver about the prescribed drug. (See *Teaching a patient about class III antiarrhythmics.*)

CLASS IV ANTIARRHYTHMICS

The calcium channel blockers diltiazem and verapamil make up the class IV antiarrhythmics. Because these drugs have antiarrhythmic properties, they're used to treat supraventricular arrhythmias with rapid ventricular response rates, which is a rapid heart rate with a rhythm that originates above the ventricles.

Like the other calcium channel blockers, diltiazem and verapamil also are used to treat angina and hypertension. (For details, see "Calcium channel blockers" and "Vasodilators" later in this chapter.)

Key nursing actions
◆ Monitor ECG tracings.
◆ Watch for evidence of pulmonary toxicity if the patient receives amiodarone.
◆ Check vital signs often.

Features of class IV antiarrhythmics
◆ Block calcium channels
◆ Are used for angina, hypertension, and supraventricular arrhythmias with rapid ventricular response rates

WARNING

Contraindications and precautions for adenosine

The antiarrhythmic adenosine is contraindicated in patients with second- or third-degree atrioventricular block, sick sinus syndrome, atrial flutter, atrial fibrillation, or ventricular tachycardia.

The drug should be used cautiously in patients with asthma because adenosine may induce bronchoconstriction.

ADENOSINE

An injectable antiarrhythmic, adenosine is indicated for the acute treatment of PSVTs, including those related to accessory bypass tracts as in Wolff-Parkinson-White syndrome.

Pharmacokinetics

After I.V. administration, adenosine probably is distributed rapidly throughout the body and metabolized in RBCs as well as in vascular endothelial cells.

Pharmacodynamics

Adenosine depresses the SA node's pacemaker activity, reducing the heart rate and the AV node's ability to conduct impulses from the atria to the ventricles.

Pharmacotherapeutics

Adenosine is especially effective against reentry tachycardias that involve the AV node. This drug also is effective with more than 90% of PSVTs. It's particularly useful in treating arrhythmias related to accessory bypass tracts as in Wolff-Parkinson-White (or preexcitation) syndrome. In this syndrome, strands of heart tissue abnormally connect structures, such as the atria and ventricles, bypassing normal conduction. Certain patients shouldn't receive this drug or may receive it only with caution. (See *Contraindications and precautions for adenosine.*)

Interactions

✦ A methylxanthine or caffeine can antagonize adenosine's effects, requiring larger doses of adenosine.
✦ Dipyridamole can potentiate adenosine's effects, requiring smaller doses of adenosine.
✦ When adenosine is used with carbamazepine, the risk of heart block increases.

Adverse reactions

Adverse reactions, including facial flushing, shortness of breath, dyspnea, and chest discomfort, may occur in more than 5% of patients.

Nursing considerations

✦ Give adenosine as a rapid I.V. bolus only. If the drug must be given through an I.V. line, give it as close as possible to the I.V. injection site and follow with a rapid saline flush.

Features of adenosine
✦ Depresses pacemaker activity in the SA node
✦ Reduces the heart rate and conduction of impulses from the atria to the ventricles
✦ Is used for acute PSVTs, including those related to accessory bypass tracts

Possible drug interactions
✦ Caffeine
✦ Carbamazepine
✦ Dipyridamole
✦ Methylxanthines

Adverse reactions to watch for
✦ Chest discomfort
✦ Dyspnea
✦ Facial flushing
✦ Shortness of breath

+ Continuously monitor the patient's respiratory rate and pattern to detect changes during adenosine administration.
+ Continuously monitor the patient's ECG tracings during adenosine therapy. New rhythms may appear on the ECG during conversion to sinus rhythm. These rhythms usually last for only a few seconds and don't require treatment. However, be prepared to treat heart block if it develops and persists. Be especially alert for heart block in a patient who also is receiving carbamazepine.
+ Use smaller doses of adenosine if the patient also is receiving dipyridamole; higher doses if he also is taking a methylxanthine.
+ Don't give additional doses of adenosine to a patient who develops high-degree heart block after a single dose of the drug.
+ Teach the patient and his caregiver about the prescribed drug. (See *Teaching a patient about adenosine*.)

ANTIANGINALS

To pump effectively, the heart needs its own blood supply, which the coronary arteries provide. These arteries originate from the aorta at the ostia situated above the cusps of the aortic valve (the sinus of Valsalva). From there, the arteries branch out to cover and penetrate all parts of the cardiac muscle, or myocardium. After delivering oxygen and nutrients throughout the myocardium, the blood moves through large coronary veins and returns to the right atrium via the coronary sinus. The myocardium can't extract oxygen from blood inside the heart's chambers; instead, it depends on blood from the coronary arteries for its supply of oxygen and nutrients.

Even when the body is at rest, the percentage of oxygen extracted from coronary arterial blood by the myocardium is about 80%. During exercise or other exertion, the amount of blood flowing through the coronary arteries must increase significantly to meet the increased myocardial demand for oxygen. This additional oxygen normally is provided by an increase in aortic blood pressure and by local factors that dilate the coronary arteries during a process called autoregulation.

When the myocardial oxygen demand exceeds the myocardial oxygen supply, areas become ischemic, causing chest pain. When the patient experiences symptoms of this myocardial ischemia, the condition is known as angina or angina pectoris.

Angina usually takes one of three main forms:

Key nursing actions
+ Monitor the respiratory rate and pattern.
+ Monitor ECG tracings continuously.
+ Don't give another dose of adenosine if high-degree heart block develops after one dose.

Elements of angina
+ When myocardial oxygen demand exceeds supply, the muscle becomes ischemic, causing chest pain.
+ In stable angina, pain occurs at predictable levels of exertion and builds gradually.
+ In unstable angina, pain is unpredictable and more severe.
+ In Prinzmetal's angina, pain usually occurs at rest and resembles that of unstable angina.

EYE ON DRUG ACTION

How antianginals work

Angina occurs when the coronary arteries, the heart's primary source of oxygen, supply insufficient oxygen to the myocardium. This increases the heart's workload, increasing heart rate, preload, afterload, and force of myocardial contractility. Antianginals relieve angina by decreasing one or more of these four factors. This diagram summarizes how antianginals affect the cardiovascular system.

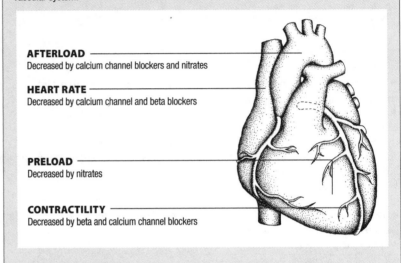

AFTERLOAD
Decreased by calcium channel blockers and nitrates

HEART RATE
Decreased by calcium channel and beta blockers

PRELOAD
Decreased by nitrates

CONTRACTILITY
Decreased by beta and calcium channel blockers

♦ Stable angina (also called predictable or chronic angina), in which pain occurs at a predictable level of physical or emotional stress, builds gradually, and reaches maximum intensity quickly.

♦ Unstable angina (also called preinfarction or crescendo angina, acute coronary insufficiency, or impending MI), in which pain takes an unpredictable course and is more severe than in stable angina.

♦ Prinzmetal's angina (also called variant angina), in which pain usually occurs while the patient is at rest and resembles that of unstable angina. Occasionally, a patient may have stable and Prinzmetal's angina.

Although angina's principal symptom is chest pain, the drugs used to treat angina aren't analgesics. They're nitrates, beta blockers, and calcium channel blockers. These antianginals treat angina by reducing myocardial oxygen demand, by increasing myocardial oxygen supply, or both. (See *How antianginals work*.)

Combination drug therapy

Combination therapy with drugs from different antianginal classes is indicated when symptoms persist despite therapy with one or more drugs from a single class. Combining drugs from different classes provides antianginal effects from different mechanisms of action and reduces the risk of adverse reactions from high dosages of any one drug.

This therapy also is used to control different types of angina occurring in one patient. For example, a patient might take a beta blocker or calcium channel block-

Reviewing combination therapy

♦ Antianginal drugs from different classes may be combined if symptoms persist with single-drug therapy.

♦ Combining drugs from different classes provides antianginal effects from differing mechanisms of action and allows lower doses of each drug.

♦ Combination therapy may be used to control different types of angina in the same patient.

er for long-term treatment of angina and supplement this therapy with rapid-acting nitrates for unusual, strenuous demands. Beta blockers prevent the reflex tachycardia sometimes reported with nitrates. Nitrates, in turn, prevent the increased preload from beta blockers. Calcium channel and beta blockers together more effectively treat Prinzmetal's angina that's unresponsive to beta blockers alone.

NITRATES

Nitrates include isosorbide and nitroglycerin. These antianginals act mainly as vasodilators, working directly on vascular smooth muscle to reduce vasoconstriction. They work primarily on venous, but also on arterial, smooth muscle.

Pharmacokinetics

Nitrates can be given in various ways. When given sublingually, buccally, as chewable tablets, or as lingual aerosols, nitrates are absorbed almost completely. That's because the oral mucous membranes have a rich blood supply. When swallowed as capsules, nitrates are absorbed through the mucous membranes of the GI tract. Only about half of the dose enters circulation.

Transdermal nitrates are absorbed slowly and in varying amounts, depending on the quantity of drug applied, the location of the applied patch, the surface area of skin used, and the circulation to the skin.

Once in the body, nitrates are distributed widely; nitroglycerin is about 60% bound to plasma proteins. Nitrate metabolism occurs partly in the blood but mainly in the liver. Metabolite excretion occurs via the kidneys.

Pharmacodynamics

Nitrates cause the smooth muscle of the veins and, to a lesser extent, the arteries to relax and dilate. When the veins dilate, less blood returns to the heart. This reduces preload. By reducing preload, nitrates reduce ventricular size and ventricular wall tension. (The left ventricle doesn't have to stretch as much to pump blood.) This, in turn, reduces the heart's oxygen requirements.

The arterioles provide the most resistance to the blood pumped by the left ventricle. Nitrates decrease afterload by dilating the arterioles, reducing resistance, easing the heart's workload, and easing the demand for oxygen.

Pharmacotherapeutics

Nitrates are used for immediate relief of angina, prevention of angina when an attack is expected, and long-term prevention of chronic angina. These drugs work synergistically with some beta blockers and calcium channel blockers. However, certain conditions call for their cautious use or contraindicate their use. (See *Contraindications and precautions for nitrates*, page 180.)

Interactions

✦ When nitrates are taken with alcohol, severe hypotension can result.
✦ An anticholinergic may delay absorption of a sublingual nitrate.
✦ Together, a calcium channel blocker and a nitrate may cause marked orthostatic hypotension with light-headedness, fainting, or blurred vision.

 CLINICAL ALERT When sildenafil (Viagra), tadalafil (Cialis), or vardenafil (Levitra) is taken within 24 hours of a nitrate, severe, life-threatening hypotension may occur.

Features of nitrates

✦ Reduce preload by relaxing the smooth muscles of the veins and, to a lesser degree, the arteries
✦ Reduce ventricular size and ventricular wall tension
✦ Reduce afterload by dilating arterioles and reducing resistance, oxygen demand, and the heart's workload
✦ Relieve and prevent angina

Possible drug interactions

✦ Alcohol
✦ Anticholinergics
✦ Calcium channel blockers
✦ Sildenafil
✦ Tadalafil
✦ Vardenafil

Adverse reactions to watch for

+ Alcohol intoxication
+ Blurred vision
+ Dry mouth
+ Flushing of the face and neck
+ Headache
+ Hypotension
+ Increased peripheral edema
+ Methemoglobinemia

Understanding nitrate tolerance

+ A patient who takes a nitrate for a long time, especially at high doses, may develop tolerance not only to that drug but to the entire class.
+ To minimize tolerance, therapy should be tailored to the individual, using the lowest effective dose and an intermittent dosage schedule.

Adverse reactions

Most adverse reactions to nitrates are caused by changes in the cardiovascular system. These reactions usually disappear when the dosage is reduced.

The decreased afterload produced by arteriolar dilation can cause hypotension, which may be compounded by reduced cardiac output after decreased preload. Hypotension is most noticeable when the patient stands up because blood pressure is insufficient to perfuse the brain adequately. In addition to a systolic blood pressure of less than 90 mm Hg, signs and symptoms of hypotension include syncope, dizziness, weakness, clammy skin, nausea, and vomiting. To compensate for this hypotension, the heart rate may increase to 150 beats/minute or more.

Although rare, complete cardiovascular collapse can occur even with normal doses. Signs of this adverse reaction include thready or absent peripheral pulses, loss of blood pressure, loss of consciousness, and incontinence.

Headache, the most common adverse reaction, probably is caused by blood vessel dilation in the meningeal layers between the brain and the cranium. The pain may be severe and persistent but usually disappears after several days of nitrate administration. Headache may be relieved by acetaminophen. For a patient wearing a transdermal patch, the application site doesn't affect the likelihood of headache.

Transdermal application occasionally causes local skin irritation. Many patients report a stinging sensation from sublingual tablets, but the effect is not objectionable and may even indicate that the tablets are fresh. A few patients taking nitrates experience transient flushing of the face and neck.

Tolerance to nitrates may develop over time, especially with high-dose, long-term therapy. Patients appear to develop tolerance not only to the prescribed nitrate, but also to the entire class. To minimize tolerance, nitrate therapy should be individualized, using the lowest effective dose and an intermittent dosage schedule.

I.V. nitroglycerin can produce alcohol intoxication when large doses are given for long periods. This reaction results from the alcohol used to preserve nitroglycerin in ampules or vials from which I.V. infusions are prepared. The most prominent signs of alcohol intoxication are an additive hypotensive effect and depression of myocardial contractility.

Other reactions may include blurred vision, dry mouth, increased peripheral edema, and methemoglobinemia, which occur with large, continuous doses of nitrates.

PATIENT TEACHING

Teaching a patient about nitrates

Whenever a nitrate is prescribed, teach the patient and his family the drug's name, dose, frequency, action, and adverse effects. Also take the following actions.

◆ Instruct the patient to store sublingual (S.L.) nitroglycerin tablets in the original container away from heat, including body heat. Advise him to discard the cotton filler after opening the container, because cotton may absorb some of the drug. Also instruct him to replace the tablets with fresh ones every 3 months and to discard any unused tablets.

◆ Instruct the patient to go to the nearest emergency department if angina isn't relieved by three tablets taken 5 minutes apart while resting. Explain that the pain may indicate an acute myocardial infarction.

◆ Inform the patient using a lingual aerosol not to inhale the spray.

◆ Suggest that the patient use plastic wrap to cover a transdermal patch because nitroglycerin ointment may stain clothing.

◆ Instruct the patient using long-acting patches to change them at the same time every day; for example, right after showering.

◆ Encourage the patient to avoid drinking alcoholic beverages during nitrate therapy.

◆ Instruct the patient to take nitrate tablets or capsules 30 minutes before or 1 hour after meals, for better absorption.

◆ Teach the patient with dry mouth to take a few sips of water before taking sublingual or buccal tablets because a dry mouth can inhibit absorption.

◆ Instruct the patient not to stop taking the nitrate without consulting his prescriber because vasospasm may follow abrupt discontinuation.

◆ Instruct the patient to take an S.L. dose a few minutes before engaging in activities known or expected to induce angina.

◆ Inform the patient that the stinging sensation from S.L. nitroglycerin tablets is normal and indicates drug freshness.

◆ Advise the patient with local skin irritation to apply transdermal nitrate patches in a different location until the irritation disappears.

◆ Teach the patient to recognize and report signs and symptoms of hypotension. Also describe how to minimize the effects of orthostatic hypotension.

◆ Instruct the patient to relieve nitrate-induced headache with a mild analgesic, such as acetaminophen.

◆ Reassure the patient that, although headache pain may be severe and persistent, it usually disappears after several days of nitrate administration.

◆ Instruct the patient to notify the prescriber if adverse reactions occur or if the drug is ineffective.

◆ Tell a male patient not to take erectile dysfunction drugs, such as sildenafil, tadalafil, or vardenafil, to avoid a serious decrease in blood pressure.

Nursing considerations

◆ Teach the patient and his caregiver about the prescribed drug. (See *Teaching a patient about nitrates.*)

◆ Don't give isosorbide mononitrate to relieve acute angina.

◆ With the patient sitting or lying down, take his pulse and blood pressure before giving the first nitrate dose and again at the onset of action.

◆ Repeat the isosorbide dinitrate dose two times at 5- to 10-minute intervals (for a total of three doses) if acute angina pain isn't relieved, or plan to repeat the dose of sublingual or spray nitroglycerin up to three times.

◆ Don't give more than 5 mg of chewable isosorbide dinitrate as an initial dose.

Key nursing actions

◆ Monitor the blood pressure and pulse every 5 to 15 minutes during nitroglycerin infusion and every hour thereafter.

◆ Watch for evidence of alcohol intoxication.

◆ Have the patient sit up briefly before standing to minimize orthostatic hypotension.

◆ Check vital signs regularly.

◆ If the patient is hypotensive, position him to enhance venous return.

◆ Assess for headache.

✦ Place a nitroglycerin sustained-release tablet between the patient's upper gum and lips.

✦ Apply a subsequent dose of nitroglycerin ointment by removing the ointment remaining from the preceding dose and selecting a new administration site to avoid skin irritation.

✦ Remove a transdermal patch before electrical cardioversion to prevent arcing that can damage the paddles and burn the patient.

✦ Prepare I.V. nitroglycerin infusions cautiously. Mix the drug with dextrose 5% in water or normal saline solution in a glass bottle. Use administration tubing supplied by the manufacturer, if available, because nitroglycerin readily migrates into standard polyvinyl chloride tubing, greatly reducing the amount administered.

✦ Monitor the patient's blood pressure and pulse every 5 to 15 minutes while titrating the I.V. nitroglycerin dosage and every hour thereafter, or according to facility policy. Use an infusion pump.

✦ Monitor the patient closely for signs of alcohol intoxication, such as hypotension or depressed myocardial contractility, during high-dosage, long-term I.V. therapy with nitroglycerin.

✦ Have the patient sit up for a few minutes before standing to minimize the effects of orthostatic hypotension.

✦ Take the patient's vital signs regularly and monitor closely for signs and symptoms of hypotension, such as a systolic blood pressure below 90 mm Hg, syncope, dizziness, weakness, clammy skin, nausea, vomiting, or tachycardia of at least 150 beats/minute.

✦ Position a hypotensive patient to promote venous return, such as in a supine position or legs-elevated position, and recheck his blood pressure. If hypotension persists, remove the nitrate ointment or slow the I.V. infusion rate, notify the prescriber, and continue to monitor the patient's heart rate and blood pressure every 5 to 15 minutes.

✦ Monitor the patient for headache during nitrate therapy. Give acetaminophen or another analgesic in case headache occurs.

BETA BLOCKERS

Also called beta-adrenergic receptor antagonists, beta blockers are used for long-term prevention of angina and for treatment of hypertension. Among the beta blockers, atenolol, carvedilol, metoprolol, nadolol, and propranolol commonly are used as antianginals.

Pharmacokinetics

Carvedilol, metoprolol, and propranolol are absorbed almost entirely from the GI tract, whereas less than half the dose of atenolol or nadolol is absorbed. These beta blockers are distributed widely. Carvedilol and propranolol are highly protein-bound; the others are poorly protein-bound.

Atenolol and nadolol aren't metabolized and are excreted unchanged in urine and stool. Carvedilol is metabolized by aromatic ring oxidation and glucuronidation; its metabolites are primarily excreted via bile in feces. Metoprolol and propranolol are metabolized in the liver, and their metabolites are excreted in urine.

Pharmacodynamics

Beta blockers decrease blood pressure and block beta-adrenergic receptor sites in the heart muscle and conduction system, decreasing the heart rate and the force of cardiac contractions, which reduces the demand for oxygen.

Features of beta blockers

✦ Antagonize beta-adrenergic receptors in the heart muscle and conduction system
✦ Decrease the blood pressure, heart rate, and force of contraction
✦ Are used for long-term prevention of angina and treatment of hypertension

WARNING

Contraindications and precautions for beta blockers

Beta blockers are contraindicated in patients who are hypersensitive to them. These drugs also are contraindicated in patients with cardiogenic shock, sinus bradycardia, heart block greater than first degree, bronchial asthma, and heart failure unless the failure was caused by a tachyarrhythmia that's treatable with propranolol.

Use beta blockers cautiously in patients with nonallergic bronchospastic disorders, diabetes mellitus, or impaired hepatic or renal function.

Pharmacotherapeutics

Beta blockers are indicated for long-term prevention or treatment of angina. Because these drugs can reduce blood pressure, they're also prescribed to treat hypertension. In addition, carvedilol and metoprolol are used to treat heart failure. For some patients, however, these drugs aren't appropriate or require cautious use. (See *Contraindications and precautions for beta blockers.*)

Interactions

◆ An antacid may delay absorption of a beta blocker.
◆ An NSAID can decrease a beta blocker's hypotensive effects.
◆ When lidocaine is given with a beta blocker, lidocaine toxicity may occur.
◆ A beta blocker can alter the requirements for insulin or an oral antidiabetic drug.
◆ A nonselective beta blocker (such as carvedilol, nadolol, or propranolol) can impair theophylline's ability to produce bronchodilation.

Adverse reactions

The most common adverse reactions to beta blockers involve the cardiovascular system and occur during the initial administration. Because these drugs inhibit sinus node stimulation, they can cause bradycardia and hypotension with peripheral vascular insufficiency. Angina, syncope, or shock may accompany these reactions. Fluid retention and peripheral edema may also occur.

Decreased force of myocardial contractility and increased preload may cause or worsen heart failure. Arrhythmias, especially AV block, may also occur.

Rapid discontinuation of a beta blocker may precipitate angina, hypertension, arrhythmias, or acute MI.

Adverse CNS reactions include dizziness, fatigue, lethargy, confusion or depression (especially in geriatric patients), and decreased libido. These reactions occur most commonly with propranolol therapy. GI reactions, such as nausea, vomiting, and diarrhea, usually are transient.

Significant bronchoconstriction is more likely to occur with the nonselective beta blockers carvedilol, nadolol, and propranolol. However, it also can occur with high doses of atenolol and metoprolol.

Rarely, rashes, blood dyscrasias, depression, and vivid dreams occur.

Possible drug interactions

◆ Antacids
◆ Insulin
◆ Lidocaine
◆ NSAIDs
◆ Oral antidiabetic drugs
◆ Theophylline

Adverse reactions to watch for

◆ Angina
◆ Arrhythmias
◆ Bradycardia
◆ Bronchoconstriction
◆ Confusion, decreased libido, depression, dizziness, fatigue, lethargy
◆ Diarrhea, nausea, vomiting
◆ Fluid retention
◆ Hypotension with peripheral vascular insufficiency
◆ New or worsened heart failure
◆ Peripheral edema
◆ Shock
◆ Syncope

Key nursing actions
- Check vital signs regularly.
- If the patient is diabetic, monitor his glucose level carefully.
- Auscultate the lungs frequently.
- Watch for evidence of excess fluid volume.

Nursing considerations
- Monitor the patient closely for adverse reactions, especially for cardiovascular dysfunction during the initial administration.
- Regularly measure the patient's vital signs, particularly noting decreased blood pressure or heart rate or an irregular rhythm. Withhold the dose and notify the prescriber if the patient's apical pulse is less than 60 beats/minute or his systolic blood pressure is less than 90 mm Hg.
- Monitor the diabetic patient's glucose level regularly. Adjust the insulin or oral antidiabetic dose, as needed.
- Auscultate the patient's lungs frequently and assess his ease of breathing to detect bronchoconstriction. Notify the prescriber if bronchoconstriction occurs; prepare to give bronchodilator and oxygen therapy.
- Assess the patient for signs of fluid volume excess, such as crackles, increasing dyspnea, elevated blood pressure, peripheral edema, and jugular vein distention. Notify the prescriber if fluid volume excess occurs; prepare to give a diuretic as prescribed and take other measures to reduce fluid overload.
- Teach the patient and his caregiver about the prescribed drug. (See *Teaching a patient about beta blockers*.)

CALCIUM CHANNEL BLOCKERS

This class is extensive, comprehensive, and inclusive of many common drugs. Selected calcium channel blockers—amlodipine, diltiazem, nicardipine, nifedipine, and verapamil—are used to prevent angina that's unresponsive to other antianginals. Some calcium channel blockers (diltiazem and verapamil) also are used as antiarrhythmics. Others (felodipine and isradipine) serve as antihypertensives. (For details, see "Class IV antiarrhythmics" and "Vasodilators" elsewhere in this chapter.)

Pharmacokinetics
When given orally, calcium channel blockers are absorbed quickly and almost completely. Because of the first-pass effect, however, their bioavailability is relatively

How calcium channel blockers work

Calcium channel blockers increase the myocardial oxygen supply and slow the heart rate. It seems that the drugs produce these effects by blocking the slow calcium channel. This action inhibits the influx of extracellular calcium ions across myocardial and vascular smooth muscle cell membranes. Calcium channel blockers achieve this blockade without changing the calcium level.

This calcium blockade causes the coronary arteries (and, to a lesser extent, the peripheral arteries and arterioles) to dilate, decreasing afterload and increasing myocardial oxygen supply. The blockade also slows sinoatrial and atrioventricular node conduction, slightly reducing the heart rate.

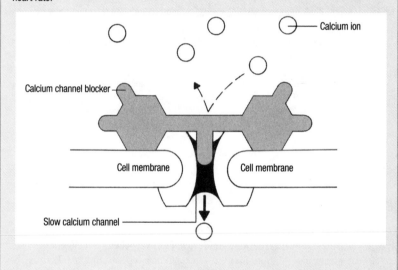

low. Calcium channel blockers are highly bound to plasma proteins. They're metabolized rapidly and almost completely in the liver.

Pharmacodynamics

Calcium channel blockers prevent calcium ions from passing across the membranes of myocardial cells and vascular smooth muscle cells. This causes the coronary and peripheral arteries to dilate, which decreases the force of cardiac contractions and reduces the heart's workload. (See *How calcium channel blockers work.*) By preventing arterioles from constricting, calcium channel blockers also reduce afterload, which decreases the heart's oxygen demands.

Diltiazem and verapamil also reduce the heart rate by slowing conduction through the SA and AV nodes. A slower heart rate reduces the heart's need for additional oxygen.

Pharmacotherapeutics

Drugs from this class are prescribed to manage chronic stable angina and are particularly effective in Prinzmetal's angina. Oral verapamil is used to treat unstable

Features of calcium channel blockers

+ Prevent calcium ions from crossing myocardial and vascular smooth muscle cell membranes
+ Decrease the force of contractions, afterload, and cardiac workload
+ Reduce the heart rate by slowing conduction through the SA and AV nodes
+ Are used to manage stable, unstable, and Prinzmetal's angina and to prevent angina unresponsive to other antianginals
+ Also are used as antiarrhythmics

WARNING

Contraindications for calcium channel blockers

All calcium channel blockers are contraindicated in patients who are hypersensitive to them or their components. These drugs also are contraindicated in patients with sick sinus syndrome or second- or third-degree AV block unless they have a functioning pacemaker. Other contraindications depend on the specific drug.

✦ Diltiazem, and verapamil are contraindicated when the patient's systolic blood pressure is less than 90 mm Hg.

✦ Diltiazem is contraindicated in patients with acute myocardial infarction and pulmonary congestion.

✦ Nicardipine is contraindicated in patients with advanced aortic stenosis.

✦ Verapamil is contraindicated in patients with severe left ventricular dysfunction; with cardiogenic shock and severe heart failure unless it's secondary to a supraventricular tachycardia that's responsive to verapamil treatment, or with atrial flutter or fibrillation and an accessory bypass tract.

✦ Intravenous (I.V.) verapamil is contraindicated within a few hours of use of an I.V. beta blocker because both drugs may depress myocardial contractility and atrioventricular node conduction. I.V. verapamil also is contraindicated in ventricular tachycardia because this use may cause hemodynamic deterioration and ventricular fibrillation.

Possible drug interactions

✦ Calcium
✦ Carbamazepine
✦ Digoxin
✦ Nondepolarizing blockers
✦ Rifampin
✦ Vitamin D

Adverse reactions to watch for

✦ Arrhythmias
✦ Diarrhea, nausea, vomiting
✦ Dizziness, flushing, headache, persistent peripheral edema, weakness
✦ Mood changes
✦ Muscle fatigue and cramps
✦ Nasal congestion
✦ New or worsened heart failure
✦ Orthostatic hypotension
✦ Photosensitivity
✦ Pruritus
✦ Skin eruptions
✦ Undesirable cardiovascular changes
✦ Worsened angina

angina. Specific calcium channel blockers shouldn't be given to certain patients. (See *Contraindications for calcium channel blockers.*)

Interactions

✦ Calcium and vitamin D reduce a calcium channel blocker's effectiveness.
✦ When given with a calcium channel blocker, a nondepolarizing blocker may have enhanced muscle relaxant effects.
✦ Diltiazem and verapamil increase the risk of digoxin toxicity.
✦ Diltiazem and verapamil enhance carbamazepine action.
✦ Rifampin may decrease the effectiveness of oral verapamil.

Adverse reactions

Undesirable changes in the cardiovascular system are the most common and most serious adverse reactions to calcium channel blockers. Because these drugs decrease afterload and the force of ventricular contraction, they sometimes cause a decrease in blood pressure, including orthostatic hypotension. Arrhythmias, such as bradycardia, sinus block, and AV block, result from inhibition of the sinus and AV nodes, especially by diltiazem and verapamil. The depressant action on myocardial contractility may account for the onset or worsening of heart failure.

Vasodilation can produce dizziness, headache, flushing, weakness, and persistent peripheral edema, especially with amlodipine, nicardipine, and nifedipine. Other adverse reactions include GI disturbances, such as nausea, vomiting, and diarrhea, as well as muscle fatigue and cramps, worsening of angina and skin eruptions, photosensitivity, pruritus, nasal congestion, and mood changes.

Teaching a patient about calcium channel blockers

Whenever a calcium channel blocker is prescribed, teach the patient and his family the drug's name, dose, frequency, action, and adverse effects. Also take the following actions.
✦ Demonstrate how to take a pulse, and tell the patient to take his pulse before each dose. Advise him to delay the dose and notify the prescriber if his pulse is less than 60 beats/minute.
✦ Teach the patient to recognize and report signs of fluid retention, such as peripheral edema and increasing shortness of breath.
✦ Emphasize that calcium channel blockers can't relieve acute angina. If acute chest pain occurs, advise the patient to notify the prescriber immediately or go to the nearest emergency department.
✦ Teach the patient how to manage orthostatic hypotension.
✦ Advise the patient not to perform activities that require alertness if dizziness occurs.
✦ Instruct the patient to report nausea, vomiting, or diarrhea.
✦ Instruct the patient to take diltiazem before meals.
✦ Instruct the patient to take a once-daily sustained-release tablet in the morning.
✦ Advise a woman of childbearing age to tell the prescriber if she is pregnant or plans to become pregnant during therapy.
✦ Advise the patient with headaches or muscle cramps to take an analgesic.

Nursing considerations

✦ Regularly measure the patient's vital signs and monitor his ECG tracings for arrhythmias. Also assess him for fluid retention. If the patient's heart rate is less than 60 beats/minute or if his systolic blood pressure is less than 90 mm Hg, withhold the dose and notify the prescriber.
✦ Have the patient sit up for a few minutes before standing to minimize the effects of orthostatic hypotension.
✦ Give the once-daily dose of a sustained-release tablet in the morning. Give diltiazem before meals.
✦ Monitor the patient for headache or muscle cramps.
✦ Teach the patient and his caregiver about the prescribed drug. (See *Teaching a patient about calcium channel blockers.*)

ANTIHYPERTENSIVES

Antihypertensives, which reduce blood pressure, are used to treat hypertension, a disorder characterized by an elevation in systolic pressure, diastolic pressure, or both. Hypertension can occur in varying degrees. The Joint National Committee on Detection, Evaluation, and Treatment of High Blood Pressure of the National Institutes of Health has devised a classification system for hypertension. This system describes three stages of hypertension. (See *Classification of blood pressure,* page 188.)

All stages of hypertension are linked to an increased risk of cardiovascular and renal disease. The goal of antihypertensive therapy is to reduce cardiovascular and renal morbidity and mortality. In most patients, the target blood pressure is less

Key nursing actions
✦ Check vital signs regularly.
✦ Monitor ECG tracings.
✦ Assess for fluid retention.
✦ Have the patient sit up briefly before standing to minimize orthostatic hypotension.
✦ Monitor the patient for headache and muscle cramps.

Reviewing hypertension
✦ Hypertension can occur in varying degrees and is classified in three stages.
✦ All stages are linked to an increased risk of cardiovascular and renal disease.

Classification of blood pressure

For adults age 18 and older, use the following chart to classify blood pressure. Treatment is determined by the highest blood pressure category.

CLASSIFICATION	SYSTOLIC BLOOD PRESSURE	DIASTOLIC BLOOD PRESSURE
Normal blood pressure	< 120 mm Hg and	< 80 mm Hg
Prehypertension	120 to 139 mm Hg or	80 to 89 mm Hg
Stage 1 hypertension	140 to 159 mm Hg or	90 to 99 mm Hg
Stage 2 hypertension	≥ 160 mm Hg or	≥ 100 mm Hg

Based on recommendations of the *Seventh Report of the Joint National Committee on Prevention, Detection, Evaluation, and Treatment of High Blood Pressure.* (NIH Publication 03-5233, May 2003).

Understanding hypertensive therapy

✦ Antihypertensive therapy aims to reduce cardiovascular and renal effects.

✦ Lifestyle efforts are integral to antihypertensive therapy and may include weight reduction, a low-sodium diet, regular exercise, and moderation of alcohol consumption.

✦ Choice of antihypertensive drug is based in part on preexisting conditions, such as heart failure, diabetes, chronic kidney disease, recent MI, high coronary risk level, or the need to prevent stroke.

✦ For therapy to succeed, the patient must not only adhere to drug therapy but also make and maintain needed lifestyle changes and return for follow-up care.

than 140/90 mm Hg, which reduces the risk of cardiovascular disease. In patients with diabetes or renal disease, the target is 130/80 mm Hg.

Lifestyle modifications, such as weight reduction, use of a low-sodium diet, regular exercise, and moderate alcohol consumption, help prevent hypertension and are an integral part of its management.

When antihypertensive therapy becomes necessary, a thiazide diuretic may be used alone or with a drug from another antihypertensive class, such as a sympatholytic, vasodilator, angiotensin-converting enzyme (ACE) inhibitor, or angiotensin II receptor blocker. In some patients, a preexisting condition (such as heart failure, diabetes, chronic kidney disease, recent MI, high coronary risk, or need to prevent recurrent stroke) becomes a compelling indication and determines the choice of antihypertensive. (See *Which class of antihypertensive is right for your patient?*)

Because most patients with hypertension need more than one drug to reach their blood pressure goal, the prescriber should use a treatment algorithm to ensure effective drug selection and combination. (See *Ensuring effective drug selection,* page 190.)

As with most treatments, antihypertensive therapy can be successful only if the patient is compliant, taking the drugs as prescribed, adhering to lifestyle modifications, and returning for follow-up appointments. Educating the patient thoroughly and establishing trust can help the patient to stay motivated, comply with treatment, and achieve his treatment goal.

SYMPATHOLYTICS

The sympatholytic class includes groups of drugs that reduce blood pressure by inhibiting or blocking motor and secretory actions in the sympathetic nervous system. These drugs are classified by their site or mechanism of action as:

✦ central-acting sympathetic nervous system inhibitors, such as clonidine.

✦ alpha-adrenergic blockers, such as doxazosin, phentolamine, prazosin, and terazosin.

✦ beta blockers, such as acebutolol, atenolol, carteolol, metoprolol, nadolol, propranolol, and timolol.

Which class of antihypertensive is right for your patient?

Certain conditions determine the choice of antihypertensive drug class in patients with hypertension. As shown in the table below, these deciding indications direct the use of diuretics, beta blockers (a group of sympatholytics), ACE inhibitors, angiotensin II receptor blockers, calcium channel blockers (a group of vasodilators), and aldosterone antagonists (a group of potassium-sparing diuretics).

INDICATION	Diuretics	Beta blockers	ACE inhibitors	Angiotensin II receptor blockers	Calcium channel blockers	Aldosterone antagonists
Heart failure	•	•	•	•		•
Myocardial infarction (MI) recovery		•	•			•
High risk of coronary disease	•	•	•		•	
Diabetes mellitus	•	•	•	•	•	
Chronic renal disease			•	•		
Prevention of stroke recurrence	•		•			

Based on recommendations of the *Seventh Report of the Joint National Committee on Prevention, Detection, Evaluation, and Treatment of High Blood Pressure.* (NIH Publication 03-5233, May 2003).

♦ mixed alpha-adrenergic and beta blockers such as labetalol.

Pharmacokinetics

Most sympatholytics are absorbed well from the GI tract, distributed widely, metabolized in the liver, and excreted primarily in urine.

Pharmacodynamics

All sympatholytics inhibit the stimulation of the sympathetic nervous system. This causes dilation of the peripheral blood vessels or decreases cardiac output, thereby reducing blood pressure.

Pharmacotherapeutics

Although sympatholytics are used to treat hypertension, they aren't first-line drugs.

Interactions

♦ Use of clonidine with a tricyclic antidepressant may increase blood pressure.
♦ Together, clonidine and a CNS depressant may worsen CNS depression.
♦ The combination of prazosin with a beta blocker or verapamil may increase the risk of first-dose orthostatic hypotension.

Features of sympatholytics

♦ May be central-acting sympathetic nervous system inhibitors, alpha-adrenergic blockers, beta blockers, or mixed alpha-adrenergic and beta blockers
♦ Reduce blood pressure by inhibiting stimulation of the sympathetic nervous system
♦ Dilate peripheral blood vessels or decrease cardiac output
♦ Are used to treat hypertension but aren't first choice

Ensuring effective drug selection

The flowchart below is based on the approach to antihypertensive therapy endorsed by the Joint National Committee on the Detection, Evaluation, and Treatment of High Blood Pressure.

Step 1

✦ Obtain baseline blood pressure readings.
✦ Instruct patient in lifestyle modifications (weight reduction, moderate alcohol intake, regular physical activity, reduction of sodium intake, smoking cessation).

Adequate response? — No

Yes

Continue to monitor and reinforce instructions.

Step 2

✦ Continue instructions for lifestyle modifications; enlist aid of family members and support groups.
✦ Prepare patient to begin drug therapy.
✦ Anticipate use of thiazide-type diuretics, ACE inhibitor, angiotensin receptor blocker (ARB), beta blocker (BB), calcium channel blocker (CCB), or a combination for stage 1 hypertension in the absence of compelling indications (see below).
✦ Instruct patient in drug regimen.
✦ Continue monitoring blood pressure.
✦ Assess for signs and symptoms of adverse effects.
✦ Anticipate use of a two-drug combination (usually a thiazide-type diuretic and an ACE inhibitor, ARB, BB, or CCB) for stage 2 hypertension in the absence of compelling indications (see below).
✦ Anticipate use of the following drugs if the patient has any of these compelling indications: heart failure—diuretic, BB, ACE inhibitor, ARB, or aldosterone antagonist; post MI—BB, ACE inhibitor, or aldosterone antagonist; high coronary disease risk—diuretic, BB, ACE inhibitor, or CCB; diabetes, BB, ACE inhibitor, ARB, or CCB; chronic kidney disease—ACE inhibitor or ARB; recurring stroke prevetion—diuretic or ACE inhibitor.

Step 3

✦ Anticipate change in drug therapy regimen (addition of second or third antihypertensive, addition of diuretic if not already prescribed)
✦ Instruct patient in new drug regimen; reinforce previous instructions.
✦ Continue monitoring blood pressure.
✦ Assess for signs and symptoms of adverse effects.

Adequate response? — No

Yes

Continue therapy and monitoring.

Based on recommendations of *The Seventh Report of the Joint National Committee on Detection, Evaluation, and Treatment of High Blood Pressure* (NIH Publication 03-5233, May 2003).

✦ Indomethacin may decrease prazosin's antihypertensive action.
✦ Verapamil may increase the prazosin level.

Adverse reactions

Many sympatholytics cause adverse reactions in the CNS and cardiovascular system. Additional reactions affecting other body systems vary with each drug.

Central-acting inhibitors typically produce CNS effects, such as sedation, drowsiness, and depression. Other common reactions include forgetfulness, inability to concentrate, and vivid dreams, which usually diminish after 2 to 3 weeks of therapy. Additional adverse reactions include sodium and water retention, edema, hepatic dysfunction, vertigo, paresthesia, weakness, fever, nasal congestion, and dry mouth. These drugs may decrease libido and result in impotence, limiting their usefulness in men. They may also produce lactation in both sexes. Other adverse reactions vary with the specific drug. For example, clonidine may cause dry mouth or rebound hypertension when the drug is stopped.

Because of their ability to penetrate the blood-brain barrier, beta blockers can produce the same CNS effects as the central-acting inhibitors. Adverse cardiovascular reactions may include bradycardia, hypotension, heart failure, and exacerbation of peripheral vascular disease (PVD). Beta blockers may also reduce the high-density lipoprotein (HDL) level and increase triglyceride, total cholesterol, low-density lipoprotein (LDL), and very-low-density lipoprotein (VLDL) levels.

Other adverse reactions to beta blockers include nausea, vomiting, diarrhea, nightmares, depression, insomnia, hallucinations, dry eyes, paresthesia, transient thrombocytopenia, agranulocytosis, sore throat, fever, and breathing difficulty.

In a patient with intermittent claudication or PVD, beta blockers may produce further symptoms of arterial insufficiency. In an insulin-dependent diabetic patient, these drugs can mask the early warning signs of hypoglycemia and, rarely, produce hyperglycemia. They may also alter test results for alkaline phosphatase, BUN, LDL, creatinine, potassium, transaminase, triglyceride, uric acid, and glucose levels.

Alpha-adrenergic blockers tend to produce different adverse reactions than beta blockers do. For example, doxazosin and prazosin produce orthostatic hypotension more commonly than beta blockers do. They also produce first-dose syncope. Terazosin produces a few mild adverse reactions, including orthostatic hypotension and dizziness. Phentolamine can precipitate anginal attacks from rebound tachycardia and may produce hypotension as well as dizziness, weakness, flushing, palpitations, diarrhea, nausea, vomiting, and nasal congestion.

Adverse reactions to the mixed alpha-adrenergic and beta blocker labetalol resemble those of the beta blockers. Other reactions may include scalp tingling, alopecia, orthostatic hypotension, intermittent claudication, bronchospasm, drug-induced lupus erythematosuslike syndrome, eye irritation, myalgia, and rash.

Nursing considerations

✦ Obtain baseline data before beginning sympatholytic therapy. Assess the patient's blood pressure and pulses in the sitting, standing, and lying positions. Monitor and record the patient's blood pressure and pulse when starting drug therapy, before giving each dose, and at peak level.
✦ Monitor the patient's vital signs. For example, expect to monitor the patient's blood pressure and pulse every 15 to 30 minutes for at least the first 2 hours during initial administration of an alpha-adrenergic blocker.
✦ Assess the patient's hepatic and renal function before and regularly during beta blocker therapy. If the BUN or creatinine level is elevated, notify the prescriber.

Possible drug interactions
✦ Beta blockers
✦ CNS depressants
✦ Indomethacin
✦ Tricyclic antidepressants
✦ Verapamil

Adverse reactions to watch for
✦ Agranulocytosis, transient thrombocytopenia
✦ Alopecia, scalp tingling
✦ Bradycardia
✦ Breathing difficulty
✦ Bronchospasm
✦ Decreased libido, impotence
✦ Depression, drowsiness, forgetfulness, hallucinations, inability to concentrate, insomnia, nightmares, sedation, vertigo, vivid dreams, weakness
✦ Diarrhea, nausea, vomiting
✦ Dry and irritated eyes
✦ Dry mouth, nasal congestion
✦ Edema, sodium and water retention, worsening of PVD
✦ Fever
✦ First-dose syncope
✦ Heart failure
✦ Hepatic dysfunction
✦ Hypotension
✦ Increased triglyceride, total cholesterol, LDL, and VLDL levels; decreased HDL level
✦ Intermittent claudication
✦ Lupuslike syndrome
✦ Myalgia
✦ Orthostatic hypotension
✦ Paresthesia
✦ Rash
✦ Sore throat

Key nursing actions

- ✦ Assess blood pressure and pulse with the patient lying, sitting, and standing.
- ✦ Document blood pressure and pulse before each dose and at peak level.
- ✦ Check vital signs regularly.
- ✦ Assess hepatic and renal function before and regularly throughout beta blocker therapy.
- ✦ Watch closely for syncope.
- ✦ If the patient is diabetic, monitor his glucose level carefully.
- ✦ Closely supervise a patient with a history of depression.
- ✦ Discontinue beta blocker therapy gradually.

Reviewing vasodilators

- ✦ Come in two types: direct vasodilators and calcium channel blockers
- ✦ Decrease systolic and diastolic blood pressure by relaxing arteriolar smooth muscle, which decreases peripheral resistance
- ✦ Acts on arteries, veins, or both (direct vasodilators)
- ✦ Relaxes arterioles (calcium channel blockers)
- ✦ Are rarely used alone to treat hypertension, but may be used with other drugs for moderate to severe hypertension

PATIENT TEACHING

Teaching a patient about sympatholytics

Whenever a sympatholytic is prescribed, teach the patient and his family the drug's name, dose, frequency, action, and adverse effects. Also take the following actions.
- ✦ Inform the patient taking clonidine that vivid dreams may occur.
- ✦ Reassure the patient receiving a central-acting inhibitor that adverse CNS reactions usually diminish after 2 to 3 weeks of therapy.
- ✦ Advise the patient that methyldopa may darken the urine.
- ✦ Instruct the patient to take the first dose of doxazosin, prazosin, or terazosin at bedtime or to remain lying down for at least 3 hours after taking it to prevent severe first-dose orthostatic hypotension.
- ✦ Inform the patient and family about possible depression. Describe the early signs of depression, which may not occur until 6 months after therapy begins, and the signs of suicidal behavior if severe depression occurs.
- ✦ Alert the patient on a sodium-restricted diet that not complying may cause fluid retention and edema.

✦ Observe the patient closely for syncope when giving the first dose of doxazosin, prazosin, or terazosin. To prevent severe first-dose orthostatic hypotension, have the patient lie down for at least 3 hours after taking the dose.

✦ Monitor a diabetic patient's glucose level carefully, especially during beta blocker therapy.

✦ Give labetalol between meals. If sedation occurs with a central-acting inhibitor, give the drug in the evening. If the dosage is increased, start with an evening dose to minimize sedative effects.

✦ Closely supervise a patient with a history of depression, because it may recur during antihypertensive therapy.

✦ Discontinue a beta blocker gradually over 3 to 14 days. During this time, the patient should avoid vigorous physical activity to prevent overtaxing his heart.

✦ Teach the patient and his caregiver about the prescribed drug. (See *Teaching a patient about sympatholytics.*)

VASODILATORS

The two types of vasodilators are direct vasodilators and calcium channel blockers. Both types of vasodilators decrease systolic and diastolic blood pressure by relaxing arteriolar smooth muscle, which dilates the arterioles and decreases peripheral resistance.

Direct vasodilators act on arteries, veins, or both. They include diazoxide, hydralazine, minoxidil, and nitroprusside. Hydralazine and minoxidil usually are used to treat resistant or refractory hypertension. Diazoxide and nitroprusside are reserved for managing hypertensive crisis.

Calcium channel blockers relax the arterioles. They include amlodipine, diltiazem, felodipine, isradipine, nicardipine, nifedipine, and verapamil. In addition to serving as antihypertensives, many calcium channel blockers also are used as antiarrhythmics and antianginals. (For details on these uses, see "Class IV antiarrhythmics" and "Calcium channel blockers" earlier in this chapter.)

Pharmacokinetics

Most vasodilators are absorbed rapidly and distributed well. Typically, they're metabolized in the liver and excreted by the kidneys.

Pharmacodynamics

Direct vasodilators relax peripheral vascular smooth muscles, causing the blood vessels to dilate. This lowers blood pressure by increasing the diameter of the blood vessels, reducing total peripheral resistance. Calcium channel blockers relax the arterioles by preventing calcium ions from entering cells, thus reducing the mechanical activity of vascular smooth muscle.

Pharmacotherapeutics

Vasodilators rarely are used alone to treat hypertension. Usually, they're used with other drugs to treat patients with moderate to severe hypertension. Calcium channel blockers may be used alone to treat mild to moderate hypertension.

Interactions

✦ When given with another antihypertensive, hydralazine and minoxidil have increased antihypertensive effects.
✦ Therapy with a vasodilator and a nitrate, such as isosorbide dinitrate or nitroglycerin, may produce additive effects.
✦ Grapefruit juice may inhibit the metabolism of diltiazem, felodipine, nifedipine, or nicardipine, increasing the drug's effects.

Adverse reactions

Direct vasodilators commonly produce adverse reactions related to reflex activation of the sympathetic nervous system: palpitations, angina, tachycardia, increased myocardial workload, ECG changes, edema, breast tenderness, fatigue, headache, and rash. Severe pericardial effusions may develop. Alkaline phosphatase, BUN, and creatinine levels may increase. Unlike direct vasodilators, calcium channel blockers don't produce rebound tachycardia or significant edema. Other adverse reactions depend on the specific drug used.

   Hypersensitivity reactions (urticaria, rash, pruritus, fever, chills, arthralgia, eosinophilia, and, rarely, obstructive jaundice and hepatitis) and blood dyscrasias (leukopenia, agranulocytosis, and thrombocytopenia) may also occur with some vasodilators.

Nursing considerations

✦ Prevent orthostatic hypotension by having the patient lie down for 15 to 30 minutes after giving diazoxide or hydralazine.
✦ Obtain baseline blood pressure and pulse rates before giving diazoxide or hydralazine. While giving the drug, monitor the blood pressure and pulse every 5 minutes for the first 30 minutes, and then every 15 minutes for 2 hours after each dose is given and until the blood pressure stabilizes.
✦ During nitroprusside therapy, monitor the patient's blood pressure continuously by an arterial line or every 5 minutes if an arterial line isn't available.

 CLINICAL ALERT Monitor for signs and symptoms of cerebral ischemia and impaired renal blood flow. These effects are most likely to occur when a vasodilator reduces the blood pressure too rapidly. If any signs or symptoms appear, help the patient to lie down, elevate his legs, and notify the prescriber immediately.

Possible drug interactions
✦ Antihypertensives
✦ Nitrates

Adverse reactions to watch for
✦ Angina, ECG changes, increased myocardial workload, palpitations, tachycardia
✦ Blood dyscrasias
✦ Breast tenderness
✦ Edema
✦ Fatigue, headache
✦ Hypersensitivity reactions
✦ Rash
✦ Severe pericardial effusion

Key nursing actions
✦ Obtain baseline blood pressure and pulse rate before giving diazoxide or hydralazine.
✦ Have the patient lie down for 15 to 30 minutes after giving diazoxide or hydralazine to prevent orthostatic hypotension.
✦ Monitor blood pressure continuously throughout nitroprusside therapy.

Teaching a patient about vasodilators

Whenever a vasodilator is prescribed, teach the patient and his family the drug's name, dose, frequency, action, and adverse effects. Also take the following actions.
- ✦ Teach the patient to take the drug exactly as prescribed, even if he feels better.
- ✦ Advise the patient to swallow felodipine or nifedipine capsules whole.
- ✦ Instruct the patient to take a missed dose as soon as possible, unless it's almost time for his next dose. Warn him never to take a double dose.
- ✦ Caution the patient not to stop taking the drug suddenly because doing so can produce serious adverse reactions.
- ✦ Urge the patient to report irregular heartbeat, shortness of breath, swelling of the hands or feet, dizziness, constipation, or nausea.
- ✦ Instruct the patient to rise slowly from a lying position and to sit for a few moments before standing to reduce the chance of dizziness.
- ✦ Warn the patient not to take diltiazem, felodipine, nicardipine, or nifedipine with grapefruit juice.

✦ Monitor a diabetic patient for increases in the glucose level for up to 1 week after diazoxide administration.

✦ Observe for early signs of drug-induced lupus erythematosuslike syndrome, such as myalgia, arthralgia, and pleuritis, when the hydralazine dosage exceeds 200 mg daily.

✦ Don't crush felodipine tables.

✦ Give sustained-release verapamil with food.

✦ Give diazoxide via a peripheral vein to prevent arrhythmias.

✦ Ask the patient to report headache, angina, or muscle cramps.

✦ Teach the patient and his caregiver about the prescribed drug. (See *Teaching a patient about vasodilators.*)

ACE INHIBITORS

Angiotensin-converting enzyme (ACE) inhibitors reduce blood pressure by interrupting the renin-angiotensin-aldosterone system. Commonly prescribed ACE inhibitors include benazepril, captopril, enalapril, enalaprilat, fosinopril, lisinopril, moexipril, quinapril, ramipril, and trandolapril.

Pharmacokinetics

After oral administration, ACE inhibitors are absorbed from the GI tract, distributed to most body tissues, metabolized somewhat in the liver, and excreted by the kidneys. Ramipril also is excreted in stool.

Pharmacodynamics

In the renin-angiotensin-aldosterone system, the kidneys normally maintain blood pressure by releasing the hormone renin. Renin acts on the plasma protein angiotensinogen to form angiotensin I. Angiotensin I is then converted to angiotensin II. Angiotensin II, a potent vasoconstrictor, increases peripheral resistance and promotes the excretion of aldosterone. Aldosterone, in turn, promotes the retention of sodium and water, increasing the volume of blood the heart needs to pump.

Features of ACE inhibitors

- ✦ Interrupt the renin-angiotensin-aldosterone system
- ✦ Promote sodium and water excretion
- ✦ Reduce blood pressure
- ✦ May be used alone or with other drugs to treat hypertension or various aspects of heart failure
- ✦ Improve survival for patients who have left-ventricular dysfunction or previous MI

LIFESPAN

Using ACE inhibitors safely

For patients at different developmental stages, therapy with an angiotensin-converting enzyme (ACE) inhibitor requires special considerations for safe use.

✦ For a woman of childbearing age, instruct her to report suspected pregnancy immediately to her prescriber. High risks of fetal morbidity and mortality are linked to ACE inhibitor use, especially in the second and third trimesters.

✦ For a breast-feeding woman, explain that some ACE inhibitors appear in breast milk. To avoid adverse reactions in the infant, instruct her to stop breast-feeding during therapy.

✦ For a child, give an ACE inhibitor only if its potential benefits outweigh the risks because the safety and efficacy haven't been established in children.

✦ For a geriatric patient, reduce the ACE inhibitor dose if needed because drug clearance is likely to be lessened.

ACE inhibitors interfere with this system. They work by preventing the conversion of angiotensin I to angiotensin II. As angiotensin II is reduced, arterioles dilate, reducing peripheral vascular resistance. By reducing aldosterone secretion, ACE inhibitors promote sodium and water excretion, reducing the amount of blood the heart needs to pump and resulting in decreased blood pressure.

Pharmacotherapeutics

All ACE inhibitors may be used alone or with other drugs, such as thiazide diuretics, to treat hypertension. Captopril, enalapril, fosinopril, lisinopril, quinapril, ramipril, and trandolapril also are indicated in heart failure to:

✦ treat left-ventricular systolic failure, unless contraindications or intolerance exists.

✦ treat left-ventricular systolic dysfunction without symptoms of heart failure.

✦ reduce mortality after an acute MI, especially in patients with prior myocardial injury.

✦ prevent or delay development of left ventricular dilation and overt heart failure in patients with recent or remote left ventricular dysfunction.

✦ produce complementary effects when combined with beta blockers.

✦ prevent fluid retention when combined with diuretics in patients with fluid retention or a history of it.

Lisinopril, ramipril, and trandolapril also are indicated to improve survival in patients who have had an MI. These drugs can reduce morbidity and mortality in patients with symptomatic or asymptomatic left-ventricular dysfunction.

In patients with vascular disease or diabetes, ramipril also can be used to prevent major cardiovascular events and reduce the risk of death, nonfatal MI, nonfatal stroke, and vascular complications of diabetes.

For patients at certain developmental stages, ACE inhibitor therapy requires special consideration. (See *Using ACE inhibitors safely*.)

Interactions

✦ An ACE inhibitor can enhance the hypotensive effects of a diuretic, beta blocker, or other antihypertensive.

✦ An ACE inhibitor can increase the lithium level, possibly resulting in lithium toxicity.

Possible drug interactions

✦ Antacids
✦ Antihypertensives
✦ Beta blockers
✦ Diuretics
✦ Lithium
✦ NSAIDs
✦ Potassium-sparing diuretics
✦ Tetracycline

✦ When an ACE inhibitor is used with a potassium-sparing diuretic, potassium supplement, or salt substitute containing potassium, hyperkalemia may occur.
✦ When taken with an NSAID, captopril, enalapril, or lisinopril may become less effective.
✦ An antacid may impair fosinopril absorption.
✦ Quinapril may reduce tetracycline absorption.

Adverse reactions

ACE inhibitors can produce a wide range of mild to severe adverse reactions. Severe adverse reactions, such as proteinuria, neutropenia, agranulocytosis, rash, and loss of taste, occur most commonly with captopril and may limit its use. Some of these reactions may be dose-related and may disappear during the first few weeks of therapy. The initial dose may cause profound hypotension or a severe allergic reaction.

CNS reactions, which may be related to lower blood pressure, can occur with all ACE inhibitors. These reactions may include headache, dizziness, fatigue, and syncope. GI reactions, such as abdominal pain, nausea, vomiting, and diarrhea, also can occur.

All ACE inhibitors may cause transient elevations of BUN and creatinine levels, especially in patients with hypertension caused by blood volume depletion or with renal or cardiovascular disease. The potassium level commonly increases, especially in patients with reduced renal function.

All ACE inhibitors can produce tickling in the throat and a dry, nonproductive, persistent cough. The cough, which occurs in about 15% of patients receiving these drugs, usually occurs in the first week of therapy and resolves with drug discontinuation.

Angioedema may occur with all ACE inhibitors, producing flushing or pallor and swelling of the face, arms, legs, lips, tongue, glottis, or larynx.

Adverse reactions to watch for

✦ Abdominal pain, diarrhea, nausea, vomiting
✦ Agranulocytosis, neutropenia, proteinuria
✦ Angioedema
✦ Dizziness, fatigue, headache, syncope
✦ Dry cough, tickle in throat
✦ Hypotension
✦ Increased potassium level
✦ Loss of taste
✦ Rash
✦ Transient increase in BUN and creatinine levels

Nursing considerations

✦ Obtain a baseline blood pressure and pulse rate before beginning ACE inhibitor therapy for later comparisons. Check the patient for hypotension when an ACE inhibitor is given for the first time with a diuretic.

 CLINICAL ALERT Observe for signs of angioedema. If angioedema occurs, withhold the drug, notify the prescriber, and begin emergency treatment, as indicated.

✦ Give a potassium supplement cautiously because ACE inhibitors may cause potassium retention.
✦ Monitor the patient's liver function test results and BUN, creatinine, and potassium levels before treatment begins and monthly for the first 3 months of therapy.
✦ Periodically monitor the patient's white blood cell (WBC) count.
✦ Teach the patient and his caregiver about the prescribed drug. (See *Teaching a patient about ACE inhibitors.*)

ANGIOTENSIN II RECEPTOR BLOCKERS

Angiotensin II receptor blockers lower blood pressure by blocking the vasoconstrictive effects of angiotensin II. Drugs in this class include candesartan, eprosartan, irbesartan, losartan, olmesartan, telmisartan, and valsartan.

Pharmacokinetics

Although these drugs vary greatly in their pharmacokinetic properties, all of them are highly bound to plasma proteins.

Pharmacodynamics

Angiotensin II receptor blockers interfere with the renin-angiotensin-aldosterone system. They selectively block the binding of angiotensin II to angiotensin$_1$ (AT$_1$) receptors. This leads to a blocking of the vasoconstriction and aldosterone-secreting action of angiotensin II, a potent vasoconstrictor. These drugs don't inhibit ACE, which is responsible for converting angiotensin I to angiotensin II, nor do they cause a breakdown in bradykinin (a vasodilator).

Pharmacotherapeutics

Used alone or with other drugs, such as diuretics, angiotensin II receptor blockers are prescribed to treat hypertension. Valsartan may also be used as an alternative — or adjunct — to ACE inhibitors for managing heart failure. Irbesartan and losartan are indicated for their renal protective effects in patients with type 2 diabetes mellitus. All drugs in this class require cautious use in certain patients. (See *Precautions for angiotensin II receptor blockers,* page 198.)

Interactions

✦ Fluconazole may increase the losartan level, leading to increased hypotensive effects.
✦ An NSAID may reduce the antihypertensive effects of any angiotensin II receptor blocker.
✦ Rifampin may increase losartan's metabolism and decrease its antihypertensive effects.
✦ When given with an angiotensin II receptor blocker, a potassium supplement can increase the risk of hyperkalemia.

Key nursing actions

✦ Obtain a baseline blood pressure and pulse rate before starting an ACE inhibitor.
✦ Watch for evidence of angioedema.
✦ Monitor liver function test results and BUN, creatinine, and potassium levels.
✦ Check the WBC count periodically.

Features of angiotensin II receptor blockers

✦ Reduce blood pressure by blocking the vasoconstrictive effects of angiotensin II
✦ Interfere with the renin-angiotensin-aldosterone system by blocking the binding of angiotensin II to AT$_1$ receptors
✦ Are used to treat hypertension

Possible drug interactions

✦ Fluconazole
✦ NSAIDs
✦ Potassium supplements
✦ Rifampin

Precautions for angiotensin II receptor blockers

Angiotensin II receptor blockers shouldn't be used in patients with heart failure or renal artery stenosis. In these patients, drug use may cause renal function to deteriorate, progressing from oliguria to azotemia, renal failure, and death.

These antihypertensive also should be avoided in pregnant women. The use of these drugs during the second or third trimester can result in fetal injury or death.

Adverse reactions to watch for

- Abdominal pain, diarrhea
- Altered renal function, hematuria
- Arthralgia, back pain, headache
- Bronchitis, pharyngitis, rhinitis, sinusitis, upper respiratory infection
- Depression, dizziness, fatigue
- Hypotension

Key nursing actions

- Monitor blood pressure closely.
- If hypotension develops, have the patient lie down; give volume expanders.
- Watch for evidence of angioedema.
- Correct intravascular volume depletion before starting antihypertensive therapy.

Adverse reactions

All angiotensin II receptor blockers may cause symptomatic hypotension, back pain, dizziness, upper respiratory infection (URI), pharyngitis, and rhinitis. Because the drugs act directly on the renin-angiotensin-aldosterone system, effects on renal function may be significant, especially in patients with heart failure or renal artery stenosis.

Other adverse effects of these drugs may include abdominal pain, arthralgia, fatigue, depression, headache, bronchitis, diarrhea, hematuria, and sinusitis.

Nursing considerations

- Monitor the patient's blood pressure closely. Symptomatic hypotension may occur.
- If hypotension occurs, have the patient lie down and give fluid volume expanders.
- Monitor the patient for signs and symptoms of angioedema.
- In a patient with intravascular volume depletion, correct the depletion before starting treatment.
- Teach the patient and his caregiver about the prescribed drug. (See *Teaching a patient about angiotensin II receptor blockers.*)

Teaching a patient about angiotensin II receptor blockers

Whenever an angiotensin II receptor blocker is prescribed, teach the patient and his family the drug's name, dose, frequency, action, and adverse effects. Also take the following actions.

- Instruct a woman of childbearing age to immediately notify the prescriber if she is, suspects she is, or plans to become pregnant.
- Advise the patient to avoid using a potassium supplement or salt substitute that contains potassium, unless approved by the prescriber.
- Instruct the patient to report light-headedness or fainting.

THIAZIDE AND THIAZIDE-LIKE DIURETICS

Diuretics are used to promote water and electrolyte excretion by the kidneys. By doing so, diuretics play a major role in treating hypertension and other cardiovascular conditions.

Thiazide and thiazide-like diuretics are sulfonamide derivatives. Thiazide diuretics include bendroflumethiazide, benzthiazide, chlorothiazide, hydrochlorothiazide, hydroflumethiazide, methyclothiazide, polythiazide, and trichlormethiazide.

Thiazide-like diuretics include chlorthalidone, indapamide, metolazone, and quinethazone.

Pharmacokinetics

After oral administration, thiazide diuretics are absorbed rapidly but incompletely from the GI tract. These drugs cross the placenta and appear in breast milk. They differ in how well they're metabolized, but are excreted primarily in urine.

Thiazide-like diuretics are absorbed from the GI tract. Indapamide is distributed widely into body tissues and metabolized in the liver. Chlorthalidone is 90% bound to RBCs. Little is known about chlorthalidone metabolism. These drugs are excreted primarily in urine.

Pharmacodynamics

Thiazide and thiazide-like diuretics work by preventing sodium reabsorption in the kidneys. As sodium is excreted, it pulls water along with it. These diuretics also increase the excretion of chloride, potassium, and bicarbonate, which can result in electrolyte imbalances.

Initially, these drugs decrease the circulating blood volume, leading to a reduced cardiac output. However, if therapy continues, cardiac output stabilizes, but fluid volume decreases.

Pharmacotherapeutics

Thiazide and thiazide-like diuretics are used for long-term treatment of hypertension and for treatment of edema caused by mild or moderate heart failure, liver disease, kidney disease, or corticosteroid or estrogen therapy.

Because these drugs decrease the calcium level in urine, they're also used alone or with other drugs to prevent the development and recurrence of calcium renal calculi. In patients with diabetes insipidus, thiazides paradoxically decrease urine volume, possibly through sodium depletion and extracellular volume reduction. In patients with certain disorders, however, thiazides should be avoided or used cautiously. (See *Contraindications and precautions for thiazide diuretics,* page 200.)

Interactions

For thiazide and thiazide-like diuretics, drug interactions typically result in altered fluid volume, blood pressure, and serum electrolyte levels.
+ A thiazide or thiazide-like diuretic may increase the need for insulin or an oral antidiabetic by increasing the glucose level.
+ When used with a thiazide or thiazide-like diuretic, a corticosteroid, corticotropin, or amphotericin may cause hypokalemia.
+ A thiazide or thiazide-like diuretic may increase the lithium level.
+ A thiazide or thiazide-like diuretic may increase the response to a skeletal muscle relaxant.
+ A cycloxygenase-2 (COX-2) inhibitor or other NSAID may reduce the antihypertensive effects of a thiazide or thiazide-like diuretic.

Features of thiazide and thiazide-like diuretics
+ Promote water and electrolyte excretion
+ Play a major role in treating hypertension and other cardiovascular conditions
+ Are sulfonamide derivatives
+ Prevent sodium reabsorption in the kidneys and increase excretion of water, chloride, potassium, and bicarbonate
+ Initially decrease cardiac output, which eventually stabilizes with reduced fluid volume
+ Are used for long-term treatment of hypertension and edema from heart failure, liver disease, kidney disease, or estrogen or corticosteroid therapy
+ Are also used to prevent renal calculi and to increase urine volume in patients with diabetes insipidus

Possible drug interactions
+ Amphotericin
+ Corticosteroids
+ Corticotropin
+ COX-2 inhibitors
+ Insulin
+ Lithium
+ NSAIDs
+ Oral antidiabetics
+ Skeletal muscle relaxants

Contraindications and precautions for thiazide diuretics

Thiazides are contraindicated in patients with anuria and in those who are allergic to thiazides or sulfonamides.

These diuretics require cautious use in patients with severe renal disease, impaired hepatic function, or progressive liver disease.

Adverse reactions to watch for

+ Anorexia, nausea, pancreatitis
+ Blood volume depletion, orthostatic hypotension
+ Glucose intolerance
+ Hypercalcemia, hyperuricemia
+ Hypersensivity reactions
+ Hypokalemia, hyponatremia, hypophosphatemia

Key nursing actions

+ Be alert for changes in sodium and potassium levels.
+ Watch for evidence of hyponatremia and hypokalemia.
+ Give a potassium supplement.
+ Weigh the patient daily under controlled conditions.
+ Document fluid intake and output.
+ Give the diuretic in the morning or early afternoon, if possible, to prevent nocturia.

Adverse reactions

Numerous adverse reactions to thiazide and thiazide-like diuretics can occur. The most common are blood volume depletion, orthostatic hypotension, hyponatremia, and hypokalemia. Others include glucose intolerance, hypercalcemia, and hypophosphatemia, which may occur with prolonged therapy; hyperuricemia; and GI reactions, such as anorexia, nausea, and pancreatitis.

Hypersensitivity reactions may take the form of purpura, photosensitivity, rash, urticaria, necrotizing vasculitis, or blood abnormalities, such as leukopenia, thrombocytopenia, aplastic anemia, or granulocytopenia, especially in patients who are allergic to sulfa drugs.

Nursing considerations

+ Be especially alert for changes in the patient's sodium and potassium levels. Also observe for signs and symptoms of hyponatremia, such as anxiety, hypotension, and nausea; and of hypokalemia, such as drowsiness, paresthesia, muscle cramps, and hyporeflexia.
+ Give a potassium supplement to maintain an adequate potassium level. Give normal or half-normal saline solution I.V. to correct hyponatremia.
+ Monitor a diabetic patient's glucose level during long-term therapy with a thiazide or thiazide-like diuretic because these drugs can cause glucose intolerance.
+ Weigh the patient daily under controlled conditions: at the same time each morning, after the patient voids, before the patient eats, with the patient wearing similar clothing each morning, and on the same scale.
+ Don't give chlorothiazide by the I.M. or subcutaneous (S.C.) routes.
+ Anticipate delayed diuresis in a patient with heart failure, impaired renal function, or another disorder that reduces renal blood flow.
+ Switch the patient to metolazone if his glomerular filtration rate falls below 20 ml/minute.
+ Document the patient's fluid intake and output.
+ If possible, give the diuretic in the morning or early afternoon to prevent nocturia from upsetting the patient's normal sleep pattern. Keep a urinal or bedpan within reach for a bedridden patient; ensure that the bathroom is easily accessible for an ambulatory patient.
+ Teach the patient and his caregiver about the prescribed drug. (See *Teaching a patient about thiazide and thiazide-like diuretics.*)

LOOP DIURETICS

Loop diuretics are highly potent drugs. They include bumetanide, ethacrynate sodium, ethacrynic acid, furosemide, and torsemide.

Pharmacokinetics

Usually, loop diuretics are absorbed well and distributed rapidly. These drugs are highly protein-bound. For the most part, they undergo partial or complete metabolism in the liver, except for furosemide, which is excreted mainly unchanged. Primarily, the kidneys excrete loop diuretics.

Pharmacodynamics

As the most potent diuretics available, loop diuretics produce the greatest volume of diuresis. They also have a high potential for causing severe adverse reactions. Bumetanide, the shortest-acting loop diuretic, is 40 times more potent than furosemide.

Loop diuretics receive their name because they act primarily on the thick ascending loop of Henle to increase sodium, chloride, and water secretion. These drugs may also inhibit sodium, chloride, and water reabsorption.

Features of loop diuretics

✦ Are very potent; produce the greatest volume of diuresis

✦ Have a high risk of adverse reactions

✦ Act mainly on the ascending loop of Henle to increase sodium, chloride, water secretion

✦ May inhibit sodium, chloride, water reabsorption

✦ Are used to treat hypertension (usually with a potassium-sparing diuretic or potassium supplement) or edema from heart failure, liver disease, or nephrotic syndrome

LIFESPAN

Avoiding the dangers of loop diuretics in geriatric patients

During loop diuretic therapy, geriatric patients and debilitated patients are at high risk for drug-induced diuresis. In these patients, excessive diuresis can quickly lead to dehydration, hypovolemia, hypokalemia, and hyponatremia and may cause circulatory collapse. To prevent these dangerous adverse reactions, closely monitor the patient's fluid intake and output, vital signs, and electrolyte levels. If you detect any abnormalities, notify the prescriber immediately. The diuretic dosage may need to be reduced, or fluid volume expanders may need to be ordered.

Also be aware that drug-induced transient deafness and auditory changes in geriatric patients can easily be mistaken for natural effects of aging. To determine the cause, ask about the onset of the auditory problems. The patient may need auditory testing.

Possible drug interactions

- Aminoglycosides
- Cisplatin
- Digoxin
- Lithium
- Oral antidiabetics

Adverse reactions to watch for

- Abdominal discomfort or pain, diarrhea
- Asymptomatic hyperuricemia
- Blood volume depletion
- Dermatitis
- Fluid and electrolyte imbalances
- Hepatic dysfunction
- Hypocalcemia, hypochloremia, hypochloremic alkalosis, hypokalemia, hyponatremia, hypomagnesemia
- Impaired glucose tolerance
- Orthostatic hypotension
- Paresthesia
- Thrombocytopenia
- Transient deafness

Pharmacotherapeutics

Loop diuretics are used to treat hypertension, usually with a potassium-sparing diuretic or a potassium supplement to prevent hypokalemia. These drugs sometimes are called high-ceiling diuretics because they produce a peak diuresis greater than that produced by other classes of diuretics.

Loop diuretics also are used to treat edema caused by heart failure, liver disease, or nephrotic syndrome.

Interactions

◆ Together, a loop diuretic (especially furosemide) and an aminoglycoside or cisplatin can increase the risk of ototoxicity.

◆ A loop diuretic can reduce an oral antidiabetic's hypoglycemic effect, possibly resulting in hyperglycemia.

◆ A loop diuretic may increase the risk of lithium toxicity.

◆ When digoxin is used with a loop diuretic, the interaction increases the risk of electrolyte imbalances that can trigger arrhythmias.

Adverse reactions

With loop diuretics, adverse reactions may be severe because these drugs have potent effects. The most common, severe reactions involve fluid and electrolyte imbalances, which can be especially dangerous in geriatric and debilitated patients. (See *Avoiding the dangers of loop diuretics in geriatric patients.*)

Other common adverse reactions include blood volume depletion, orthostatic hypotension, hypokalemia, hypochloremia, hypochloremic alkalosis, asymptomatic hyperuricemia, hyponatremia, hypocalcemia, and hypomagnesemia. Transient deafness, diarrhea, abdominal discomfort or pain, impaired glucose tolerance, dermatitis, paresthesia, hepatic dysfunction, and thrombocytopenia also can occur. Furosemide toxicity may produce such adverse reactions as tinnitus, abdominal pain, sore throat, and fever.

Hypersensitivity reactions include purpura, photosensitivity, rash, pruritus, urticaria, necrotizing angiitis, exfoliative dermatitis, allergic interstitial nephritis, and erythema multiforme. Agranulocytosis also can occur.

Teaching a patient about loop diuretics

Whenever a loop diuretic is prescribed, teach the patient and his family the drug's name, dose, frequency, action, and adverse effects. Also take the following actions.

✦ Advise a woman of childbearing age to tell her prescriber if she is pregnant or plans to become pregnant during therapy.

✦ Inform the patient that blood tests must be performed periodically to detect imbalances caused by drug therapy.

✦ Teach the patient to recognize and report the signs of hypokalemia.

✦ Explain the importance of taking a potassium supplement and eating a potassium-rich diet. Give the patient a list of potassium-rich foods.

✦ Teach the patient who also takes digoxin to identify the signs of digoxin toxicity, such as gastrointestinal, cardiac, and neurologic disturbances.

✦ Instruct the diabetic patient to monitor his glucose level closely. Advise him that diabetes treatment may require adjustment during loop diuretic therapy.

✦ Instruct the patient to take the diuretic in the morning or early afternoon, if possible, to avoid having to urinate at night.

✦ Teach the patient weigh himself daily under the same conditions every time and to notify the prescriber of any sudden weight gain of more than 2 pounds in 1 day, peripheral edema, or shortness of breath.

✦ Tell the patient how to minimize the effects of orthostatic hypotension.

✦ Advise the patient to expect an increase in urinary frequency and quantity.

✦ Instruct the patient taking furosemide to report any signs of furosemide toxicity, such as ringing in the ears, abdominal pain, sore throat, and fever.

✦ Instruct the patient to store furosemide tablets in light-resistant containers to prevent discoloration.

✦ Tell the patient not to stop taking the drug without first consulting his prescriber.

Nursing considerations

CLINICAL ALERT Be especially alert for changes in the patient's sodium and potassium levels. Also observe for signs and symptoms of hyponatremia, such as anxiety, hypotension, and nausea; and of hypokalemia, such as drowsiness, paresthesia, muscle cramps, hyporeflexia, and tachycardia or bradycardia.

✦ Teach the patient and his caregiver about the prescribed drug. (See *Teaching a patient about loop diuretics.*)

✦ Give a potassium supplement to maintain an adequate potassium level. Give normal or half-normal saline solution I.V. to correct hyponatremia.

✦ Weigh the patient daily under controlled conditions: at the same time each morning, after the patient voids, before the patient eats, with the patient wearing similar clothing each morning, and on the same scale.

✦ Carefully monitor a diabetic patient's glucose level.

CLINICAL ALERT Check the bumetanide (Bumex) dosage with extreme care; this drug is 40 times more potent than furosemide. Don't confuse it with Buprenex.

✦ Don't give ethacrynate sodium I.M. or S.C. to avoid tissue irritation.

✦ Give I.M. furosemide using the Z-track method to minimize tissue irritation.

Key nursing actions

✦ Watch for changes in sodium and potassium levels.

✦ Give a potassium supplement as needed.

✦ Weigh the patient daily under controlled conditions.

✦ Give an I.V. drug slowly over 1 to 2 minutes.

✦ Give the drug in the morning or early afternoon, if possible, to prevent nocturia.

✦ Watch for evidence of dehydration.

✦ Document fluid intake and output.

◆ Give an I.V. loop diuretic slowly over 1 to 2 minutes to prevent adverse reactions.
◆ Store oral furosemide tablets and injectable furosemide in light-resistant containers to prevent discoloration. Refrigerate oral furosemide solutions to ensure stability. Don't use yellow injectable furosemide solutions.
◆ Give the loop diuretic in the morning or early afternoon, if possible, to prevent nocturia from disturbing the patient's normal sleep pattern.
◆ Monitor the patient for signs of dehydration, such as poor skin turgor and dry oral mucous membranes. Check his vital signs to detect signs of hypovolemia, such as tachycardia, hypotension, and dyspnea. If you detect these findings, notify the prescriber.
◆ Record the patient's fluid intake and output. If extreme discrepancies occur, notify the prescriber and decrease the diuretic dosage.

POTASSIUM-SPARING DIURETICS

Compared to other diuretics, potassium-sparing diuretics have weaker diuretic and antihypertensive effects. However, they have the advantage of conserving potassium. Drugs in this diuretic class include amiloride, spironolactone, and triamterene.

Pharmacokinetics

After oral administration, potassium-sparing diuretics are absorbed in the GI tract. They're metabolized in the liver (except for amiloride, which isn't metabolized) and excreted primarily in urine and bile.

Pharmacodynamics

By acting directly on the distal tubule of the kidneys, potassium-sparing diuretics increase urinary excretion of sodium and water as well as chloride and calcium ions. They also decrease the excretion of potassium and hydrogen ions. These effects reduce blood pressure and increase the potassium level.

Spironolactone is structurally similar to aldosterone and acts as an aldosterone antagonist. Aldosterone promotes the retention of sodium and water and loss of potassium. Spironolactone counteracts these effects by competing with aldosterone for receptor sites. As a result, sodium, chloride, and water are excreted and potassium is retained.

Pharmacotherapeutics

Potassium-sparing diuretics commonly are used with other diuretics to potentiate their action or counteract their potassium-wasting effects. These diuretics are used to treat hypertension, edema, heart failure, cirrhosis, nephrotic syndrome, and diuretic-induced hypokalemia in patients with heart failure.

Spironolactone also is used to treat hyperaldosteronism and hirsutism, including hirsutism caused by polycystic ovary syndrome.

Interactions

Few drugs interact with amiloride, spironolactone, and triamterene. Those interactions that do occur aren't related to the drug itself, but to its potassium-sparing effects.

Adverse reactions

Potassium-sparing diuretics produce few adverse reactions. However, their potassium-sparing effects can lead to hyperkalemia, especially if a potassium-sparing diuretic is taken with a potassium supplement or a high-potassium diet.

Features of potassium-sparing diuretics
◆ Have relatively weak diuretic and antihypertensive effects
◆ Act directly on distal tubule of the kidney to increase excretion of sodium, water, chloride, calcium ions
◆ Decrease excretion of potassium and hydrogen ions
◆ Increase the potassium level
◆ Are commonly used with potassium-wasting diuretics for hypertension, edema, heart failure, cirrhosis, nephrotic syndrome, diuretic-induced hypokalemia

Adverse reactions to watch for
◆ Abdominal pain or cramps, anorexia, constipation, diarrhea, nausea, vomiting
◆ Acidosis
◆ Agranulocytosis
◆ Blood volume depletion

Teaching a patient about potassium-sparing diuretics

Whenever a potassium-sparing diuretic is prescribed, teach the patient and his family the drug's name, dose, frequency, action, and adverse effects. Also take the following actions.
- ✦ Instruct the patient to expect an increase in urinary frequency and quantity.
- ✦ Advise a woman of childbearing age to tell the prescriber if she is pregnant or plans to become pregnant during diuretic therapy.
- ✦ Inform the patient that blood tests must be performed periodically to identify imbalances caused by the potassium-sparing diuretic.
- ✦ Teach the patient to recognize and report the signs of hyperkalemia.
- ✦ Advise the patient to avoid eating potassium-rich foods because these diuretics conserve potassium.
- ✦ Instruct the patient to take the diuretic in the morning or early afternoon, if possible, to avoid having to urinate at night.
- ✦ Teach the patient to weigh himself daily under the same conditions every time and to notify the prescriber of any sudden weight gain of more than 2 pounds in 1 day, peripheral edema, or shortness of breath.
- ✦ Tell the patient how to minimize the effects of orthostatic hypotension.
- ✦ Teach the patient how to manage minor adverse reactions, such as dry mouth (by chewing sugarless gum or sucking on sugarless hard candy) and constipation (by increasing fiber intake and exercise).
- ✦ Inform the patient that amiloride may cause impotence that should subside when the drug is stopped.

Other dose-related reactions to these diuretics include megaloblastic anemia (especially with triamterene), dizziness, orthostatic hypotension, sore throat, dry mouth, nausea, and vomiting.

Amiloride may produce headache, nausea, vomiting, anorexia, diarrhea, muscle cramps, abdominal pain, constipation, impotence, and metabolic disturbances, including blood volume depletion, hyponatremia, a transient rise in the BUN level, and acidosis. Spironolactone may produce headache, abdominal cramps, diarrhea, gynecomastia in men, breast soreness and menstrual abnormalities in women, and rarely, agranulocytosis.

Hypersensitivity reactions to potassium-sparing diuretics include urticaria, pruritus, erythematous eruptions, rash, photosensitivity, and anaphylaxis.

Nursing considerations
- ✦ Teach the patient and his caregiver about the prescribed drug. (See *Teaching a patient about potassium-sparing diuretics.*)
- ✦ Monitor the patient for signs and symptoms of hyperkalemia, such as confusion, hyperexcitability, muscle weakness, paresthesia, flaccid paralysis, arrhythmias, abdominal distention, diarrhea, and intestinal colic. Also monitor the patient's electrolytes for imbalances.
- ✦ Weigh the patient daily under controlled conditions: at the same time each morning, after he voids and before he eats, wearing similar clothing, and on the same scale.
- ✦ Store spironolactone in a light-resistant container.

Adverse reactions to watch for
(continued)
- ✦ Breast soreness and menstrual abnormalities in women
- ✦ Dizziness, headache, orthostatic hypotension
- ✦ Dry mouth, sore throat
- ✦ Gynecomastia in men
- ✦ Hyperkalemia
- ✦ Hypersensitivity reactions
- ✦ Hyponatremia
- ✦ Impotence
- ✦ Megaloblastic anemia
- ✦ Muscle cramps
- ✦ Transient rise in BUN level

Key nursing actions
- ✦ Watch for evidence of hyperkalemia.
- ✦ Weigh the patient daily under controlled conditions.

Key nursing actions
(continued)

+ Give the drug in the morning or early afternoon, if possible, to prevent nocturia.
+ Assess for evidence of dehydration.

✦ Give a potassium-sparing diuretic in the morning or early afternoon, if possible, to avoid nocturia.

✦ Give amiloride with food.

✦ Observe the patient with nausea, vomiting, or diarrhea for signs of dehydration.

✦ Notify the prescriber if the patient's condition doesn't improve or if he experiences adverse reactions, such as GI distress. Give an antiemetic or antidiarrheal, as needed.

ANTILIPEMICS

Antilipemics are used to lower abnormally high blood levels of lipids, such as cholesterol, triglycerides, and phospholipids. The risk of developing coronary artery disease (CAD) increases when lipid levels are elevated. To reduce lipid levels, drug therapy is combined with lifestyle changes, such as proper diet, weight loss, exercise, and treatment of any underlying disorder.

Classes of antilipemic drugs include bile-sequestering drugs, fibric acid derivatives, hydroxymethylglutaryl-coenzyme A (HMG-CoA) reductase inhibitors, cholesterol absorption inhibitors, and nicotinic acid.

BILE-SEQUESTERING DRUGS

The bile-sequestering drugs — cholestyramine, colesevelam, and colestipol — are resins that remove excess bile acids from the fat depots under the skin.

Pharmacokinetics

After oral administration, bile-sequestering drugs aren't absorbed from the GI tract. Instead, they remain in the intestine, where they combine with bile acids for about 5 hours. Eventually, they're excreted in stool.

Pharmacodynamics

The bile-sequestering drugs lower LDL levels. These drugs combine with bile acids to form an insoluble compound that is excreted in stool. The decreasing level of bile acid in the gallbladder triggers the liver to synthesize more bile acids from their precursor, cholesterol.

As cholesterol leaves the bloodstream and other storage areas to replace the lost bile acids, cholesterol levels decrease. Because the small intestine needs bile acids to emulsify lipids and form chylomicrons, absorption of all lipids and lipid-soluble drugs decreases until the bile acids are replaced.

Features of bile-sequestering drugs

+ Remove excess bile acids from fat depots under the skin
+ Combine with bile acids to form an insoluble compound excreted in stool
+ Lower the LDL levels
+ Are the treatment of choice for patients unable to lower their LDL levels through diet alone

Pharmacotherapeutics

Bile-sequestering drugs are the treatment of choice for type IIa hyperlipoproteinemia (familial hypercholesterolemia) in patients who can't lower their LDL level with dietary changes alone. A patient whose cholesterol level indicates a severe risk of CAD is likely to require one of these drugs to supplement his diet.

Possible drug interactions

+ Anticoagulants
+ Aspirin
+ Clindamycin
+ Digoxin
+ Furosemide
+ Glipizide
+ Hydrocortisone
+ Imipramine
+ Methyldopa
+ Nicotinic acid
+ Penicillins

Interactions

✦ In the GI tract, a bile-sequestering drug may bind with and decrease the absorption and effectiveness of other drugs, especially aspirin, clindamycin, digoxin, furosemide, glipizide, hydrocortisone, imipramine, methyldopa, nicotinic acid, propranolol, tetracyclines, thiazide diuretics, phenytoin, penicillins, or thyroid hormones or derivatives.

PATIENT TEACHING

Teaching a patient about bile-sequestering drugs

Whenever a bile-sequestering drug is prescribed, teach the patient and his family the drug's name, dose, frequency, action, and adverse effects. Also take the following actions.

✦ Advise the patient to have his cholesterol level checked every 3 to 6 months to evaluate the effectiveness of therapy.

✦ Advise the patient not to take the drug in its powder form. Demonstrate how to mix it in a suitable liquid, fruit, or other food.

✦ If dizziness or weakness occurs, advise the patient not to drive or perform activities that require alertness.

✦ Instruct the patient taking a drug that binds with the prescribed bile-sequestering drug to take it 1 hour before or 6 hours after taking the bile-sequestering drug.

✦ Instruct the patient to inform all other prescribers about bile-sequestering drug therapy; the dosages of other drugs may need to be adjusted.

✦ Teach the patient how to prevent constipation.

✦ Reassure the patient that adverse GI reactions usually diminish as therapy continues.

✦ A bile-sequestering drug may reduce the absorption of a lipid-soluble vitamin, such as vitamins A, D, E, and K. Poor absorption of vitamin K can significantly affect the prothrombin time and increase the risk of bleeding.

✦ Cholestyramine may decrease the therapeutic effects of an anticoagulant.

Adverse reactions

With short-term use, bile-sequestering drugs produce relatively mild adverse reactions.

With long-term therapy, these drugs may cause more severe reactions. For example, they commonly produce adverse GI effects, which can be minimized by introducing and adjusting the drugs slowly to a maximum dosage. Constipation may occur but usually isn't serious. Severe fecal impaction, however, may occur. Other adverse GI effects may include abdominal pain, abdominal distention, flatulence, belching, nausea, vomiting, diarrhea, or hemorrhoid irritation. Rarely, peptic ulceration and bleeding, cholelithiasis, and cholecystitis occur.

Miscellaneous reactions to bile-sequestering drugs include headache, dizziness, anorexia, weakness, and fatigue.

Nursing considerations

✦ Teach the patient and his caregiver about the prescribed drug. (See *Teaching a patient about bile-sequestering drugs.*)

✦ Obtain baseline cholesterol levels before therapy begins. Then monitor cholesterol levels every 3 to 6 months for a patient receiving long-term therapy.

✦ Introduce and adjust drug slowly to minimize adverse GI reactions.

✦ Give drugs that bind with bile-sequestering drugs 1 hour before or 6 hours after giving the bile-sequestering drug.

 CLINICAL ALERT Don't stop the drug suddenly if a significantly bound drug was adjusted to a maintenance dosage during antilipemic therapy. Such discontinuation could be dangerous, even toxic.

Possible drug interactions
(continued)

✦ Phenytoin
✦ Propranolol
✦ Tetracyclines
✦ Thiazide diuretics
✦ Thyroid hormones or derivatives
✦ Vitamins A, D, E, and K

Adverse reactions to watch for

✦ Abdominal pain or distention, anorexia, diarrhea, nausea, vomiting
✦ Belching, flatulence
✦ Constipation, fecal impaction
✦ Dizziness, headache, fatigue, weakness
✦ Hemorrhoid irritation

Key nursing actions

✦ Obtain baseline cholesterol levels.
✦ Monitor cholesterol levels every 3 to 6 months during therapy.
✦ Introduce and adjust the drug slowly to minimize GI reactions.
✦ Don't stop the drug abruptly.
✦ Assess regularly for constipation.
✦ Urge the patient to drink 2 to 3 L of fluid daily and to increase his fiber intake.

✦ Mix the powder form with 120 to 180 ml (4 to 6 ounces) of liquid, such as water, carbonated beverage, or soup, or a pulpy fruit with a high moisture content, such as applesauce. Never give the dry powder because the patient may inhale it accidentally.
✦ Monitor the patient's bowel habits throughout therapy to detect constipation.
✦ Encourage the patient to drink 2 to 3 L (8 to 12 8-ounce glasses) of fluid daily, increase his dietary fiber intake (unless contraindicated), and get plenty of exercise to prevent constipation.

FIBRIC ACID DERIVATIVES

Several fungi produce fibric acid. Two derivatives of this acid, fenofibrate and gemfibrozil, are used to reduce a high triglyceride level and, to a lesser extent, a high LDL level.

Pharmacokinetics

Fenofibrate and gemfibrozil are absorbed readily from the GI tract and are highly protein-bound. Fenofibrate undergoes rapid hydrolysis, and gemfibrozil undergoes extensive metabolism in the liver. Both drugs are excreted in urine.

Pharmacodynamics

Although the exact mechanism of action for these drugs isn't known, researchers believe that fibric acid derivatives may:
✦ reduce cholesterol production early in its formation.
✦ mobilize cholesterol from tissues.
✦ increase cholesterol excretion.
✦ decrease lipoprotein synthesis and secretion.
✦ decrease triglyceride synthesis.
    Gemfibrozil also increases the HDL level and the capacity to dissolve additional cholesterol.

Pharmacotherapeutics

Fibric acid derivatives are used primarily to reduce triglyceride and VLDL levels. They're also used to reduce cholesterol levels. Because of their ability to reduce triglyceride levels, these drugs are prescribed to treat patients with types II, III, IV, and mild-type V hyperlipoproteinemia.

Interactions

✦ When taken with an oral anticoagulant, a fibric acid derivative increases the risk of bleeding.
✦ Rhabdomyolysis may occur when fenofibrate or gemfibrozil is given with HMG-CoA reductase inhibitors.

Adverse reactions

The most common reactions to fibric acid derivatives are adverse GI effects, which resemble those of the bile-sequestering drugs. Several studies show that these drugs increase the risk of cholelithiasis and the need for cholecystectomy.
    Fibric acid derivatives may produce a wide range of hypersensitivity reactions. These may include rash, alopecia, urticaria, dry skin, brittle hair, hepatomegaly, impotence, decreased libido, leukopenia, weight gain, muscle pain, and abnormal liver function test results.

Features of fibric acid derivatives

✦ Reduce triglyceride and LDL levels
✦ Reduce cholesterol production, mobilize it from tissues, increase its excretion, and decrease lipoprotein and triglyceride synthesis
✦ Are prescribed for people with types II, III, IV, and mild V hyperlipoproteinemia

Possible drug interactions

✦ HMG-CoA reductase inhibitors
✦ Oral anticoagulants

Adverse reactions to watch for

✦ Adverse GI effects
✦ Cholelithiasis
✦ Hypersensitivity reactions: abnormal liver function test results, alopecia, brittle hair, decreased libido, dry skin, hepatomegaly, impotence, leukopenia, muscle pain, rash, urticaria, weight gain

Teaching a patient about fibric acid derivatives

Whenever a fibric acid derivative is prescribed, teach the patient and his family the drug's name, dose, frequency, action, and adverse effects. Also take the following actions.

✦ Stress the importance of having regular liver function studies and triglyceride and cholesterol level tests. Explain the purpose of these tests and tell the patient that they require fasting after midnight with a blood sample to be drawn the following morning.

✦ Tell the patient to report any unusual symptoms to the prescriber.

✦ Advise the patient that GI disturbances are the most common adverse reactions. Teach the patient how to manage these reactions. For example, urge him to increase fluid and fiber intake and amount of exercise to relieve constipation.

✦ Instruct the patient who also takes an anticoagulant to notify the prescriber about fibric acid derivative therapy because the anticoagulant dosage may need to be reduced to prevent bleeding. Teach the patient to take bleeding precautions, such as avoiding cuts and bruises, using a soft toothbrush, and using an electric razor when shaving.

✦ Instruct the patient with a decreased white blood cell count to prevent infection by avoiding crowds and people who are ill and by getting plenty of rest.

✦ Advise the patient to take gemfibrozil in two divided doses, 30 minutes before his morning and evening meals.

✦ Instruct the patient to report biliary colic, which typically appears as abdominal pain or nausea and vomiting that subsides, with or without treatment, after several hours. Explain that diagnostic tests may be needed to check for gallstones.

✦ Instruct the patient to report leg pain when walking or pain, swelling, or redness that develops in either calf. Tell the patient to go to the nearest emergency department if shortness of breath suddenly develops.

Nursing considerations

✦ Monitor the patient's liver function test results and WBC counts to detect abnormalities. Check his triglyceride and cholesterol levels to assess the drug's effectiveness.

✦ Give gemfibrozil in two divided doses daily, 30 minutes before morning and evening meals.

✦ Notify the prescriber if biliary colic occurs, and give an analgesic, if needed.

✦ Teach the patient and his caregiver about the prescribed drug. (See *Teaching a patient about fibric acid derivatives*.)

Key nursing actions

✦ Monitor liver function test results and WBC counts.

✦ Notify the prescriber about biliary colic; give an analgesic, if needed.

HMG-CoA REDUCTASE INHIBITORS

Also known as *statins*, HMG-CoA reductase inhibitors lower lipid levels by interfering with cholesterol synthesis. These drugs include atorvastatin, fluvastatin, lovastatin, pravastatin, and simvastatin.

Pharmacokinetics

Except for pravastatin, these drugs are highly bound to plasma proteins. All of them undergo extensive first-pass metabolism; however, plasma levels don't correlate with the drugs' ability to lower cholesterol. Their specific pharmacokinetic properties vary slightly.

Features of HMG-CoA reductase inhibitors

+ Are also known as *statins*
+ Lower LDL and total cholesterol levels by interfering with cholesterol synthesis
+ Increase HDL level slightly
+ Are used to treat primary hypercholesterolemia (types IIa and IIb) and prevent cardiovascular events

Possible drug interactions

+ Bile-sequestering drugs
+ Clarithromycin
+ Cyclosporine
+ Erythromycin
+ Fluconazole
+ Gemfibrozil
+ Itraconazole
+ Ketoconazole
+ Niacin
+ Warfarin

Adverse reactions to watch for

+ Abdominal pain, constipation, diarrhea, dyspepsia, flatulence, heartburn, nausea, vomiting
+ Alopecia, pruritus, rash
+ Altered liver function tests
+ Angina, chest pain, hypertension
+ Arthralgia, asthenia, back or shoulder pain, dizziness, fatigue, headache, muscle cramps, myalgia, myopathy, rhabdomyolysis
+ Bronchitis, cough, pharyngitis, rhinitis, sinusitis, upper respiratory infection
+ Cholestatic jaundice, cirrhosis, hepatitis, pancreatitis
+ Erectile dysfunction, gynecomastia, libido changes, sexual dysfunction

Pharmacodynamics

HMG-CoA reductase inhibitors reduce cholesterol levels by inhibiting enzyme activity. This interferes with an early step of cholesterol synthesis, thereby reducing LDL synthesis and enhancing LDL breakdown.

Pharmacotherapeutics

Drugs in this class are used primarily to reduce the LDL level and also to reduce total cholesterol levels. These drugs also produce a mild increase in the HDL level.

Because of their ability to lower cholesterol levels, these drugs are used to treat primary hypercholesterolemia (types IIa and IIb). As a result of their effect on LDL and total cholesterol levels, they're indicated for primary and secondary prevention of cardiovascular events. However, all HMG-CoA reductase inhibitors are contraindicated in pregnant and breast-feeding women.

Interactions

+ Atorvastatin, lovastatin, or simvastatin, may increase the risk of myopathy or rhabdomyolysis when used with niacin, erythromycin, clarithromycin, cyclosporine, fluconazole, gemfibrozil, itraconazole, or ketoconazole.
+ A bile-sequestering drug may bind with and reduce the effectiveness of an HMG-CoA reductase inhibitor.
+ When given with warfarin, lovastatin or simvastatin may increase the risk of bleeding.
+ St. John's wort may decrease the cholesterol-lowering effects of lovastatin or simvastatin.
+ Grapefruit juice may inhibit the first-pass metabolism of atorvastatin, increasing the drug level and the risk of adverse reactions.

Adverse reactions

HMG-CoA reductase inhibitors may alter liver function test results, increasing AST, ALT, alkaline phosphatase, and bilirubin levels. Other hepatic effects may include pancreatitis, hepatitis, cholestatic jaundice, and cirrhosis.

Myalgia is the most common adverse musculoskeletal effect of these drugs. Arthralgia, back pain, shoulder pain, muscle cramps, leg cramps, arthritis and myositis may also occur. Myopathy and rhabdomyolysis are severe, potentially fatal adverse reactions that may occur rarely with these drugs.

Adverse GI reactions may include diarrhea, abdominal pain, flatulence, nausea, vomiting, constipation, dyspepsia, and heartburn. Other adverse effects may include URI, pharyngitis, rhinitis, sinusitis, bronchitis, cough, rash, pruritus, and alopecia.

The most frequent nervous system effect is headache. Asthenia, fatigue, and dizziness may also occur.

Additional adverse effects may include chest pain, hypertension, angina, libido changes, sexual dysfunction, erectile dysfunction, and gynecomastia.

Nursing considerations

+ Advise the patient to begin or continue lifestyle changes, including dietary management, weight control, and exercise because they're crucial to successful treatment.
+ Perform liver function tests before and at 6 to 12 weeks after therapy begins.
+ Monitor the patient's cholesterol levels to assess the drug's effectiveness.
+ Give lovastatin with the evening meal to enhance absorption.

✦ Give pravastatin at bedtime to a geriatric patient or one with primary hypercholesterolemia and significant renal or hepatic dysfunction.

✦ Give simvastatin in the evening.

✦ If therapy also includes a bile-sequestering drug, give the HMG-CoA reductase inhibitor 1 hour before or 6 hours after it.

✦ Teach the patient and his caregiver about the prescribed drug. (See *Teaching a patient about HMG-CoA reductase inhibitors.*)

CHOLESTEROL ABSORPTION INHIBITORS

Drugs in this new class of antilipemics work by inhibiting the absorption of cholesterol and related phytosterols from the intestine. Ezetimibe is a cholesterol absorption inhibitor.

Pharmacokinetics

Ezetimibe is absorbed and extensively conjugated to an active form that is highly bound to plasma proteins. The drug is metabolized primarily in the small intestine and is excreted by biliary and renal routes.

Pharmacodynamics

Cholesterol absorption inhibitors work at the brush border of the small intestine to inhibit cholesterol absorption. This decreases the delivery of intestinal cholesterol to the liver, reducing hepatic cholesterol stores and increasing cholesterol clearance from the blood. Ultimately, this reduces cholesterol levels.

Pharmacotherapeutics

As an adjunct to dietary changes, ezetimibe may be given alone to treat primary hypercholesterolemia and homozygous sitosterolemia. The drug also can be used with an HMG-CoA reductase inhibitor to treat primary hypercholesterolemia and homozygous familial hypercholesterolemia. Ezetimibe further reduces total cholesterol and LDL levels and further increases the HDL level in patients who

Key nursing actions

✦ Urge the patient to start or continue lifestyle changes.

✦ Assess liver function test results before and at 6 to 12 weeks after therapy starts.

✦ Monitor cholesterol levels.

Features of cholesterol absorption inhibitors

✦ Inhibit absorption of cholesterol and related phytosterols at the brush border of the small intestine

✦ Decrease the delivery of intestinal cholesterol to the liver, reducing hepatic cholesterol stores and increasing cholesterol clearance from the blood

✦ Are used to treat primary hypercholesterolemia and homozygous sitosterolemia

✦ May be given with an HMG-CoA reductase inhibitor

Possible drug interactions

+ Cholestyramine
+ Cyclosporine
+ Fenofibrate
+ Gemfibrozil

Adverse reactions to watch for

+ Abdominal pain, diarrhea
+ Arthralgia, back pain, myalgia
+ Chest pain
+ Cough
+ Dizziness, fatigue, headache
+ Pharyngitis, sinusitis, upper respiratory tract infection

Key nursing actions

+ Place the patient on a diet for lowering cholesterol before therapy starts, and urge him to continue it during therapy.
+ If the drug is given with an HMG-CoA reductase inhibitor, assess liver function test results before therapy starts and periodically thereafter.

WARNING

Contraindications for cholesterol absorption inhibitors

The cholesterol absorption inhibitor ezetimibe is contraindicated in patients who are hypersensitive to any component of the drug. Use of ezetimibe with a hydroxymethylglutaryl-coenzyme A (HMG-CoA) reductase inhibitor is contraindicated in patients with active liver disease or unexplained persistent liver enzyme elevations.

can't achieve their antilipemic goals with the maximum dosage of an HMG-CoA reductase inhibitor.

In some patients, however, this drug should be avoided or used with caution. (See *Contraindications for cholesterol absorption inhibitors.*)

Interactions

+ Cholestyramine may reduce ezetimibe's effectiveness.
+ Cyclosporine, fenofibrate, or gemfibrozil may increase the ezetimibe level.

Adverse reactions

The most common adverse reactions to ezetimibe monotherapy include fatigue, abdominal pain, diarrhea, pharyngitis, sinusitis, arthralgia, back pain, and cough.

When the drug is given with an HMG-CoA reductase inhibitor, the most common adverse reactions are chest pain, dizziness, fatigue, headache, abdominal pain, diarrhea, pharyngitis, sinusitis, upper respiratory tract infection, arthralgia, back pain, and myalgia.

Nursing considerations

+ Before treatment, place the patient on a standard cholesterol-lowering diet. Urge him to continue the diet during treatment.
+ If ezetimibe is given with an HMG-CoA reductase inhibitor, perform liver function studies before therapy begins and then periodically based on recommendations for the HMG-CoA reductase inhibitor.
+ Teach the patient and his caregiver about the prescribed drug. (See *Teaching a patient about cholesterol absorption inhibitors.*)

NICOTINIC ACID

Also known as *niacin,* nicotinic acid is a water-soluble vitamin that decreases triglyceride and apolipoprotein B-100 levels and increases the HDL level. The drug is available in immediate-release and extended-release tablets.

Pharmacokinetics

Nicotinic acid is moderately bound to plasma proteins; its overall binding ranges from 60% to 70%. The drug undergoes rapid metabolism by the liver to active and inactive metabolites. About 75% of the drug is excreted in urine.

Pharmacodynamics

The way that nicotinic acid lowers triglyceride and apolipoprotein levels is unknown. However, it may work by inhibiting hepatic synthesis of lipoproteins that contain apolipoprotein B-100, promoting lipoprotein lipase activity, reducing free fatty acid mobilization from adipose tissue, and increasing fecal elimination of sterols.

Pharmacotherapeutics

Nicotinic acid is used primarily as an adjunct to lower triglyceride levels in patients with type IV or V hyperlipidemia who are at high risk for pancreatitis. The drug may also be used to lower cholesterol and LDL levels in patients with hypercholesterolemia. It's frequently used with other antilipemics to meet LDL goals and to increase the HDL level for patients in whom it's below the desired level.

This antilipemic is contraindicated in patients who are hypersensitive to nicotinic acid and in those with hepatic dysfunction, active peptic ulcer disease, or arterial bleeding.

Interactions

+ Together, nicotinic acid and an HMG-CoA reductase inhibitor may increase the risk of muscle wasting and weakness, or myopathy, or life-threatening breakdown of skeletal muscle, causing renal failure or rhabdomyolysis.
+ A bile-sequestering drug, such as cholestyramine or colestipol, can bind with nicotinic acid and decrease its effectiveness.
+ When given with nicotinic acid, kava may increase the risk of hepatotoxicity.

Adverse reactions

High doses of nicotinic acid may produce vasodilation and cause flushing. Extended-release forms tend to produce less severe vasodilation than immediate-release forms. To help minimize flushing, 325 mg of aspirin may be given 30 minutes before nicotinic acid, or the extended-release form may be given at night.

Nicotinic acid can cause hepatotoxicity; the risk of this adverse reaction is greater with extended-release forms. To help prevent this reaction, monitor the patient's liver function test results periodically and assess him for signs and symptoms of liver failure.

Nursing considerations

+ Don't confuse the extended-release form of nicotinic acid with the immediate-release form.
+ Monitor the patient's liver function test results every 6 to 12 weeks for the first year of therapy, then about every 6 months thereafter.

Features of nicotinic acid

+ Is a vitamin, niacin
+ Decreases triglyceride and apolipoprotein B-100 levels; increases the HDL level
+ May inhibit hepatic synthesis of lipoproteins, promote lipoprotein lipase activity, reduce free fatty acid mobilization from fat, and increase the sterol level in feces
+ Are used mainly as an adjunct to lower triglyceride levels in patients with type IV or V hyperlipidemia who are at risk for pancreatitis
+ Are often used with other antilipemics

Possible drug interactions

+ HMG-CoA reductase inhibitors
+ Bile-sequestering drugs

Adverse reactions to watch for

+ Flushing
+ Hepatotoxicity
+ Vasodilation

Key nursing actions

✦ Monitor liver function test results every 6 to 12 weeks for the first year of therapy, about every 6 months thereafter.
✦ Watch for evidence of liver failure.

Teaching a patient about nicotinic acid

Whenever nicotinic acid is prescribed, teach the patient and his family the drug's name, dose, frequency, action, and adverse effects. Also take the following actions.
◆ Warn the patient not to substitute the extended-release form for the immediate-release form.
◆ Tell the patient that nicotinic acid may cause flushing of the face and upper body, possibly accompanied by itching, tingling, or headache. Explain that these effects usually subside with therapy, but that the patient should notify his prescriber if they become bothersome. Suggest that he take aspirin 30 minutes before nicotinic acid to lessen the reaction.
◆ Tell the patient not to take the drug with hot liquids or alcohol because these beverages may exacerbate the flushing.
◆ Remind the patient to have blood tests performed regularly throughout the first year of therapy and periodically thereafter to monitor his liver function.
◆ Tell the patient to take nicotinic acid with meals if gastrointestinal distress occurs.
◆ Advise the patient not to crush, break or chew the extended-release form.
◆ Tell a patient with diabetes to monitor his glucose level carefully and to notify his prescriber if the level changes.
◆ Caution the patient not to take vitamins or other nutritional supplements containing niacin without consulting his prescriber.

✦ Don't crush or break the extended-release form.
✦ Give the drug with meals if GI distress occurs.
✦ Monitor the patient for signs and symptoms of liver failure.
✦ Give nicotinic acid and a bile-sequestering drug at least 4 hours apart.
✦ Teach the patient and his caregiver about the prescribed drug. (See *Teaching a patent about nicotinic acid*.)

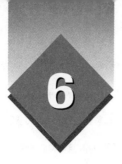

6

Respiratory drugs

In the respiratory system, common disorders range from severe asthma and chronic obstructive pulmonary disease (COPD) to mild cough and congestion. To help patients cope with these disorders, various respiratory drugs are available, including beta$_2$ agonists, corticosteroids, mast cell stabilizers, leukotriene modifiers, methylxanthines, expectorants, antitussives, mucolytics, and decongestants. Antihistamines also are used to treat respiratory disorders. (For details, see "Antihistamines" in chapter 13, Immunomodulation drugs.) Safe, effective therapy with these drugs requires an understanding of their actions — and of the respiratory system.

ANATOMY AND PHYSIOLOGY

The respiratory system, which extends from the nose to the pulmonary capillaries, performs the essential function of gas exchange between the body and its environment. It oxygenates tissue, removes carbon dioxide, regulates acid-base balance, and provides defense against infection.

Oxygen-carbon dioxide exchange

Air flows into the lungs via the conduction airways (from the nose to bronchioles) and reaches the alveoli, where gas exchange occurs. Oxygen diffuses from the alveoli into the pulmonary capillaries, where most of the oxygen is bound to hemoglobin in red blood cells (RBCs). Only a small percentage is dissolved in the plasma.

Then the RBCs are transported to all tissues, where oxygen is diffused from the blood into cells for cellular metabolism. Carbon dioxide, a by-product of cellular metabolism, is returned to the lungs to be eliminated. After diffusing from the blood into the alveoli, carbon dioxide is exhaled from the lungs. (See *Structures of the respiratory system*, page 216.)

Such conditions as mucosal edema, alveolar damage, bronchoconstriction, or a disrupted mucociliary clearance mechanism affect the integrity of the respiratory structures and can alter oxygen-carbon dioxide exchange.

Anatomy and physiology highlights

+ The respiratory system transfers oxygen from the environment to the body, removes carbon dioxide from the body, regulates acid-base balance, and defends against infection.
+ Air enters the lungs through conduction airways and moves through progressively smaller airways to the alveoli, where gas exchange takes place between the alveoli and adjacent pulmonary capillaries.
+ Oxygen binds to the hemoglobin in RBCs and is then carried to the tissues.
+ Carbon dioxide diffuses from the blood into the alveoli and is exhaled.

Structures of the respiratory system

The respiratory system consists of the organs responsible for external respiration and gas exchange in the lungs.

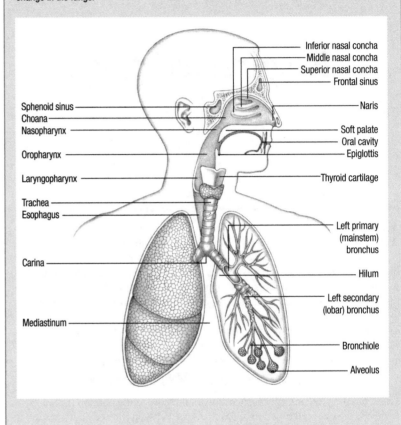

The basics of acid-base balance

◆ The respiratory, blood-buffer, and renal systems regulate acid-base balance.

◆ Normal arterial pH is 7.35 to 7.45.

◆ The body balances blood pH by retaining or secreting hydrogen and bicarbonate ions.

◆ If altered respiratory function causes carbon dioxide retention, blood pH declines and respiratory acidosis develops.

◆ If too much carbon dioxide is released, blood becomes more alkaline and respiratory alkalosis develops.

Acid-base balance

Along with the blood-buffer system and the kidneys, the respiratory system regulates acid-base balance. Normal arterial blood pH ranges from 7.35 to 7.45; blood pH can be lowered or raised by the retention or excretion of hydrogen (H) ions and bicarbonate (HCO_3) ions. Carbon dioxide (CO_2) and water (H_2O) combine in the presence of carbonic anhydrase (a catalyst) to form carbonic acid (H_2CO_3), as follows:

$$CO_2 + H_2O = H_2CO_3 = H + HCO_3$$

This reaction, which is reversible, is affected by respiratory and renal function. In patients with compromised respiratory function, carbon dioxide retention increases the hydrogen ion level in the blood, thereby decreasing the blood pH; this state is known as respiratory acidosis. Similarly, carbon dioxide elimination by the respiratory system causes the blood to become more alkaline; this is known as respiratory alkalosis. Alterations in the carbon dioxide level are regulated by the respiratory rate and depth, which is measured as minute ventilation. The respiratory system can restore normal arterial blood pH in minutes. However, a respiratory dysfunction can cause an acid-base imbalance.

Defense mechanisms

The nose filters, humidifies, and warms air during inhalation. It also traps particles in the mucosa to prevent their deposition lower in the respiratory tract. The mucosa and its secretions are influenced by the parasympathetic and sympathetic nervous systems. Sympathetic stimulation causes vasoconstriction of the nasal vascular structures and decreased mucus production. Parasympathetic stimulation has the opposite effect: it narrows the airway by vascular engorgement of mucosal tissues and increases mucus production.

Cilia are hairlike projections from the columnar epithelial cells that line the nasal and tracheal passageways. The cilia move respiratory secretions, mucus, and particles toward the oropharynx to be coughed out or swallowed. Respiratory tract mucus, produced by goblet cells, contains lysosomes and other elements that fight invading bacteria.

Coughing is a protective mechanism that rapidly expels air and particles from the airways. Sneezing clears the nasal passageway. If particles manage to get past these mechanisms, alveolar macrophages can phagocytize and detoxify them.

INHALED BETA$_2$ AGONISTS

As bronchodilators, beta$_2$ agonists are used to treat the signs and symptoms of asthma and COPD. Short-acting beta$_2$ agonists include albuterol, bitolterol, epinephrine, isoetharine, isoproterenol, metaproterenol, pirbuterol, and terbutaline. Long-acting drugs include salmeterol. Although many of these drugs are available in oral or parenteral forms, this section focuses on inhaled forms because they're preferred.

Pharmacokinetics

Upon inhalation, these drugs exert their effects locally. They aren't well absorbed or distributed systemically.

Pharmacodynamics

Beta$_2$ agonists increase the level of cyclic adenosine monophosphate by stimulating beta$_2$ receptors in bronchial smooth muscles, resulting in bronchodilation. At higher doses, these drugs may lose their selectivity, which can increase the risk of toxicity. Because inhaled forms act locally in the lungs, they produce fewer adverse effects than — and are preferred over — systemic forms.

Pharmacotherapeutics

Short-acting inhaled beta$_2$ agonists are prescribed for rapid relief of asthma symptoms. They're primarily used on an as-needed basis for asthma and COPD and also are effective for exercise-induced asthma. Some patients with COPD may use these drugs around-the-clock on a specified schedule.

Long-acting drugs usually are used with anti-inflammatory drugs, especially inhaled corticosteroids, to help control asthma. Because their onset is prolonged, they

Features of inhaled beta$_2$ agonists

+ Cause bronchodilation by stimulating beta$_2$ receptors in bronchial smooth muscle, which increases the cyclic adenosine monophosphate level
+ Act locally, producing fewer adverse effects than systemic forms
+ May lose selectivity at high doses, increasing the risk of toxicity
+ Are used for rapid asthma relief and for COPD (short-acting forms)
+ Are used with anti-inflammatory drugs to help control asthma (long-acting forms)
+ Don't affect chronic inflammation caused by asthma

PATIENT TEACHING

Teaching a patient about inhaled beta$_2$ agonists

Whenever an inhaled beta$_2$ agonist is prescribed, teach the patient and his family the drug's name, dose, frequency, action, and adverse effects. Also take the following actions.

✦ Teach the patient how to properly inhale the drug.

✦ Tell the patient that dry mouth and throat may occur but that rinsing with water after each dose may help.

✦ Instruct the patient to wait 5 minutes after using the beta$_2$ agonist before using a corticosteroid inhaler.

✦ Advise the patient to notify the prescriber if the drug loses effectiveness. Tell him not to increase the drug dosage or frequency, unless prescribed, because doing so may lead to serious adverse effects.

✦ Teach the patient the difference between short-acting and long-acting beta$_2$ agonists. Tell him to take the short-acting drug to treat acute symptoms and to use the long-acting drug for prevention — not treatment — of acute symptoms.

Adverse reactions to watch for

✦ Bronchospasm
✦ Cough
✦ Dizziness
✦ ECG changes, palpitations, tachycardia
✦ Headache
✦ Nausea
✦ Nervousness
✦ Tremor

Key nursing actions

✦ Make sure the patient doesn't use a long-acting beta$_2$ agonist for acute asthma symptoms.
✦ Monitor the use of a short-acting drug; excessive use may indicate poor control of asthma.
✦ Monitor for paradoxical bronchospasm.

must be given on a scheduled basis. They're especially helpful in patients who have asthma symptoms at night.

These drugs don't affect the chronic inflammation caused by asthma.

Interactions

As inhaled drugs, beta$_2$ agonists don't commonly cause interactions.

Adverse reactions

Most adverse reactions to beta$_2$ agonists are dose-related and characteristic of sympathomimetics. These reactions may include tremor, nervousness, dizziness, headache, nausea, tachycardia, palpitations, electrocardiogram (ECG) changes, bronchospasm, and cough.

Nursing considerations

CLINICAL ALERT Make sure that the patient doesn't use a long-acting beta$_2$ agonist for acute symptoms. Its onset of action isn't fast enough to provide immediate relief.

✦ Monitor the patient's use of a short-acting beta$_2$ agonist; excessive use may indicate poor asthma control, requiring reassessment of his therapeutic regimen.

✦ Monitor the patient for paradoxical bronchospasm.

✦ Be aware that a beta$_2$ agonist may reduce the sensitivity of spirometry in the diagnosis of asthma.

✦ Teach the patient and his caregiver about the prescribed drug. (See *Teaching a patient about inhaled beta$_2$ agonists.*)

CORTICOSTEROIDS

These anti-inflammatory drugs are used in inhaled and systemic forms to achieve short-term and long-term control of asthma symptoms. Many corticosteroids are

LIFESPAN

Managing corticosteroid effects on growth

In studies with intranasal corticosteroid therapy, pediatric patients have demonstrated reduced growth. Researchers don't yet know if the drug affects final adult height or if "catch-up growth" occurs after drug discontinuation.

To help minimize possible adverse effects on growth, monitor the growth of children and adolescents who receive a corticosteroid by any route. Also, adjust the drug regimen to the lowest effective dose.

---

available in different potencies. For treating respiratory disorders, common inhaled corticosteroids include beclomethasone, budesonide, dexamethasone, flunisolide, fluticasone, and triamcinolone. Common systemic corticosteroids include betamethasone, methylprednisolone, and prednisone.

Pharmacokinetics

After oral administration, corticosteroids are readily absorbed and distributed to the muscles, liver, skin, intestines, and kidneys. Betamethasone is weakly bound to plasma proteins; prednisone is highly bound. All corticosteroids are metabolized in the liver and excreted through the kidneys.

Inhaled corticosteroids are minimally absorbed. However, absorption increases as the dose increases.

Pharmacodynamics

Although their mechanism of action isn't fully understood, corticosteroids work by suppressing or preventing cell-mediated immune reactions; reducing the levels of leukocytes, monocytes, and eosinophils; decreasing immunoglobulin binding to receptors on cell surfaces; and inhibiting interleukin synthesis.

These drugs also prevent plasma leakage from capillaries, suppress leukocyte migration, and inhibit phagocytosis. In addition, they decrease antibody formation in injured or infected tissues and disrupt histamine synthesis, fibroblast development, collagen deposition, capillary dilation, and capillary permeability.

Pharmacotherapeutics

Corticosteroids are the most effective drugs for the long-term treatment and prevention of asthma exacerbations. Systemic forms usually are reserved for moderate to severe acute exacerbations, but also are used for severe asthma that doesn't respond to other treatments. To prevent adverse reactions, systemic corticosteroids should be used at the lowest effective dose and for the shortest time possible.

Inhaled corticosteroids remain the foundation of therapy for preventing exacerbations in most patients with mild to severe asthma. For many patients, their use reduces the need for systemic corticosteroids — and the risk of serious long-term adverse reactions. (See *Managing corticosteroid effects on growth*.)

Interactions

Inhaled corticosteroids usually don't cause interactions. However, systemic forms may interact with various drugs.

Features of corticosteroids

- ✦ Suppress or prevent cell-mediated immune reactions
- ✦ Reduce levels of leukocytes, monocytes, and eosinophils
- ✦ Decrease binding of immunoglobulins to receptors on cell surfaces
- ✦ Inhibit interleukin synthesis
- ✦ Prevent plasma leakage from capillaries
- ✦ Suppress leukocyte migration
- ✦ Inhibit phagocytosis
- ✦ Decrease antibody formation in injured or infected tissues
- ✦ Disrupt histamine synthesis, fibroblast development, collagen deposition, and capillary dilation
- ✦ Are most effective drugs for long-term management of asthma symptoms
- ✦ Should be used at the lowest possible dose and for the shortest possible time to prevent adverse reactions

Possible drug interactions

+ Barbiturates
+ Cholestyramine
+ Hormonal contraceptives
+ Ketoconazole
+ Phenytoin

Adverse reactions to watch for

Inhaled forms

+ Adrenal insufficiency after abrupt withdrawal of long-term therapy
+ Cushingoid effects
+ Dizziness, headache
+ Dry mouth, hoarseness, throat and nose irritation
+ Fungal infections of the mouth or throat
+ Osteoporosis
+ Serious respiratory reactions: bronchospasm, dyspnea, wheezing
+ Suppressed hypothalamic-pituitary-adrenal function

Systemic forms

+ Adrenal insufficiency after abrupt withdrawal of long-term therapy
+ Cushingoid effects
+ Euphoria
+ Insomnia
+ Osteoporosis
+ Peptic ulceration

Key nursing actions

+ Use the lowest effective dose.
+ Watch for evidence of oropharyngeal fungal infection.
+ Monitor the patient for cushingoid effects.

PATIENT TEACHING

Teaching a patient about corticosteroids

Whenever an inhaled or systemic corticosteroid is prescribed, teach the patient and his family the drug's name, dose, frequency, action, and adverse effects. Also take the following actions.
+ Inform the patient that the drug doesn't relieve acute asthma attacks.
+ Caution the patient not to use the drug more often than prescribed because severe adverse reactions may occur.
+ Teach the patient how to administer the inhaled form properly via inhalation.
+ Advise the patient to prevent oral fungal infections by gargling or rinsing his mouth with water after each dose of an inhaled corticosteroid. Remind the patient not to swallow the water.
+ Teach the patient to recognize early signs and symptoms of adrenal insufficiency, including fatigue, muscle weakness, joint pain, fever, anorexia, nausea, dyspnea, dizziness, and fainting. If they occur, tell him to notify his prescriber.
+ Instruct the patient to carry or wear medical identification indicating that he takes a corticosteroid.

+ Ketoconazole, a macrolide antibiotic, or a hormonal contraceptive can increase the corticosteroid's activity and may require a decrease in its dosage.
+ Barbiturates, cholestyramine, or phenytoin can decrease the corticosteroid's effectiveness and may require an increase in its dosage.

Adverse reactions

Inhaled corticosteroids may cause hoarseness, throat and nose irritation, dry mouth, and headache or dizziness. Fungal infections of the mouth or throat may occur. Serious respiratory reactions may include dyspnea, wheezing, or bronchospasm. Some inhaled corticosteroids may also suppress hypothalamic-pituitary-adrenal function. Adrenal insufficiency may occur after abrupt withdrawal with long-term therapy. Corticosteroids may produce cushingoid effects and cause osteoporosis.

Systemic corticosteroids may produce euphoria, insomnia, or peptic ulceration. They also may produce cushingoid effects and cause osteoporosis, especially with high doses of the drug and in geriatric patients. After abrupt withdrawal of long-term therapy, adrenal insufficiency may occur.

Nursing considerations

+ Use the lowest effective dose to reduce the risk of adverse reactions.
+ Monitor the patient for signs and symptoms of oropharyngeal fungal infection.
+ Observe the patient for adverse reactions to a systemic corticosteroid.
+ Monitor the patient for cushingoid effects, such as moon face, buffalo hump, central obesity, thinning hair, hypertension, and increased susceptibility to infection.
+ For a geriatric patient, suggest ways to prevent osteoporosis, such as increased calcium intake and weight-bearing exercise.
+ Teach the patient and his caregiver about the prescribed drug. (See *Teaching a patient about corticosteroids*.)

MAST CELL STABILIZERS

Mast cell stabilizers are used to prevent asthma attacks, especially in children and those with mild disease. Cromolyn sodium is the most widely used drug in this class and has several other indications. Nedocromil is used only in the preventive management of asthma.

Pharmacokinetics

Because mast cell stabilizers are inhaled and work locally, they aren't well absorbed or distributed systemically. These drugs aren't metabolized and are primarily excreted in urine.

Pharmacodynamics

Although its mechanism of action isn't fully understood, cromolyn inhibits the release of inflammatory mediators by stabilizing mast cell membranes. It may achieve this by indirectly preventing calcium ions from entering mast cells.

Nedocromil also inhibits mediator release from various types of inflammatory cells, including eosinophils, neutrophils, macrophages, mast cells, monocytes, and platelets.

Pharmacotherapeutics

Based on their anti-inflammatory effects, mast cell stabilizers are used for the prevention and long-term control of asthma symptoms. They're also used to prevent exercise-induced asthma. In addition, cromolyn is prescribed to prevent exercise-induced bronchospasm and allergic rhinitis. Its off-label use is the reduction or prevention of systemic reactions to food allergies.

Interactions

Interactions rarely occur because these drugs are inhaled and act locally.

Adverse reactions

Adverse reactions may include bad taste, cough, headache, sore throat, and nausea. Severe reactions, such as wheezing or bronchospasm, may result from inhalation of the powder.

Nursing considerations

+ Don't use these drugs for an acute asthma attack.
+ Use the drug with an inhaled beta$_2$ agonist or inhaled corticosteroid.
+ Reduce the dosage gradually to the lowest effective dosage.
+ Ensure that the patient knows how to use the product properly.
+ Teach the patient and his caregiver about the prescribed drug. (See *Teaching a patient about mast cell stabilizers*, page 222.)

LEUKOTRIENE MODIFIERS

Drugs in this class are used for the prevention and long-term control of asthma. They include montelukast, zafirlukast, and zileuton.

Features of mast cell stabilizers

+ Inhibit the release of inflammatory mediators by stabilizing mast cell membranes
+ Are used for prevention and long-term control of asthma symptoms and prevention of exercise-induced asthma

Adverse reactions to watch for

+ Cough
+ Headache
+ Nausea
+ Sore throat
+ Unpleasant taste
+ Wheezing or bronchospasm from powder inhalation

Key nursing actions

+ Don't use these drugs for acute asthma attacks.
+ Use with an inhaled beta$_2$ agonist or inhaled corticosteroid.
+ Reduce the dosage gradually to reach the lowest effective dosage.

Features of leukotriene modifiers

✦ Inhibit leukotrienes (which contract smooth muscles in airways) by keeping them from interacting with their receptors or by blocking an enzyme critical to leukotriene formation
✦ Are used to prevent and control asthma attacks in patients with mild to moderate disease
✦ May reduce the need for corticosteroids

Possible drug interactions

✦ Aspirin
✦ Carbamazepine
✦ Erythromycin
✦ Phenobarbital
✦ Phenytoin
✦ Propranolol
✦ Theophylline
✦ Tolbutamide
✦ Warfarin

Pharmacokinetics

All leukotriene modifiers are rapidly absorbed and more than 90% protein bound. Because food decreases zafirlukast absorption, the drug should be given 1 hour before or 2 hours after a meal.

Montelukast is extensively metabolized in the liver by cytochrome P450 (CYP) 2C9 and 3A4 enzymes. With therapeutic doses, however, plasma levels of its metabolites are undetectable. The drug is excreted primarily in feces. The CYP 2C9 enzyme extensively metabolizes zafirlukast into inactive metabolites. It's also excreted primarily in feces. CYP 1A2, 2C9, and 3A4 enzymes oxidatively metabolize zileuton, which is primarily excreted via metabolism.

Zafirlukast inhibits CYP 2C9 and 3A4 enzymes. Zileuton inhibits CYP 3A4 and 1A2. Metabolism by, or inhibition of, CYP enzymes is responsible for most of these drugs' interactions.

Pharmacodynamics

When mast cells, eosinophils, and basophils release leukotrienes, these substances can lead to smooth muscle contraction in the airways, increased vascular permeability and secretions, and activation of other inflammatory mediators.

Leukotriene modifiers inhibit leukotrienes in two ways. Two drugs that block leukotriene receptors, montelukast and zafirlukast, competitively inhibit leukotriene D4 and E4 receptors. This prevents leukotrienes from interacting with their receptors, which blocks their action. A drug that prevents leukotrienes from forming, zileuton, inhibits the production of 5-lipoxygenase (an enzyme that's critical to leukotriene production).

Pharmacotherapeutics

Leukotriene modifiers are primarily used to prevent and control asthma exacerbations in patients with mild to moderate disease. In some patients, these drugs also may be used to reduce the need for corticosteroids.

Interactions

✦ Zafirlukast may increase carbamazepine, phenytoin, and tolbutamide levels.
✦ Aspirin may increase the zafirlukast level.
✦ Erythromycin may decrease the zafirlukast level by about 40%.
✦ Zafirlukast or zileuton may decrease warfarin clearance, which increases the prothrombin time, the international normalized ratio, and the risk of bleeding.
✦ Zileuton may increase the theophylline level, requiring a theophylline dosage reduction of 50%.

◆ Zileuton may increase the propranolol level, increasing its beta-blocking activity and possibly requiring a dosage reduction.
◆ Phenobarbital may decrease the montelukast level,

Adverse reactions

The most common adverse reaction to leukotriene modifiers is headache. Asthenia, dizziness, dyspepsia, gastroenteritis, and fever may also occur. Zileuton also can cause musculoskeletal effects, such as myalgia, arthralgia, and hypertonia, as well as hematologic effects, such leukopenia. Zafirlukast and zileuton may produce elevated liver enzyme levels.

Nursing considerations

◆ Don't use a leukotriene modifier to treat acute bronchospasm.
◆ Use the drug with a corticosteroid and other antiasthmatics.
◆ For a patient with hepatic impairment, reduce the zafirlukast dosage and monitor him closely for adverse reactions.
◆ Monitor the patient's liver enzyme levels during zafirlukast or zileuton therapy.
◆ Teach the patient and his caregiver about the prescribed drug. (See *Teaching a patient about leukotriene modifiers.*)

METHYLXANTHINES

Also called xanthines, methylxanthines are used to treat asthma, chronic bronchitis, emphysema, and neonatal apnea. These drugs include theophylline, its salts and derivatives (aminophylline, dyphylline, and oxtriphylline), and caffeine. Theophylline is the most commonly used methylxanthine for respiratory disorders.

Pharmacokinetics

The pharmacokinetics of methylxanthines vary with the drug, dosage form, and administration route that's used.

When theophylline is given as an oral solution or a rapid-release tablet, it's absorbed rapidly and completely. Absorption of some slow-release forms depends on gastric pH and the presence of food in the stomach. High-fat meals can increase the theophylline level—and the risk of toxicity.

Theophylline is about 40% protein-bound. It readily crosses the placental barrier and appears in breast milk. This drug is metabolized primarily in the liver by the CYP 1A2 enzyme. In adults and children, about 10% of a dose is excreted un-

Adverse reactions to watch for
◆ Asthenia, dizziness
◆ Dyspepsia, gastroenteritis
◆ Elevated liver enzyme levels
◆ Fever
◆ Headache (most common)
◆ Zileuton: arthralgia, hypertonia, leukopenia, myalgia

Key nursing actions
◆ Don't use these drugs for acute bronchospasm.
◆ Give with a corticosteroid and other antiasthmatics.
◆ Monitor liver enzyme levels during zafirlukast or zileuton therapy.

Features of methylxanthines

+ Decrease airway reactivity and relieve bronchospasm by relaxing bronchial smooth muscles
+ May inhibit phosphodiesterase (theophylline)
+ May stimulate the respiratory drive by increasing the sensitivity of the respiratory center in the brain to carbon dioxide
+ Are used to treat asthma, chronic bronchitis, emphysema, and neonatal apnea
+ Decrease diaphragm fatigue and improve ventricular function (chronic bronchitis)

Possible drug interactions

+ Adrenergic stimulants
+ Antithyroid drugs
+ Caffeine
+ Charcoal
+ CYP 1A2 inducers (carbamazepine, phenobarbital, phenytoin, rifampin)
+ CYP 1A2 inhibitors (cimetidine, ciprofloxacin, clarithromycin, erythromycin, fluvoxamine, isoniazid, ketoconazole, hormonal contraceptives, ticlopidine, zileuton)
+ Enflurane, halothane, isoflurane, methoxyflurane
+ Lithium
+ Thyroid hormones

Adverse reactions to watch for

+ Abdominal cramping, anorexia, diarrhea, epigastric pain, nausea, vomiting
+ Anxiety, dizziness, headache, insomnia, irritability, restlessness

changed in urine. In infants, up to 50% a dose may be excreted unchanged in urine; this occurs because their livers are immature and have reduced metabolic function.

Pharmacodynamics

Methylxanthines decrease airway reactivity and relieve bronchospasm by relaxing bronchial smooth muscles. Theophylline may inhibit phosphodiesterase, resulting in smooth muscle relaxation and bronchodilation and a reduction in inflammatory mediators, such as mast cells, T-cells, and eosinophils. In nonreversible obstructive airway disease (chronic bronchitis, emphysema, and apnea), methylxanthines appear to increase the sensitivity of the brain's respiratory center to carbon dioxide and to stimulate the respiratory drive.

In chronic bronchitis and emphysema, these drugs decrease diaphragm fatigue. They also improve ventricular function and, therefore, the heart's pumping action.

Pharmacotherapeutics

Methylxanthines are used for long-term control and prevention of the signs and symptoms of asthma, chronic bronchitis, and emphysema. Although theophylline is effective as a bronchodilator, its narrow therapeutic index, strict monitoring requirements, and increased risk of adverse reactions make it a second-line drug compared to inhaled beta$_2$ agonists and corticosteroids.

Interactions

+ Use of an adrenergic stimulant or beverages with caffeine may cause additive adverse reactions to theophylline or methylxanthine toxicity.
+ Charcoal may decrease the theophylline level.
+ Use of enflurane, halothane, isoflurane, or methoxyflurane with theophylline or a theophylline derivative increases the risk of cardiac toxicity.
+ Theophylline or any of its derivatives may increase lithium's rate of excretion and reduce its effects.
+ A thyroid hormone may reduce the theophylline level.
+ An antithyroid drug may increase the theophylline level.
+ A CYP 1A2 inhibitor, such as cimetidine, ciprofloxacin, clarithromycin, erythromycin, fluvoxamine, isoniazid, ketoconazole, hormonal contraceptive, ticlopidine, or zileuton may decrease theophylline metabolism, increasing its level and the risk of adverse reactions and toxicity.
+ A CYP 1A2 inducer, such as carbamazepine, phenobarbital, phenytoin, rifampin, St. John's wort, or charbroiled meat, may increase theophylline metabolism, possibly reducing its effectiveness and requiring an increase in the theophylline dosage.
+ Smoking cigarettes or marijuana increases theophylline elimination, decreasing its level and effectiveness.

Adverse reactions

Adverse reactions to methylxanthines can be transient or symptomatic of toxicity. Reactions may appear shortly after giving the first dose and can affect the GI tract and the central nervous system (CNS). GI tract irritation and increased gastric acid secretion may cause nausea, vomiting, abdominal cramping, epigastric pain, anorexia, or diarrhea. Adverse CNS effects include headache, irritability, restlessness, anxiety, insomnia, and rarely dizziness.

Methylxanthines also can produce adverse reactions when drug use produces a high level (usually above 20 mcg/ml for theophylline). These reactions include nausea, vomiting, diarrhea, and such CNS effects as irritability, insomnia, anxiety, headache, and seizures (with a very high level).

Teaching a patient about methylxanthines

Whenever a methylxanthine is prescribed, teach the patient and his family the drug's name, dose, frequency, action, and adverse effects. Also take the following actions.

✦ Stress the importance of having regular blood tests to determine if the drug has reached a therapeutic level.

✦ Advise the patient to consult his prescriber if adverse reactions occur.

✦ Warn the patient to take the drug regularly, but only as directed. Patients tend to want to take extra pills.

✦ Teach the patient who misses a dose or vomits shortly after taking a dose to consult his prescriber for instructions.

✦ Tell the patient to take an oral methylxanthine with 8 oz (240 ml) of water, preferably on an empty stomach.

✦ Advise the patient not to chew or crush a sustained-release methylxanthine.

✦ For a patient who can't swallow pills whole, instruct him to open the capsule and sprinkle its contents over soft food.

✦ Tell a smoker to inform his prescriber if he quits smoking. He may need a dosage reduction to prevent toxicity.

Drugs in this class also can irritate the myocardium, producing cardiovascular effects, such as tachycardia, palpitations, extrasystoles, and arrhythmias. Also, these drugs can cause peripheral vasodilation and hypotension.

Although hypersensitivity reactions can occur, they are extremely rare and typically occur with the base in theophylline salts. Shortly after receiving the drug, the patient may display severe signs and symptoms of theophylline toxicity, which include nausea, vomiting, diarrhea, headache, and occasionally anxiety and dizziness; this indicates intolerance.

Nursing considerations

✦ Monitor the patient for adverse CNS, cardiovascular, and GI reactions, especially when the theophylline level exceeds 20 mcg/ml, when therapy begins or restarts, or when the dosage is changed.

✦ Monitor the theophylline level regularly during treatment and whenever a drug is added to or removed from the patient's regimen. Theophylline has a narrow therapeutic index, which is why it may be involved in serious drug interactions.

✦ Monitor a neonate's theophylline and caffeine levels because theophylline is metabolized to caffeine in these patients.

✦ Give an oral form with a full glass of water on an empty stomach or with a small amount of food. Open bead-filled capsules and scatter their contents on a small amount of soft food for a patient who can't swallow tablets.

✦ Ensure that the patient doesn't chew or crush a slow-release product.

✦ Assess the patient with adverse GI reactions for signs of fluid volume deficit, such as poor skin turgor, dry mucous membranes, and decreased urine volume.

✦ Teach the patient and his caregiver about the prescribed drug. (See *Teaching a patient about methylxanthines.*)

Adverse reactions to watch for
(continued)

✦ Arrhythmias, extrasystoles, palpitations, tachycardia

✦ Peripheral vasodilation and hypotension

✦ Toxicity: anxiety, diarrhea, headache, insomnia, irritability, nausea, seizures, vomiting

Key nursing actions

✦ Watch for adverse CNS, cardiovascular, and GI effects, especially when the theophylline level exceeds 20 mcg/ml, therapy starts or resumes, or the dosage changes.

✦ Monitor the theophylline level regularly during treatment and whenever a drug is added to or removed from the regimen.

✦ If the patient has GI reactions, watch for evidence of fluid volume deficit.

Features of expectorants

✦ Promote a more productive cough by increasing the production of respiratory tract fluids, which helps liquefy mucus
✦ Soothe mucous membranes in the respiratory tract
✦ Are used to relieve unproductive cough and related symptoms

Adverse reactions to watch for

✦ Abdominal pain, diarrhea, nausea, vomiting
✦ Drowsiness
✦ Iodide expectorants: thyroid adenoma, goiter, myxedema, hypersensitivity reactions (angioneurotic edema, arthralgia, fever, enlarged lymph nodes, eosinophilia)

EXPECTORANTS

Expectorants promote a more productive cough and soothe mucous membranes in the respiratory tract. The most commonly used expectorant is guaifenesin. Other expectorants include iodides, such as iodinated glycerol and potassium iodide. However, these iodide products are infrequently used because they pose a greater risk of adverse reactions.

Pharmacokinetics

Guaifenesin is absorbed through the GI tract, metabolized by the liver, and excreted primarily by the kidneys.

Iodides are absorbed as iodinated amino acids and distributed extracellularly to the thyroid gland and to gastric and salivary secretions. They're excreted primarily by the kidneys.

Pharmacodynamics

By increasing the production of respiratory tract fluids, expectorants reduce the thickness, adhesiveness, and surface tension of mucus, making it easier to clear from airways. These drugs also provide a soothing effect on mucous membranes of the respiratory tract.

Pharmacotherapeutics

Guaifenesin is used to relieve unproductive cough and related symptoms.

Interactions

No interactions are known to occur with expectorant use.

Adverse reactions

Guaifenesin rarely or infrequently causes adverse reactions. However, the drug may produce vomiting if taken in doses larger than needed to cause expectoration. Diarrhea, drowsiness, nausea, vomiting, and abdominal pain may also occur.

The use of iodide expectorants may cause thyroid adenoma, goiter, or myxedema. They also may produce hypersensitivity reactions, including angioneurotic edema, fever, arthralgia, enlarged lymph nodes, and eosinophilia.

PATIENT TEACHING

Teaching a patient about expectorants

Whenever an expectorant is prescribed, teach the patient and his family the drug's name, dose, frequency, action, and adverse effects. Also take the following actions.

✦ Stress the importance of taking the drug exactly as prescribed.
✦ Advise family members who give guaifenesin to a child to check with the pharmacist or prescriber if they don't understand the pediatric dosage.
✦ Instruct the patient to avoid activities that require alertness if drowsiness occurs.
✦ Encourage the patient to increase his fluid intake, unless contraindicated.
✦ Teach the patient to perform deep-breathing exercises and change positions frequently to help clear mucus from his airways.

Nursing considerations

✦ Monitor the patient for dyspnea or ineffective cough. Keep suction equipment readily available during expectorant therapy.

✦ Teach the patient and his caregiver about the prescribed drug. (See *Teaching a patient about expectorants.*)

ANTITUSSIVES

Antitussives suppress or inhibit coughing. They're typically used to treat dry, non-productive cough. Major drugs in this class are benzonatate, codeine, dextromethorphan, and hydrocodone combination products.

Pharmacokinetics

Antitussives are absorbed well through the GI tract, metabolized in the liver, and excreted in urine.

Pharmacodynamics

Different antitussives act in slightly different ways. Benzonatate acts by anesthetizing stretch receptors throughout the bronchi, alveoli, and pleura. Codeine, dextromethorphan, and hydrocodone suppress the cough reflex by acting directly on the cough center in the medulla of the brain.

Pharmacotherapeutics

Therapeutic uses of these drugs vary slightly, but each can be used to treat a serious, nonproductive cough that interferes with a patient's ability to rest or carry out activities of daily living. Benzonatate relieves cough caused by pneumonia, bronchitis, the common cold, and chronic pulmonary diseases, such as emphysema. It also is used during bronchial diagnostic tests, such as bronchoscopy, when the patient must avoid coughing.

Dextromethorphan is the most widely used antitussive because it's highly effective but produces few adverse reactions. Opioid antitussives, such as codeine and hydrocodone, are reserved for treating intractable cough. Except for dextromethorphan, antitussives sometimes require cautious use. (See *Contraindications and precautions for antitussives.*)

WARNING

Contraindications and precautions for antitussives

Benzonatate is contraindicated in patients who are hypersensitive to it or to related compounds. Severe hypersensitivity reactions to benzonatate — including bronchospasm, laryngospasm, and cardiovascular collapse — have occurred. These reactions may result from local anesthesia caused by sucking or chewing liquid-filled capsules rather than swallowing them whole.

Opioid antitussives require cautious use in patients with opioid addiction or a history of it. They also should be used cautiously in patients with such respiratory disorders as chronic obstructive pulmonary disease or asthma.

Key nursing actions

✦ Monitor the patient for dyspnea and ineffective cough.

✦ Keep suction equipment readily available.

Features of antitussives

✦ Suppress or inhibit coughing

✦ May anesthetize stretch receptors in bronchi, alveoli, and pleura or act directly on the cough center in the medulla

✦ Are used to treat dry, nonproductive cough caused by the common cold, pneumonia, bronchitis, chronic pulmonary diseases

✦ Are used for bronchial diagnostic tests when the patient must avoid coughing

✦ Used for intractable cough (opioids)

Possible drug interactions

+ CNS depressants
+ MAO inhibitors

Adverse reactions to watch for

benzonatate

+ Burning eyes, nasal congestion
+ Chilly sensation, skin eruptions, pruritus, rash
+ Constipation, GI upset, nausea
+ Dizziness, headache, sedation
+ Numbness in the chest

dextromethorphan

+ Drowsiness
+ GI upset

opioids

+ Agitation, constipation, dizziness, excessive perspiration, nausea, palpitations, pruritus, sedation, vomiting
+ Hydrocodone: constipation, dizziness, dysphoria, euphoria, nausea, pruritus, rash, sedation, vomiting
+ Physical dependence (long-term use)
+ Reduced alertness or coordination
+ Toxicity: bradycardia, circulatory collapse, constricted pupils, hypotension, narcosis, respiratory arrest, seizures, tachycardia

PATIENT TEACHING

Teaching a patient about antitussives

Whenever an antitussive is prescribed, teach the patient and his family the drug's name, dose, frequency, action, and adverse effects. Also take the following actions.
+ Stress the importance of taking the drug exactly as prescribed. To prevent toxicity, tell the patient not to exceed the prescribed or recommended dosage.
+ If sedation or dizziness occurs, caution the patient not to perform activities that require alertness.
+ Inform the patient that prolonged use of codeine can cause physical dependence.
+ Teach the patient to recognize the signs of toxicity and, if they occur, to notify the prescriber before taking another antitussive dose.
+ Instruct the patient to swallow benzonatate capsules whole and not chew them because the release of benzonatate in the mouth may numb the mouth and throat and compromise his airway.
+ Instruct the patient to report a cough that lasts longer than 7 days or that changes from nonproductive to productive.
+ Advise the patient to keep the drug out of the reach of children.
+ Warn the patient about the potentially fatal additive effects of central nervous system depressants, such as alcohol, when combined with an antitussive.
+ Teach the patient how to prevent constipation.

Interactions

+ Use of dextromethorphan with a monoamine oxidase (MAO) inhibitor may produce excitation, fever, hypotension, and coma. Don't use dextromethorphan within 14 days of an MAO inhibitor.
+ Use of codeine with another CNS depressant (such as alcohol, a barbiturate, a sedative-hypnotic, or a phenothiazine) may cause increased CNS depression, such as drowsiness, lethargy, stupor, respiratory depression, coma, and death.

Adverse reactions

Benzonatate can cause dizziness, sedation, headache, nasal congestion, burning in the eyes, nausea, GI upset, constipation, and skin rash. A vague chilly sensation, skin eruptions, pruritus, and numbness in the chest also have been reported.

At recommended doses, adverse reactions rarely occur with dextromethorphan. Patients most commonly report drowsiness and GI upset.

Toxic doses of the opioid antitussives can produce constricted pupils, bradycardia, tachycardia, hypotension, narcosis, seizures, circulatory collapse, and respiratory arrest. Antitussive doses of codeine seldom cause respiratory depression. However, the patient may experience an impaired ability to perform activities that require alertness or coordination. Repeated doses of codeine increase the risk of nausea, vomiting, constipation, dizziness, sedation, palpitations, pruritus, excessive perspiration, and agitation. Long-term use of codeine may result in physical dependence. Antitussive doses of hydrocodone bitartrate usually don't produce adverse reactions. However, some patients experience dizziness, sedation, nausea, and vomiting. Rash, pruritus, constipation, euphoria, and dysphoria also can occur with hydrocodone bitartrate use.

Hypersensitivity reactions to hydrocodone bitartrate can occur. Hypersensitivity reactions to benzonatate, codeine, and dextromethorphan are rare; however, urticaria, pruritus, rash, and facial swelling can result from codeine use.

Nursing considerations

 CLINICAL ALERT Give codeine cautiously to a patient who also is receiving a CNS depressant because this combination can be fatal. Closely monitor the patient's consciousness level to detect increased CNS depression.

✦ During codeine therapy, monitor the patient for signs of respiratory depression, such as decreased respiratory rate, respiratory depth, and level of consciousness.
✦ During codeine or hydrocodone bitartrate therapy, monitor the patient for signs and symptoms of hypersensitivity reaction and opioid toxicity.
✦ Encourage the patient to increase his fluid and dietary fiber intake and to exercise regularly to prevent constipation.
✦ If constipation occurs, give a laxative.
✦ Teach the patient and his caregiver about the prescribed drug. (See *Teaching a patient about antitussives.*)

MUCOLYTICS

Mucolytics act directly on mucus, breaking down sticky, thick secretions so they're easier to eliminate. Acetylcysteine is the major mucolytic in the United States.

Pharmacokinetics

When inhaled, acetylcysteine is absorbed from the pulmonary epithelium. When taken orally, the drug is absorbed from the GI tract. It's metabolized in the liver, and its excretion is unknown.

Pharmacodynamics

Acetylcysteine decreases the thickness of respiratory tract secretions by altering the molecular composition of mucus. It also irritates the mucosa to encourage clearance. In addition, the drug restores glutathione, a substance that plays an important role in oxidation-reduction processes.

Pharmacotherapeutics

Mucolytics are used with other therapies to treat patients with abnormal or thick mucous secretions. They may benefit patients with bronchitis, pulmonary complications of cystic fibrosis, or atelectasis caused by mucous obstruction, which may occur in pneumonia, bronchiectasis, or chronic bronchitis. These drugs may also be used to prepare patients for bronchial studies. However, they require cautious use in some patients. (See *Precautions for mucolytics*, page 230.)

Acetylcysteine is the antidote for acetaminophen overdose. However, it doesn't fully protect against the liver damage caused by acetaminophen toxicity.

Interactions

✦ Activated charcoal decreases acetylcysteine's effectiveness, requiring charcoal removal from the stomach before acetylcysteine administration to treat acetaminophen overdose.

WARNING

Precautions for mucolytics

Acetylcysteine appears to have a wide margin of safety, but requires cautious use in asthmatic patients because bronchospasm may occur. If bronchospasm occurs, administer a bronchodilator by nebulization. If it progresses, discontinue acetylcysteine immediately.

Adverse reactions

Acetylcysteine provides a wide margin of safety. Nausea may result from the drug's rotten-egg smell. With prolonged or persistent use, acetylcysteine may produce stomatitis, nausea, vomiting, drowsiness, and severe rhinorrhea.

Hypersensitivity reactions rarely occur; however, a rash can develop with prolonged or frequent use of acetylcysteine. Patients may have excessive secretion of bronchial mucus, which may cause increased airway obstruction for those who can't expectorate effectively. Bronchospasm can occur, particularly in asthmatic patients. The frequency of this adverse reaction increases with the 20% solution. Because bronchospasm can occur unpredictably, the patient must be monitored closely during inhalation therapy.

Nursing considerations

+ Prepare the patient for the drug's rotten-egg smell, which may cause nausea.
+ Give acetylcysteine by nebulizer. Because the drug reacts with iron, copper, and rubber, frequently monitor the patient's nebulizer equipment for reactive effects. The drug doesn't react with glass, plastic, aluminum, or stainless steel.

 CLINICAL ALERT Be prepared to give an inhaled beta$_2$ agonist if the patient experiences bronchospasm. Inhaled forms act locally rather than systemically, which reduces the risk of adverse reactions.

+ Use the 10% or 20% acetylcysteine solution undiluted. If further dilution is needed, use normal saline solution or sterile water for injection. During continuous nebulization with dry gas, when 3/4 of the initial volume has been nebulized, dilute the remaining solution with an equal volume of sterile water for injection.
+ Avoid contamination of the solution and refrigerate an opened vial; acetylcysteine doesn't contain an antimicrobial. Discard opened vials after 4 days.
+ Assess the patient's respiratory status before and after each dose, particularly noting breathing difficulty, ineffective cough, or dyspnea. Follow acetylcysteine administration with chest physiotherapy and postural drainage and encourage coughing and deep breathing to facilitate removal of respiratory secretions.
+ Keep suction equipment nearby, especially for a patient with a weak cough reflex. Suction him as needed to help clear the increased volume of bronchial secretions produced by the drug.
+ Have the patient gargle after administration to relieve the unpleasant odor and dryness. Wash the patient's face to eliminate stickiness caused by the drug.
+ When treating acetaminophen overdose, remove previously administered activated charcoal by gastric lavage before giving acetylcysteine. If the patient vomits within 1 hour of acetylcysteine administration, repeat the dose.

Teaching a patient about mucolytics

Whenever a mucolytic is prescribed, teach the patient and his family the drug's name, dose, frequency, action, and adverse effects. Also take the following actions.
◆ Advise the patient not to perform activities that require alertness.
◆ Show the patient how to use and maintain the nebulizer.
◆ Teach the patient and family how to avoid contamination of acetylcysteine solution. Tell them that the solution may discolor to a light purple, but is still usable. Instruct the patient and his family to refrigerate an open vial and to discard it after 4 days.
◆ Stress the importance of gargling after treatment to relieve the drug's odor. Inform the patient about effective coughing before and after each treatment. Teach him and his family to perform chest physiotherapy and postural drainage after acetylcysteine administration.
◆ Teach the patient to recognize signs and symptoms of stomatitis and, if they occur, to manage them appropriately.
◆ Instruct the patient to seek medical help if his respiratory condition worsens or if adverse reactions occur.

◆ Monitor the patient closely for signs of stomatitis, such as papulovesicular ulcers in the mouth and throat, malaise, irritability, fever, and swollen, tender gums that bleed easily.
◆ Rinse the patient's mouth with a warm, water-based oral solution if stomatitis occurs. Avoid antiseptic mouthwashes, which are irritating. Give a topical anesthetic to relieve mouth ulcer pain. Switch the patient to a bland or liquid diet until symptoms subside.
◆ If stomatitis occurs, notify the prescriber because acetylcysteine therapy may need to be discontinued.
◆ Teach the patient and his caregiver about the prescribed drug. (See *Teaching a patient about mucolytics*.)

DECONGESTANTS

As sympathomimetic amines, decongestants may be systemic or topical. Systemic decongestants activate the sympathetic division of the autonomic nervous system to reduce swelling of the respiratory tract's vascular network. Topical decongestants are powerful vasoconstrictors that provide immediate relief from nasal congestion and swollen mucous membranes when applied directly to the nasal mucosa.

Major systemic decongestants include ephedrine and pseudoephedrine. Major topical decongestants include epinephrine, naphazoline, phenylephrine, tetrahydrozoline, and xylometazoline.

Pharmacokinetics

Decongestants vary in their pharmacokinetic properties. After oral administration, systemic decongestants are absorbed readily from the GI tract and widely distributed into various tissues and fluids, including the cerebrospinal fluid, placenta, and breast milk. They're slowly and incompletely metabolized by the liver and excreted largely unchanged in urine within 24 hours of administration.

Features of decongestants
◆ May be systemic or topical
◆ Systemic: activate the sympathetic division of the autonomic nervous system to reduce swelling of the respiratory vascular network
◆ Topical: cause vasoconstriction and immediate relief from nasal congestion and swollen mucous membranes
◆ Reduce blood supply to the nose by stimulating alpha-adrenergic receptors in blood vessels (systemic) or nose (topical)
◆ Cause contraction of GI and urinary sphincters, dilation of pupils, decreased secretion of insulin (systemic forms)
◆ Are used to relieve swollen nasal membranes caused by hay fever, allergic rhinitis, vasomotor rhinitis, sinusitis, the common cold

Topical decongestants act directly on alpha-adrenergic receptors in the vascular smooth muscle of the nose, causing the arterioles to constrict. Because of this direct vasoconstriction, only a small amount of drug is absorbed.

Pharmacodynamics

The actions of systemic and topical decongestants vary slightly. Systemic decongestants cause vasoconstriction by stimulating alpha-adrenergic receptors in blood vessels. This reduces the blood supply to the nose, which decreases nasal mucosal edema. These drugs also cause contraction of urinary and GI sphincters, pupil dilation, and decreased insulin secretion. They may also act indirectly; this action results in the release of norepinephrine from storage sites in the body, which causes peripheral vasoconstriction.

Topical decongestants stimulate alpha-adrenergic receptors in the smooth muscle of the blood vessels in the nose, which causes vasoconstriction. The combination of reduced blood flow to the nasal mucous membranes and decreased capillary permeability reduces swelling. This action improves respiration by helping to drain sinuses, clear nasal passages, and open eustachian tubes.

Pharmacotherapeutics

Systemic and topical decongestants are used to relieve the signs and symptoms of swollen nasal membranes caused by hay fever, allergic rhinitis, vasomotor rhinitis, sinusitis, and the common cold. In some patients, however, systemic decongestants may require cautious use. (See *Precautions for decongestants*.)

Interactions

Because topical decongestants are minimally absorbed, they seldom cause drug interactions. Systemic decongestants, however, may interact with other drugs.

✦ When a systemic decongestant is taken with another sympathomimetic, like dobutamine, dopamine, epinephrine, isoproterenol, metaproterenol, norepinephrine, phenylephrine, terbutaline, or tyramine, increased CNS stimulation may occur.

✦ Use of a systemic decongestant with an MAO inhibitor may cause severe hypertension or hypertensive crisis, which can be fatal.

✦ An alkalinizing drug may reduce urinary excretion of pseudoephedrine and increase its effects.

✦ Use of a topical decongestant with an MAO inhibitor can cause severe headache, hypertension, and possibly hypertensive crisis.

✦ Use of a topical decongestant with a beta blocker can cause initial hypertension followed by bradycardia.

✦ Use of a topical decongestant with methyldopa may cause or increase the pressor response.

Adverse reactions

The risk and severity of adverse reactions depends primarily on the patient's sensitivity to decongestants and, with topical decongestants, on the duration of action and frequency of drug use. Patients who are hypersensitive to other sympathomimetic amines may be hypersensitive to decongestants as well.

For nonsensitive patients, the risk of adverse reactions to systemic decongestants is low. The most common adverse reactions result from CNS stimulation and include nervousness, restlessness, and insomnia. Nausea, palpitations, difficult urination, and dose-related elevations in blood pressure occasionally occur.

Possible drug interactions

✦ Alkalinizing drugs
✦ Beta blockers
✦ MAO inhibitors
✦ Methyldopa
✦ Sympathomimetics (dobutamine, dopamine, epinephrine, isoproterenol, metaproterenol, norepinephrine, phenylephrine, terbutaline, tyramine)

Adverse reactions to watch for

✦ First-time hypersensitivity reactions
✦ Hallucinations, headache, seizures
✦ Irregular heartbeat, tachycardia, tightness in the chest
✦ Teratogenic effects
✦ Very high blood pressure

Systemic forms
✦ Difficult urination
✦ Dose-related elevations in blood pressure
✦ Insomnia, nervousness, palpitations, restlessness
✦ Nausea

Topical forms
✦ Mucosal dryness or ulceration
✦ Rebound nasal congestion
✦ Sneezing
✦ Transient burning and stinging of the nasal mucosa

When topical decongestants are used for more than 3 to 5 days, the most common adverse reaction is rebound nasal congestion. The disorder is characterized by hyperemia of the nasal mucosa, which appears red, boggy, and swollen. Rebound nasal congestion usually resolves spontaneously within a few days after stopping the topical decongestant.

The second most frequent adverse reaction to topical decongestants is transient burning and stinging of the nasal mucosa upon application. Patients also report sneezing and mucosal dryness or ulceration. Less common adverse reactions result from CNS stimulation and include nervousness, restlessness, and insomnia. Occasionally, nausea, palpitations, difficult urination, and dose-related elevations in blood pressure occur.

Other adverse reactions to systemic and topical decongestants may include first-time drug hypersensitivity reactions, irregular heartbeat or tachycardia, feeling of tightness in the chest, hallucinations, seizures, headache, very high blood pressure, and teratogenic effects.

Nursing considerations

✦ Discourage the use of over-the-counter decongestants in a patient who is hypersensitive to other sympathomimetic amines. Such a patient may also be hypersensitive to decongestants.

✦ Monitor the patient's blood pressure, pulse, and ECG tracing, particularly noting hypertension and an irregular heartbeat or tachycardia.

✦ Determine if the patient uses drugs that alter urine pH. Alkaline urine increases renal tubular reabsorption of sympathomimetic amines, which increases the risk of toxic effects. Acidic urine may increase the elimination of the decongestant, which can reduce its therapeutic effects.

✦ Don't give an MAO inhibitor, a beta blocker, or methyldopa with a decongestant. Use with an MAO inhibitor can cause severe headache and hypertension, possibly hypertensive crisis. Beta blockers may cause initial hypertension followed by bradycardia, and methyldopa may increase pressor response.

✦ Warn the patient that transient burning and stinging of the nasal mucosa may occur with use of a topical decongestant.

✦ For a patient receiving a topical decongestant, inspect the nasal mucosa for signs of rebound nasal congestion, such as redness, swelling, and bogginess. If rebound nasal congestion occurs, notify the prescriber. The patient may need to switch to a normal saline nasal spray.

✦ Encourage the patient to report difficulty urinating, which is especially common in patients with prostatic hypertrophy.

Key nursing actions

✦ Monitor the blood pressure, pulse, and ECG tracing, looking for hypertension, an irregular heartbeat, or tachycardia.

✦ Determine whether the patient takes drugs that alter urine pH.

✦ If the patient uses a topical decongestant, inspect his nasal mucosa for rebound congestion and his oral and nasal mucosa for ulcers.

✦ Urge the patient to report difficulty urinating.

Teaching a patient about decongestants

Whenever a decongestant is prescribed, teach the patient and his family the drug's name, dose, frequency, action, and adverse effects. Also take the following actions.

✦ Teach the patient to recognize and report adverse reactions.

✦ Remind the patient not to exceed the recommended amount and frequency or duration of use of topical decongestants because rebound nasal congestion may occur after the vasoconstrictor effect subsides. Warn him that increasing the amount or frequency of use may increase the severity or frequency of adverse reactions or worsen rebound nasal congestion.

✦ Caution the patient to avoid over-the-counter products, including herbal remedies, which may interact with a systemic decongestant.

✦ Inform the patient that a systemic decongestant may interfere with sleep. Suggest that he take the drug a few hours before bedtime to minimize insomnia.

✦ Instruct the patient to take the drug in its complete form when using sustained-release capsules or long-acting tablets. Tell him not to break, cut, crush, or chew the capsule or tablet.

✦ To minimize central nervous system stimulation, teach the patient how to take his topical decongestant properly: in the lateral head-low position for drops, in the upright position for sprays.

✦ Instruct the patient who uses a decongestant for relieving blocked eustachian tubes to lie on the side opposite the affected ear. Tell him to gently pull the top of the ear up and back to straighten the ear canal. (For a child under age 3, pull the ear lobe down and back.) To avoid discomfort, advise the patient to let the drops run down the side of the ear canal, instead of dropping them directly onto the eardrum. Instruct him to remain on his side for 5 minutes. If both sides require treatment, advise the patient to repeat the procedure on the other side after the 5-minute wait.

✦ Instruct the patient to use a humidifier if nasal dryness occurs.

✦ If a topical decongestant is used, inspect the patient's oral and nasal mucosa regularly for ulcers.

✦ If nasal dryness occurs, encourage the patient to use a humidifier.

✦ Teach the patient and his caregiver about the prescribed drug. (See *Teaching a patient about decongestants.*)

Gastrointestinal drugs

For most GI disorders, treatment is conservative, symptomatic, and supportive. Typically, it begins with diet therapy, rest, and stress management. If these measures aren't effective, it may require drug therapy or surgery. Drug therapy may be used to:

✦ treat a specific disease, such as a digestive enzyme deficiency, hepatic encephalopathy, acute poisoning, peptic ulcer disease, or gastroesophageal reflux.

✦ control the signs and symptoms of a disease, such as nausea, vomiting, epigastric pain, dyspepsia, flatulence, diarrhea, and constipation.

Depending on the disorder, the prescriber may select from peptic ulcer drugs; adsorbents, antiflatulents, and digestants; antidiarrheals and laxatives; and antiemetics. Because many of these agents are available over the counter (OTC), the patient may also self-medicate with them. For any of them, you can help achieve treatment goals by applying an understanding of the GI system.

ANATOMY AND PHYSIOLOGY

The GI tract has three major functions: digestion of foods and fluids, absorption of foods and fluids, and excretion of metabolic waste. In the GI tract, various hormones and enzymes break down food into particles that are small enough to permeate cell membranes and be used for cellular energy. The GI tract itself helps prevent infection by maintaining mucous membrane integrity, secreting immunoglobulins, and destroying pathogens. (See *Structures of the GI system,* page 236.)

By altering any of these functions, GI disorders can disrupt activities of daily living, interrupt work schedules, and lead to hospital admissions. They may result from such diseases as benign or malignant tumors, peptic ulcer disease, gastroesophageal reflux, Crohn's disease, ulcerative colitis, malabsorption, intestinal obstruction, or diverticulosis, or they may stem from stress or other psychological problems. No matter what the cause, however, GI disorders usually produce similar signs and symptoms that typically are so vague and nonspecific that many patients delay seeking treatment.

Anatomy and physiology highlights

✦ The GI tract digests and absorbs food and fluids and excretes metabolic waste.

✦ Hormones and enzymes break food into particles small enough to permeate cell membranes and provide cellular energy.

✦ The GI tract helps prevent infection by maintaining mucous membrane integrity, secreting immunoglobulins, and destroying pathogens.

✦ GI disorders may involve benign or malignant tumors, peptic ulcer disease, gastroesophageal reflux, Crohn's disease, ulcerative colitis, malabsorption, intestinal obstruction, diverticulosis, stress, or other physical or psychological problems.

ANATOMY & PHYSIOLOGY

Structures of the GI system

To understand GI disorders and visualize the actions of GI drugs, you need a working knowledge of the GI system's major anatomical structures, as illustrated below.

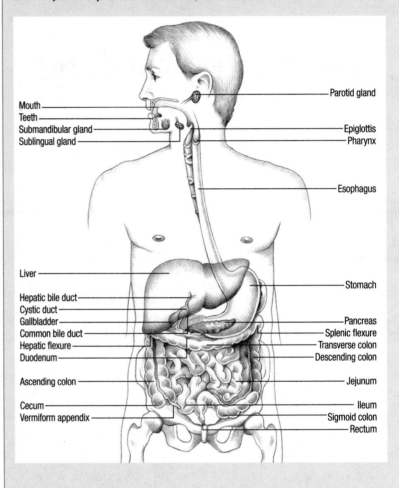

Common signs and symptoms of GI disorders

- Abdominal distention
- Abscesses or fistulas
- Altered body image
- Anorexia
- Constipation
- Diarrhea
- Dyspepsia
- Dysphagia
- Epigastric or abdominal pain
- Extended areas of inflammation or infection
- Flatulence
- Fluid and electrolyte imbalances that lead to arrhythmias and hypovolemia
- Malnutrition
- Nausea, vomiting
- Perforation that results in peritonitis
- Rectal bleeding

Common signs and symptoms of GI disorders include anorexia, dysphagia, nausea, vomiting, dyspepsia, epigastric or abdominal pain, abdominal distention, flatulence, diarrhea, constipation, and rectal bleeding. These findings can have many possible causes. GI disorders may cause fluid and electrolyte imbalances that lead to arrhythmias and hypovolemia, extended areas of inflammation or infection, abscesses or fistulas, malnutrition, structure perforation that results in peritonitis, and altered body image.

PEPTIC ULCER DRUGS

A peptic ulcer is a circumscribed lesion in the mucosal membrane of the lower esophagus, stomach, duodenum, or jejunum. Peptic ulcer disease may result from:

✦ bacterial infection with *Helicobacter pylori*.

✦ use of nonsteroidal anti-inflammatory drugs (NSAIDs).

✦ a hypersecretory state, such as Zollinger-Ellison syndrome, a condition caused by excessive gastric acid secretion.

Peptic ulcer disease may also have a genetic link: 20% to 50% of patients with the disease have a family history of it.

Peptic ulcer drugs aim to eradicate *H. pylori* or restore the balance between acid and pepsin secretions and the GI mucosal defense. These drugs include systemic antibiotics, antacids, histamine-2 (H_2) receptor antagonists, proton-pump inhibitors, and misoprostol and sucralfate.

SYSTEMIC ANTIBIOTICS

H. pylori is a gram-negative bacteria that is thought to cause peptic ulcers and gastritis. Eradication of the bacteria promotes ulcer healing and decreases recurrence.

Successful ulcer treatment involves the use of two or more antibiotics with other drugs. Antibiotics used for this purpose include amoxicillin, clarithromycin, metronidazole, and tetracycline. A combination drug of metronidazole, tetracycline, and bismuth (an antacid) is available.

Pharmacokinetics

Systemic antibiotics vary in their absorption from the GI tract. Food — especially dairy products — decreases tetracycline absorption, but doesn't significantly delay the absorption of other antibiotics.

All of these antibiotics are distributed widely. Amoxicillin is partially metabolized. Clarithromycin and metronidazole are metabolized to active metabolites. Tetracycline doesn't undergo metabolism. All of these drugs are excreted primarily in urine.

Pharmacodynamics

Antibiotics act by treating *H. pylori* infection. They're usually combined with an H_2-receptor antagonist or a proton-pump inhibitor to decrease stomach acid and promote further healing.

Pharmacotherapeutics

Various combinations of antibiotics are used with an H_2-receptor antagonist or a proton-pump inhibitor to treat *H. pylori* infection and promote ulcer healing.

Interactions

✦ When used with digoxin, tetracycline can increase the digoxin level.

✦ When used with methoxyflurane, tetracycline increases the risk of nephrotoxicity.

✦ When given with an oral anticoagulant, metronidazole and tetracycline increase the risk of bleeding.

Teaching a patient about systemic antibiotics

Whenever a systemic antibiotic is prescribed, teach the patient and his family the drug's name, dose, frequency, action, and adverse effects. Also take the following actions.

◆ If the patient is age 18 or younger, teach him and his family to stop taking an antibiotic containing bismuth and notify the prescriber if he experiences signs and symptoms of a viral infection.

◆ Teach the patient that his mouth, tongue, and stools may become black during therapy with an antibiotic containing bismuth. Reassure him that these changes are temporary.

◆ Instruct the patient and family to report tinnitus, which may occur with use of an antibiotic that contains bismuth.

◆ Teach the patient to avoid products that contain aspirin during treatment with an antibiotic that contains bismuth.

◆ Advise the patient that food — and some dairy products — can inhibit the absorption of a tetracycline, except for doxycycline and minocycline. To avoid problems, tell the patient to take the drug 1 hour before or 2 hours after meals.

◆ Warn the patient that clarithromycin can cause disturbances in taste.

◆ Urge the patient to notify his prescriber if diarrhea, nausea, or vomiting occurs.

◆ Advise the patient to avoid consuming alcohol during metronidazole treatment.

Adverse reactions to watch for

◆ Blackened tongue and stool
◆ Diarrhea
◆ Mild GI disturbances
◆ Superinfection
◆ Taste disturbances
◆ Tinnitus

Key nursing actions

◆ Watch for evidence of superinfection.
◆ Assess the patient for evidence of bismuth toxicity.

Adverse reactions

Amoxicillin may cause diarrhea. The bismuth in combination drugs temporarily turns the tongue and stool black and may cause tinnitus. Bismuth toxicity can lead to encephalopathy and osteodystrophy. Clarithromycin, metronidazole, and tetracycline commonly produce mild GI disturbances. Clarithromycin may also cause taste disturbances. Antibiotic use also can lead to superinfection.

Nursing considerations

◆ Use a systemic antibiotic cautiously in a patient with hepatic or renal insufficiency.
◆ Avoid the use of salicylates, such as aspirin, during combination therapy that contains bismuth.
◆ Monitor the patient for signs and symptoms of superinfection during antibiotic therapy.
◆ Monitor the patient for signs of bismuth toxicity, including tinnitus, encephalopathy, and osteodystrophy.
◆ Give tetracycline on an empty stomach with plenty of water.
◆ Teach the patient and his caregiver about the prescribed drug. (See *Teaching a patient about systemic antibiotics.*)

ANTACIDS

These OTC drugs are used alone or with other drugs to treat peptic ulcer disease. Antacids include aluminum carbonate and hydroxide; calcium carbonate; magaldrate; magnesium carbonate, hydroxide, and oxide; and sodium carbonate. Some OTC products combine several antacids and may add simethicone.

Pharmacokinetics

Antacids don't need to be absorbed to treat peptic ulcers. They work locally in the stomach, dissolving in gastric acid. These drugs are distributed throughout the GI tract, undergo no metabolism, and are eliminated primarily in feces.

Pharmacodynamics

These drugs neutralize gastric acid, which reduces the total amount of acid in the GI tract and gives peptic ulcers time to heal.

Because pepsin acts more effectively when stomach acidity is high, pepsin action decreases as acidity decreases. Contrary to popular belief, antacids don't work by coating peptic ulcers or the lining of the GI tract.

Pharmacotherapeutics

Used alone or with other drugs, antacids primarily are prescribed to relieve pain in peptic ulcer disease. They're also used to relieve symptoms of acid indigestion, heartburn, dyspepsia, or gastroesophageal reflux disease (GERD). Antacids that contain calcium usually aren't recommended for treatment of peptic ulcer disease, but are recommended as short-term therapy for other GI conditions.

In critically ill patients, antacids may be used to prevent stress ulcers and GI bleeding during times of severe physical stress. In patients with renal failure, calcium carbonate antacids may be used to control hyperphosphatemia because their calcium binds with phosphate in the GI tract, preventing phosphate absorption.

Interactions

✦ An antacid can interfere with the absorption of any oral drug given at the same time.
✦ An antacid can reduce the absorption of digoxin, an iron salt, isoniazid, a quinolone, phenytoin, ketoconazole, or a tetracycline given within 2 hours of antacid administration.

Adverse reactions

Adverse reactions to antacids are dose related. The most common reactions occur in the GI tract. Diarrhea and constipation commonly result from long-term antacid use. Aluminum hydroxide is particularly constipating. Constipation can be severe and, if accompanied by dehydration or fluid restriction, may lead to intestinal obstruction. Hemorrhoids, rectal fissures, and fecal impaction may occur from hard stools. Conversely, antacids containing magnesium produce a laxative effect and, with frequent use, can produce diarrhea and electrolyte abnormalities. Aluminum hydroxide and antacids containing magnesium are usually prescribed together, which typically produces a mild laxative effect.

Most antacids contain sodium, and those with more than 0.2 mEq of sodium per dose must be labeled with the amount. Patients with dietary restrictions should check the product label. The use of sodium-containing antacids should be restricted in patients with heart failure, renal failure, cirrhosis, or edema.

In patients with renal failure, antacids containing aluminum may produce hyperaluminemia, in which aluminum accumulates in bones, lungs, and nerve tissue and can lead to osteomalacia and dementia. Hypophosphatemia, characterized by anorexia, malaise, and muscle weakness, may also occur from prolonged use of antacids containing aluminum.

In patients with renal failure, antacids containing magnesium may cause hypermagnesemia, characterized by hypotension, nausea, vomiting, electrocardiogram (ECG) changes, respiratory or mental depression, and coma.

Features of antacids

✦ Work locally in the stomach, dissolving in stomach acid
✦ Neutralize gastric acid, reducing the total acid in the GI tract and allowing ulcers to heal
✦ Don't work by coating ulcers or the lining of the GI tract
✦ Relieve pain, symptoms of acid indigestion, heartburn, dyspepsia, GERD
✦ May be used to control hyperphosphatemia in patients with renal failure (antacids containing calcium)
✦ Are used to prevent stress ulcers and GI bleeding during times of severe physical stress

Adverse reactions to watch for

aluminum
✦ Constipation
✦ Fecal impaction, hemorrhoids, and rectal fissures from hard stools
✦ Hyperaluminemia and possible osteomalacia and dementia in patients with renal failure
✦ Hypophosphatemia (anorexia, malaise, muscle weakness)

magnesium
✦ Diarrhea, electrolyte abnormalities
✦ Hypermagnesemia (hypotension, nausea, vomiting, ECG changes, respiratory or mental depression, coma) in patients with renal failure

calcium
✦ Acid rebound
✦ Milk-alkali syndrome (hypercalcemia, metabolic alkalosis, renal impairment)

Teaching a patient about antacids

Whenever an antacid is prescribed, teach the patient and his family the drug's name, dose, frequency, action, and adverse effects. Also take the following actions.
+ Reassure the patient that antacid therapy normally makes stools appear speckled or whitish.
+ Teach the patient when and how to take the antacid.
+ Stress the importance of taking the antacid exactly as prescribed for maximum effectiveness.
+ To prevent hypermagnesemia, instruct the patient with renal failure not to take an antacid containing magnesium.
+ Advise the patient who must restrict his sodium intake to avoid antacids that contain more than 0.2 mEq of sodium per dose. Otherwise, sodium and fluid retention may occur or increase.
+ Instruct the patient who must restrict his potassium intake to read antacid labels carefully because some antacids have a high potassium content.
+ Teach the patient how to prevent constipation during antacid therapy.
+ Instruct the patient to report adverse reactions.

Key nursing actions

+ If the patient has renal failure and takes an aluminum antacid, monitor for evidence of hyperaluminemia.
+ Watch for evidence of hypophosphatemia with aluminum antacid use.
+ Assess the patient for constipation.
+ Urge the patient to drink plenty of fluid and eat a high-fiber diet.

When calcium carbonate is used, gastric hypersecretion and acid rebound occur. Calcium carbonate may also cause milk-alkali syndrome, characterized by hypercalcemia, metabolic alkalosis, and renal impairment.

Nursing considerations
+ Avoid giving calcium carbonate for long-term treatment of peptic ulcer disease because gastric hypersecretion and acid rebound may occur.
+ Monitor a patient with renal failure for signs of hyperaluminemia, which can result in osteomalacia and dementia, during therapy with an antacid containing aluminum.
+ Monitor the patient for symptoms of hypophosphatemia, such as anorexia, malaise, and muscle weakness, during long-term therapy with an antacid containing aluminum. If hypophosphatemia is suspected, withhold the drug and notify the prescriber.
+ Shake the suspension well and give it with a small amount of water. Have the patient drink 6 to 8 oz (180 to 240 ml) of water after swallowing the suspension.
+ Don't give another oral drug within 2 hours of antacid administration because the antacid may impair its absorption.
+ Separate the administration of an antacid and an enteric-coated drug by 1 hour because the antacid may cause premature release of the enteric-coated drug in the stomach.
+ Monitor the patient for constipation, which may become severe, especially with aluminum hydroxide use.
+ Place the patient on a high-fiber diet and encourage him to drink plenty of fluid to help prevent constipation.
+ Teach the patient and his caregiver about the prescribed drug. (See *Teaching a patient about antacids*.)

H$_2$-RECEPTOR ANTAGONISTS

For treating peptic ulcer disease, commonly prescribed H$_2$-receptor antagonists include cimetidine, famotidine, nizatidine, and ranitidine.

Pharmacokinetics

Cimetidine, nizatidine, and ranitidine are absorbed rapidly and completely from the GI tract. Famotidine isn't absorbed completely. Food and antacids may reduce the absorption of H$_2$-receptor antagonists.

These drugs are distributed widely throughout the body, metabolized by the liver, and excreted primarily in urine.

Pharmacodynamics

Acid secretion in the stomach depends on the binding of gastrin, acetylcholine, and histamine to receptors on the parietal cells. If the binding of any one of these substances is blocked, acid secretion is reduced. By binding with H$_2$ receptors, the H$_2$-receptor antagonists block histamine from binding to those receptors and from stimulating the parietal cells that secrete acid, thereby creating less acid in the stomach. (See *How H$_2$-receptor antagonists work,* page 242.)

Pharmacotherapeutics

H$_2$-receptor antagonists are used therapeutically to:
✦ promote healing of duodenal and gastric ulcers.
✦ provide long-term treatment of GI hypersecretory disorders, such as Zollinger-Ellison syndrome.
✦ reduce gastric acid production and prevent stress ulcers in severely ill patients and in those with reflux esophagitis or upper GI bleeding.

Interactions

✦ An antacid can reduce the absorption of cimetidine, famotidine, nizatidine, or ranitidine.
✦ Cimetidine may increase the levels of benzodiazepines, calcium channel blockers, carbamazepine, cyclosporine, lidocaine, opioid analgesics, oral anticoagulants, phenytoin, procainamide, propranolol and other beta blockers, quinidine, theophylline, and tricyclic antidepressants by reducing their metabolism and subsequent excretion.
✦ When used with carmustine, cimetidine increases the risk of bone marrow toxicity.
✦ Cimetidine inhibits alcohol metabolism in the stomach, which increases the alcohol level.

Adverse reactions

Adverse reactions may occur in patients receiving H$_2$-receptor antagonists, especially in geriatric patients and those with altered hepatic or renal function.

Cimetidine and ranitidine may produce headache, dizziness, malaise, myalgia, nausea, diarrhea or constipation, rash, pruritus, loss of libido, and impotence; cimetidine, however, is more likely to produce these adverse reactions. Famotidine and nizatidine produce few adverse reactions. Headache is the most common reaction and occurs in about 2% of patients, followed by constipation or diarrhea and rash. Reversible confusion, agitation, depression, and hallucinations may also occur; these reactions are more common in patients receiving cimetidine, especially in severely ill or elderly patients with decreased renal function.

Featureas of H$_2$-receptor antagonists

✦ Bind with H$_2$ receptors and prevent histamine from binding to receptors and stimulating parietal cells, which secrete acid
✦ Are used to promote healing of duodenal and gastric ulcers, provide long-term treatment of GI hypersecretory disorders, reduce gastric acid production, and prevent stress ulcers

Possible drug interactions

✦ Alcohol
✦ Antacids
✦ Benzodiazepines
✦ Beta blockers
✦ Calcium channel blockers
✦ Carbamazepine
✦ Carmustine
✦ Cyclosporine
✦ Lidocaine
✦ Opioid analgesics
✦ Oral anticoagulants
✦ Phenytoin
✦ Procainamide
✦ Quinidine
✦ Theophylline
✦ Tricyclic antidepressants

Adverse reactions to watch for

✦ Constipation, diarrhea, nausea
✦ Dizziness
✦ Headache
✦ Impotence, loss of libido
✦ Malaise
✦ Myalgia
✦ Pruritus, rash
✦ Reversible agitation, confusion, depression, hallucinations

EYE ON DRUG ACTION

How H$_2$-receptor antagonists work

These illustrations show how histamine-2 (H$_2$) receptor antagonists reduce the release of gastric acid.

To stimulate gastric acid secretion, certain endogenous substances—primarily histamine, but also acetylcholine and gastrin—attach to receptors on the surface of parietal cells. These substances activate the enzyme adenyl cyclase, which converts adenosine triphosphate (ATP) to the intracellular catalyst cyclic adenosine monophosphate (cAMP).

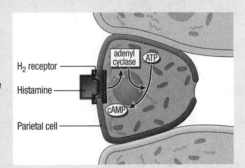

The cAMP ultimately stimulates proton-pump (H/K ATPase) activity. The pump catalyzes the exchange of extracellular potassium (K) ions for intracellular hydrogen (H) ions. When the H+ ions combine with extracellular chloride (Cl) ions excreted by gastric cells at a different site, the result is hydrochloric (HCl), or gastric, acid.

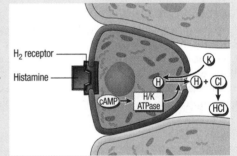

H$_2$-receptors antagonists competitively bind to H$_2$-receptor sites on the surface of parietal cells and inhibit the common pathway that histamine and the other substances must travel to stimulate proton-pump activity and promote gastric acid secretion.

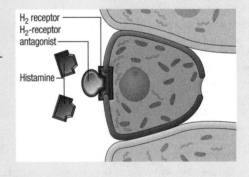

When given by rapid I.V. injection, H$_2$-receptor antagonists can produce profound bradycardia and other cardiotoxic effects. Pain at the injection site occasionally occurs.

H$_2$-receptor antagonists seldom cause hypersensitivity reactions. Some patients have increased liver enzyme levels, but this reaction is rare. Gynecomastia has been reported in patients taking cimetidine for 1 month or longer.

Nursing considerations

✦ Don't give an antacid within 1 hour of H₂-receptor antagonist administration because absorption of the H₂-receptor antagonist may decrease.

✦ Monitor the patient for profound bradycardia and other cardiotoxic effects when giving an H₂-receptor antagonist by rapid I.V. injection.

✦ Give an I.V. H₂-receptor antagonist to a critically ill patient to prevent GI bleeding.

✦ Give the H₂-receptor antagonist without regard to meals.

✦ Dilute cimetidine, famotidine, and ranitidine before I.V. administration. Dilute cimetidine in at least 50 ml, famotidine in at least 100 ml, and ranitidine in at least 20 ml of a compatible I.V. solution, such as normal saline solution or dextrose 5% in water (D₅W).

✦ During cimetidine or ranitidine therapy, encourage the patient to express concerns about adverse genitourinary effects, such as loss of libido and impotence.

✦ If the patient experiences sexual dysfunction, consult the prescriber about substituting a different H₂-receptor antagonist.

✦ Teach the patient and his caregiver about the prescribed drug. (See *Teaching a patient about H₂-receptor antagonists.*)

Key nursing actions

✦ Give an H₂-receptor antagonist I.V. to a critically ill patient to prevent GI bleeding.

✦ If giving the drug by rapid I.V. injection, monitor the patient for profound bradycardia and other cardiotoxic effects.

✦ If the patient receives cimetidine or ranitidine, discuss his concerns about impotence or reduced libido.

PROTON-PUMP INHIBITORS

Proton-pump inhibitors disrupt chemical binding in stomach cells to reduce acid production, which lessens irritation and allows peptic ulcers to heal better. Drugs in this class include esomeprazole, lansoprazole, omeprazole, pantoprazole, and rabeprazole.

Pharmacokinetics

Because these drugs are unstable in acid, they're available only in enteric-coated forms. After oral administration, the enteric-coated drugs bypass the stomach. Upon reaching the small intestine, they dissolve and are absorbed rapidly. These drugs are highly protein-bound, extensively metabolized by the liver to inactive compounds, and then eliminated in urine.

Features of proton-pump inhibitors

+ Reduce stomach acid production by combining with hydrogen, potassium, and adenosine triphosphate in parietal cells of stomach to block the last step in gastric acid secretion
+ Are used with antibiotics to treat active peptic ulcers caused by *H. pylori* infection
+ Are used alone for short-term treatment of gastric ulcers, duodenal ulcers, erosive esophagitis, symptomatic GERD
+ May be used for long-term treatment of hypersecretory conditions

Adverse reactions to watch for

esomeprazole
+ Abdominal pain, constipation, diarrhea, flatulence, nausea
+ Dry mouth
+ Headache

lansoprazole
+ Diarrhea, minor GI complaints
+ Headache

omeprazole
+ Asthenia
+ Cough
+ Diarrhea, vomiting
+ Dizziness
+ Headache
+ Upper respiratory tract infection

pantoprazole
+ Abdominal pain, diarrhea
+ Abnormal liver function tests
+ Headache
+ Hyperglycemia

rabeprazole
+ Headache

Pharmacodynamics

Proton-pump inhibitors block the last step in gastric acid secretion by combining with hydrogen, potassium, and adenosine triphosphate in the parietal cells of the stomach.

Pharmacotherapeutics

When used with antibiotics, proton-pump inhibitors are indicated for treatment of active peptic ulcers caused by *H. pylori* infection. They also can be used alone for short-term treatment of active gastric ulcers, active duodenal ulcers, erosive esophagitis, and symptomatic GERD that doesn't respond to other therapies. In addition, they can be used for long-term treatment of hypersecretory disorders, such as Zollinger-Ellison syndrome.

Interactions

+ A proton-pump inhibitor may interfere with diazepam, phenytoin, or warfarin metabolism, increasing the half-life and serum level of these drugs.
+ A proton-pump inhibitor may interfere with the absorption of drugs that depend on gastric pH for absorption, such as ampicillin, digoxin, iron salts, and ketoconazole.
+ When used with a proton-pump inhibitor, enteric-coated aspirin may dissolve more rapidly, increasing its adverse GI reactions.
+ A proton-pump inhibitor may reduce indinavir's antiviral activity.

Adverse reactions

Common adverse reactions to esomeprazole include headache, diarrhea, nausea, flatulence, abdominal pain, constipation, and dry mouth.

Lansoprazole and omeprazole are usually tolerated well even in the higher dosages used to treat hypersecretory disorders. The most common adverse reactions are diarrhea and headaches. Lansoprazole may produce only minor GI complaints. Omeprazole may cause vomiting, headache, asthenia, upper respiratory tract infection, cough, and dizziness.

The most common adverse reactions to pantoprazole include diarrhea, hyperglycemia, headache, abdominal pain, and abnormal liver function test results. Headache is the only noteworthy reaction to rabeprazole.

Nursing considerations

✦ Give an antacid with the proton-pump inhibitor to relieve GI discomfort.

✦ For a patient who can't swallow capsules, open esomeprazole or lansoprazole capsules, sprinkle the contents on soft food, and have the patient swallow it immediately.

✦ Don't open omeprazole capsules.

✦ Teach the patient and his caregiver about the prescribed drug. (See *Teaching a patient about proton-pump inhibitors.*)

MISOPROSTOL AND SUCRALFATE

Misoprostol and sucralfate are the most recent additions to the arsenal of drugs used to treat peptic ulcer disease.

Pharmacokinetics

After an oral dose, misoprostol is absorbed extensively and rapidly. It's metabolized to its active metabolite, misoprostol acid, which is clinically active (able to produce a pharmacologic effect). Misoprostol acid is highly protein-bound and is excreted primarily in urine.

Sucralfate is minimally absorbed from the GI tract and is excreted in feces.

Pharmacodynamics

As a synthetic prostaglandin E_1 analogue, misoprostol protects against peptic ulcers by reducing gastric acid secretion, increasing bicarbonate production, and boosting production of gastric mucus, a natural defense against peptic ulcers.

Sucralfate works locally in the stomach, rapidly reacting with hydrochloric acid to form a thick, pasty substance that adheres to the gastric mucosa, especially to ulcers. By binding to the ulcer, sucralfate protects the ulcer from the damaging effects of acid and pepsin, promoting healing.

Pharmacotherapeutics

Misoprostol is used to prevent NSAID-induced gastric ulcers in patients at high risk for complications. Sucralfate is to be used no longer than 8 weeks for treatment of duodenal or gastric ulcers and for prevention of recurrent ulcers or stress ulcers.

Interactions

✦ An antacid, and possibly food, may bind with misoprostol or decrease its absorption; however, this effect may not be significant because misoprostol's therapeutic action appears to be local rather than systemic.

✦ Sucralfate may bind with some drugs, such as quinidine and digoxin, in the GI tract, decreasing their absorption.

✦ Sucralfate may decrease the absorption of diclofenac, oral phenytoin, or warfarin by a mechanism that isn't fully understood.

✦ An antacid may reduce the binding of sucralfate to the GI mucosa, reducing its effectiveness.

Adverse reactions

Misoprostol commonly causes adverse GI reactions. Diarrhea occurs in up to 40% of patients. It may be followed by abdominal pain, flatulence, dyspepsia, nausea, and vomiting. Because misoprostol is a prostaglandin, it may also affect the uterus, causing spotting, cramps, hypermenorrhea, and other menstrual disorders. In a

Features of misoprostol and sucralfate

misoprostol

✦ Protects against peptic ulcers by reducing gastric acid secretion and increasing bicarbonate and gastric mucus production

✦ Is used to prevent NSAID-induced gastric ulcers

sucralfate

✦ Works locally in the stomach

✦ Reacts rapidly with hydrochloric acid to form a thick, pasty substance that adheres to the mucosa and ulcers, protecting ulcers from acid and pepsin

✦ Is used no longer than 8 weeks for treating duodenal or gastric ulcers or preventing recurrent ulcers or stress ulcers

Possible drug interactions

✦ Antacids
✦ Diclofenac
✦ Digoxin
✦ Food
✦ Oral phenytoin
✦ Quinidine
✦ Warfarin

Adverse reactions to watch for

misoprostol

✦ Abdominal pain, diarrhea, dyspepsia, flatulence, nausea, vomiting

✦ Menstrual disorders: cramping, hypermenorrhea, spotting

sucralfate

✦ Back pain

✦ Constipation, diarrhea, dry mouth, indigestion, metallic taste, nausea

✦ Dizziness, sleepiness, vertigo

Dangers of misoprostol use during pregnancy

Use of misoprostol during pregnancy can lead to premature birth, birth defects, and abortion. When the drug is used after the 8th week of pregnancy to induce labor or abortion, it has caused uterine rupture. Misoprostol-induced abortions may be incomplete. For these reasons, the drug is contraindicated for gastric ulcer prevention during pregnancy.

pregnant patient, misoprostol therapy may induce spontaneous abortion. (See *Dangers of misoprostol use during pregnancy.*)

Usually, sucralfate is tolerated well. Although typically minor, adverse reactions may become bothersome for the patient. Constipation is the most common dose-related adverse reaction, occurring in about 2% of all patients. Nausea and a metallic taste may also accompany the use of sucralfate. Less common reactions to this drug include diarrhea, indigestion, dry mouth, back pain, dizziness, sleepiness, and vertigo. Rarely, sucralfate may cause rash and pruritus.

Nursing considerations

✦ Don't give an antacid with misoprostol or sucralfate because it may decrease the peptic ulcer drug's activity.
✦ Give sucralfate 2 hours before or after any other oral drug to reduce the risk of binding with them and reducing their effects.
✦ Give misoprostol with food. Give sucralfate at least 1 hour before meals and at bedtime for best results.
✦ Monitor the patient's bowel function to detect diarrhea, especially during misoprostol therapy.
✦ If the patient develops diarrhea, monitor his hydration and give an antidiarrheal, if needed.
✦ If diarrhea becomes severe, consult the prescriber about stopping the drug.
✦ Teach the patient and his caregiver about the prescribed drug. (See *Teaching a patient about misoprostol and sucralfate.*)

Key nursing actions

✦ Monitor the patient's bowel function, especially during misoprostol therapy.
✦ If diarrhea develops, monitor hydration and give an antidiarrheal, if needed.
✦ If diarrhea becomes severe, consult the prescriber about stopping the drug.

ADSORBENTS, ANTIFLATULENTS, AND DIGESTANTS

Natural and synthetic adsorbents are used to manage toxin ingestion, which may cause poisoning or overdose. These toxins include poisonous mushrooms and drugs such as amphetamines, aspirin, barbiturates, cocaine, morphine, opium, and tricyclic antidepressants.

Antiflatulents and digestants are used to relieve two major disturbances of digestion in the GI tract. Antiflatulents are indicated for gastric bloating with or without flatulence. Digestants are used to compensate for inadequate or incomplete digestion.

Teaching a patient about misoprostol and sucralfate

Whenever misoprostol or sucralfate is prescribed, teach the patient and his family the drug's name, dose, frequency, action, and adverse effects. Also take the following actions.

✦ Teach the patient how to manage adverse reactions, such as constipation, diarrhea, and dry mouth.

✦ Advise the patient not to perform any activity that requires alertness if dizziness, sleepiness, or vertigo occurs.

✦ Instruct the patient not to take an antacid with misoprostol or sucralfate.

✦ Tell the patient to take sucralfate 2 hours before or after cimetidine.

✦ Alert the patient that nausea and a metallic taste may accompany sucralfate use.

✦ Provide verbal and written warnings to a woman of childbearing age that misoprostol may induce miscarriage. Advise her to obtain a pregnancy blood test 2 weeks before beginning therapy, to use effective contraception during treatment, and to notify her prescriber if she is pregnant or plans to become pregnant. If pregnancy is suspected, tell her to stop taking misoprostol immediately.

ADSORBENTS

An adsorbent is a drug that attracts molecules of a liquid, gas, or dissolved substance to its surface. Adsorbents are prescribed in acute poisonings to prevent the absorption of drugs or other toxins from the GI tract. In this class, the most commonly used drug is activated charcoal, a black powder residue obtained from the distillation of organic materials.

Pharmacokinetics

Activated charcoal must be given soon after toxic ingestion because it can only bind with drugs or other toxins that haven't yet been absorbed by the GI tract. After initial absorption, some toxins move back into the intestines, where they're reabsorbed. Activated charcoal may be given repeatedly to break this cycle.

Activated charcoal isn't absorbed or metabolized by the body. It's excreted unchanged in feces.

Pharmacodynamics

Because adsorbents attract and bind toxins in the intestine, they inhibit toxins from being absorbed from the GI tract. However, this binding doesn't change any toxic effects caused by earlier absorption of the toxin.

Pharmacotherapeutics

Activated charcoal is a general-purpose antidote used for many types of acute oral poisoning. It isn't indicated in acute poisoning from cyanide, ethanol, inorganic acids, iron, methanol, organic solvents, or sodium chloride alkalies.

Interactions

✦ Ipecac syrup may decrease the efficacy of activated charcoal by causing emesis.

✦ Milk, ice cream, or sherbet can decrease the absorptive capacity of activated charcoal.

Features of activated charcoal

✦ Must be given soon after ingestion because it can bind only with unabsorbed substances

✦ Binds with toxins, inhibiting them from being absorbed from the GI tract

✦ Is a general-purpose antidote used for many types of acute oral poisoning

✦ Isn't indicated for cyanide, ethanol, inorganic acids, iron, methanol, organic solvents, sodium chloride alkalies

Adverse reactions to watch for
+ Black stools
+ Bowel obstruction
+ Constipation

Key nursing actions
+ Give large doses to treat poisoning if the patient has food in his stomach.
+ For maximum effectiveness, give the drug within 30 minutes of poisoning but after ipecac-induced vomiting has stopped.
+ Give a laxative, such as sorbitol, to prevent constipation.
+ Don't mix activated charcoal with milk, ice cream, or sherbet.

Features of antiflatulents
+ Provide an antifoaming effect in the GI tract
+ Disperse mucus-enclosed gas pockets and help prevent their formation
+ Are used for disorders that create excess gas

Adverse reactions

Adverse reactions to activated charcoal administration include black stools and constipation. Bowel obstruction can occur with overdose. A laxative, such as sorbitol, is usually given with activated charcoal to prevent constipation and improve the taste. No known hypersensitivity reactions exist.

Nursing considerations
+ Give large doses of activated charcoal to treat poisoning if food is present in the patient's stomach.
+ Add grape juice to the charcoal-and-water mixture to make it more palatable.
+ For maximum effectiveness, give activated charcoal within 30 minutes of the poisoning but after ipecac-induced vomiting has ceased.
+ Plan to give multiple doses of activated charcoal to treat severe poisoning by drugs that undergo enterohepatic or enteroenteric recycling, such as acetaminophen, digoxin, phenobarbital, phenytoin, and theophylline. Multiple doses also may be used to treat life-threatening overdoses of carbamazepine, dapsone, or quinidine.
+ Give a laxative, such as sorbitol, to prevent constipation caused by the adsorbent.
+ Don't give activated charcoal to a child younger than age 1.
+ Don't mix activated charcoal with milk, ice cream, or sherbet. This decreases the drug's capacity to adsorb toxins.
+ Teach the patient and his caregiver about the prescribed drug. (See *Teaching a patient about adsorbents*.)

ANTIFLATULENTS

Antiflatulents, which disperse gas pockets in the GI tract, are available alone or with antacids. The major antiflatulent is simethicone.

Pharmacokinetics
Drugs in this class aren't absorbed from the GI tract. They're distributed only in the intestinal lumen, undergo no metabolism, and are eliminated intact in feces.

Pharmacodynamics
Antiflatulents provide an antifoaming action in the GI tract. By producing a film in the intestines, simethicone disperses mucus-enclosed gas pockets and helps prevent their formation.

Teaching a patient about antiflatulents

Whenever simethicone is prescribed, teach the patient and his family the drug's name, dose, frequency, action, and adverse effects. Also take the following actions.
+ Instruct the patient to take simethicone after meals and at bedtime.
+ Teach the patient to shake the simethicone suspension before taking the dose.
+ Advise the patient that chewable tablets must be chewed thoroughly before swallowing.
+ Encourage a patient with functional gastric bloating to increase his physical activity and exercise, unless contraindicated.
+ Instruct the patient to notify the prescriber if simethicone is ineffective.
+ Advise the patient not to exceed the recommended dose.

Pharmacotherapeutics

Antiflatulents are prescribed to treat disorders characterized by excess gas, such as functional gastric bloating, postoperative gaseous bloating, diverticular disease, spastic or irritable colon, and air swallowing.

Interactions

Simethicone doesn't interact significantly with other drugs.

Adverse reactions

Simethicone causes no known adverse reactions.

Nursing considerations

+ Periodically assess the patient's degree of GI discomfort.
+ To ensure adequate mixing, shake a simethicone suspension before giving it.
+ Use a calibrated dropper to give liquid simethicone.
+ Give simethicone after each meal and at bedtime for maximum effectiveness.
+ Teach the patient and his caregiver about the prescribed drug. (See *Teaching a patient about antiflatulents.*)

DIGESTANTS

Drugs in this class aid digestion by replacing missing enzymes or other substances needed to digest food. Digestants may function in the GI tract, liver, or pancreas. These drugs include the pancreatic enzymes pancreatin and pancrelipase, and dehydrocholic acid, a synthetic bile acid.

Pharmacokinetics

Digestants aren't absorbed or metabolized. They act locally in the GI tract and are excreted in feces.

Pharmacodynamics

The action of digestants resembles the action of the body substances they replace. The bile acid dehydrocholic acid increases bile output in the liver. Pancreatin and pancrelipase replace normal pancreatic enzymes.

Key nursing actions
+ Periodically assess the patient's level of GI distress.
+ Give simethicone after each meal and at bedtime.

Features of digestants
+ Aid digestion by replacing missing enzymes or other substances needed to digest food
+ May function in the GI tract, liver, or pancreas
+ Act like the substance being replaced
+ Increase bile output in the liver and ease constipation; are used to treat nonmechanical biliary stasis (dehydrocholic acid)

Features of digestants
(continued)
✦ Replace pancreatic enzymes; are used for pancreatitis, cystic fibrosis, steatorrhea (pancreatin and pancrelipase)

Adverse reactions to watch for

dehydrocholic acid
✦ Abdominal cramps
✦ Diarrhea

pancreatic enzymes
✦ Abdominal cramps
✦ Diarrhea
✦ Nausea

Pancreatic enzymes also contain amylase to digest carbohydrates, lipase to digest fats, and trypsin to digest proteins. The drugs act in the duodenum and upper jejunum of the upper GI tract.

Pharmacotherapeutics
Dehydrocholic acid provides temporary relief from constipation and promotes the flow of bile. It's used to treat biliary stasis that isn't caused by mechanical obstruction of the hepatic or common bile duct.

Pancreatic enzymes are given to patients with insufficient levels of pancreatic enzymes, such as those with pancreatitis and cystic fibrosis. They may also be used to treat steatorrhea, a disorder of fat metabolism characterized by fatty, foul-smelling stools.

Interactions
✦ An antacid can reduce the effects of pancreatin or pancrelipase and shouldn't be given with either digestant.
✦ Pancreatin or pancrelipase may decrease the absorption of folic acid or iron.

Adverse reactions
Dehydrocholic acid can produce abdominal cramps and diarrhea. If a dislodged gallstone is obstructing a biliary duct, this digestant also can produce biliary colic.

Pancreatic enzymes typically cause nausea, abdominal cramps, and diarrhea. They may produce allergic reactions in patients who are sensitive to trypsin.

Nursing considerations
✦ Monitor the patient for adverse reactions and drug interactions during digestant therapy.
✦ Give pancrelipase and pancreatin with meals and dehydrocholic acid after meals.

✦ Don't give an antacid with pancreatin or pancrelipase because it can negate the digestant's effects.
✦ Teach the patient and his caregiver about the prescribed drug. (See *Teaching a patient about digestants.*)

ANTIDIARRHEALS AND LAXATIVES

Diarrhea and constipation are the two major symptoms of disturbances in the large intestine. To manage these symptoms, prescribers rely on antidiarrheals and laxatives, respectively. To control diarrhea, antidiarrheals may act systemically, as with the opioid-related antidiarrheals, or locally, as with kaolin and pectin.

Laxatives are used to stimulate defecation. Major classes of laxatives include dietary fiber and related bulk-forming laxatives as well as hyperosmolar, emollient, stimulant, and lubricant laxatives.

OPIOID-RELATED ANTIDIARRHEALS

These antidiarrheals produce their effects by decreasing intestinal peristalsis. They include difenoxin and diphenoxylate (combination drugs that include atropine) as well as loperamide and opium tincture.

Pharmacokinetics
Difenoxin and diphenoxylate are readily absorbed from the GI tract. In contrast, loperamide isn't absorbed well after oral administration. Opium tincture is variably absorbed.

Difenoxin, diphenoxylate, and loperamide are distributed in serum, metabolized in the liver, and excreted primarily in feces. Diphenoxylate is metabolized to difenoxin, its biologically active major metabolite. Although opium alkaloids are distributed widely in the body, the low doses used to treat diarrhea act primarily in the GI tract. Opium is rapidly metabolized in the liver and excreted in urine.

Pharmacodynamics
Opioid-related antidiarrheals slow GI motility by depressing circular and longitudinal muscle action, also called peristalsis, in the large and small intestines. These drugs also decrease expulsive contractions throughout the colon.

Pharmacotherapeutics
Difenoxin, diphenoxylate, loperamide, and opium tincture are used to treat acute, nonspecific diarrhea. Loperamide also is used to treat chronic diarrhea, although a pediatric dosage for chronic diarrhea hasn't been established. None of these drugs is recommended for children younger than age 2. (See *Minimizing the risks of opioid-related antidiarrheals in children,* page 252.)

Interactions
✦ Difenoxin, diphenoxylate, loperamide, or opium tincture may enhance the depressant effects of alcohol or a barbiturate, opiate, sedative, or tranquilizer.
✦ Opium tincture may antagonize the effects of metoclopramide.

Adverse reactions
Reactions to opioid-related antidiarrheals include nausea, vomiting, abdominal discomfort, drowsiness, fatigue, central nervous system (CNS) depression, tachy-

Features of opioid-related antidiarrheals
✦ Slow GI motility by depressing peristalsis in the small and large intestines
✦ Decrease expulsive contractions in the colon
✦ Are used for acute, nonspecific diarrhea
✦ Are used for chronic diarrhea (loperamide only)

Possible drug interactions
✦ Alcohol
✦ Barbiturates
✦ Metoclopramide
✦ Opiates
✦ Sedatives
✦ Tranquilizers

Minimizing the risks of opioid-related antidiarrheals in children

The opioid-related antidiarrheals diphenoxylate and loperamide require cautious use in pediatric patients because young children respond to these drugs differently than adults do. For example, dehydration from diarrhea may predispose children to diphenoxylate or loperamide intoxication. Also by inhibiting peristalsis, these drugs may cause fluid retention in the intestines, which can exacerbate a child's dehydration and electrolyte imbalances.

Adverse reactions to watch for

✦ Abdominal discomfort, nausea, paralytic ileus, vomiting
✦ CNS depression, drowsiness, fatigue
✦ Physical dependence
✦ Tachycardia

Key nursing actions

✦ Stop the drug if diarrhea lasts more than 48 hours or symptoms worsen during therapy.
✦ Monitor the fluid and electrolyte status.
✦ Consider the risk of physical dependence.

cardia, and paralytic ileus. With prolonged use, opium preparations may produce physical dependence. Diphenoxylate also may produce physical dependence if used at high doses for a prolonged time. At doses used to treat acute diarrhea, however, these drugs pose a low risk of physical dependence.

Nursing considerations

✦ Teach the patient and his caregiver about the prescribed drug. (See *Teaching a patient about opioid-related antidiarrheals.*)
✦ Stop the drug if diarrhea persists for more than 48 hours or if symptoms worsen during drug therapy.
✦ Monitor the patient's fluid and electrolyte status, which may be altered by diarrhea. Replace fluids and electrolytes, as needed.
✦ Consider the risk of dependence on diphenoxylate if the patient receives high doses of it for a prolonged time. Or consider the risk of dependence on opium tincture during prolonged therapy.

Teaching a patient about opioid-related antidiarrheals

Whenever an opioid-related antidiarrheal is prescribed, teach the patient and his family the drug's name, dose, frequency, action, and adverse effects. Also take the following actions.
✦ Instruct the patient not to exceed the recommended dosage.
✦ Urge the patient to notify the prescriber if diarrhea continues for more than 48 hours or worsens with treatment.
✦ Caution the patient to avoid activities that require mental alertness until the drug's CNS effects are known.
✦ Inform the patient that the drug may cause dry mouth. Advise him to drink plenty of clear fluids to help relieve this adverse effect and prevent dehydration, which may accompany diarrhea.

KAOLIN AND PECTIN

As combination drugs, kaolin and pectin mixtures are local-acting OTC antidiarrheals. They work by adsorbing irritants and soothing the intestinal mucosa.

Pharmacokinetics

Kaolin and pectin aren't absorbed and, therefore, aren't distributed throughout the body. They undergo no metabolism and are excreted in feces.

Pharmacodynamics

These antidiarrheals act as adsorbents, binding with bacteria, toxins, and other irritants on the intestinal mucosa. Pectin decreases the pH in the intestinal lumen and soothes the irritated mucosa.

Pharmacotherapeutics

Kaolin and pectin are used to relieve mild to moderate acute diarrhea. They may also be used to temporarily relieve chronic diarrhea until the cause has been determined, and definitive treatment begun.

Interactions

✦ Kaolin and pectin can interfere with the absorption of digoxin or other drugs from the intestinal mucosa if administered at the same time.
✦ Allopurinol may have decreased therapeutic effects if given up to 3 hours before the antidiarrheal.

Adverse reactions

Constipation may occur—especially in geriatric or debilitated patients or with overdose or prolonged use—but it's usually mild and transient. Rarely, fecal impaction occurs in infants and debilitated patients.

Nursing considerations

✦ Teach the patient and his caregiver about the prescribed drug. (See *Teaching a patient about kaolin and pectin.*)

Features of kaolin and pectin

✦ Act as adsorbents, binding with bacteria, toxins, other irritants on the intestinal mucosa
✦ Relieve mild to moderate acute diarrhea
✦ May be used temporarily for chronic diarrhea
✦ Decrease the pH in the intestinal lumen and soothe irritated mucosa

Adverse reactions to watch for

✦ Constipation
✦ Fecal impaction (rare) in infants and debilitated patients

PATIENT TEACHING

Teaching a patient about kaolin and pectin

Whenever a kaolin and pectin mixture is prescribed, teach the patient and his family the drug's name, dose, frequency, action, and adverse effects. Also take the following actions.
◆ Advise the patient not to self-medicate for longer than 48 hours. Instruct him to consult his prescriber if diarrhea persists.
◆ Instruct the patient who takes other drugs to consult his prescriber because kaolin and pectin can interfere with the absorption of other drugs, making them less effective.
◆ Tell the patient to drink 8 to 13 8-oz (240-ml) glasses of fluid daily to replace lost fluids.
◆ Instruct the patient to take kaolin and pectin as prescribed; for example, a dose of kaolin and pectin after each loose bowel movement, but not more than eight doses per day. Tell the patient who experiences more than eight bowel movements per day to consult his prescriber.

✦ Monitor the patient closely for constipation during kaolin and pectin therapy. Be aware that fecal impaction can result from severe constipation, especially in an infant or debilitated patient.

✦ If the patient develops constipation, withhold the kaolin and pectin and notify the prescriber.

DIETARY FIBER AND BULK-FORMING LAXATIVES

A high-fiber diet is the most natural way to prevent or treat constipation. Dietary fiber refers to the parts of plants that aren't digested in the small intestine.

Bulk-forming laxatives resemble dietary fiber. They contain natural and semi-synthetic polysaccharides and cellulose and include methylcellulose, polycarbophil, and psyllium hydrophilic mucilloid.

Pharmacokinetics

Dietary fiber and bulk-forming laxatives aren't absorbed systemically. The polysaccharides in these substances are converted by intestinal bacterial flora into osmotically active metabolites that draw water into the intestines. Dietary fiber and bulk-forming laxatives are excreted in feces.

Pharmacodynamics

Dietary fiber and related laxatives increase stool mass and water content, promoting peristalsis.

Pharmacotherapeutics

Along with dietary fiber, bulk-forming laxatives are used to treat simple constipation, especially constipation caused by a low-fiber or low-fluid diet. They're also used to help patients avoid Valsalva's maneuver by maintaining soft feces during recovery from acute myocardial infarction (MI) or cerebral aneurysm. In addition, they're prescribed to manage irritable bowel syndrome and diverticulosis.

Interactions

✦ Dietary fiber or a bulk-forming laxative can decrease the absorption of digoxin, warfarin, or a salicylate if they're taken within 2 hours of laxative administration.

Adverse reactions

Reactions include flatulence, a sensation of abdominal fullness, intestinal obstruction, fecal impaction, esophageal obstruction (if sufficient liquid hasn't been given with the drug), and severe diarrhea. Hypersensitivity reactions rarely occur.

Nursing considerations

✦ Monitor the patient closely for adverse GI reactions.

✦ Evaluate the effects of dietary fiber intake or bulk-forming laxative use on the patient's bowel pattern. Notify the prescriber if these measures are ineffective.

✦ Give a bulk-forming laxative with 8 oz (240 ml) of water to prevent esophageal obstruction. Ensure that the patient follows each dose of psyllium hydrophilic mucilloid with another 8 oz of water.

✦ Monitor the patient for diarrhea, which may become severe. Also monitor for laxative dependence.

Teaching a patient about dietary fiber and bulk-forming laxatives

Whenever dietary fiber or a bulk-forming laxative is prescribed, teach the patient and his family appropriately. For a bulk-forming laxative, discuss the drug's name, dose, frequency, action, and adverse effects. Also take the following actions.

✦ Inform the patient and family about dietary sources of fiber, such as bran, whole grain cereals, fresh fruits and vegetables, and legumes. Tell the patient to consume 6 to 11 servings (about 25 mg) of dietary fiber daily to prevent constipation, but to increase consumption slowly to minimize GI upset.

✦ Advise the patient with restricted sugar and salt intake to avoid frequent use of a bulk-forming laxative because most of these drugs contain sugar and salt. Recommend a sugar-free laxative to a diabetic patient.

✦ Teach the patient to take each dose of a bulk-forming laxative with an 8-oz (240-ml) glass of water and to increase fluid intake during the day to prevent fecal impaction. Also tell the patient to follow each dose of psyllium hydrophilic mucilloid with a second 8-oz glass of water.

✦ Instruct the patient with chronic constipation to take additional measures to correct constipation.

✦ Explain that the patient may experience flatulence or a sensation of abdominal fullness when taking dietary fiber or a bulk-forming laxative.

✦ If the patient develops diarrhea, monitor his hydration, temporarily withhold the dietary fiber or bulk-forming laxative, and notify the prescriber.

✦ Teach the patient and his caregiver about the prescribed fiber or drug. (See *Teaching a patient about dietary fiber and bulk-forming laxatives.*)

HYPEROSMOLAR LAXATIVES

These laxatives work by drawing water into the intestines, which promotes bowel distention and peristalsis. Drugs in this class include glycerin, lactulose, polyethylene glycol (PEG), and saline compounds, such as magnesium salts, sodium biphosphate, and sodium phosphate.

Pharmacokinetics

With rectal administration, glycerin is poorly absorbed, distributed locally, and excreted in feces.

After oral administration, lactulose enters the GI tract and is minimally absorbed. As a result, it's distributed only in the intestines. It's metabolized by bacteria in the colon and excreted in feces.

PEG is a nonabsorbable solution that acts as an osmotic drug but doesn't alter electrolyte balance. Because the drug isn't absorbed, it can't be distributed or metabolized. It's excreted by the GI tract.

After oral or rectal administration, saline compounds undergo absorption of some ions into the GI tract. Absorbed ions are excreted in urine; unabsorbed drug, in feces.

Features of hyperosmolar laxatives

✦ Draw water into the intestines, which promotes bowel distention and peristalsis

✦ Are helpful in bowel retraining (glycerin)

✦ Are used for constipation and to help reduce ammonia production and absorption in liver disease (lactulose)

✦ Are used for bowel cleansing before internal GI examination (PEG)

✦ Are used for prompt, complete bowel evacuation (saline compounds)

Pharmacodynamics

Hyperosmolar laxatives produce bowel movements by drawing water into the intestines. Fluid accumulation distends the bowel and promotes peristalsis and bowel movement.

Pharmacotherapeutics

The uses of hyperosmolar laxatives vary. Glycerin is helpful in bowel retraining. Lactulose is used to treat constipation and help reduce ammonia production and absorption from the intestines in liver disease. PEG is used for bowel cleansing before internal GI examination. Saline compounds are prescribed when prompt, complete bowel evacuation is required.

Interactions

Except for PEG, hyperosmolar laxatives don't interact significantly with other drugs.

An oral drug given 1 hour before PEG may be flushed from the GI tract unabsorbed.

Adverse reactions

With hyperosmolar laxatives, adverse reactions involve fluid and electrolyte imbalances. Glycerin administration may also cause weakness and fatigue; rarely, it may produce severe diarrhea and hypovolemia.

Adverse reactions to lactulose include abdominal distention, flatulence, and abdominal cramps in about 20% of patients taking full doses. Other reactions include nausea, vomiting, diarrhea, hypokalemia, hypovolemia, increased blood glucose level in patients with impaired glucose tolerance, and increased hepatic encephalopathy in patients with severe liver dysfunction.

The most common adverse reactions to PEG include nausea, abdominal fullness, and bloating.

Adverse reactions to saline compounds include weakness, lethargy, dehydration from hypernatremia and resultant hypovolemia, hypermagnesemia, hyperphosphatemia, hypocalcemia, arrhythmias from electrolyte imbalances, and hypovolemic shock.

Nursing considerations

+ Closely monitor the patient for fluid and electrolyte imbalances.
+ Perform a neurologic assessment regularly to detect the CNS effects of an electrolyte imbalance.
+ During lactulose therapy, monitor the patient's glucose level once every shift or as prescribed for a patient with impaired glucose tolerance. Also observe for signs and symptoms of hyperglycemia, such as polyuria, polydipsia, polyphagia, and weakness.
+ Dilute lactulose with water or unsweetened juice before administration to reduce the sweetness and prevent nausea.
+ Store lactulose below 86° F (30° C), but don't allow the drug to freeze.
+ Encourage the patient to drink at least 3 L of fluid daily during saline compound therapy.
+ Periodically monitor the patient's bowel pattern to assess the drug's effectiveness or detect diarrhea.
+ If nausea, vomiting, or diarrhea occurs, monitor the patient's hydration.
+ Prepare PEG solution with tap water and shake it vigorously to dissolve the powdered drug. Store the solution under refrigeration for up to 48 hours.

Teaching a patient about hyperosmolar laxatives

Whenever a hyperosmolar laxative is prescribed, teach the patient and his family the drug's name, dose, frequency, action, and adverse effects. Also take the following actions.

◆ Describe the proper use of laxatives and caution the patient about laxative dependence.

◆ Discuss additional measures the patient can take to prevent constipation.

◆ Teach the patient with chronic constipation about bowel retraining, if prescribed.

◆ Stress the importance of taking the hyperosmolar laxative exactly as prescribed to help prevent fluid and electrolyte imbalances.

◆ Teach the patient to recognize the signs and symptoms of fluid and electrolyte imbalances and, if they occur, to withhold the drug and notify the prescriber.

◆ Advise the patient to avoid activities that require mental alertness if weakness, drowsiness, or lethargy occurs.

◆ Instruct the patient with impaired glucose tolerance to be alert for signs and symptoms of hyperglycemia and to monitor his glucose level regularly during lactulose therapy.

◆ Instruct the patient to drink at least 3 L (3¼ quarts) of fluid daily during saline compound therapy.

◆ Instruct the patient who experiences diarrhea to withhold the drug, notify the prescriber, and increase his fluid intake (unless contraindicated).

◆ Advise the patient to take oral drugs more than 1 hour before taking polyethylene glycol (PEG) for proper absorption.

◆ Inform the patient that PEG is best tolerated when chilled. If signs of hypothermia occur, tell him to contact the prescriber.

◆ Administer PEG after at least 3 hours of fasting.

◆ Encourage the patient to drink the prescribed 4 L of PEG solution rapidly (240 ml every 10 minutes) rather than drinking small amounts continuously.

◆ Give chilled PEG solution with caution. Although chilling enhances the flavor, it can lead to hypothermia after ingestion of a large amount of solution.

◆ Teach the patient and his caregiver about the prescribed drug. (See *Teaching a patient about hyperosmolar laxatives.*)

EMOLLIENT LAXATIVES

Also known as *stool softeners,* emollients include the calcium, potassium, and sodium salts of docusate.

Pharmacokinetics

After oral administration, emollients are absorbed and excreted through bile in feces.

Pharmacodynamics

Emollients soften the stool and make bowel movements easier by emulsifying the fat and water components of feces in the small and large intestines. This detergent action allows water and fats to penetrate the stool, making it softer and easier to eliminate. Emollients also stimulate electrolyte and fluid secretion from intestinal mucosal cells.

Features of emollient laxatives

◆ Are also known as *stool softeners*

◆ Emulsify the fat and water components of feces (a detergent action) in the small and large intestine so fat and water can better penetrate and soften stool

◆ Stimulate electrolyte and fluid secretion from intestinal mucosal cells

◆ Are used for patients who should avoid straining at stool, such as those with a recent MI or surgery or those with anal or rectal disease, increased ICP, or a hernia

Possible drug interactions
+ Mineral oil
+ Vitamin A
+ Vitamin B
+ Vitamin E
+ Vitamin K

Adverse reactions to watch for
+ Bitter taste
+ Diarrhea
+ Throat irritation
+ Mild abdominal cramping

Key nursing actions
+ Monitor the patient's hydration.
+ Notify the prescriber if diarrhea develops.
+ Replace fluid and electrolytes lost through diarrhea.

Features of stimulant laxatives
+ Are also known as *irritant cathartics*

Pharmacotherapeutics
These laxatives are used to soften stools in patients who should avoid straining during a bowel movement, including those who have recently had an MI or surgery or who have an anal or rectal disease, increased intracranial pressure (ICP), or a hernia.

Interactions
+ When given together orally, an emollient increases the systemic absorption of mineral oil, may result in the formation of tumor-like deposits in tissues, and may interfere with the absorption of vitamins A, D, E, and K and other nutrients.

 CLINICAL ALERT An emollient can increase the absorption of many oral drugs. Use caution when giving an emollient with a drug that has a narrow therapeutic index.

Adverse reactions
Although adverse reactions to emollients seldom occur, they may include a bitter taste, diarrhea, throat irritation, and mild, transient abdominal cramps.

Nursing considerations
+ Store the emollient laxative at 59° to 86° F (15° to 30° C). Protect liquid preparations from light.
+ Give a liquid emollient in milk or fruit juice to mask the bitter taste.
+ Monitor the patient's hydration and notify the prescriber if diarrhea occurs.
+ Replace fluid and electrolytes lost through diarrhea.
+ Teach the patient and his caregiver about the prescribed drug. (See *Teaching a patient about emollient laxatives.*)

STIMULANT LAXATIVES
Sometimes called *irritant cathartics,* stimulant laxatives include bisacodyl, cascara sagrada, castor oil, and senna.

Pharmacokinetics
Stimulant laxatives are minimally absorbed and are metabolized in the liver. The metabolites are excreted in urine and feces.

Teaching a patient about stimulant laxatives

Whenever a stimulant laxative is prescribed, teach the patient and his family the drug's name, dose, frequency, action, and adverse effects. Also take the following actions.

✦ Inform the patient that the herbal remedies cascara sagrada and senna may discolor his urine reddish pink or brown.

✦ Instruct the patient to take the stimulant laxative exactly as prescribed to prevent dependence, chronic use, and cathartic colon with atony and dilation.

✦ Teach the patient how to administer and store the drug.

✦ Instruct the patient not to chew bisacodyl tablets because they're coated to prevent GI irritation. Also, advise him not to take them with antacids.

Pharmacodynamics

These laxatives stimulate peristalsis and produce bowel movement by irritating the intestinal mucosa or stimulating nerve endings of the intestinal smooth muscle. Castor oil also increases peristalsis in the small intestine.

Pharmacotherapeutics

Stimulant laxatives are used to empty the bowel before general surgery, sigmoidoscopy or proctoscopy, and radiologic procedures, such as barium studies of the GI tract. They also are used to treat constipation caused by prolonged bed rest, neurologic colon dysfunction, and constipating drugs.

Interactions

✦ When given at the same time, a stimulant laxative can reduce the absorption of other oral drugs, especially sustained-release ones.

Adverse reactions

Adverse reactions to stimulant laxatives include weakness, nausea, abdominal cramps, and mild proctitis. Rectal administration of bisacodyl can produce a burning sensation. Cascara sagrada and senna cause a reddish pink or brown urine discoloration. Castor oil may cause pelvic congestion in menstruating women.

With long-term use or overdose, stimulant laxatives may cause electrolyte imbalances, including hypokalemia, hypocalcemia, metabolic alkalosis, or metabolic acidosis. Malabsorption and weight loss may also occur. Habitual use may lead to cathartic colon with atony and dilation.

Stimulant laxatives can cause hypersensitivity reactions, such as rash and pruritus.

Nursing considerations

✦ Teach the patient and his caregiver about the prescribed drug. (See *Teaching a patient about stimulant laxatives.*)

✦ Monitor the patient's fluid and electrolyte levels, and notify the prescriber if an imbalance occurs.

✦ Monitor the patient's bowel evacuation pattern.

Features of stimulant laxatives
(continued)

✦ Stimulate peristalsis and produce bowel movement by irritating the intestinal mucosa or stimulating nerve endings in intestinal smooth muscles

✦ Are used to empty the bowel before general surgery or procedures involving the GI tract

✦ Used to treat constipation from prolonged bed rest, neurologic colon dysfunction, constipating drugs

Adverse reactions to watch for

✦ Abdominal cramps, mild proctitis, nausea

✦ Long-term use or overdose: cathartic colon with atony and dilation, electrolyte imbalances (hypokalemia, hypocalcemia, metabolic alkalosis, metabolic acidosis), malabsorption, weight loss

✦ Pelvic congestion in menstruating women (castor oil)

✦ Rectal burning (bisacodyl)

✦ Reddish pink or brown urine (cascara sagrada, senna)

✦ Weakness

Key nursing actions

✦ Monitor the fluid and electrolyte levels.

✦ Monitor the bowel evacuation pattern.

✦ Stop the drug and notify the prescriber if rash or pruritus develops.

Using mineral oil safely in geriatric patients

During treatment with mineral oil, geriatric patients are at high risk for aspiration. To help make therapy as safe as possible, don't give mineral oil at bedtime to a geriatric patient. Instead, give the drug — preferably on an empty stomach — when he's awake, alert, and if possible ambulatory.

♦ Stop the drug and notify the prescriber if rash or pruritus develops.
♦ Give castor oil on an empty stomach for best results.
♦ Mix castor oil with juice or a carbonated beverage to mask the preparation's oily taste. Tell the patient to hold ice in his mouth before taking castor oil to help decrease the taste.
♦ Store castor oil below 104° F (40° C), but don't freeze; shake well before giving.

LUBRICANT LAXATIVES

Mineral oil is the main lubricant laxative in use.

Pharmacokinetics

In its nonemulsified form, mineral oil is minimally absorbed; the emulsified form is about 50% absorbed. Absorbed mineral oil is distributed to the mesenteric lymph nodes, intestinal mucosa, liver, and spleen. Then it's metabolized by the liver and excreted in feces.

Pharmacodynamics

Mineral oil lubricates the stool and the intestinal mucosa and prevents water reabsorption from the lumen of the bowel. The increased fluid content of feces increases peristalsis. Rectal administration by enema also produces distention.

Pharmacotherapeutics

Mineral oil is used to treat constipation and maintain soft stools when straining is contraindicated, such as after a recent MI (to avoid Valsalva's maneuver), eye surgery (to prevent increased pressure in the eye), or cerebral aneurysm repair (to avoid increased ICP). In older patients, use of this drug requires certain precautions. (See *Using mineral oil safely in geriatric patients.*)

Given orally or by enema, this lubricant laxative may also be given to patients with fecal impaction.

Interactions

♦ Mineral oil may impair the absorption of many oral drugs, including fat-soluble vitamins, hormonal contraceptives, and anticoagulants.
♦ Mineral oil may interfere with the bactericidal activity of nonabsorbable sulfonamides.

Adverse reactions

Reactions to mineral oil include nausea, vomiting, diarrhea, and abdominal cramps. Seepage from the rectum after rectal administration may result in anal irri-

Features of lubricant laxatives

♦ Prevent water reabsorption from the bowel lumen
♦ Increase fluid content of feces, which stimulates peristalsis
♦ Are used to treat constipation and maintain soft stools when straining is contraindicated

Possible drug interactions

♦ Many oral drugs, including fat-soluble vitamins, hormonal contraceptives, and anticoagulants
♦ Nonabsorbable sulfonamides

tation, pruritus ani, infection, and impaired healing of lesions in the area. Long-term oral use of nonemulsified mineral oil may impair absorption of fat-soluble vitamins, causing vitamin deficiencies. Lipid pneumonitis may result from aspiration of oral mineral oil.

   Systemic absorption of emulsified mineral oil can lead to granulomatous reactions in the mesenteric lymph nodes, liver, and spleen.

Nursing considerations

✦ Give mineral oil cautiously to prevent aspiration.

✦ Monitor the patient's hydration status. If he experiences nausea, vomiting, or diarrhea, withhold the next dose of mineral oil and notify the prescriber.

✦ Avoid giving mineral oil with other oral drugs because it may impair their absorption.

✦ Monitor the patient for decreased effectiveness of fat-soluble vitamins, anticoagulants, and nonabsorbable sulfonamides during mineral oil therapy.

✦ Mix mineral oil with fruit juice or a carbonated beverage to disguise its taste.

✦ During long-term mineral oil therapy, monitor the patient for early signs of fat-soluble vitamin deficiencies: night blindness (vitamin A deficiency); profuse sweating, restlessness, and irritability (vitamin D deficiency); muscle weakness or intermittent claudication (vitamin E deficiency); and abnormal bleeding tendency (vitamin K deficiency).

✦ Withhold mineral oil and notify the prescriber if you suspect a fat-soluble vitamin deficiency.

✦ Don't give mineral oil with or shortly after meals or with fat-soluble vitamins because it can interfere with vitamin absorption.

✦ Teach the patient and his caregiver about the prescribed drug. (See *Teaching a patient about lubricant laxatives*.)

Adverse reactions to watch for

✦ Abdominal cramps, diarrhea, nausea, vomiting

✦ Anal irritation and infection, impaired healing of anal lesions, pruritus ani

✦ Granulomatous reactions in the mesenteric lymph nodes, liver, and spleen (systemic absorption of emulsified mineral oil)

✦ Lipid pneumonitis (aspiration of oral mineral oil)

✦ Vitamin deficiencies from impaired absorption of fat-soluble vitamins (long-term oral use of nonemulsified mineral oil)

Key nursing actions

✦ Give mineral oil cautiously to prevent aspiration.

✦ Mix mineral oil with fruit juice or a carbonated beverage to mask its taste.

✦ Monitor the patient's hydration.

✦ During long-term therapy, monitor the patient for evidence of fat-soluble vitamin deficiency.

ANTIEMETICS

Antiemetics decrease nausea, which reduces the urge to vomit. Antiemetic classes include:
+ antihistamines, such as buclizine, cyclizine, dimenhydrinate, diphenhydramine, hydroxyzine, meclizine, and trimethobenzamide.
+ phenothiazines, such as chlorpromazine, perphenazine, prochlorperazine, and promethazine.
+ serotonin-receptor antagonists, such as dolasetron, granisetron, and ondansetron.

Although many drugs are used to prevent or halt vomiting, one drug is commonly used to induce vomiting. (See *Using ipecac syrup effectively.*)

Pharmacokinetics

Oral antihistamine antiemetics are absorbed well from the GI tract and are metabolized primarily by the liver. Their inactive metabolites are excreted in urine.

Phenothiazine antiemetics and serotonin-receptor antagonists are absorbed well, extensively metabolized by the liver, and excreted in urine and feces.

Pharmacodynamics

For antihistamines, the mechanism of action that produces antiemesis is unclear.

Phenothiazines produce antiemesis by blocking the dopaminergic receptors in the chemoreceptor trigger zone of the brain. This area of the brain, near the medulla, stimulates the vomiting center in the medulla and causes vomiting. These drugs may also directly depress the vomiting center.

Serotonin-receptor antagonists block serotonin stimulation centrally in the chemoreceptor trigger zone and peripherally in vagal nerve terminals, both of which stimulate vomiting.

Pharmacotherapeutics

Except for trimethobenzamide, antihistamine antiemetics are specifically used for nausea and vomiting caused by inner ear stimulation. As a result, these drugs prevent or treat motion sickness. They usually prove most effective when given before activities that produce motion sickness and are much less effective when nausea or vomiting has already begun.

Phenothiazines and serotonin-receptor antagonists control severe nausea and vomiting from various causes. They're used when vomiting becomes severe and potentially hazardous, such as postsurgical or viral nausea and vomiting. Both types of drugs also are prescribed to control nausea and vomiting caused by cancer chemotherapy and radiotherapy.

Interactions

+ An antihistamine or phenothiazine can produce additive CNS depression and sedation when taken with a CNS depressant, such as alcohol or an antidepressant, barbiturate, opioid, or tranquilizer.
+ An antihistamine can cause additive anticholinergic effects, such as constipation, dry mouth, vision problems, and urine retention, when taken with an anticholinergic, such as an antiparkinsonian, phenothiazine, or tricyclic antidepressant.
+ Together, an anticholinergic and a phenothiazine can cause increased anticholinergic effects and decreased antiemetic effects.

Features of antiemetics

+ Types of antiemetics: antihistamines, phenothiazines, serotonin-receptor antagonists
+ Antihistamines: action unclear; used for nausea and vomiting caused by inner ear stimulation (motion sickness)
+ Phenothiazines: block dopaminergic receptors in chemoreceptor trigger zone of brain and may directly depress vomiting center; used for severe nausea and vomiting
+ Serotonin-receptor antagonists: block serotonin stimulation in chemoreceptor trigger zone (central) and vagal nerve terminals (peripheral); used for severe nausea and vomiting

Possible drug interactions

+ Anticholinergics
+ CNS depressants
+ Droperidol
+ Lithium

Using ipecac syrup effectively

At times, you may need to induce vomiting, such as when treating drug overdoses or certain poisonings. To induce vomiting, administer ipecac syrup after contacting the prescriber or a poison control center. Ipecac syrup causes vomiting by exerting a local irritant effect on the GI mucosa and stimulating the chemoreceptor trigger zone. In most cases, the patient vomits within 30 minutes of receiving an adequate dose.

For safe, effective treatment with ipecac syrup, follow these guidelines:

✦ Don't use ipecac syrup in a semiconscious or unconscious patient.
✦ Avoid using ipecac syrup in a patient who has ingested strychnine, a corrosive (such as an alkali or strong acid), or a petroleum distillate.
✦ If activated charcoal and ipecac syrup are used to treat poisoning, give the charcoal after the patient vomits. Otherwise, the charcoal can adsorb the ipecac syrup, making it ineffective.
✦ Use activated charcoal to treat ipecac syrup overdose; ipecac can be cardiotoxic if it's absorbed.

✦ When taken with lithium, a phenothiazine may increase the risk of neurologic toxicity.
✦ The combination of droperidol and a phenothiazine can increase the risk of extrapyramidal effects.

Adverse reactions

Antihistamine and phenothiazine antiemetics produce some drowsiness. Antihistamines may cause paradoxical CNS stimulation, which is more common in children than adults. Signs and symptoms of paradoxical CNS stimulation may range from restlessness, insomnia, and euphoria to tremors and seizures. Other adverse CNS reactions to antihistamine antiemetics include dizziness, headache, and lethargy. Adverse CNS reactions to phenothiazine and serotonin-receptor antagonists include confusion, anxiety, euphoria, agitation, depression, headache, insomnia, restlessness, and weakness. Rarely, high doses or abrupt dosage changes of phenothiazines may increase the risk of electroencephalogram changes and seizures.

The anticholinergic effects of antiemetics may cause constipation, dry mouth and throat, dysuria, urine retention, impotence, and vision and auditory disturbances, such as blurred vision or tinnitus.

Antihistamine antiemetics may cause mild nausea, epigastric distress, or anorexia. Hypotension and orthostatic hypotension with tachycardia, syncope, and dizziness are common adverse reactions to the phenothiazine antiemetics. Trimethobenzamide and phenothiazine antiemetics may also produce extrapyramidal symptoms, such as acute dystonia and dyskinesia, that require drug discontinuation.

Hypersensitivity reactions, manifested by rashes and photosensitivity, may occur with antihistamine antiemetics but rarely occur with phenothiazine antiemetics. Rarely, such blood dyscrasias as granulocytopenia, hemolytic anemia, leukopenia, thrombocytopenia, and pancytopenia may also occur. Rarely, serotonin-receptor antagonists may cause a rash.

Adverse reactions to watch for

✦ Acute dystonia and dyskinesia
✦ Agitation, anxiety, confusion, depression, euphoria, headache, insomnia, restlessness, weakness
✦ Anorexia, epigastric distress, nausea
✦ Constipation, dry mouth and throat, dysuria, impotence, urine retention, vision and hearing changes
✦ Dizziness, headache, lethargy
✦ Drowsiness
✦ Hypersensitivity reactions
✦ Hypotension, orthostatic hypotension with tachycardia, syncope, dizziness
✦ Paradoxical CNS stimulation

Teaching a patient about antiemetics

Whenever an antiemetic is prescribed, teach the patient and his family the drug's name, dose, frequency, action, and adverse effects. Also take the following actions.

✦ Describe the drug's sedative effects and advise the patient not to drive or perform other activities that require mental alertness. Urge him not to drink alcohol or take other central nervous system (CNS) depressants; doing so can increase the sedative effects.

✦ Teach the patient how to relieve the drug's anticholinergic effects, such as constipation and dry mouth.

✦ Reassure the patient that vision and hearing disturbances are dose-related and should disappear when the drug is stopped.

✦ Inform the male patient that impotence may occur.

✦ Instruct the patient to avoid prolonged exposure to sunlight or to wear protective clothing and a sunscreen because the antiemetic may cause photosensitivity.

✦ Advise the patient to notify his prescriber if he experiences urinary frequency and a sense of fullness in the lower abdomen.

✦ Advise family members that paradoxical CNS stimulation may occur in a child who receives an antihistamine antiemetic.

✦ Instruct the patient to notify the prescriber if anorexia or a weight loss of more than 1½ kg (3 lb) in 1 week occurs during long-term antihistamine antiemetic therapy.

✦ Instruct the patient to take the prescribed antihistamine antiemetic with milk or food to minimize adverse GI effects.

✦ Advise the patient to ingest an antihistamine antiemetic 30 to 60 minutes before the activity that may produce motion sickness.

✦ Advise the patient that phenothiazine antiemetics aren't effective for motion sickness.

✦ Inform the patient about the risk of hypotension with a phenothiazine antiemetic; instruct him to remain lying down for 30 to 60 minutes after taking the drug.

✦ Explain that a phenothiazine antiemetic may make the patient's urine pink or reddish brown but that this discoloration is harmless.

✦ Inform the seizure-prone patient that a phenothiazine antiemetic can lower the seizure threshold. Instruct him to notify the prescriber if a seizure occurs because the drug may need to be stopped.

✦ Advise the patient to stop taking trimethobenzamide or a phenothiazine antiemetic and to notify the prescriber if he experiences extrapyramidal symptoms, such as slow, involuntary movements of large muscles in the limbs, trunk, and neck.

✦ Advise the patient to notify the prescriber if adverse reactions occur or if the antiemetic is ineffective.

✦ Advise the patient that a serotonin-receptor antagonist may cause taste disturbances. If these occur and affect his appetite, tell him to notify the prescriber.

Key nursing actions

✦ Take seizure precautions if giving a phenothiazine antiemetic to a patient prone to seizures.

✦ If giving an antihistamine to a child, watch for evidence of paradoxical CNS stimulation.

✦ Observe the patient for extrapyramidal symptoms.

✦ Evaluate hematologic test results for signs of blood dyscrasias.

✦ Assess the patient regularly for vision and hearing changes.

Nursing considerations

CLINICAL ALERT Take seizure precautions when giving a phenothiazine antiemetic to a patient who is predisposed to seizures. These drugs can lower the seizure threshold.

✦ Monitor a child for signs of paradoxical CNS stimulation during antihistamine therapy and notify the prescriber if paradoxical CNS stimulation occurs.

✦ Observe the patient for extrapyramidal symptoms during trimethobenzamide or phenothiazine therapy.

✦ Evaluate the patient's hematologic test results for signs of blood dyscrasias. Alert the prescriber if abnormalities occur.

✦ Avoid skin contact with oral solutions and injections when preparing or giving these drugs because they can cause dermatologic effects.

✦ Give an antihistamine with food or milk to minimize epigastric distress and nausea.

✦ Inject an intramuscular drug deep in the upper outer quadrant of the gluteus muscle.

✦ Assess the patient regularly for vision and auditory disturbances.

✦ Teach the patient and his caregiver about the prescribed drug. (See *Teaching a patient about antiemetics*.)

Psychotropic drugs

Usually, psychotropic drugs are used with other treatments, such as psychotherapy. These drugs may be prescribed for sleep disorders and various psychogenic disorders. They include sedatives and hypnotics, anxiolytics, antidepressants and mood disorder drugs, antipsychotic drugs, and central nervous system (CNS) stimulants.

When caring for a patient who is receiving a drug to promote sleep or alter psychogenic behavior, keep in mind that it's likely to be prescribed for long-term therapy. Because of this and because the drug may cause intolerable adverse reactions, plan to monitor the patient closely for adverse reactions, check the drug level regularly, and watch for signs of noncompliance, such as a recurrence of symptoms. Because some psychotropic drugs are addictive, also look for signs of dependence and, when the drug is stopped, for withdrawal symptoms.

SEDATIVES AND HYPNOTICS

Sedatives act to reduce activity or excitement, thereby calming a patient. Some degree of drowsiness commonly accompanies sedative use. When given in large doses, sedatives are considered hypnotics, which induce a state resembling natural sleep.

Drugs from several classes are used therapeutically as sedatives and hypnotics: benzodiazepines, barbiturates, and nonbenzodiazepines-nonbarbiturates.

BENZODIAZEPINES

Benzodiazepines offer many therapeutic effects. They are used to produce sedation before anesthesia, induce sleep, relieve anxiety and tension, relax skeletal muscles, and treat seizures. Commonly used benzodiazepines include alprazolam, chlordiazepoxide, clonazepam, diazepam, estazolam, flurazepam, lorazepam, midazolam, oxazepam, temazepam, and triazolam.

Pharmacokinetics

After oral administration, benzodiazepines are absorbed rapidly and completely from the GI tract. They're distributed widely in the body and penetrate into the brain rapidly. Some benzodiazepines also can be given parenterally. When given I.M., chlordiazepoxide and diazepam are absorbed erratically and slowly; lorazepam is absorbed completely and rapidly.

The absorption rate determines how quickly the drug produces its effects. Rapidly absorbed flurazepam and triazolam have the fastest onset. The extent of distribution determines the duration of action. Triazolam, which is highly lipophilic and widely distributed, has a short duration.

All benzodiazepines are metabolized in the liver and excreted primarily in urine. Some of these drugs have active metabolites that give them a longer duration of action. Lorazepam and oxazepam have relatively short half-lives and may be preferred for geriatric patients and those with liver impairment.

Pharmacodynamics

Benzodiazepines may work by stimulating gamma-aminobutyric acid (GABA) receptors in the ascending reticular activating system of the brain. The reticular activating system is linked to wakefulness and attention and includes the cerebral cortex and limbic, thalamic, and hypothalamic levels of the CNS. (See *How benzodiazepines work,* page 268.)

At low dosages, benzodiazepines decrease anxiety by acting on the limbic system and other areas of the brain that help regulate emotional activity. The drugs usually can calm or sedate the patient without causing drowsiness.

At higher dosages, benzodiazepines induce sleep, probably because they depress the reticular activating system. These drugs increase total sleep time and produce a reduced number of awakenings. In most cases, they don't decrease the time spent in rapid-eye-movement (REM) sleep, the sleep stage in which the brain activity resembles the activity it shows when awake, the muscles relax, and the eyes move rapidly. This gives benzodiazepines a significant advantage over barbiturates.

Pharmacotherapeutics

Clinical indications for benzodiazepines include relaxing the patient before surgery, inducing general anesthesia, treating insomnia, treating alcohol withdrawal symptoms, treating anxiety and seizure disorders, and producing skeletal muscle relaxation.

Interactions

✦ Erythromycin, ketoconazole, or another drug that inhibits the cytochrome P450 (CYP) 3A4 enzyme system may increase and prolong the alprazolam or triazolam level and related CNS depression and psychomotor impairment.

✦ When a benzodiazepine is taken with a CNS depressant, such as alcohol or an anticonvulsant, sedation and CNS depression increase, which may cause decreased consciousness level, reduced muscle coordination, respiratory depression, and death.

✦ Hormonal contraceptives may reduce flurazepam metabolism and increase the risk of toxicity.

✦ St. John's wort may induce the enzymes involved in the hepatic and intestinal metabolism of alprazolam, diazepam, midazolam, or triazolam, which can reduce their therapeutic effects.

✦ By acting on the same CNS receptors, kava may increase the adverse CNS effects of chlordiazepoxide, clonazepam, diazepam, and oxazepam.

Features of benzodiazepines

✦ May work by stimulating GABA receptors in the ascending reticular activating system
✦ At low doses, decrease anxiety by acting on the limbic system and other brain areas that control emotions; usually calm or sedate a patient without drowsiness
✦ At higher doses, induce sleep, probably by depressing the reticular activating system; increase sleep time and decrease awakenings
✦ Are used to relax patients before surgery, produce skeletal muscle relaxation, and treat insomnia, alcohol withdrawal, anxiety, and seizure disorders

Possible drug and herb interactions

✦ CNS depressants
✦ Drugs that inhibit the cytochrome P450 (CYP) 3A4 enzyme system, such as erythromycin and ketoconazole
✦ Hormonal contraceptives
✦ Kava
✦ St. John's wort

EYE ON DRUG ACTION

How benzodiazepines work

These illustrations show how impulses normally are transmitted and how benzodiazepines work at the cellular level.

CHLORIDE ION MOVEMENT
The speed of impulses from a presynaptic neuron across a synapse is influenced by the amount of chloride ions in the postsynaptic neuron. The passage of chloride ions into the postsynaptic neuron depends on the inhibitory neurotransmitter gamma-aminobutyric acid (GABA).

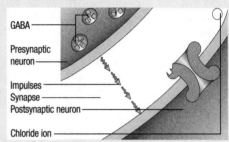

GABA BINDING
When GABA is released from the presynaptic neuron, it travels across the synapse and binds to GABA receptors on the postsynaptic neuron. This binding opens the chloride channels, which allows chloride ions to flow into the postsynaptic neuron and slow the nerve impulses.

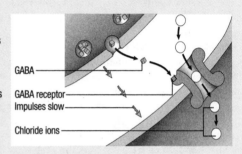

DRUG ENHANCES GABA EFFECTS AND CHLORIDE MOVEMENT
Benzodiazepines bind to receptors on or near GABA receptors, enhancing the effect of GABA and allowing more chloride ions to flow into the postsynaptic neuron. This depresses the nerve impulses, causing them to slow or stop.

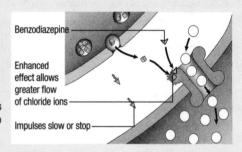

Adverse reactions to watch for

- ✦ Amnesia
- ✦ Ataxia, dizziness, muscle weakness
- ✦ Daytime sedation, fatigue, hangover effect, respiratory depression
- ✦ Dependence (physical and psychological, with high doses and prolonged use)
- ✦ Dry mouth, nausea, vomiting
- ✦ Rebound insomnia
- ✦ Weakness, delirium, tonic-clonic seizures (with abrupt withdrawal)

Adverse reactions

Benzodiazepines cause few adverse reactions. The most common adverse reactions are daytime sedation and hangover effect. Rebound insomnia may occur, especially with short-acting drugs, such as triazolam. Some benzodiazepines may cause amnesia. Dose-related dizziness and ataxia may also occur. Geriatric patients, debilitated patients, and patients with liver disease are more likely to experience dose-related adverse reactions to benzodiazepines. (See *Benzodiazepine's effects in a geriatric patient.*)

Fatigue, muscle weakness, mouth dryness, nausea, and vomiting occasionally result from benzodiazepine use. Respiratory depression is more common in geriatric or debilitated patients, patients with limited ventilatory reserve, and patients re-

LIFESPAN

Benzodiazepine's effects in a geriatric patient

During benzodiazepine therapy, a geriatric patient is at high risk for experiencing dose-related adverse effects. He's also particularly susceptible to rare idiosyncratic reactions, such as nervousness, restlessness, talkativeness, apprehension, euphoria, and excitement. These effects occur because benzodiazepines with long half-lives or active metabolites are likely to accumulate in a geriatric patient.

To minimize such adverse effects in a geriatric patient, use a lower starting dose and increase the dosage gradually.

ceiving other CNS depressants. Signs and symptoms of psychological and physical dependence may occur with prolonged use and high dosages, but rarely with usual dosages. If a patient becomes physically dependent, sudden withdrawal of the benzodiazepine may cause weakness, delirium, and tonic-clonic seizures.

Rare and usually mild allergic reactions include rash, pruritus, urticaria, burning eyes, and photosensitivity.

Nursing considerations

✦ Monitor the patient regularly for adverse reactions and interactions, especially if he's elderly or debilitated or has liver disease.

 CLINICAL ALERT Consult the prescriber if other CNS depressants also are prescribed during benzodiazepine therapy; this combination may cause lethal depressant effects.

✦ Stop benzodiazepine therapy in a hallucinating and violent patient.
✦ Assist with gastric lavage, respiratory support, and other supportive measures, such as I.V. fluid or drug administration, if overdose occurs. Frequently monitor the patient's vital signs and fluid intake and output. Give flumazenil as the antidote for benzodiazepine overdose.
✦ Keep epinephrine and a corticosteroid readily available for emergency care of a patient who experiences a hypersensitivity reaction to the drug.
✦ Plan care and give drugs based on the patient's daily routines and bedtime rituals. Don't wake a patient to give a benzodiazepine.
✦ Watch the patient take the drug to prevent drug hoarding.
✦ Monitor the patient's vital signs frequently, particularly noting signs of respiratory depression, such as decreased number of respirations or respiratory pattern changes.
✦ Perform a respiratory assessment before and after giving each dose of the drug.
✦ Withhold the dose and notify the prescriber if respiratory depression occurs.
✦ Reduce the dosage for a patient receiving another CNS depressant because of the risk of increased respiratory depression.
✦ Position the debilitated patient to maximize respiratory function. For example, help the patient into a semi-Fowler's or high Fowler's position.
✦ Teach the patient and his caregiver about the drug. (See *Teaching a patient about benzodiazepines*, page 270.)

Key nursing actions
✦ Consult the prescriber if other CNS depressants are ordered during benzodiazepine therapy.
✦ Stop benzodiazepine therapy if the patient hallucinates or becomes violent.
✦ Keep epinephrine and a corticosteroid readily available in case of hypersensitivity.
✦ Watch the patient take the drug to prevent hoarding.
✦ Check vital signs frequently.
✦ Perform respiratory assessments before and after each dose.
✦ Position a debilitated patient to maximize respiratory function.

Features of barbiturates

✦ Reduce overall CNS alertness and produce drowsiness, sedation, and hypnosis by depressing the sensory cortex of the brain, decreasing motor activity, and altering cerebral function
✦ Are particularly active in the reticular activating system of the brain, although they seem to act throughout the CNS
✦ In low doses, depress the sensory and motor cortex of brain, causing drowsiness
✦ In high doses, depress all levels of the CNS and may cause respiratory depression and death
✦ Are used for insomnia, preoperative sedation and anesthesia, anxiety, seizures, and short-term daytime sedation

Possible drug interactions

✦ Acetaminophen
✦ Beta blockers
✦ Chloramphenicol
✦ CNS depressants
✦ Corticosteroids
✦ Cyclosporine
✦ Doxycycline
✦ Hormonal contraceptives
✦ Hydantoins
✦ MAO inhibitors
✦ Metronidazole
✦ Oral anticoagulants
✦ Quinidine
✦ Theophylline
✦ Tricyclic antidepressants
✦ Valproic acid

BARBITURATES

The major action of barbiturates is to reduce overall CNS alertness. In low doses, these drugs depress the sensory and motor cortex in the brain, causing drowsiness. In high doses, they can cause respiratory depression and death because they can depress all levels of the CNS.

Barbiturates include amobarbital, butabarbital, mephobarbital, pentobarbital, phenobarbital, and secobarbital.

Pharmacokinetics

Barbiturates are absorbed well from the GI tract, distributed rapidly, metabolized by the liver, and excreted in urine.

Pharmacodynamics

As sedative-hypnotics, barbiturates depress the sensory cortex of the brain, decrease motor activity, alter cerebral function, and produce drowsiness, sedation, and hypnosis.

These drugs appear to act throughout the CNS. However, the reticular activating system of the brain, which is responsible for wakefulness, is particularly sensitive to these drugs.

Pharmacotherapeutics

Barbiturates have many indications, including insomnia, preoperative sedation and anesthesia, anxiety, seizures, and short-term, daytime sedation for periods of typically less than 2 weeks.

Interactions

✦ A barbiturate may reduce the effects of a corticosteroid, chloramphenicol, cyclosporine, doxycycline, metronidazole, an oral anticoagulant, a hormonal contraceptive, quinidine, theophylline, a tricyclic antidepressant, and a beta blocker, such as metoprolol and propranolol.

✦ A hydantoin, such as phenytoin, may reduce phenobarbital metabolism and increase its toxic effects.
✦ Together, a barbiturate and another CNS depressant may cause excessive CNS depression.
✦ Valproic acid may increase the barbiturate level.
✦ A monoamine oxidase (MAO) inhibitor can inhibit barbiturate metabolism and increase its sedative effects.
✦ When taken with acetaminophen, a barbiturate increases the risk of liver toxicity.

Adverse reactions

The most common adverse reactions to barbiturates relate to the CNS and include drowsiness, lethargy, headache, depression, and vertigo.

Idiosyncratic reactions include paradoxical anxiety, agitation, restlessness, and rage or paradoxical excitement. These reactions occur most commonly among geriatric patients and those with severe uncontrolled pain. (See *Adverse reactions to barbiturates in a geriatric patient.*)

The patient can experience serious adverse respiratory reactions, including hypoventilation, laryngospasm, bronchospasm, and severe respiratory depression, especially when large I.V. doses are given too rapidly. Large dosages of barbiturates suppress the hypoxic and chemoreceptor drive of the respiratory system, resulting in decreased respiratory rate and rhythm.

The patient also can sustain adverse cardiovascular reactions, such as mild bradycardia and hypotension. Less common adverse reactions to barbiturates affect the GI tract, resulting in nausea, vomiting, diarrhea, and epigastric pain.

 CLINICAL ALERT Acute barbiturate toxicity causes overdose symptoms, which can be severe. The symptoms are characterized by CNS and respiratory depression and can lead to respiratory failure, cardiac arrest, and death.

With prolonged use, the patient can develop drug tolerance as well as psychological and physical dependence on the barbiturate. Withdrawal symptoms resemble those of chronic alcoholism and occur with sudden discontinuation after long-term use.

Allergic reactions mainly involve the skin and mucous membranes and occur more commonly in patients with past allergies or asthma. Allergic reactions include various rashes, urticaria, angioedema, and fever. Rarely, photosensitivity also has

Adverse reactions to watch for

✦ Allergic reactions: angioedema, fever, rash, skin reactions, urticaria
✦ Bradycardia
✦ Bronchospasm, laryngospasm
✦ Decreased respiratory rate and rhythm (large doses)
✦ Depression
✦ Drowsiness, headache, lethargy, vertigo
✦ Drug dependence or tolerance
✦ Hypotension
✦ Hypoventilation, respiratory depression
✦ Idiosyncratic reactions: agitation, anxiety, excitement, rage, restlessness
✦ Toxicity: CNS and respiratory depression that can lead to respiratory failure, cardiac arrest, and death
✦ Withdrawal symptoms: like those of chronic alcoholism, from an abrupt end to long-term therapy

Teaching a patient about barbiturates

Whenever a barbiturate is prescribed, teach the patient and his family the drug's name, dose, frequency, action, and adverse effects. Also take the following actions.

✦ Advise the patient not to discontinue the barbiturate suddenly without consulting the prescriber because withdrawal symptoms may occur.

✦ Instruct the patient not to drive or engage in other activities that require mental alertness until the drug's central nervous system effects are known.

✦ Instruct the patient not to drink alcohol during drug therapy because respiratory depression can occur.

✦ Advise the patient to consult the prescriber before taking any tranquilizers, opioids, or other prescription pain relievers or any herbal remedies.

✦ Counsel the patient not to give any of the prescribed drug to family members or friends.

✦ Advise the patient to keep this drug and all others out of the reach of children.

✦ Encourage the patient to be honest about barbiturate use because dependence can occur with long-term use.

---

been reported. Other allergic reactions include rare blood dyscrasias, such as pancytopenia, leukopenia, granulocytopenia, thrombocytopenia, and megaloblastic anemia caused by folic acid depletion.

Nursing considerations

✦ Monitor the patient periodically for adverse reactions and interactions. Be alert for idiosyncratic reactions, such as paradoxical anxiety or excitement, in a geriatric patient or a patient with severe, uncontrolled pain.

✦ Reduce the dosage for a geriatric or debilitated patient.

✦ Discontinue the barbiturate gradually after long-term therapy to prevent rebound REM sleep.

✦ Monitor the prothrombin time for a patient who also receives an anticoagulant. Keep in mind that abrupt withdrawal of a barbiturate may cause serious bleeding. Adjust the anticoagulant dosage as needed.

✦ Rotate — don't shake — the amobarbital ampule and mix the solution with sterile water only. Discard a solution that doesn't become clear in 5 minutes.

✦ Use the solution within 30 minutes after opening to minimize deterioration, and inject it slowly and deeply into a large muscle mass when using the intramuscular (I.M.) route.

✦ Don't use a cloudy pentobarbital, phenobarbital, or secobarbital solution; don't mix the solution with other drugs; use the solution within 30 minutes after opening to minimize deterioration; and inject it into a large muscle mass when using the I.M. route of administration.

 CLINICAL ALERT Don't stop therapy abruptly. Otherwise, the patient receiving long-term therapy may develop withdrawal symptoms similar to those of alcohol abuse.

✦ Alert the prescriber if you suspect barbiturate dependence.

✦ Teach the patient and his caregiver about the prescribed drug. (See *Teaching a patient about barbiturates.*)

Key nursing actions

✦ Monitor the prothrombin time if the patient also receives an anticoagulant.

✦ Don't stop barbiturates abruptly after long-term therapy.

NONBENZODIAZEPINES-NONBARBITURATES

Drugs in this class are used as hypnotics only for short-term treatment of simple insomnia because they lose their effectiveness by the end of the second week. They offer no advantages over other sedatives and hypnotics. Nonbenzodiazepines-nonbarbiturates include chloral hydrate, glutethimide, paraldehyde, zaleplon, and zolpidem.

Pharmacokinetics

Nonbenzodiazepines-nonbarbiturates are absorbed rapidly from the GI tract, metabolized in the liver, and excreted in urine.

Pharmacodynamics

The mechanism of action for nonbenzodiazepines-nonbarbiturates isn't fully known, but they produce depressant effects similar to barbiturates.

Pharmacotherapeutics

Typically, nonbenzodiazepines-nonbarbiturates are used for short-term treatment of simple insomnia, sedation before surgery, and sedation before electroencephalogram (EEG) tests.

Interactions

✦ When used with another CNS depressant, a nonbenzodiazepine-nonbarbiturate can cause additive CNS depression, resulting in drowsiness, respiratory depression, stupor, coma, and death.
✦ When given with an oral anticoagulant, chloral hydrate may increase the risk of bleeding.
✦ Use of chloral hydrate with I.V. furosemide may produce sweating, flushing, blood pressure fluctuations, and uneasiness.
✦ Taking zaleplon or zolpidem with meals may delay the onset of sleep.
✦ Cimetidine may inhibit the enzymes needed for zaleplon metabolism, requiring the zaleplon dose to be reduced to 5 mg during combined therapy.

Adverse reactions

The most common dose-related adverse reactions to nonbenzodiazepines-nonbarbiturates include GI symptoms and hangover effect. Adverse GI reactions include nausea, vomiting, and some gastric irritation. Adverse CNS reactions, which occur especially with hypnotic dosages, include the hangover effect. Particularly in geriatric patients, the nonbenzodiazepine-nonbarbiturate hangover occurs less commonly than the barbiturate and benzodiazepine hangovers.

At high dosages, the drugs can produce CNS depression of the respiratory center, thereby causing respiratory depression, respiratory failure, and death — especially in geriatric patients. Habitual use can cause tolerance and dependence. Chronic and acute toxicity can occur, and abrupt withdrawal from large dosages may cause dangerous symptoms similar to those seen in barbiturate withdrawal.

Rare and mild hypersensitivity reactions include rash and urticaria. Also rare, idiosyncratic reactions can include marked excitement, hysteria, prolonged hypnosis, profound muscle weakness, and syncope without marked hypotension.

Nursing considerations

✦ Give a lower dosage to a geriatric or debilitated patient.

Features of nonbenzodiazepines-nonbarbiturates

✦ Produce effects similar to barbiturates by an unknown mechanism
✦ Lose effectiveness by the end of the second week of therapy
✦ Are used for short-term treatment of simple insomnia and for sedation before surgery or EEG tests

Possible drug interactions

✦ Cimetidine
✦ CNS depressants
✦ I.V. furosemide
✦ Oral anticoagulants

Adverse reactions to watch for

✦ Dangerous symptoms similar to those of barbiturate withdrawal (abrupt withdrawal of large doses)
✦ Dependence, tolerance (habitual use)
✦ Gastric irritation, nausea, vomiting
✦ Hangover effect
✦ Respiratory depression, respiratory failure, death (high doses)

Key nursing actions
✦ Check vital signs frequently, especially noting evidence of respiratory depression.
✦ Perform respiratory assessments before and after each dose.
✦ Position a debilitated patient to maximize respiratory function.

✦ Minimize gastric irritation from the liquid or capsule form of chloral hydrate by giving the drug after meals. Dilute liquid chloral hydrate with a fluid that minimizes its unpleasant taste, such as juice or soda. Store chloral hydrate in a light-resistant container, and refrigerate suppositories.
✦ Frequently monitor the patient's vital signs, particularly noting signs of respiratory depression, such as decreased number of respirations or respiratory pattern changes.
✦ Perform a respiratory assessment before and after giving each dose of the prescribed nonbenzodiazepine-nonbarbiturate.
✦ Withhold the prescribed dose and notify the prescriber if respiratory depression occurs.
✦ Position the debilitated patient to maximize respiratory function. For example, help the patient into a semi-Fowler's or high Fowler's position.
✦ Teach the patient and his caregiver about the prescribed drug. (See *Teaching a patient about nonbenzodiazepines-nonbarbiturates*.)

Features of buspirone
✦ Has a different structure and action than other anxiolytics
✦ Offers advantages over other anxiolytics: less sedation; no increased CNS depression when taken with alcohol, sedatives, or hypnotics; less potential for abuse
✦ Produces varied effects in the midbrain and acts as midbrain modulator, possibly from the high affinity for serotonin receptors
✦ Is used for generalized anxiety but, because of its slow onset, isn't useful for quick relief

ANXIOLYTICS

Anxiolytics, or antianxiety drugs, are among the most commonly prescribed drugs in the United States. They're used primarily to treat anxiety disorders. The three main classes of antianxiety drugs are benzodiazepines, barbiturates, and buspirone. (For details on the first two classes, see "Benzodiazepines" and "Barbiturates" earlier in this chapter.)

BUSPIRONE

Because buspirone is an azaspirodecanedione derivative, its structure and mechanism of action differ from those of the other anxiolytics. Also, buspirone offers several advantages over those drugs; less sedation; no increase in CNS depression when taken with alcohol, a sedative, or a hypnotic; and less potential for abuse.

Pharmacokinetics
Buspirone is absorbed rapidly, undergoes extensive first-pass effect, and is metabolized in the liver to at least one active metabolite. The drug is eliminated in urine and feces.

PATIENT TEACHING

Teaching a patient about buspirone

Whenever buspirone is prescribed, teach the patient and his family the drug's name, dose, frequency, action, and adverse effects. Also take the following actions.

✦ Inform the patient that buspirone's therapeutic effects may not be noticeable for several weeks.

✦ Caution the patient not to abruptly stop taking buspirone because of the risk of withdrawal symptoms.

✦ Tell the patient to avoid alcohol use during drug therapy.

✦ Instruct the patient to take safety precautions at home. Tell family members to supervise his walking if dizziness or light-headedness occurs.

✦ Instruct the patient to prevent insomnia by taking the last daily dose of buspirone several hours before bedtime. Also suggest alternative methods for getting to sleep if insomnia occurs.

✦ Advise the patient to ask the prescriber to recommend an analgesic if headaches occur.

✦ Instruct the patient to notify her prescriber if she becomes pregnant or plans to breast-feed her infant.

Pharmacodynamics

Although buspirone's mechanism of action isn't clear, the drug doesn't affect GABA receptors like benzodiazepines do. Instead, buspirone seems to produce various effects in the midbrain and acts as a midbrain modulator, possibly because of its high affinity for serotonin receptors.

Pharmacotherapeutics

Buspirone is used to treat generalized anxiety. Patients who haven't received benzodiazepines seem to respond better to buspirone. Because of its slow onset of action, however, buspirone is ineffective for quick relief from anxiety.

Interactions

Unlike other anxiolytics, buspirone doesn't interact with alcohol or other CNS depressants.

✦ When buspirone is used with an MAO inhibitor, hypertensive reactions may occur.

✦ Erythromycin, itraconazole, or nefazodone can increase the buspirone level, requiring a reduction in the initial buspirone dose during combined therapy.

✦ Buspirone may increase the haloperidol level.

Adverse reactions

The most common reactions to buspirone include dizziness, light-headedness, insomnia, tachycardia, palpitations, and headache. Buspirone appears to have no abuse potential, and no deaths from overdose have been reported.

Nursing considerations

✦ Teach the patient and his caregiver about the prescribed drug. (See *Teaching a patient about buspirone.*)

✦ Switch a patient from long-term benzodiazepine therapy to buspirone therapy by tapering off the benzodiazepine dosage to avoid a withdrawal reaction.

Possible drug interactions

✦ Erythromycin
✦ Haloperidol
✦ Itraconazole
✦ MAO inhibitors
✦ Nefazodone

Adverse reactions to watch for

✦ Dizziness
✦ Headache
✦ Insomnia
✦ Light-headedness
✦ Palpitations
✦ Tachycardia

Key nursing actions

✦ Switch from long-term benzodiazepine to buspirone therapy by tapering the benzodiazepine to avoid withdrawal symptoms.

✦ Prevent insomnia by giving the last buspirone dose of the day several hours before bedtime.

✦ Help the patient find ways to induce sleep, such as a warm bath or quiet meditation. Give a hypnotic as needed.

✦ Prevent insomnia by giving the last daily dose of buspirone several hours before bedtime, if possible.

✦ Help the patient explore alternative methods for inducing sleep if insomnia occurs, such as a warm bath or quiet meditation. Give a hypnotic as needed.

ANTIDEPRESSANTS AND MOOD DISORDER DRUGS

Antidepressants and mood disorder drugs are used to treat affective disorders — disturbances in mood, characterized by depression or elation. These drugs include selective serotonin reuptake inhibitors (SSRIs), tricyclic antidepressants, MAO inhibitors, other antidepressants, and the mood disorder drug lithium.

SELECTIVE SEROTONIN REUPTAKE INHIBITORS

SSRIs were developed to treat depression with fewer adverse reactions than with tricyclic antidepressants and MAO inhibitors. Commonly used SSRIs include citalopram, escitalopram, fluoxetine, fluvoxamine, paroxetine, and sertraline.

Pharmacokinetics

After oral administration, SSRIs are absorbed almost completely and are highly protein bound. They're primarily metabolized in the liver and excreted in urine.

Pharmacodynamics

SSRIs inhibit the neuronal reuptake of the neurotransmitter serotonin. This increases the amount of circulating serotonin, which relieves depression.

Pharmacotherapeutics

Used to treat the same major depressive episodes as tricyclic antidepressants, SSRIs have the same degree of effectiveness. Fluoxetine, fluvoxamine, paroxetine, and sertraline also are used to treat obsessive-compulsive disorder. In addition, paroxetine is indicated for social anxiety disorder; fluoxetine and sertraline are approved for premenstrual dysphoric disorder.

SSRIs may also be useful in treating panic, eating, personality, impulse control, and anxiety disorders as well as posttraumatic stress disorder.

Interactions

✦ Use of an SSRI with another drug that's metabolized by the CYP 2D6 enzyme, including carbamazepine, flecainide, metoprolol, tricyclic antidepressants, and antipsychotics, such as clozapine and thioridazine, may increase the level of the interacting drug and the risk of toxicity.

✦ Use of an SSRI with an MAO inhibitor can cause serious, potentially fatal reactions.

✦ Use of citalopram or paroxetine with warfarin may lead to increased bleeding.

✦ Carbamazepine may increase citalopram clearance.

✦ Fluoxetine can increase the half-life of diazepam and displace other highly protein-bound drugs, leading to toxicity.

✦ Together, fluvoxamine and diltiazem may cause bradycardia.

✦ Use of an SSRI with a dietary supplement or herbal product that contains L-tryptophan may cause symptoms of central and peripheral toxicity.

Features of SSRIs

✦ Treat depression with fewer adverse effects than tricyclic antidepressants and MAO inhibitors
✦ Inhibit the neuronal uptake of serotonin, increasing the amount of circulating serotonin
✦ Are as effective as tricyclic antidepressants for major depressive episodes
✦ Are also used to treat obsessive-compulsive disorder, social anxiety disorder, premenstrual dysphoric disorder
✦ May be useful for treating panic, eating, personality, impulse control, anxiety, and posttraumatic stress disorders

Possible drug and herb interactions

✦ Cimetidine
✦ Diazepam
✦ Diltiazem
✦ Drugs that are highly protein-bound
✦ Drugs metabolized by CYP 2D6 enzyme, such as carbamazepine, flecainide, metoprolol, tricyclic antidepressants, antipsychotics
✦ MAO inhibitors
✦ Phenobarbital
✦ Phenytoin
✦ Procyclidine
✦ St. John's wort
✦ Sumatriptan
✦ Warfarin

> **WARNING**
>
> ## SSRI discontinuation syndrome
>
> Sudden discontinuation of a selective serotonin reuptake inhibitor (SSRI) may cause SSRI discontinuation syndrome. This syndrome may cause physical effects, such as dizziness, vertigo, ataxia, nausea, vomiting, muscle pains, tremor, and migraine. It also may produce psychological effects, such as anxiety, irritability, sadness, and vivid dreams.
> To prevent this syndrome, gradually taper off the patient's SSRI doses over several weeks.

✦ Paroxetine may increase the procyclidine level, causing increased anticholinergic effects.

✦ Cimetidine, phenobarbital, or phenytoin may reduce paroxetine metabolism by the liver, increasing the risk of toxicity.

✦ Paroxetine or sertraline may interact with other highly protein-bound drugs, causing adverse reactions to either drug.

✦ Use of sumatriptan or possibly another selective 5-HT_1-receptor agonist with SSRIs may cause serotonin syndrome (shivering, increased muscle tone, myoclonus, CNS irritability, and altered level of consciousness).

✦ Use of St. John's wort with an SSRI may increase serotonin reuptake inhibition, leading to increased sedative-hypnotic effects.

Adverse reactions

Citalopram commonly produces somnolence, insomnia, dry mouth, nausea, and increased sweating. The most common adverse reaction to escitalopram is nausea.

The most common adverse reactions to fluoxetine are headache, nervousness, anxiety, insomnia, nausea, anorexia, diarrhea, and diaphoresis. Rash may also occur.

During clinical trials, at least 10% of patients reported these adverse reactions to fluvoxamine and sertraline: dry mouth, headache, dizziness, diarrhea, nausea, and insomnia or somnolence. Tremor, sexual dysfunction in men, and fatigue also were reported with sertraline.

Paroxetine may produce adverse CNS reactions, including somnolence, dizziness, and insomnia. It may also cause adverse GI reactions, such as nausea, dry mouth, constipation, and diarrhea. Other reactions may include headache, asthenia, sweating, and ejaculatory and other disorders of the male genitalia.

Anorgasmia and delayed ejaculation may occur in patients taking an SSRI. Skin rash may also occur. Abrupt withdrawal of an SSRI can lead to significant adverse reactions. (See *SSRI discontinuation syndrome.*)

Nursing considerations

✦ Give the SSRI before bedtime or with food to minimize anticholinergic effects.

✦ Give a reduced paroxetine dosage to a patient with renal or hepatic impairment.

✦ Give a fluoxetine dosage that exceeds 20 mg daily in two divided doses — in the morning and at noon.

✦ Withhold fluoxetine and notify the prescriber if the patient develops a rash.

✦ Don't withdraw an SSRI suddenly.

✦ Teach the patient and his caregiver about the prescribed drug. (See *Teaching a patient about SSRIs,* page 278.)

Adverse reactions to watch for

✦ Anorgasmia, delayed ejaculation
✦ Rash

citalopram
✦ Dry mouth, nausea
✦ Insomnia, somnolence
✦ Sweating

escitalopram
✦ Nausea

fluoxetine
✦ Anorexia, diarrhea, nausea
✦ Anxiety, headache, insomnia, nervousness
✦ Rash
✦ Sweating

fluvoxamine
✦ Diarrhea, nausea
✦ Dizziness, dry mouth, headache, insomnia, somnolence

sertraline
✦ Diarrhea, nausea
✦ Dizziness, dry mouth, headache, insomnia, somnolence
✦ Fatigue
✦ Tremor
✦ Sexual dysfunction in men

paroxetine
✦ Asthenia
✦ Constipation, diarrhea, nausea
✦ Dizziness, dry mouth, headache, insomnia, somnolence
✦ Ejaculatory and other genital disorders in men
✦ Sweating

Key nursing actions

✦ Give the SSRI before bedtime or with food to minimize anticholinergic effects.
✦ Withhold fluoxetine and notify the prescriber if the patient develops a rash.
✦ Don't withdraw SSRIs abruptly.

Teaching a patient about SSRIs

Whenever a selective serotonin reuptake inhibitor (SSRI) is prescribed, teach the patient and his family the drug's name, dose, frequency, action, and adverse effects. Also take the following actions.

◆ Inform the patient that the drug may take a few weeks to produce its full therapeutic benefits. Advise him to take the drug as prescribed and, if a dose is missed, not to double the dose.

◆ Advise the patient to avoid operating a motor vehicle or dangerous machinery because sedation may occur.

◆ Teach the patient to take most of the daily dosage at bedtime if sedation is a problem.

◆ Instruct the patient to take the drug with meals or a snack to enhance absorption and to decrease dizziness.

◆ Tell the patient to consult his prescriber before taking an herbal remedy.

◆ Instruct the patient to notify her prescriber if she becomes pregnant or plans to become pregnant.

Features of tricyclic antidepressants

◆ May increase norepinephrine, serotonin, or both by preventing their reuptake into storage granules in presynaptic nerves

◆ Block acetylcholine and histamine receptors

◆ Are used to treat major depression, particularly with weight loss, anorexia, or insomnia

◆ May relieve physical effects in 1 to 2 weeks; psychological effects in 2 to 4 weeks

◆ Are used to prevent migraines and treat phobias, urinary incontinence, ADHD, diabetic neuropathy, some chronic pain, enuresis

---

TRICYCLIC ANTIDEPRESSANTS

These antidepressants include amitriptyline, amoxapine, clomipramine, desipramine, doxepin, imipramine, nortriptyline, protriptyline, and trimipramine.

Pharmacokinetics

All tricyclic antidepressants are active pharmacologically, and some of their metabolites are also active. They're absorbed completely when taken orally but undergo first-pass effect.

With first-pass effect, a drug passes from the GI tract to the liver, where it's partially metabolized before entering the circulation. Tricyclic antidepressants are metabolized extensively in the liver and eventually excreted as inactive compounds in urine.

The extreme lipid solubility of these drugs accounts for their wide distribution throughout the body, slow excretion, and long half-lives.

Pharmacodynamics

Tricyclic antidepressants probably increase the amount of either neurotransmitter norepinephrine or serotonin, or both, by preventing their reuptake into the storage granules in the presynaptic nerves. They also block acetylcholine and histamine receptors. After a neurotransmitter has performed its job, it can undergo reuptake, rapidly reentering the neuron from which it was released. By preventing reuptake, tricyclic antidepressants increase the levels of these neurotransmitters in the synapses, relieving depression.

Pharmacotherapeutics

These antidepressants are used to treat episodes of major depression. They're especially effective in treating depression of insidious onset when the depression is accompanied by weight loss, anorexia, or insomnia. Physical signs and symptoms may respond after 1 to 2 weeks of therapy; psychological symptoms, after 2 to 4 weeks.

LIFESPAN

Cardiovascular risks of tricyclic antidepressants

Tricyclic antidepressants pose cardiovascular risks, especially for geriatric and pediatric patients. To help avoid these risks in a geriatric patient, use a tricyclic antidepressant with caution and obtain an electrocardiogram (ECG) tracing before drug therapy begins. During therapy, monitor the patient closely for cardiovascular effects.

Because desipramine may cause sudden death in children and adolescents, also obtain an ECG tracing before beginning therapy with a tricyclic antidepressant in a child.

For any patient taking a tricyclic antidepressant, monitor for palpitations, tachycardia, and ECG changes.

Tricyclic antidepressants are much less effective in patients with hypochondriasis, atypical depression, or depression accompanied by delusions. However, they may be helpful in treating acute episodes of depression.

The drugs are also used in preventing migraine headaches and in treating phobias, urinary incontinence, attention deficit hyperactivity disorder (ADHD), diabetic neuropathy, certain types of chronic pain, and enuresis.

Interactions

✦ A tricyclic antidepressant can increase the catecholamine effect of an amphetamine or sympathomimetic, which can lead to hypertension.
✦ A barbiturate can increase the metabolism — and decrease the level — of a tricyclic antidepressant.
✦ Cimetidine can impair hepatic metabolism of a tricyclic antidepressant, increasing the risk of toxicity.
✦ Use of a tricyclic antidepressant with an MAO inhibitor may cause extreme elevation of body temperature, excitation, and seizures.
✦ When taken with an anticholinergic, a tricyclic antidepressant can increase anticholinergic effects, such as dry mouth, urine retention, and constipation.
✦ A tricyclic antidepressant can reduce clonidine's antihypertensive effects.
✦ St. John's wort may reduce the tricyclic antidepressant level.

Adverse reactions

Orthostatic hypotension commonly results from tricyclic antidepressant therapy. When it occurs, the dosage may be reduced or the drug changed to nortriptyline — especially for geriatric patients — because it's less likely to cause this adverse reaction.

A conduction delay, demonstrated by a widened QT interval, may also occur with tricyclic antidepressant therapy. This adverse reaction can exacerbate heart failure or an existing bundle-branch block. (See *Cardiovascular risks of tricyclic antidepressants.*)

Adverse anticholinergic reactions commonly occur with tricyclic antidepressant therapy, but they may diminish or disappear as treatment continues. Reactions include blurred vision, urine retention, dry mouth, and constipation.

At high dosages, these antidepressants can cause seizures. Other adverse reactions include sedation, jaundice, a fine resting tremor, decreased libido, inhibited ejaculation, transient eosinophilia and leukopenia and, rarely, granulocytopenia.

Possible interactions

✦ Amphetamines
✦ Anticholinergics
✦ Barbiturates
✦ Cimetidine
✦ Clonidine
✦ MAO inhibitors
✦ St. John's wort
✦ Sympathomimetics

Adverse reactions to watch for

✦ Anticholinergic reactions: blurred vision, constipation, dry mouth, urine retention
✦ Decreased libido, inhibited ejaculation
✦ Fine resting tremor
✦ Jaundice
✦ Mania
✦ Orthostatic hypotension
✦ Photosensitivity reactions
✦ Psychosis in susceptible patients
✦ Rash
✦ Sedation
✦ Seizures (high doses)
✦ Transient eosinophilia, granulocytopenia (rare), leukopenia
✦ Widened QT interval (conduction delay)

PATIENT TEACHING

Teaching a patient about tricyclic antidepressants

Whenever a tricyclic antidepressant is prescribed, teach the patient and his family the drug's name, dose, frequency, action, and adverse effects. Also take the following actions.

✦ Caution the patient not to stop taking the tricyclic antidepressant abruptly after long-term use; abrupt withdrawal can produce nausea, headache, and malaise.

✦ Advise the patient not to operate a motor vehicle or dangerous machinery if blurred vision or sedation occurs.

✦ Inform the patient that urine retention may occur.

✦ Teach the patient to identify high-fiber foods and include them in his diet to prevent constipation.

✦ Teach the patient how to manage orthostatic hypotension.

✦ Inform the patient that decreased libido may occur. Tell a man that inhibited ejaculation may also occur. Provide reassurance that drug-induced decreased libido and inhibited ejaculation should resolve when the tricyclic antidepressant is discontinued.

✦ Alert the patient that a full therapeutic response may take up to 30 days for most drugs in this class or 10 to 14 days with amitriptyline use.

✦ Instruct the patient to take the entire daily dosage at bedtime to avoid sedation and anticholinergic effects, unless otherwise prescribed.

✦ Warn the patient that the use of alcohol or other central nervous system depressants may increase sedation.

✦ Reassure the patient that adverse anticholinergic reactions may diminish or disappear as therapy continues.

✦ Tell the patient to keep tricyclic antidepressants out of the reach of children.

Rash may occur during the first 2 months of therapy, particularly with amitriptyline and imipramine. It usually is mild and doesn't require drug discontinuation. Photosensitivity reactions may also occur. Tricyclic antidepressant use may trigger manic episodes in patients with or without bipolar disorder and may exacerbate psychotic symptoms in susceptible patients.

Key nursing actions

✦ Switch to a different tricyclic antidepressant if the patient develops intolerable adverse effects, which can differ markedly among these drugs.

✦ Notify the prescriber if the QT interval widens.

✦ Monitor a suicidal patient closely until the drug takes effect.

Nursing considerations

✦ Switch the patient to a different tricyclic antidepressant if intolerable adverse reactions occur because adverse reactions can differ markedly among these drugs.

✦ If adverse reactions occur, divide a once-daily dose to decrease the risk of their occurrence.

✦ Notify the prescriber if the QT interval widens.

✦ Monitor a suicidal patient closely until the drug takes full effect.

✦ Teach the patient and his caregiver about the prescribed drug. (See *Teaching a patient about tricyclic antidepressants.*)

MAO INHIBITORS

Based on chemical structure, MAO inhibitors are divided into two classifications: hydrazines (isocarboxazid and phenelzine) and nonhydrazines (tranylcypromine). All of these drugs are used to treat depression.

Pharmacokinetics

MAO inhibitors are absorbed rapidly and completely from the GI tract and are metabolized in the liver to inactive metabolites. These metabolites are excreted mainly by the GI tract and to a lesser degree by the kidneys.

Pharmacodynamics

MAO inhibitors appear to work by inhibiting MAO, the enzyme that normally metabolizes many neurotransmitters, including norepinephrine and serotonin, making more norepinephrine and serotonin available to the receptors and thereby relieving the symptoms of depression.

Pharmacotherapeutics

These drugs are used for treating typical depression when it doesn't respond to other therapies or when other therapies are contraindicated. Isocarboxazid shouldn't be used in patients who are newly diagnosed with depression.

MAO inhibitors also have been investigated in the treatment of panic disorder with agoraphobia, eating disorders, posttraumatic stress disorder, pain disorder, and atypical depression.

Interactions

✦ Use of an MAO inhibitor with an amphetamine, levodopa, methylphenidate, a nonamphetamine appetite suppressant, or a sympathomimetic may increase catecholamine release, which may cause hypertension.
✦ Use of an MAO inhibitor with citalopram, clomipramine, fluoxetine, fluvoxamine, paroxetine, sertraline, trazodone, or a tricyclic antidepressant may result in elevated body temperature, excitation, and seizures.

 CLINICAL ALERT To prevent elevated body temperature, excitation, and seizures, withhold an MAO inhibitor for 2 weeks before starting the patient on an alternative antidepressant.

✦ When taken with doxapram, an MAO inhibitor may cause hypertension and arrhythmias and may increase adverse reactions to doxapram.
✦ An MAO inhibitor may enhance the hypoglycemic effects of an antidiabetic.
✦ Use of an MAO inhibitor with meperidine may result in excitation, hypertension or hypotension, extremely elevated body temperature, and coma.
✦ Tyramine-rich foods can interact with MAO inhibitors and produce hypertensive crisis.

Adverse reactions

The most serious adverse reaction to MAO inhibitors is hypertensive crisis, which can lead to death. Increased blood pressure, severe headache, palpitations, nausea, vomiting, neck stiffness or soreness, fever, clammy skin, mydriasis, and photophobia or other vision disturbances characterize hypertensive crisis. It may also include tachycardia or bradycardia, constricting chest pain, or intracranial hemorrhage.

The most common adverse reactions are restlessness, drowsiness, dizziness, headache, insomnia, constipation, anorexia, nausea, vomiting, weakness, arthralgia, dry mouth, blurred vision, peripheral edema, urine retention, transient impotence, rash, and purpura. Orthostatic hypotension is also common, especially in geriatric patients, and may lead to syncope with high dosages. Orthostatic hypotension usually occurs in patients with preexisting hypertension, although it may also occur in patients with normal blood pressure.

Features of MAO inhibitors

✦ Appear to inhibit MAO, an enzyme that metabolizes many neurotransmitters
✦ Are used for typical depression that hasn't responded to other therapies or when other therapies are contraindicated
✦ May be used for panic disorder with agoraphobia, eating disorders, posttraumatic stress disorder, pain disorder, atypical depression
✦ May cause fever, excitation, seizures if a different antidepressant is given within 2 weeks of stopping an MAO inhibitor

Possible interactions

✦ Amphetamines
✦ Antidiabetics
✦ Citalopram
✦ Clomipramine
✦ Doxapram
✦ Fluoxetine
✦ Fluvoxamine
✦ Levodopa
✦ Meperidine
✦ Methylphenidate
✦ Nonamphetamine appetite suppressants
✦ Paroxetine
✦ Sertraline
✦ Sympathomimetics
✦ Trazodone
✦ Tricyclic antidepressants
✦ Tyramine-rich foods

Adverse reactions to watch for

+ Agitation, hyperexcitability, hypomania, mania, schizophrenia (high doses)
+ Anorexia, constipation, increased appetite, nausea, vomiting, weight gain
+ Arthralgia, dry mouth, blurred vision, peripheral edema, urinary frequency, urine retention, transient impotence
+ Dizziness, drowsiness, headache, insomnia, restlessness
+ Fever, flushing, clammy skin, sweating
+ Hyperreflexia, muscle spasms, myoclonic jerks, numbness, paresthesia, tremor
+ Hypertensive crisis: severe headache, palpitations, stiff or sore neck, nausea, vomiting, ocular disturbances, tachycardia or bradycardia, constricting chest pain, intracranial hemorrhage
+ Increased blood pressure
+ Orthostatic hypotension
+ Purpura, rash
+ Weakness

Key nursing actions

+ Monitor for evidence of hypertensive crisis; prepare for emergency interventions if it develops.
+ Give the drug in the early evening if it causes drowsiness; in the morning if it causes insomnia.
+ Continue monitoring the patient for 7 to 10 days after therapy stops.
+ Document fluid intake and output.

PATIENT TEACHING

Teaching a patient about MAO inhibitors

Whenever a monoamine oxidase (MAO) inhibitor is prescribed, teach the patient and his family the drug's name, dose, frequency, action, and adverse effects. Also take the following actions.
+ Teach the patient which drugs and foods to avoid during MAO inhibitor therapy and provide him with a written list.
+ Teach the patient and family to recognize the signs and symptoms of hypertensive crisis, such as severe headache, sudden vision changes, and dizziness.
+ Instruct the patient to inform other prescribers about MAO inhibitor therapy.
+ Caution the patient not to stop taking the MAO inhibitor abruptly, and explain that the drug should be tapered off as prescribed.
+ Instruct the patient to take the drug at bedtime if it produces drowsiness or to take the last daily dose in the afternoon if it causes insomnia.
+ Inform a man that impotence may occur during MAO inhibitor therapy but should subside when the drug is stopped.
+ Teach the patient to recognize and report the symptoms of urine retention, such as urinary hesitancy, frequent voiding of small amounts, and a sensation of fullness in the lower abdomen.

Other adverse reactions to MAO inhibitors include urinary frequency, increased appetite, weight gain, increased perspiration, flushing, numbness, paresthesia, muscle spasms, tremor, myoclonic jerks, and hyperreflexia. With high dosages, these drugs may cause hyperexcitability, agitation, mania, and hypomania and may activate latent schizophrenic disorder. Such reactions require a dosage reduction or use of a phenothiazine.

Rare reactions include amblyopia, aggravation of glaucoma, vision disturbances, impaired water excretion, leukopenia, granulocytopenia, thrombocytopenia, and normocytic or normochromic anemia.

With high dosages of tranylcypromine, dependence and addiction may occur. When this drug is stopped, the patient may display anxiety, depression, confusion, hallucinations, diarrhea, and other withdrawal symptoms.

Nursing considerations

+ Monitor the patient for signs and symptoms of hypertensive crisis, such as increased blood pressure, severe headache, palpitations, neck stiffness or soreness, nausea, and vomiting.
+ Prepare for emergency interventions if hypertensive crisis occurs. For example, stop the MAO inhibitor immediately and give appropriate treatment.
+ Switch the patient to a different MAO inhibitor or adjust the dosage if adverse reactions don't diminish with time.
+ Change the administration time to the early evening or the morning if drowsiness or insomnia occurs.
+ Don't stop tranylcypromine abruptly. If discontinuation is needed, taper off the dosage over 2 weeks to prevent withdrawal reactions, such as anxiety, depression, confusion, and hallucinations.
+ Continue to monitor the patient for 7 to 10 days after discontinuation of the MAO inhibitor because of its long-lasting effects.
+ Record the patient's fluid intake and output to help detect urine retention.

✦ Teach the patient and his caregiver about the drug. (See *Teaching a patient about MAO inhibitors*.)

OTHER ANTIDEPRESSANTS

Miscellaneous drugs used as antidepressants include bupropion, maprotiline, mirtazapine, nefazodone, trazodone, and venlafaxine.

Pharmacokinetics

These antidepressants take different paths through the body. Bupropion is well absorbed from the GI tract and metabolized by the liver. The drug's metabolites are excreted by the kidneys.

Maprotiline and mirtazapine are absorbed from the GI tract, distributed widely in the body, metabolized by the liver, and excreted by the kidneys.

Nefazodone is rapidly and completely absorbed but, because of extensive metabolism, only about 20% of the drug is available. It's almost completely bound to plasma proteins and is excreted in urine.

Trazodone is well absorbed from the GI tract, distributed widely in the body, metabolized by the liver, and about 75% is excreted in urine. The remainder is excreted in feces.

After oral administration, venlafaxine is rapidly absorbed, partially bound to plasma proteins, metabolized in the liver, and excreted in urine.

Pharmacodynamics

The actions of these drugs aren't yet fully understood. Bupropion was once thought to inhibit the reuptake of the neurotransmitter dopamine. However, its action is more likely on noradrenergic receptors.

In the CNS, maprotiline and mirtazapine probably increase the amount of norepinephrine, serotonin, or both by blocking reuptake by presynaptic neurons.

Nefazodone's action isn't precisely defined. It inhibits neuronal uptake of serotonin and norepinephrine. It also is a serotonin antagonist, which explains its effectiveness in treating anxiety.

Although its effect is unknown, trazodone is thought to inhibit the reuptake of norepinephrine and serotonin in the presynaptic neurons.

Venlafaxine may potentiate neurotransmitter activity in the CNS by inhibiting the neural reuptake of serotonin and norepinephrine.

Pharmacotherapeutics

These miscellaneous drugs are used to treat depression. Trazodone may also be effective in treating aggressive behavior and panic disorder.

Interactions

✦ When combined with an MAO inhibitor, any of these antidepressants may produce serious, potentially fatal reactions.
✦ Use of bupropion with levodopa, a phenothiazine, or a tricyclic antidepressant can increase the risk of adverse reactions, including seizures.
✦ Use of maprotiline, mirtazapine, nefazodone, or trazodone with a CNS depressant can cause added CNS depression.
✦ Nefazodone or trazodone may increase the digoxin level.
✦ Trazodone may increase the phenytoin level.
✦ Use of trazodone with an antihypertensive may cause increased hypotensive effects.

Features of other antidepressants

✦ Aren't fully understood but may act by increasing levels of norepinephrine and serotonin
✦ Are used to treat depression
✦ May be useful in treating aggression and panic disorder (trazodone)

Possible drug interactions

✦ Antihypertensives
✦ CNS depressants
✦ Digoxin
✦ Levodopa
✦ MAO inhibitors
✦ Phenothiazines
✦ Phenytoin
✦ Tricyclic antidepressants

Adverse reactions to watch for

bupropion
+ Hallucinations
+ Insomnia
+ Psychotic episodes
+ Restlessness
+ Seizures

maprotiline
+ ECG changes
+ Orthostatic hypotension
+ Seizures
+ Tachycardia

mirtazapine
+ Confusion
+ Constipation
+ Nausea
+ Tremors

nefazodone and venlafaxine
+ Dizziness
+ Headache
+ Nausea
+ Somnolence

trazodone
+ Dizziness
+ Drowsiness

Key nursing actions

+ Take seizure precautions.
+ Give the drug before bedtime or with food to minimize anticholinergic effects.
+ Start bupropion with small doses and increase them gradually if the patient also takes levodopa.

Adverse reactions

Bupropion causes dose-related CNS stimulation, including restlessness, hallucinations, seizures, insomnia, and psychotic episodes. This distinguishes bupropion from other antidepressants, which commonly produce sedation. Bupropion produces fewer cardiovascular and anticholinergic symptoms than other antidepressants.

Maprotiline may cause seizures, orthostatic hypotension, tachycardia, and electrocardiogram (ECG) changes. Mirtazapine may cause tremors, confusion, nausea, and constipation.

Nefazodone and venlafaxine may cause headache, somnolence, dizziness, and nausea. Trazodone may cause drowsiness and dizziness.

Nursing considerations

+ Take seizure precautions, such as padding the bed rails, during therapy with bupropion, maprotiline, or mirtazapine in a patient who has a history of a seizure disorder or is receiving high doses of bupropion. Also, give less than the maximum dosage of bupropion or maprotiline to prevent seizures.
+ Give the antidepressant before bedtime or with food to minimize anticholinergic effects.
+ Begin bupropion therapy with small doses and increase them gradually in a patient who also receives levodopa.
+ Teach the patient and his caregiver about the prescribed drug. (See *Teaching a patient about other antidepressants.*)

LITHIUM

Lithium is used to prevent or treat mania and bipolar disorder (mood disorder in which depression alternates with mania).

Pharmacokinetics

When taken orally, lithium is absorbed rapidly and completely and is distributed to body tissues. An active drug, lithium isn't metabolized and is excreted from the body unchanged.

Pharmacodynamics

In mania, the patient experiences excessive catecholamine stimulation. In bipolar disorder, the patient is affected by swings between the excessive catecholamine stimulation of mania and the diminished catecholamine stimulation of depression.

Lithium may regulate catecholamine release in the CNS by increasing norepinephrine and serotonin uptake, reducing norepinephrine release from synaptic vesicles where neurotransmitters are stored in presynaptic neurons, and inhibiting norepinephrine's action in postsynaptic neurons.

Pharmacotherapeutics

Lithium is used primarily to treat acute episodes of mania and to prevent relapses of bipolar disorders.

Interactions

Lithium's narrow therapeutic range accounts for its serious interactions with other drugs.
+ When lithium is taken with a thiazide or loop diuretic or a nonsteroidal anti-inflammatory drug, the risk of lithium toxicity increases.
+ Use of lithium with carbamazepine, haloperidol, or a phenothiazine may increase the risk of neurotoxicity.
+ Lithium may increase the hypothyroid effects of potassium iodide.
+ Sodium bicarbonate may increase lithium excretion and reduce its effects.
+ Theophylline can reduce lithium's effects.

Adverse reactions

Adverse reactions to lithium may occur in any phase of therapy and usually are dose-related. Because GI effects are related to an increase in the lithium level, they're most common when therapy begins and when the dosage in increased. About 50% of patients experience a fine tremor that may diminish with dosage reduction and worsen with dosage increase. Polyuria of 2 to 3 L/day may appear, accompanied by polydipsia.

When the lithium level exceeds 1.5 mEq/L, toxicity may occur and produce confusion, lethargy, slurred speech, hyperreflexia, and seizures. Long-term lithium therapy may result in distal tubule atrophy and decreased glomerular filtration rate. Diabetes insipidus syndrome may occur and produce a daily urine output exceeding 3 L and having a low specific gravity. Hypothyroidism and nontoxic goiters may affect about 4% of patients. Other adverse reactions include weight gain, skin eruptions, alopecia, and leukocytosis.

Nursing considerations

+ Obtain baseline tests of the patient's thyroid and renal functions and an ECG tracing.
+ Monitor the patient's lithium level periodically during therapy and after dosage adjustments. Draw blood and evaluate the lithium level 12 hours after the last daily dose. Lithium has a narrow margin of safety. A drug level that's even slightly higher than the therapeutic level can be dangerous. Particularly note a level that exceeds 1.5 mEq/L, which may be toxic.
+ Monitor the patient's white blood cell count.
+ Monitor the patient for GI distress, especially when lithium therapy begins.
+ Give lithium with food to reduce GI distress.
+ Record the patient's fluid intake and output; polyuria of 2 to 3 L/day may occur in a patient with diabetes insipidus syndrome.

Features of lithium

+ May regulate catecholamine release in the CNS by increasing norepinephrine and serotonin uptake, reducing norepinephrine release from synaptic vesicles, and inhibiting norepinephrine's action in postsynaptic neurons
+ Is used mainly to treat acute manic episodes and prevent relapses of bipolar disorder

Possible drug interactions

+ Carbamazepine
+ Haloperidol
+ NSAIDs
+ Phenothiazines
+ Potassium iodide
+ Sodium bicarbonate
+ Theophylline
+ Thiazide or loop diuretics

Adverse reactions to watch for

+ Alopecia, skin eruptions
+ Diabetes insipidus syndrome
+ Distal tubule atrophy and decreased glomerular filtration rate
+ Fine tremor
+ Hypothyroidism, nontoxic goiter
+ Leukocytosis
+ Polydipsia and polyuria
+ Toxicity: confusion, hyperreflexia, lethargy, seizures, slurred speech
+ Weight gain

Key nursing actions

- ✦ Obtain baseline tests of thyroid and renal functions and an ECG tracing.
- ✦ Monitor the lithium level periodically during therapy and after dosage adjustments.
- ✦ Monitor the white blood cell count.
- ✦ Assess for GI distress.
- ✦ Document fluid intake and output.
- ✦ If patient has polyuria, watch for evidence of dehydration.
- ✦ Note the specific gravity and color of the patient's urine.
- ✦ Give fluids to replace loss, as needed.
- ✦ Monitor the patient's salt intake.

Features of antipsychotics

- ✦ Control psychotic symptoms (delusions, hallucinations, thought disorders) from schizophrenia, mania, other psychoses
- ✦ Help treat organic psychiatric disorders, such as dementia, delirium, and stimulant-induced psychoses
- ✦ Can sedate agitated patients
- ✦ Are used to treat movement disorders of Tourette's syndrome and Huntington's chorea
- ✦ Are used to augment the pain-relieving effects of preoperative analgesics and anesthetics
- ✦ Are used to treat nausea, vomiting, intractable hiccups, pruritus
- ✦ Are also known as *major tranquilizers* and *neuroleptics*

PATIENT TEACHING

Teaching a patient about lithium

Whenever lithium is prescribed, teach the patient and his family the drug's name, dose, frequency, action, and adverse effects. Also take the following actions.
- ✦ Advise the patient that lithium may take 1 to 3 weeks to produce a therapeutic response.
- ✦ Instruct the patient to take lithium with food to reduce gastrointestinal distress.
- ✦ Stress the importance of having blood drawn to determine the drug level and white blood cell count.
- ✦ Teach the patient and family to recognize signs and symptoms of toxicity (confusion, lethargy, slurred speech, hyperreflexia, and seizures) and to notify the prescriber if they occur before giving the next dose.
- ✦ Instruct the patient to notify other prescribers about lithium therapy to avoid serious drug interactions.
- ✦ Advise the patient to measure his fluid intake and output and to notify the prescriber if his output exceeds 3 quarts (2.8 L) daily.
- ✦ Advise the patient who develops a fine tremor that it may diminish with a dosage reduction and worsen with a dosage increase. Reassure him that the tremor will cease when lithium is stopped.
- ✦ Reassure the patient that weight gain, skin eruptions, and alopecia will cease when lithium is stopped.
- ✦ Instruct the patient to notify her prescriber if she becomes pregnant or plans to become pregnant.

✦ Monitor the patient with polyuria for signs of dehydration, such as dry mucous membranes, polydipsia, and poor skin turgor.

✦ Note the specific gravity and color of the patient's urine. With diabetes insipidus syndrome, the specific gravity is low and the urine is diluted rather than concentrated, which usually occurs in dehydration.

✦ Notify the prescriber if the patient's urine output significantly exceeds his fluid intake.

✦ Give fluids to replace fluid loss, as needed.

✦ Monitor the patient's salt intake. A patient on a severe salt-restricted diet is susceptible to lithium toxicity. On the other hand, an increased intake of sodium may reduce lithium's therapeutic effects.

✦ Teach the patient and his caregiver about the prescribed drug. (See *Teaching a patient about lithium.*)

ANTIPSYCHOTICS

Antipsychotics can control psychotic symptoms, such as delusions, hallucinations, and thought disorders that may arise from schizophrenia, mania, and other psychoses. These drugs can help treat organic psychiatric disorders, such as dementia, delirium, and stimulant-induced psychoses and can sedate agitated patients. They also are used to treat the movement disorders of Tourette's syndrome and Huntington's chorea, to augment the pain-relieving effects of preoperative analgesics and anesthetics, and to treat nausea, vomiting, intractable hiccups, and pruritus.

Antipsychotics also are called *major tranquilizers* because they can calm an agitated patient and are called *neuroleptics* because they may have adverse neurobiological effects, such as apathy or limited emotions, lack of initiative, and normalization of psychomotor activity. Antipsychotics fall into two major classes: conventional and novel antipsychotics, which have become the first-line treatment for psychoses.

CONVENTIONAL ANTIPSYCHOTICS

Conventional antipsychotics were formerly known as *typical antipsychotics*. The major antipsychotics are phenothiazines, which include chlorpromazine, fluphenazine, mesoridazine, perphenazine, prochlorperazine, promazine, thioridazine, trifluoperazine, and triflupromazine. Lesser groups of antipsychotics are thioxanthenes (thiothixene), phenylbutylpiperadines (haloperidol and pimozide), dihydroindolones (molindone), and dibenzepines (loxapine).

Pharmacokinetics

Although phenothiazines are absorbed erratically, they're highly lipid soluble and protein-bound. Therefore, they're distributed to many tissues and are highly concentrated in the brain.

Like phenothiazines, the other conventional antipsychotics are absorbed erratically, are lipid soluble, and are highly protein-bound. They're also distributed throughout the tissues and are highly concentrated in the brain.

All phenothiazines are metabolized in the liver and excreted in urine and bile. Because fatty tissues slowly release accumulated phenothiazine metabolites into the plasma, phenothiazines may produce effects up to 3 months after they're stopped.

The other conventional antipsychotics also are metabolized in the liver and excreted in urine and bile.

Pharmacodynamics

Phenothiazines probably work by blocking postsynaptic dopaminergic receptors in the brain. Their antipsychotic effects may come from receptor blockade in the limbic system; their antiemetic effects from receptor blockade in the chemoreceptor trigger zone located in the brain's medulla. Phenothiazines also stimulate the motor pathways that connect the cerebral cortex with the spinal nerve pathways, also known as the extrapyramidal system.

The mechanism of action of the other conventional antipsychotics resembles that of the phenothiazines.

Pharmacotherapeutics

Phenothiazines are used primarily to treat schizophrenia, reduce anxiety or agitation, improve a patient's thought processes, and alleviate delusions and hallucinations.

Other therapeutic uses have been found for phenothiazines. They're given to treat other psychiatric disorders, such as brief reactive psychosis, atypical psychosis, schizoaffective psychosis, autism, and major depression with psychosis. With lithium, they're used to treat bipolar disorder, until the slower-acting lithium produces its therapeutic effect. They're prescribed to quiet mentally challenged children and agitated geriatric patients, particularly those with dementia. They can be used to boost the preoperative effects of analgesics. Plus, they're helpful in managing pain, anxiety, and nausea in patients with cancer.

The other conventional antipsychotics are used to treat psychotic disorders. Haloperidol and pimozide may also be used to treat Tourette's syndrome. Thiothixene also is used to control acute agitation.

Features of conventional antipsychotics

- Were formerly known as *typical antipsychotics*
- May block postsynaptic dopaminergic receptors in the brain
- May cause antipsychotic effects from receptor blockade in the limbic system
- May cause antiemetic effects from receptor blockade in the chemoreceptor trigger zone in the medulla

phenothiazines

- Stimulate motor pathways that connect the cerebral cortex with the spinal nerve pathways
- Are used mainly for schizophrenia, reducing anxiety or agitation, improving thought processes, alleviating delusions and hallucinations
- Are also used for brief reactive psychosis, atypical psychosis, schizoaffective psychosis, autism, major depression with psychosis
- Are given with lithium for bipolar disorder until lithium action begins
- Are used to quiet mentally challenged children and agitated elderly patients, especially those with dementia
- Are helpful for managing pain, anxiety, and nausea in cancer patients

other conventional antipsychotics

- Are used for psychotic disorders, Tourette's syndrome (haloperidol, pimozide), and acute agitation (thiothixene)

Interactions

Phenothiazines interact with many different drugs and may have serious effects. Other conventional antipsychotics interact with fewer drugs.

+ When used with a CNS depressant, a phenothiazine can increase CNS depressant effects, such as stupor.
+ A CNS depressant may reduce a phenothiazine's effectiveness and may result in increased psychotic behavior or agitation.
+ Use of an anticholinergic with a phenothiazine may increase anticholinergic effects, such as dry mouth and constipation, and may increase phenothiazine metabolism and reduce antipsychotic effects.
+ A phenothiazine may reduce levodopa's antiparkinsonian effects.
+ Use of a phenothiazine with lithium increases the risk of neurotoxicity.
+ Use of a phenothiazine with droperidol increases the risk of extrapyramidal effects.
+ When taken with an anticonvulsant, a phenothiazine can lower the seizure threshold.
+ A phenothiazine may increase tricyclic antidepressant and beta blocker levels.
+ Another conventional antipsychotic can inhibit levodopa and lead to disorientation.
+ Haloperidol may boost the effects of lithium, producing encephalopathy.

Adverse reactions

Neurologic reactions are the most common and serious adverse reactions to phenothiazines. Extrapyramidal symptoms may appear after the first few days of therapy; tardive dyskinesia may occur after several years of treatment.

Neuroleptic malignant syndrome is a life-threatening condition that produces muscle rigidity, extreme extrapyramidal symptoms, severely elevated body temperature, hypertension, and rapid heart rate. If untreated, it can result in respiratory failure and cardiovascular collapse.

Most other conventional antipsychotics cause the same adverse reactions as phenothiazines. After long-term therapy, abrupt withdrawal of a conventional antipsychotic may lead to gastritis, nausea, vomiting, headache, tachycardia, insomnia, and dizziness.

Nursing considerations

+ Monitor the patient for extrapyramidal symptoms. Notify the prescriber immediately if the patient experiences acute dystonia.
+ Measure the patient's blood pressure before starting therapy. Then monitor him for orthostatic hypotension.
+ Monitor the patient for tardive dyskinesia, especially after prolonged use.
+ Don't abruptly withdraw the drug after long-term therapy.

 CLINICAL ALERT Monitor the patient for signs and symptoms of neuroleptic malignant syndrome, such as extrapyramidal symptoms, hyperthermia, and autonomic disturbances. Although rare, this adverse reaction can be fatal.

+ Teach the patient and his caregiver about the prescribed drug. (See *Teaching a patient about conventional antipsychotics.*)

NOVEL ANTIPSYCHOTICS

Originally, these drugs were called *atypical antipsychotics*. Because they're now the most typically used antipsychotics, they're currently known as *novel antipsychotics*. These drugs became more popular than conventional antipsychotics because they're less likely to cause extrapyramidal symptoms and other adverse reactions. Novel antipsychotics include dibenzodiazepines (clozapine, olanzapine, and quetiapine) and benzisoxazoles (aripiprazole, risperidone, and ziprasidone).

Pharmacokinetics

After oral administration, novel antipsychotics are rapidly absorbed. The liver metabolizes them. The action of aripiprazole and ziprasidone primarily results from the parent drug, although aripiprazole's major metabolite shows some affinity for dopamine$_2$ receptors. Metabolites of clozapine and olanzapine are inactive, whereas risperidone has an active metabolite. Novel antipsychotics are highly plasma protein-bound and eliminated in urine and feces.

Pharmacodynamics

Novel antipsychotics typically block dopamine receptors, but to a lesser extent than conventional antipsychotics do, which produces fewer extrapyramidal symptoms. Also, novel antipsychotics block serotonin receptor activity.

These combined actions account for their effectiveness in controlling the symptoms of schizophrenia with minimal extrapyramidal effects.

Pharmacotherapeutics

Novel antipsychotics are used to manage schizophrenia.

Features of novel antipsychotics

+ Were originally called *atypical antipsychotics*
+ Are more popular than conventional antipsychotics because they're less likely to cause extrapyramidal symptoms and other adverse reactions
+ Block dopamine receptors, but less than conventional antipsychotics do
+ Block serotonin receptor activity
+ Are used to manage schizophrenia

Teaching a patient about novel antipsychotics

Whenever a novel antipsychotic is prescribed, teach the patient and his family the drug's name, dose, frequency, action, and adverse effects. Also take the following actions.

◆ Caution the patient to avoid activities that require mental alertness until the drug's central nervous system effects are known.

◆ Instruct the patient to avoid alcohol while taking the drug.

◆ Suggest that the patient relieve dry mouth with sugarless gum or hard candy.

◆ Advise the patient to rise slowly to avoid orthostatic hypotension.

◆ Tell the patient to use caution in hot weather to prevent heatstroke.

◆ Instruct the patient or caregiver to notify the prescriber about other prescription or over-the-counter drugs he takes or plans to take.

Adverse reactions to watch for

◆ Agranulocytosis, seizures, weight gain (clozapine)
◆ Arrhythmias, QT prolongation (ziprasidone)
◆ Extrapyramidal effects (risperidone)
◆ Neuroleptic malignant syndrome
◆ Orthostatic hypotension
◆ Sedation (aripiprazole and quetiapine)
◆ Weight gain (olanzapine)

Key nursing actions

◆ Watch carefully for evidence of neuroleptic malignant syndrome.
◆ Measure the blood pressure at the start of therapy; monitor it throughout therapy to detect orthostatic hypotension.
◆ Monitor the complete blood count closely during clozapine therapy and for 4 weeks afterward.
◆ Watch for evidence of tardive dyskinesia, especially after prolonged use.

Interactions

◆ Any drug that induces or inhibits the CYP enzyme system can decrease or increase a novel antipsychotic's metabolism, although these effects may not be clinically significant for the benzisoxazoles.

◆ A novel antipsychotic can counteract the effects of levodopa or another dopamine agonist.

Adverse reactions

Novel antipsychotics produce fewer extrapyramidal symptoms than conventional antipsychotics do. As with any antipsychotic, however, the risk of life-threatening neuroleptic malignant syndrome exists. Although infrequent, orthostatic hypotension also can occur. Except for clozapine, novel antipsychotics have minimal risk for seizures. Clozapine may cause agranulocytosis and weight gain.

Olanzapine places the patient at minimal risk for extrapyramidal effects. Weight gain is a common reaction to olanzapine.

In high doses, risperidone has a higher risk of extrapyramidal effects than other novel antipsychotics. Quetiapine may cause sedation; aripiprazole may produce mild sedation.

 CLINICAL ALERT Because of ziprasidone's potential to cause dose-related QT prolongation and cause life-threatening arrhythmias, this drug is contraindicated in patients with a history of QT prolongation, recent acute myocardial infarction, or uncompensated heart failure.

Nursing considerations

◆ Closely monitor the patient's complete blood count during clozapine therapy and for 4 weeks after it ends. This antipsychotic poses a significant risk of agranulocytosis.

◆ Measure the patient's blood pressure before therapy begins. Then monitor the patient for orthostatic hypotension.

◆ Monitor the patient for tardive dyskinesia, especially after prolonged use.

CLINICAL ALERT Monitor the patient for signs and symptoms of neuroleptic malignant syndrome, such as extrapyramidal symptoms, hyperthermia, irregular pulse or blood pressure, tachycardia, diaphoresis, and arrhythmias. Although rare, this adverse reaction can be fatal.

✦ Teach the patient and his caregiver about the prescribed drug. (See *Teaching a patient about novel antipsychotics*.)

CNS STIMULANTS

Drugs in this class are used to treat narcolepsy, obesity, and ADHD, which is a condition characterized by inattention, impulsivity, and hyperactivity. They include amphetamine, atomoxetine, dextroamphetamine, methylphenidate, and pemoline. Except for atomoxetine, all of these drugs are controlled substances.

Pharmacokinetics
CNS stimulants are absorbed well from the GI tract and distributed widely in the body. Methylphenidate undergoes significant first-pass effect. All of these drugs are metabolized in the liver and excreted primarily in urine.

Pharmacodynamics
Stimulants probably work by increasing dopamine and norepinephrine levels. They may do this by blocking dopamine and norepinephrine reuptake, enhancing their presynaptic release, or inhibiting MAO.

Pharmacotherapeutics
For years, stimulants have been the treatment of choice for ADHD. The recent approval of atomoxetine, a selective norepinephrine reuptake inhibitor, now offers the ability to treat ADHD without using a controlled substance. Pemoline is no longer a first-line choice for ADHD because it can cause hepatotoxicity. In all children, these drugs should be used with care.

Interactions
✦ Use of a CNS stimulant with an MAO inhibitor can cause hypertensive crisis.
✦ A CNS stimulant may reverse guanethidine's hypotensive effects.
✦ A CNS stimulant may increase an SSRI's effects.
✦ A urinary alkalinizer may prolong the effects of an amphetamine. These drugs shouldn't be used together, especially in overdose.
✦ When used together, methylphenidate may increase the tricyclic antidepressant level.

Adverse reactions
Many adverse CNS reactions result from overstimulation, such as restlessness, dizziness, insomnia, and headache. Adverse cardiovascular reactions include palpitations, tachycardia, and increased blood pressure. Cardiomyopathy may occur with long-term amphetamine use.

Amphetamines can cause dry mouth, unpleasant taste, and diarrhea or constipation. Methylphenidate may cause nausea and abdominal pain. Both can cause anorexia and weight loss.

Although structurally different than amphetamines and methylphenidate, pemoline shares many of the same adverse reactions. In addition, it can cause acute

---

Features of CNS stimulants
✦ May increase dopamine and norepinephrine levels, possibly by blocking their reuptake, enhancing their presynaptic release, or inhibiting MAO
✦ Are the treatment of choice for ADHD; pemoline is no longer a first-line choice because it may cause hepatotoxicity

Adverse reactions to watch for
✦ Increased blood pressure, palpitations, tachycardia
✦ Overstimulation (restlessness, dizziness, insomnia, headache)

amphetamines
✦ Anorexia, weight loss
✦ Cardiomyopathy (long-term use)
✦ Constipation, diarrhea
✦ Dry mouth
✦ Unpleasant taste

methylphenidate
✦ Abdominal pain
✦ Anorexia, weight loss
✦ Nausea

pemoline
✦ Many of same reactions as amphetamines and methylphenidate
✦ Hepatic failure
✦ Hepatitis
✦ Risk of abuse and dependence

Key nursing actions

+ Refer the patient for psychological, educational, and social support for ADHD.
+ Measure the child's weight and height regularly during long-term therapy.
+ Check the blood pressure and pulse periodically.
+ Watch for evidence of dependence or abuse.

PATIENT TEACHING

Teaching a patient about CNS stimulants

Whenever a central nervous system (CNS) stimulant is prescribed, teach the patient and his family the drug's name, dose, frequency, action, and adverse effects. Also take the following actions.

+ Instruct the patient not to chew or crush sustained-release or long-acting tablets.
+ Inform the patient and caregiver that the drug may cause nervousness, restlessness, insomnia, dizziness, and gastrointestinal distress. Tell them to notify the prescriber if these adverse effects become bothersome.
+ Caution the patient to avoid activities that require alertness or good psychomotor coordination until the drug's CNS effects are known.
+ Warn the parent of a child with a seizure disorder that methylphenidate may decrease the seizure threshold. Instruct him to notify the prescriber if seizures occur.
+ Tell the patient to avoid caffeine while taking the CNS stimulant.
+ Instruct the patient to avoid insomnia by taking the drug late in the evening.

hepatic failure and hepatitis. Like the other CNS stimulants that are controlled substances, pemoline poses a risk of abuse and dependence.

Nursing considerations

+ Refer the patient for psychological, educational, and social support for ADHD.
+ Measure a child's weight and height regularly during long-term therapy.
+ Monitor the patient's blood pressure and pulse periodically.
+ Monitor the patient for signs of drug dependence or abuse.
+ Teach the patient and his caregiver about the prescribed drug. (See *Teaching a patient about CNS stimulants.*)

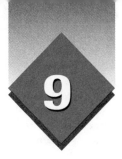

9

Anti-infective drugs

Currently available anti-infective drugs vary in their degree of effectiveness against different microorganisms. A drug's spectrum of activity refers to the number and type of organisms vulnerable to its action. Broad-spectrum anti-infective drugs affect a wide variety of pathogens; narrow-spectrum drugs affect a few. Anti-infective drugs tend to affect pathogens with similar biochemical characteristics.

The most common method used to differentiate various microorganisms is the Gram stain, which uses laboratory dyes to stain organisms; the reactions reveal chemical differences in the cell wall. Organisms that take on the Gram stain are called gram-positive; those that don't are called gram-negative.

For some bacteria, Gram staining isn't a useful analytical tool. Some of these organisms, such as mycobacteria, can be stained with carbolfuchsin and then decolorized with ethyl alcohol and hydrochloric acid. They're classified as acid-fast if they retain the stain.

Spirochetes can be visualized only by special techniques, such as dark-field examination. Other important stains used to identify bacteria include Gimenez stain for *Rickettsia,* Giemsa and Wright's stains for parasites and intracellular microorganisms, and fluorescent antibody tests for various organisms.

Organisms with similar staining properties tend to be susceptible to the same anti-infective drugs. Therefore, a drug's spectrum of activity may be described by its activity against gram-negative, gram-positive, or acid-fast bacilli.

Organisms are also classified as organisms that can live and grow in the presence of oxygen (or aerobes) or as organisms that can live or grow without oxygen (or anaerobes).

DRUG SELECTION

Selecting an appropriate drug to treat a specific infection involves several important factors. First the microorganism must be isolated and identified. Then its sus-

Features of anti-infective drugs

✦ Vary in effectiveness against different microorganisms
✦ Broad-spectrum drugs are effective against many pathogens
✦ Narrow-spectrum drugs are effective against a few pathogens
✦ May be described as effective against gram-positive, gram-negative, or acid-fast bacilli
✦ May be described as effective against aerobes (organisms that live in oxygen) or anaerobes (organisms that live without oxygen)

Elements of anti-infective drug selection

- ✦ Identification of the organism
- ✦ Susceptibility of the organism to various drugs
- ✦ Lowest anti-infective level that prevents visible growth of the organism in 18 to 24 hours
- ✦ Lowest anti-infective level that completely suppresses growth after overnight incubation
- ✦ Location of the infection
- ✦ Number of organisms contributing to the infection
- ✦ Way to deliver the appropriate anti-infective drug (or drugs) to the appropriate location
- ✦ Relative cost of the drugs
- ✦ Adverse effects of the drugs
- ✦ Patient's drug allergies

Understanding resistance

- ✦ Pathogens may develop resistance to anti-infective drugs.
- ✦ Resistance is the ability of an organism to live and grow in the presence of a bacteriostatic or bactericidal drug.
- ✦ Resistance commonly develops from genetic mutation in the organism.
- ✦ Exposing organisms to anti-infective drugs without good reason encourages the emergence of resistant strains.
- ✦ Exposing organisms to levels of anti-infective drugs inadequate to kill them encourages the emergence of resistant strains.

ceptibility to various drugs must be determined. The lowest anti-infective concentration that prevents visible growth after an 18- to 24-hour incubation period is the minimal inhibitory concentration (MIC). The minimal bactericidal concentration, or MBC, is the lowest anti-infective concentration that totally suppresses growth after overnight incubation. Because culture and sensitivity results take 48 hours, treatment usually begins based on assessment findings and is then reevaluated when test results are complete.

Another important factor in choosing an anti-infective drug is the location of the infection. For anti-infective therapy to be effective, an adequate concentration of the drug must be delivered to the infection site. That means the local anti-infective concentration should be at least equal to the MIC for the infecting organism. Other factors in selecting an anti-infective drug are the relative cost of the drug, its potential adverse effects, and the patient's allergies.

Infections caused by two or more organisms, each of which may be sensitive to different drugs, or mixed infections, respond best to treatment with a selected combination of anti-infective drugs. Examples are peritoneal or pelvic infections caused by mixed bowel flora and foot infections in diabetic patients.

The patient's condition determines when anti-infective therapy is started and how it's given. If the patient is stable, therapy may be delayed until culture and sensitivity test results are available. An unstable patient is usually treated immediately with a broad-spectrum drug. A patient with a serious infection is likely to need a higher and more predictable drug level, necessitating I.V. therapy. In a less severe infection, I.M. or oral therapy can be used. Depending on the infecting organism, the prescriber may select an antibacterial, antiviral, antituberculotic, antifungal, or drotrecogin alfa.

PREVENTING RESISTANCE

One aspect limits the usefulness of anti-infective drugs: pathogens may develop resistance to a drug's action. Resistance is the ability of organisms to live and grow in the presence of a bacteriostatic antibacterial (one that usually inhibits bacterial growth or multiplication) or a bactericidal antibacterial (one that usually kills bacteria). Resistance usually results from a genetic occurrence that leads to the development of mutant strains of the organism. These mutant strains resist a drug's activity by enhancing the action of specific enzymes that break down the drug's chemical structure, restrict its uptake, or alter cellular target sites.

Anti-infective drugs shouldn't be used indiscriminately because exposing organisms to these drugs unnecessarily encourages the emergence of resistant strains. The drugs should be reserved for patients with infections caused by susceptible organisms and should be used in high enough dosages and for a long enough time to kill all organisms. Use of subtherapeutic dosages may allow resistant mutant strains to flourish. New anti-infective drugs should be reserved for severely ill patients with serious infections that don't respond to conventional drugs.

All anti-infective drugs can produce beneficial and adverse reactions in a patient. The adverse reactions can be classified as:
- ✦ direct toxic effects on such organs as the GI tract, kidneys, and liver or the auditory, optic, and peripheral nerves.
- ✦ allergic reactions and other kinds of hypersensitivity reactions affecting the skin and other organs and structures, including the bone marrow and blood.

✦ superinfections that result from drug-induced overgrowth of resistant bacteria or fungi.

ANTIBACTERIALS

Classes of antibacterials include aminoglycosides, carbapenems, cephalosporins, clindamycin, fluoroquinolones, macrolides, monobactams, nitrofurantoin, penicillins, sulfonamides, tetracyclines, and vancomycin. These drugs are used mainly to treat systemic (rather than localized) bacterial infections.

AMINOGLYCOSIDES

Aminoglycosides are used primarily for their bactericidal activity against aerobic gram-negative bacilli. They're also used to treat some aerobic gram-positive bacteria, mycobacteria, and some protozoa.

Aminoglycosides in use include amikacin, gentamicin, kanamycin, neomycin, netilmicin, paromomycin, streptomycin, and tobramycin.

Pharmacokinetics

Because aminoglycosides are absorbed poorly from the GI tract, they're usually given parenterally. After I.V. or I.M. administration, aminoglycoside absorption is rapid and complete. The drugs are distributed widely in extracellular fluid and readily cross the placental barrier but not the blood-brain barrier. Aminoglycosides aren't metabolized and are excreted primarily by the kidneys.

Pharmacodynamics

Against susceptible organisms, aminoglycosides produce their bactericidal action by irreversibly binding to the 30S subunits of bacterial ribosomes in the organisms. This interrupts protein synthesis and causes cell death.

Bacterial resistance to an aminoglycoside may be related to: failure of the drug to cross the cell membrane, altered binding to ribosomes, or drug destruction by bacterial enzymes. Some gram-positive cocci, such as enterococci, resist aminoglycoside transport across the cell membrane. When penicillin is used with an aminoglycoside, the bacterial cell wall is altered, allowing the aminoglycoside to penetrate it. That's why combination therapy with penicillins and aminoglycosides is commonly used to increase efficacy.

Pharmacotherapeutics

Aminoglycosides are most useful in treating:
✦ infections caused by aerobic gram-negative bacilli.
✦ serious nosocomial, or hospital-acquired, infections, such as gram-negative bacteremia, peritonitis, and pneumonia, in critically ill patients.
✦ urinary tract infections (UTIs) caused by enteric bacilli that are resistant to less toxic antibiotics, such as penicillins and cephalosporins.
✦ infections of the central nervous system (CNS).
✦ eye infections, which are treated topically with eyedrops or ointments.

Aminoglycosides are used with penicillins to treat gram-positive organisms, such as staphylococcal or enterococcal infections. They're inactive against anaerobic bacteria.

Features of aminoglycosides

✦ Bind irreversibly to 30S subunits of bacterial ribosomes, which interrupts protein synthesis and kills bacterial cells
✦ Are used mainly for bactericidal action against aerobic, gram-negative bacilli
✦ Treat gram-negative bacteremia, peritonitis, pneumonia in critically ill patients; UTIs; CNS infections; eye infections
✦ Are also used against some aerobic, gram-positive bacteria, mycobacteria, and protozoa
✦ Are commonly used with penicillin because it disrupts the cell wall, allowing the aminoglycoside to enter

WARNING

Precautions for aminoglycosides

Aminoglycosides require cautious use in patients with neuromuscular disorders, such as myasthenia gravis or parkinsonian syndrome. In these patients, the drugs may increase muscle weakness and neuromuscular blockade. If an aminoglycoside must be used in such a patient, keep emergency equipment nearby.

Individual aminoglycosides may have other specific uses. Amikacin, gentamicin, netilmicin, and tobramycin are active against *Acinetobacter, Citrobacter, Enterobacter, Klebsiella, Proteus* (indole-positive and indole-negative), *Providencia, Serratia, Escherichia coli,* and *Pseudomonas aeruginosa.* Streptomycin is active against many strains of mycobacteria, including *Mycobacterium tuberculosis,* and against the gram-positive bacteria *Nocardia* and *Erysipelothrix.*

Interactions

✦ Carbenicillin, ticarcillin, and piperacillin can reduce the effects of amikacin, gentamicin, kanamycin, neomycin, netilmicin, streptomycin, or tobramycin, especially if mixed in the same container or I.V. line.
✦ When used with a cephalosporin, an aminoglycoside may increase the risk of nephrotoxicity.
✦ When given with a neuromuscular blocker, amikacin, gentamicin, kanamycin, neomycin, netilmicin, streptomycin, or tobramycin can cause increased neuromuscular blockade, such as increased muscle relaxation and respiratory distress.
✦ When an aminoglycoside is given with the anesthetic methoxyflurane, the risk of renal and neurologic toxicity increases.
✦ If amikacin, gentamicin, kanamycin, netilmicin, or tobramycin is taken with cyclosporine, amphotericin B, or acyclovir, the risk of renal toxicity increases.
✦ An antiemetic may mask the symptoms of aminoglycoside-induced ototoxicity.
✦ Use of a loop diuretic with an aminoglycoside increases the risk of ototoxicity.

Adverse reactions

Serious adverse reactions limit the use of aminoglycosides, all of which display the same spectrum of toxicity; the total dosage and duration of therapy contribute to toxicity. The most notable adverse reactions are ototoxicity and nephrotoxicity. These most often occur in geriatric patients, dehydrated patients, those with renal impairment, and those who receive ototoxic or nephrotoxic drugs.

Aminoglycosides can produce irreversible damage to cranial nerve VIII. Hearing loss of varying degrees may occur and may be irreversible. High-frequency hearing loss usually occurs before clinical hearing loss. These drugs can induce vestibular symptoms, such as dizziness, nystagmus, vertigo, and ataxia.

Aminoglycosides can produce renal tubular necrosis, resulting in elevated serum creatinine and blood urea nitrogen (BUN) levels. Nephrotoxicity is related to a high drug level and drug accumulation in the renal cortex. Renal tubular damage usually is reversible after the drug is stopped.

PATIENT TEACHING

Teaching a patient about aminoglycosides

Whenever an aminoglycoside is prescribed, teach the patient and his family the drug's name, dose, frequency, action, and adverse effects. Also take the following actions.

◆ Stress the importance of taking the drug for the prescribed length of time.

◆ Instruct a woman to alert the prescriber if she is or suspects she is pregnant during therapy.

◆ Urge the patient to have blood tests to evaluate the effectiveness of therapy and detect adverse reactions.

◆ Instruct the patient to notify the nurse immediately if breathing difficulty or irregular heartbeat occurs because neuromuscular blockade may develop.

◆ Caution the patient with vestibular toxicity not to perform any activity that requires alertness. Also instruct him to notify the prescriber if dizziness, nystagmus, vertigo, or ataxia occurs.

◆ Advise the patient receiving an oral aminoglycoside to notify the prescriber if nausea, vomiting, or diarrhea occurs and to request a prescription for an antiemetic or antidiarrheal as needed.

◆ Instruct the patient to notify the prescriber at once if he notices changes in his hearing.

◆ Instruct the patient to notify the prescriber if other adverse reactions occur or if the infection persists or worsens.

Aminoglycosides can produce neuromuscular reactions that range from peripheral nerve toxicity to neuromuscular blockade. Reactions commonly occur after local, peritoneal, pleural, or wound instillation. Neuromuscular reactions can also occur when aminoglycosides are given to patients immediately after surgery. Neomycin and netilmicin produce the most potent neuromuscular reactions. (See *Precautions for aminoglycosides.*)

The most common adverse reactions to oral aminoglycosides are nausea, vomiting, and diarrhea.

Allergic reactions to aminoglycosides are rare. Rash, urticaria, stomatitis, pruritus, generalized burning, fever, and eosinophilia occasionally occur.

Nursing considerations

◆ Teach the patient and his family about the prescribed drug. (See *Teaching a patient about aminoglycosides.*)

◆ Collect blood, urine, sputum, or wound specimens, as appropriate, for culture and sensitivity tests before aminoglycoside therapy begins.

◆ To decrease the risk of nephrotoxicity, make sure the patient is well hydrated before beginning therapy.

◆ Refrigerate a prepared aminoglycoside I.V. solution until use; infuse the solution over at least 30 minutes.

◆ Don't mix an aminoglycoside in a solution that contains a penicillin; the aminoglycoside may be inactivated.

◆ Monitor the patient's aminoglycoside level and renal function closely if therapy also includes a cephalosporin. If renal dysfunction occurs, notify the prescriber and adjust the dosage as needed.

Key nursing actions

◆ To reduce the risk of nephrotoxicity, make sure the patient is hydrated before starting therapy.

◆ Monitor the aminoglycoside level regularly.

◆ Monitor the creatinine level to assess renal function, especially if therapy includes a cephalosporin.

◆ Notify the prescriber if routine urinalysis shows casts or protein in the urine.

◆ Monitor the patient for ototoxicity.

✦ Monitor the patient for adverse reactions and drug interactions during amino-glycoside therapy. If you detect any, notify the prescriber.

✦ Regularly monitor the patient's aminoglycoside level.

✦ Immediately after drawing a serum sample for aminoglycoside assay, place it on ice and transport it to the laboratory to prevent inactivation of the drug. Notify the prescriber if the peak or trough level doesn't fall within the expected range for the prescribed aminoglycoside.

✦ Monitor the patient's creatinine level to help detect changes in renal function. For a patient with unstable renal function, monitor the level at least every other day; for a patient with normal renal function, at least once per week.

✦ Notify the prescriber if routine urinalysis indicates casts or protein in the patient's urine. These findings may indicate aminoglycoside-induced renal damage.

✦ Give an aminoglycoside and a penicillin at least 2 hours apart to prevent a decrease in the aminoglycoside level and half-life in a patient with normal renal function.

✦ Monitor the patient for ototoxicity during aminoglycoside therapy. Prepare him for audiometric testing as indicated, because high-frequency loss usually occurs before clinical hearing loss.

✦ If ototoxicity is suspected, discontinue the prescribed aminoglycoside and initiate another antibacterial.

CARBAPENEMS

This class of beta-lactam antibacterials includes ertapenem, the combination product imipenem and cilastatin, and meropenem. Imipenem and cilastatin's spectrum of activity is broader than that of any other antibacterial. Because all carbapenems have a broad spectrum of activity, their use should be reserved for serious or life-threatening infections.

Pharmacokinetics

After I.V. administration, ertapenem is completely absorbed and is more highly protein-bound than the other two carbapenems. Metabolism occurs by hydrolysis, and excretion occurs mainly in urine.

Imipenem must be given with cilastatin because imipenem alone is rapidly metabolized in the tubules of the kidneys, which renders it ineffective. After parenteral administration, imipenem and cilastatin is distributed widely. It's metabolized by several mechanisms and excreted primarily in urine.

After parenteral administration, meropenem is distributed widely, including to the CNS. Metabolism is insignificant. About 70% of the drug is excreted unchanged in urine.

Pharmacodynamics

Ertapenem, imipenem and cilastatin, and meropenem are usually bactericidal. They exert antibacterial activity by inhibiting bacterial cell-wall synthesis.

Pharmacotherapeutics

Ertapenem's spectrum of activity includes treatment of intra-abdominal, skin, urinary tract, and gynecologic infections, as well as community-acquired pneumonias from various gram-positive, gram-negative, and anaerobic organisms.

Imipenem and cilastatin has the broadest spectrum of activity among the existing beta-lactam antibiotics. It's effective against aerobic gram-positive species, such as *Streptococcus, Staphylococcus aureus,* and *Staphylococcus epidermidis.* It inhibits

---

Features of carbapenems

✦ Belong to the beta-lactam class
✦ Have a broad spectrum of activity
✦ Are reserved for serious or life-threatening infections
✦ Are usually bactericidal
✦ Inhibit bacterial cell-wall synthesis

ertapenem

✦ Is used for intra-abdominal, skin, urinary tract, and gynecologic infections and for community-acquired pneumonias from various gram-positive, gram-negative, and anaerobic organisms

imipenem and cilastatin

✦ Is the broadest spectrum beta-lactam antibiotic
✦ May be used alone for mixed aerobic and anaerobic infections, for serious nosocomial infections, or infections in immunocompromised patients

meropenem

✦ Is used for intra-abdominal infections and bacterial meningitis

most *Enterobacter* species. It also inhibits *P. aeruginosa* (including strains resistant to piperacillin and ceftazidime) and most anaerobic species, including *Bacteroides fragilis.* In addition, it may be used alone for mixed aerobic and anaerobic infections, serious nosocomial infections, or infections in immunocompromised patients.

Meropenem is indicated for treating intra-abdominal infections as well as for managing bacterial meningitis caused by susceptible organisms.

Interactions
✦ Use of probenecid with imipenem and cilastatin increases the cilastatin level, but only slightly increases the imipenem level.
✦ Probenecid may cause ertapenem or meropenem to accumulate to a toxic level.
✦ Together, imipenem and cilastatin and an aminoglycoside act synergistically against *Enterococcus faecalis.*

Adverse reactions
The most common adverse reactions to carbapenems are nausea, vomiting, and diarrhea. Geriatric patients and patients with a history of seizures, underlying CNS disease, or renal insufficiency may experience seizures; these reactions aren't as common with meropenem. In some cases, nausea is related to rapid infusion and is reduced by increasing the administration time. Pseudomembranous colitis caused by *Clostridium difficile* may also occur.

Phlebitis, thrombophlebitis, and pain may occur at the I.V. site. Pain can also occur at the injection site when the drug is given I.M. Transient elevations in liver function values, such as aspartate aminotransferase (AST), alanine aminotransferase (ALT), and lactate dehydrogenase (LDH) may occur.

Hypersensitivity reactions, such as rash, have been reported in patients who are hypersensitive to penicillins.

Nursing considerations
✦ Obtain appropriate specimens for culture and sensitivity testing before carbapenem therapy begins.
✦ Don't mix ertapenem, imipenem and cilastatin, or meropenem with or add any of them to other antibiotics.
✦ Don't give a carbapenem with probenecid.
✦ Adjust the dosage in a patient with renal impairment.
✦ Monitor the patient periodically for adverse reactions and drug interactions during therapy. Notify the prescriber if any occur.
✦ Regularly monitor the patient's liver function test results for transient elevations in AST, ALT, and LDH.
✦ Give ertapenem, imipenem and cilastatin, or meropenem by intermittent I.V. infusion over 30 minutes. Give I.M. ertapenem or imipenem and cilastatin deeply into the gluteal muscle mass or lateral part of the thigh.
✦ Maintain seizure precautions throughout therapy.
✦ Be especially alert for seizure activity in an older patient or one with a history of seizures, underlying CNS disease, or renal insufficiency.
✦ Teach the patient and his family about the prescribed drug. (See *Teaching a patient about carbapenems,* page 300.)

Adverse reactions to watch for
✦ Diarrhea, nausea, vomiting
✦ Pain at the I.M. injection site
✦ Pain, phlebitis, thrombophlebitis at the I.V. site
✦ Pseudomembranous colitis
✦ Seizures in geriatric patients and patients with a history of seizures, underlying CNS disease, or renal insufficiency
✦ Transient elevations in liver function values (AST, ALT, LDH)

Key nursing actions
✦ Monitor liver function tests regularly to detect transient elevations in liver function values.
✦ Maintain seizure precautions throughout therapy.
✦ Be especially alert for seizures if the patient is elderly or has a history of seizures, a CNS disease, or renal insufficiency.

Features of cephalosporins

+ Are categorized into four groups called *generations*
+ Vary by generation in therapeutic uses

First generation

+ Act mainly against gram-positive organisms
+ Are used to treat staphylococcal and streptococcal infections, such as pneumonia, cellulitis, osteomyelitis
+ May be used as an alternative to penicillin in patients allergic to penicillin

Second generation

+ Act against gram-negative bacteria
+ Are the only cephalosporins effective against anaerobes (cefoxitin and cefotetan)

Third generation

+ Act mainly against gram-negative organisms
+ Are the drugs of choice for infections with *Enterobacter, P. aeruginosa,* and anaerobic organisms

Fourth generation

+ Act against many gram-positive and gram-negative organisms

CEPHALOSPORINS

In recent years, cephalosporins have accounted for most of the antibacterials that have been introduced. Cephalosporins are categorized into groups called *generations*, based on their spectra of activity, their characteristics, and their development:
+ First-generation cephalosporins include cefadroxil, cefazolin, cephalexin, and cephradine.
+ Second-generation cephalosporins include cefaclor, cefprozil, and cefuroxime.
+ Third-generation cephalosporins include cefdinir, cefoperazone, cefotaxime, cefpodoxime, ceftazidime, ceftibuten, ceftizoxime, and ceftriaxone.
+ A fourth-generation cephalosporin is cefepime.
Loracarbef is a synthetic beta-lactam antibiotic that belongs to the carbacephem antibiotic class. However, because this drug is similar to second-generation cephalosporins, it's included with them.

Because penicillin and cephalosporin molecules share a similar beta-lactam molecular structure, some cross-sensitivity occurs. This means that a patient who has had a reaction to penicillin is also at risk for a reaction to a cephalosporin.

Pharmacokinetics

Many cephalosporins are given parenterally because they aren't absorbed from the GI tract. Some cephalosporins are absorbed from the GI tract and can be administered orally; food usually delays their absorption, but not the amount absorbed. Cefpodoxime and cefuroxime have increased absorption when given with food.

After absorption, cephalosporins are distributed widely, although most aren't distributed in the CNS. Cefuroxime, cefotaxime, ceftizoxime, ceftriaxone, and ceftazidime cross the blood-brain barrier. Cefepime also crosses the blood-brain barrier, but it isn't known to what extent.

Many cephalosporins, including loracarbef, aren't metabolized at all. Cephapirin and cefotaxime are metabolized to nonacetyl forms, which provide less antibacterial activity than the parent compounds. To a small extent, ceftriaxone is metabolized in the intestines to inactive metabolites, which are excreted via the biliary system.

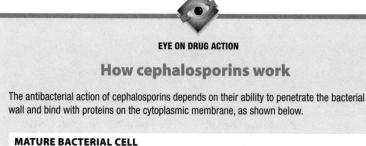

How cephalosporins work

The antibacterial action of cephalosporins depends on their ability to penetrate the bacterial wall and bind with proteins on the cytoplasmic membrane, as shown below.

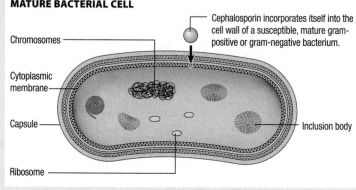

MATURE BACTERIAL CELL

Chromosomes

Cytoplasmic membrane

Capsule

Ribosome

Cephalosporin incorporates itself into the cell wall of a susceptible, mature gram-positive or gram-negative bacterium.

Inclusion body

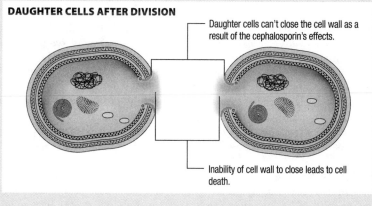

DAUGHTER CELLS AFTER DIVISION

Daughter cells can't close the cell wall as a result of the cephalosporin's effects.

Inability of cell wall to close leads to cell death.

All cephalosporins are excreted primarily unchanged by the kidneys, except for cefoperazone and ceftriaxone, which are excreted via bile in feces.

Pharmacodynamics

Like penicillins, cephalosporins inhibit cell-wall synthesis by binding to the bacterial enzymes known as penicillin-binding proteins (PBPs), located on the cell membrane. After the drug damages the cell wall by binding with the PBPs, the body's natural defense mechanisms destroy the bacteria. (See *How cephalosporins work.*)

Pharmacotherapeutics

The four generations of cephalosporins have particular therapeutic uses. First-generation cephalosporins, which act primarily against gram-positive organisms,

Features of cephalosporins

✦ Damage bacterial cell walls by binding to PBPs on cell membranes
✦ Allows the body's natural defenses to kill bacteria

may be used as alternative therapy in patients who are allergic to penicillin, depending on the seriousness of the allergy. They're also used to treat staphylococcal and streptococcal infections, including pneumonia; cellulitis, a type of skin infection; and osteomyelitis, a type of bone infection.

Second-generation cephalosporins act against gram-negative bacteria. Cefoxitin and cefotetan are the only cephalosporins effective against anaerobes.

Third-generation cephalosporins, which act primarily against gram-negative organisms, are the drugs of choice for infections caused by *Enterobacter, P. aeruginosa,* and anaerobic organisms.

Fourth-generation cephalosporins are active against a wide range of gram-positive and gram-negative bacteria.

Interactions

◆ Using alcohol with — or up to 72 hours after taking — cefotetan, cefoperazone, or cefazolin may lead to acute alcohol intolerance, which may produce headache, flushing, dizziness, nausea, vomiting, or abdominal cramps within 30 minutes of alcohol use and lasting up to 3 days after stopping the drug.

◆ A uricosuric, such as probenecid and sulfinpyrazone, can reduce renal excretion of some cephalosporins, including loracarbef.

◆ Probenecid can increase the level, and prolong the action, of a cephalosporin and may be used for that purpose.

Adverse reactions

Hypersensitivity reactions are the most common systemic adverse reactions to cephalosporins. Allergic reactions range in severity from mild to life-threatening. Usually, these reactions appear as urticaria, pruritus, morbilliform eruptions, or serum sickness. Anaphylaxis is rare. Because of the similarities between penicillins and cephalosporins, cross-sensitivity may occur. Patients with a history of penicillin reactions are at risk for developing an allergic reaction to cephalosporins.

I.M. administration of cefoxitin commonly produces pain, induration, and tenderness at the injection site.

In patients with renal impairment who receive high dosages of cephalosporins, the most common reactions are confusion and seizures. Seizures may result with high dosages of cefazolin.

Possible drug interactions

◆ Alcohol
◆ Probenecid
◆ Sulfinpyrazone

Adverse reactions to watch for

◆ Confusion, seizures in patients with renal impairment who receive high dosages
◆ Diarrhea, nausea, vomiting
◆ False-positive results on urine glucose tests using cupric sulfate solution
◆ Hypersensitivity reactions (mild to life-threatening, usually urticaria, pruritus, morbilliform eruption, or serum sickness)
◆ Pain, induration, tenderness at the cefoxitin I.M. injection site
◆ Pseudomembranous colitis

CLINICAL ALERT Cefoperazone, cefotetan, and ceftriaxone may decrease prothrombin activity, leading to an increased risk of bleeding. Patients at highest risk for this reaction include those with renal impairment, hepatic disease, or impaired vitamin K synthesis or storage.

Oral cephalosporins commonly cause nausea, vomiting, and diarrhea, which may be relieved by giving the drug with food. Pseudomembranous colitis caused by *C. difficile* may occur during cephalosporin therapy or after it's stopped, especially with the third-generation cephalosporins.

Cephalosporins may produce nephrotoxicity. (See *Precautions for cephalosporins.*)

Cephalosporin use may lead to superinfection, which could produce problems like diarrhea, sore mouth caused by oral thrush, and vaginal itching.

All cephalosporins, except cefotaxime, can cause false-positive results on urine glucose tests using cupric sulfate solution, such as Benedict's test and Clinitest. However, they don't affect the results of glucose oxidase tests, such as glucose enzymatic test strip and Clinistix.

Nursing considerations

✦ Avoid giving a cephalosporin to a patient who recently has experienced a severe, immediate reaction to a penicillin or cephalosporin. Obtain a thorough drug history, and screen the patient for possible allergy and cross-sensitivity with cephalosporins.

✦ Monitor the patient for adverse reactions and drug interactions during cephalosporin therapy. Notify the prescriber if any occur. Keep in mind that toxicity increases from the first to the third generation of these drugs.

✦ Observe the patient for hypersensitivity reactions. Keep standard emergency equipment readily available. If a hypersensitivity reaction occurs, withhold the drug and notify the prescriber.

✦ Adjust the cephalosporin dosage for a patient with renal insufficiency, unless he receives cefoperazone or ceftriaxone.

✦ Infuse an I.V. cephalosporin over 30 minutes to minimize pain and irritation at the injection site.

✦ Routinely monitor the I.V. site for signs of thrombophlebitis, such as localized redness, swelling, and pain.

✦ Reconstitute cefoxitin or ceftriaxone with a 0.5% to 1% lidocaine injection (without epinephrine) to decrease pain at the I.M. injection site.

✦ Give the prescribed cephalosporin with food to prevent or minimize GI distress. However, give loracarbef at least 1 hour before or 2 hours after meals.

✦ Monitor the patient's hydration if nausea, vomiting, or diarrhea occurs. If these adverse reactions persist or worsen, notify the prescriber, administer an antiemetic or antidiarrheal as needed, and switch the oral cephalosporin to a parenteral equivalent.

✦ Monitor the patient for signs and symptoms of pseudomembranous colitis, such as abdominal pain and diarrhea, during and after therapy with a cephalosporin, especially a third-generation cephalosporin.

✦ Teach the patient and his family about the prescribed drug. (See *Teaching a patient about cephalosporins*, page 304.)

Adverse reactions to watch for
(continued)

✦ Nephrotoxicity
✦ Superinfection, possibly with diarrhea, oral thrush, vaginal itching

Key nursing actions

✦ Don't give a cephalosporin to a patient who recently had a severe, immediate reaction to a penicillin or cephalosporin.
✦ Watch for hypersensitivity reactions.
✦ Monitor the I.V. site routinely for evidence of thrombophlebitis.
✦ Monitor hydration if the patient develops diarrhea, nausea, or vomiting.
✦ Watch for evidence of pseudomembranous colitis.

Teaching a patient about cephalosporins

Whenever a cephalosporin is prescribed, teach the patient and his family the drug's name, dose, frequency, action, and adverse effects. Also take the following actions.

✦ Stress the importance of taking the drug for the prescribed length of time.
✦ Teach the patient to recognize and immediately report the signs and symptoms of a hypersensitivity reaction.
✦ Review with the patient the signs and symptoms of a superinfection.
✦ Advise the patient to ingest yogurt or buttermilk, which replenishes normal GI flora, to prevent intestinal superinfection.
✦ Instruct the patient to take an oral cephalosporin with food to prevent GI upset. Instruct him to take loracarbef 1 hour before or 2 hours after meals.
✦ Inform the patient that I.M. cephalosporin may cause pain, inflammation, or tenderness at the injection site.
✦ Advise the patient to avoid taking cefoperazone, cefazolin, or cefotetan with alcohol or drugs that contain alcohol, such as elixirs.
✦ Advise the diabetic patient taking a cephalosporin to test his urine glucose level with glucose enzymatic test strips or Clinistix (not Clinitest).
✦ Stress the importance of keeping follow-up appointments and having laboratory tests done to evaluate drug effectiveness or detect adverse reactions.
✦ Advise the patient receiving cefotetan, ceftriaxone, or cefoperazone to take bleeding precautions, such as using an electric razor for shaving, avoiding cuts and bruises, using a soft toothbrush, and wearing shoes at all times.
✦ Instruct the patient to notify the prescriber if adverse reactions occur or if the condition persists or worsens.

Features of clindamycin

✦ Is prescribed only when no alternative exists
✦ Inhibits bacterial protein synthesis and may inhibit the binding of bacterial ribosomes
✦ Is bacteriostatic against most organisms
✦ Potent against most aerobic gram-positive organisms, including staphylococci, streptococci (except *E. faecalis*), and pneumococci
✦ Is effective against most major anaerobes
✦ Is used mainly for anaerobic intra-abdominal, pleural, or pulmonary infections caused by *B. fragilis*
✦ Is used as an alternative to penicillin for *C. perfringens* infections or for staphylococcal infections in a patient allergic to penicillin

CLINDAMYCIN

Because of its high potential for serious adverse effects, clindamycin is another antibacterial prescribed only when no therapeutic alternative exists. The drug is available as clindamycin hydrochloride, clindamycin palmitate hydrochloride, and clindamycin phosphate.

Pharmacokinetics

When taken orally, clindamycin is absorbed well and distributed widely in the body. It's metabolized by the liver and excreted by the kidney and biliary pathways.

Pharmacodynamics

Clindamycin inhibits bacterial protein synthesis. It may also inhibit the binding of bacterial ribosomes. At a therapeutic level, clindamycin is primarily bacteriostatic against most organisms.

Pharmacotherapeutics

Because of the potential for serious toxicity and pseudomembranous colitis, clindamycin use is limited to a few situations in which safer antibacterials aren't available.

The drug is potent against most aerobic gram-positive organisms, including staphylococci, streptococci (except *E. faecalis*), and pneumococci. It's effective against most of the major anaerobes and is used primarily to treat anaerobic intra-abdominal, pleural, or pulmonary infections caused by *B. fragilis*. It's also used as an alternative to penicillin in treating *Clostridium perfringens* infections. In addition, it may be used as an alternative to penicillin in treating staphylococcal infections in a patient with penicillin allergy.

Interactions
✦ Clindamycin may enhance the action of a neuromuscular blocker, blocking neuromuscular transmission and possibly leading to severe respiratory depression.

Adverse reactions
During clindamycin therapy, diarrhea occurs in about 80% of patients and is most common with oral administration. Oral administration of clindamycin may also produce stomatitis, nausea, and vomiting.

 CLINICAL ALERT **Clindamycin may cause pseudomembranous colitis, characterized by severe diarrhea, abdominal pain, fever, and mucus and blood in stools. When a patient experiences significant diarrhea that suggests pseudomembranous colitis, stop clindamycin or, if absolutely necessary, continue the drug while monitoring the patient closely. In either case, plan to replace fluids and electrolytes as needed.**

With I.V. administration, clindamycin can damage tissue. With I.M. administration, it may produce pain, induration, and sterile abscess.

Hypersensitivity reactions in the form of rash occur in about 10% of patients treated with clindamycin. The rash resembles one seen in a patient receiving ampicillin.

Stevens-Johnson syndrome occurs rarely, and in a few instances, anaphylactic reactions may occur.

Nursing considerations
✦ Don't refrigerate reconstituted oral clindamycin palmitate hydrochloride solution because it thickens and becomes difficult to measure accurately. The solution remains stable for 2 weeks at room temperature.
✦ Monitor the patient periodically for adverse reactions and drug interactions during clindamycin therapy. If you detect any, notify the prescriber.
✦ Keep standard emergency equipment nearby. Although anaphylactic reactions are rare, they may occur.
✦ Inspect the I.V. infusion site regularly for signs and symptoms of thrombophlebitis. If signs and symptoms occur, switch the infusion to another site.
✦ Observe the I.M. injection site regularly for signs of irritation, such as induration or sterile abscess.
✦ Monitor the patient for signs and symptoms of pseudomembranous colitis, such as severe diarrhea, abdominal pain, fever, and mucus and blood in stools. If they occur, promptly stop the drug and notify the prescriber.
✦ Don't give an antiperistaltic because it can aggravate pseudomembranous colitis.
✦ Give vancomycin or metronidazole to treat pseudomembranous colitis.
✦ Teach the patient and his family about the prescribed drug. (See *Teaching a patient about clindamycin,* page 306.)

Adverse reactions to watch for
✦ Diarrhea
✦ Hypersensitivity reactions (rash)
✦ Nausea, vomiting
✦ Pain, induration, sterile abscess with I.M. use
✦ Pseudomembranous colitis
✦ Stomatitis
✦ Tissue damage with I.V. use

Key nursing actions
✦ Keep emergency equipment available.
✦ Inspect the I.V. site regularly for evidence of thrombophlebitis.
✦ Inspect the I.M. site regularly for signs of irritation.
✦ Monitor the patient for signs and symptoms of pseudomembranous colitis.

Teaching a patient about clindamycin

Whenever clindamycin is prescribed, teach the patient and his family the drug's name, dose, frequency, action, and adverse effects. Also take the following actions:

✦ Stress the importance of taking the drug for the prescribed length of time.

✦ Warn the patient that the I.M. injection may be painful.

✦ Instruct the patient to notify the nurse if he feels discomfort at the I.V. infusion site.

✦ Teach the patient the importance of notifying the prescriber if he experiences adverse reactions, such as GI upset (especially diarrhea), pseudomembranous colitis, or hypersensitivity reactions.

Features of fluoroquinolones

✦ Are synthetic antibiotics

✦ Interrupt bacterial replication by inhibiting DNA gyrase, which blocks DNA synthesis

✦ Are used for a wide variety of UTIs, plus specific indications for individual drugs

✦ Ciprofloxacin is used for lower respiratory tract infections; infectious diarrhea; and skin, bone, or joint infections.

✦ Gatifloxacin is used for bronchitis, community-acquired pneumonia, UTIs, gynecologic infections.

✦ Levofloxacinis used for lower respiratory infections, skin infections, UTIs.

✦ Ofloxacin is used for selected sexually transmitted diseases, lower respiratory infections, skin and skin-structure infections, prostatitis.

Possible interactions

✦ Antacids containing aluminum or calcium

FLUOROQUINOLONES

Structurally similar synthetic antibiotics, fluoroquinolones are primarily used to treat UTIs as well as upper respiratory infections, pneumonia, and gonorrhea. Drugs in this class include ciprofloxacin, gatifloxacin, levofloxacin, lomefloxacin, moxifloxacin, norfloxacin, ofloxacin, and sparfloxacin.

Pharmacokinetics

After oral administration, fluoroquinolones are absorbed well. They aren't highly protein-bound, are minimally metabolized in the liver, and are excreted primarily in urine. Ofloxacin is excreted substantially in urine.

Pharmacodynamics

Fluoroquinolones work by interrupting deoxyribonucleic acid (DNA) synthesis during bacterial replication, through the inhibition of DNA gyrase, an essential enzyme in the process of replicating DNA. As a result, the bacteria are prevented from replicating.

Pharmacotherapeutics

Fluoroquinolones can be used to treat a wide variety of UTIs. Each drug in this class also has specific indications. For example, ciprofloxacin is used to treat lower respiratory tract infections; infectious diarrhea; and skin, bone, or joint infections.

Gatifloxacin is used to treat bronchitis and community-acquired pneumonia as well as UTIs and gynecologic infections.

Levofloxacin is indicated for the treatment of lower respiratory infections as well as skin infections and UTIs.

Ofloxacin is also used to treat selected sexually transmitted diseases, lower respiratory infections, skin and skin-structure infections, and prostatitis.

Interactions

✦ An antacid that contains magnesium or aluminum can decrease fluoroquinolone absorption.

✦ When used with aminophylline, theophylline, or another xanthine derivative, ciprofloxacin, norfloxacin, or ofloxacin may increase the theophylline level and the risk of theophylline toxicity.

✦ Probenecid can decrease renal elimination of ciprofloxacin or norfloxacin, increasing the fluoroquinolone level and half-life.

✦ When gatifloxacin or moxifloxacin is used with an antiarrhythmic or other drug that prolongs the QT interval, additive effects may further prolong the QT interval.

✦ Calcium-fortified orange juice may decrease the level of any fluoroquinolone and may reduce its therapeutic effects.

Adverse reactions

Well tolerated by most patients, fluoroquinolones produce few adverse reactions. The most common reactions affect the GI tract and include nausea, vomiting, diarrhea, and abdominal pain. About 1% of patients have developed adverse CNS reactions, such as headache, drowsiness, seizures, vision disturbances, hallucinations, depression, and agitation. Ofloxacin and levofloxacin may cause insomnia and dizziness.

Less common adverse reactions affect the integumentary system. In 1% of patients or fewer, fluoroquinolones produce hypersensitivity reactions that include urticaria, nonspecific rash, pruritus, and edema. Some patients experience transient arthralgia or myalgia.

Other rare reactions include hematologic problems, such as hemolytic anemia, that are related to glucose-6-phosphate dehydrogenase (G6PD) deficiency and glucose anomalies, such as symptomatic hyperglycemia and hypoglycemia.

 CLINICAL ALERT Moderate to severe phototoxic reactions may occur during fluoroquinolone therapy. These reactions may occur with direct and indirect sunlight and with artificial ultraviolet light, and may occur with and without sunscreen.

Nursing considerations

✦ Question the patient about a history of head trauma, seizures, or use of drugs that cause seizures before administering a fluoroquinolone.

✦ Adjust the dosage for a patient with renal impairment because the elimination rate will decrease and the half-life will increase.

✦ Give an antacid, if needed, at least 2 hours after giving a fluoroquinolone.

✦ Monitor the patient for adverse reactions and drug interactions during fluoroquinolone therapy. Alert the prescriber if any occur.

✦ Take safety precautions if the patient experiences adverse CNS reactions, such as drowsiness, vision disturbances, or dizziness. For example, place the bed in the lowest position, keep the bed rails raised, and supervise the patient's movement.

✦ Monitor the patient for seizures during fluoroquinolone therapy.

✦ Take seizure precautions, such as padding the bed rails, if needed.

✦ Notify the prescriber immediately if seizures occur.

✦ Teach the patient and his family about the prescribed drug. (See *Teaching a patient about fluoroquinolones,* page 308.)

Possible interactions
(continued)

✦ Calcium-fortified orange juice
✦ Drugs that prolong the QT interval
✦ Probenecid
✦ Xanthine derivatives

Adverse reactions to watch for

✦ Abdominal pain, diarrhea, nausea, vomiting
✦ Agitation, depression, drowsiness, hallucinations, headache, seizures, vision disturbances
✦ Dizziness, insomnia (with ofloxacin, levofloxacin)
✦ Hypersensitivity reactions (urticaria, rash, pruritus, edema)
✦ Phototoxic reactions
✦ Transient arthralgia or myalgia

Key nursing actions

✦ Give an antacid, if needed, at least 2 hours after a fluoroquinolone.
✦ Take safety precautions if the patient has CNS effects.
✦ Monitor the patient for seizures during therapy.
✦ Take seizure precautions.

MACROLIDES

Used to treat many common infections, macrolides include azithromycin, clarithromycin, dirithromycin, erythromycin, and various erythromycin salts (estolate, ethylsuccinate, gluceptate, lactobionate, and stearate).

Pharmacokinetics

Azithromycin, clarithromycin, and dithromycin are readily absorbed from the GI tract, although food may slow their absorption. All three are distributed widely. They readily penetrate cells, but not the CNS. Azithromycin and dithromycin are excreted primarily in feces; 20% of clarithromycin is excreted in urine.

Because erythromycin is acid-sensitive, it must be buffered or enteric coated to prevent destruction by gastric acid. Erythromycin is absorbed in the duodenum. It's distributed to most tissues and body fluids. Only a low level is distributed into cerebrospinal fluid.

Erythromycin is metabolized by the liver and excreted in bile in high amounts; small amounts are excreted in urine. It also crosses the placental barrier and appears in breast milk.

Pharmacodynamics

Macrolides inhibit ribonucleic acid (RNA)–dependent protein synthesis by acting on a small portion of the ribosome, much like clindamycin.

Pharmacotherapeutics

Azithromycin provides a broad spectrum of activity against gram-positive and gram-negative bacteria, including *Mycobacterium, Staphylococcus aureus, Haemophilus influenzae, Moraxella catarrhalis,* and *Chlamydia.* It's also effective against pneumococci and groups C, F, and G streptococci.

Features of macrolides

- ✦ Inhibit RNA-dependent protein synthesis by acting on a small portion of the ribosome, much like clindamycin
- ✦ Are used to treat many common infections

Clarithromycin is a broad-spectrum antibacterial that's active against gram-positive aerobes, such as *Staphylococcus aureus, Streptococcus pneumoniae,* and *Streptococcus pyogenes;* gram-negative aerobes, such as *H. influenzae* and *M. catarrhalis;* and other aerobes, such as *Mycoplasma pneumoniae.* Clarithromycin is also used with antacids, histamine (H_2)-receptor antagonists, and proton-pump inhibitors, to treat *Helicobacter pylori* infection and duodenal ulcer disease.

Dirithromycin provides broad-spectrum coverage similar to azithromycin and clarithromycin, but is also effective against *Listeria monocytogenes.* Dirithromycin shouldn't be used in patients with known, suspected, or potential bacteremia because the drug doesn't reach an adequate level to produce antibacterial effects in bacteremia.

Erythromycin has a range of therapeutic uses. It provides a broad spectrum of activity against gram-positive and gram-negative bacteria, including *Mycobacterium, Treponema, Mycoplasma,* and *Chlamydia.* It's also effective against pneumococci and group A streptococci. *S. aureus* is sensitive to erythromycin; however, resistant strains may appear during therapy. Erythromycin is the drug of choice for treating *M. pneumoniae* infections as well as pneumonia caused by *Legionella pneumophila.*

In patients who are allergic to penicillin, erythromycin is effective for infections produced by group A beta-hemolytic streptococci or *S. pneumoniae.* It may also be used to treat gonorrhea and syphilis in patients who can't tolerate penicillin G or tetracyclines. The drug may also be used to treat minor staphylococcal infections of the skin.

Interactions
+ Azithromycin, clarithromycin, or erythromycin can increase the theophylline level in a patient receiving a high theophylline dosage and can increase the risk of theophylline toxicity.
+ Clarithromycin may increase the carbamazepine level.
+ When given immediately after an antacid or H_2-receptor antagonist, dirithromycin has slightly enhanced absorption.

Adverse reactions
The most common adverse reactions to azithromycin are GI disturbances, such as nausea, vomiting, diarrhea, and abdominal pain. However, azithromycin appears to cause fewer adverse GI reactions than erythromycin. Other adverse reactions include palpitations, chest pain, vaginal candidiasis, nephritis, dizziness, headache, vertigo, somnolence, fatigue, rash, and photosensitivity. Rare but potentially serious adverse reactions include angioedema and cholestatic jaundice.

The most commonly reported adverse reactions to clarithromycin include diarrhea, nausea, abnormal taste, dyspepsia, abdominal pain or discomfort, and headache. Like azithromycin, clarithromycin also appears to cause fewer adverse GI reactions than erythromycin.

Commonly reported adverse reactions to dirithromycin include nausea and abdominal pain.

Erythromycin produces few adverse reactions. Dose-related GI reactions (epigastric distress, nausea, vomiting, and diarrhea) are most common, especially with large doses. Stomatitis, heartburn, anorexia, and melena may also occur.

Although rare, reversible sensorineural hearing loss may occur with I.V. erythromycin lactobionate. This reaction is most likely to occur in patients with renal failure who are receiving high dosages of erythromycin. Venous irritation and

Possible drug interactions
+ Antacids
+ Carbamazepine
+ H_2-receptor antagonists
+ Theophylline

Adverse reactions to watch for

azithromycin
+ Abdominal pain, diarrhea, nausea, vomiting
+ Angioedema
+ Chest pain, palpitations
+ Cholestatic jaundice
+ Dizziness, fatigue, headache, somnolence, vertigo
+ Nephritis
+ Photosensitivity, rash
+ Vaginal candidiasis

clarithromycin
+ Abdominal pain or discomfort, abnormal taste, diarrhea, dyspepsia, nausea
+ Headache

dirithromycin
+ Abdominal pain, nausea

erythromycin
+ Anorexia, diarrhea, epigastric distress, heartburn, nausea, vomiting
+ Melena
+ Stomatitis

Teaching a patient about macrolides

Whenever a macrolide is prescribed, teach the patient and his family the drug's name, dose, frequency, action, and adverse effects. Also take the following actions.
◆ Stress the importance of taking the drug for the prescribed length of time.
◆ Instruct the patient not to take erythromycin stearate with food.
◆ Instruct the patient to take azithromycin at least 1 hour before or 2 hours after a meal.
◆ Tell the patient who receives I.V. erythromycin lactobionate to notify the nurse if he notices changes in his hearing.
◆ Review the signs and symptoms of cholestatic hepatitis with the patient who receives erythromycin estolate or erythromycin ethylsuccinate. Advise him to notify the prescriber if they appear.
◆ Teach the patient on long-term macrolide therapy the importance of undergoing routine liver function tests.
◆ Instruct the patient to notify the prescriber if adverse reactions occur.

thrombophlebitis can occur after I.V. administration of erythromycin gluceptate or erythromycin lactobionate.

Allergic reactions, including rash, fever, eosinophilia, and anaphylaxis, can also occur.

Although rare, the most serious toxicity is cholestatic hepatitis, which is most commonly caused by erythromycin estolate and erythromycin ethylsuccinate. This syndrome is characterized by nausea, vomiting, and abdominal pain followed by jaundice, fever, and abnormal liver function test results that are consistent with cholestatic hepatitis. These reactions sometimes are accompanied by rash, leukocytosis, and eosinophilia. The syndrome may represent a hypersensitivity reaction to the specific structure of the estolate compound. The cholestatic jaundice and hepatocellular necrosis may resolve within days or a few weeks after stopping the drug.

Nursing considerations
◆ Don't mix I.V. erythromycin lactobionate with vitamin B complex, vitamin C, tetracycline, heparin, colistimethate sodium, furosemide, metaraminol bitartrate, or metoclopramide hydrochloride because they're incompatible.
◆ Reconstitute erythromycin solutions in normal saline solution or dextrose 5% in water and give the solution no more than 4 hours after preparation.
◆ Monitor the patient periodically for adverse reactions and drug interactions during macrolide therapy. Notify the prescriber if any occur.
◆ Observe the patient for allergic reactions and keep standard emergency equipment nearby. If allergic reactions occur, withhold the macrolide and notify the prescriber.
◆ Monitor for hearing changes in a patient receiving I.V. erythromycin lactobionate, especially in a geriatric patient or one with renal insufficiency.
◆ Observe the I.V. site for thrombophlebitis when giving erythromycin gluceptate or erythromycin lactobionate.
◆ Don't give erythromycin stearate with food.
◆ Give azithromycin at least 1 hour before or 2 hours after a meal.

Key nursing actions
◆ Watch for allergic reactions, and keep emergency equipment nearby.
◆ Assess the patient for hearing changes during therapy with I.V. erythromycin lactobionate, especially if he's elderly or has renal impairment.
◆ Inspect the I.V. site for evidence of thrombophlebitis when giving erythromycin gluceptate or lactobionate.

✦ Don't give erythromycin by I.M. injection; this injection is painful and may cause abscess or local tissue necrosis.

✦ Monitor the patient for hepatic dysfunction. If he receives long-term therapy, do frequent liver function tests and physical assessments to detect signs of liver failure.

✦ Monitor the patient for signs and symptoms of cholestatic hepatitis, such as nausea, vomiting, abdominal pain, jaundice, rash, leukocytosis, and eosinophilia, during therapy with erythromycin estolate or erythromycin ethylsuccinate.

✦ Stop erythromycin if cholestatic hepatitis occurs.

✦ Teach the patient and his family about the prescribed drug. (See *Teaching a patient about macrolides.*)

MONOBACTAMS

Aztreonam is the first member in this class of antibacterials. This synthetic monobactam has a narrow spectrum of activity and is effective against many gram-negative aerobic bacteria.

Pharmacokinetics

After parenteral administration, aztreonam is rapidly and completely absorbed and distributed widely. It's metabolized partially and excreted primarily in urine as unchanged drug.

Pharmacodynamics

Aztreonam's bactericidal activity results from inhibition of bacterial cell-wall synthesis. It preferentially binds to PBP-3 in susceptible gram-negative bacteria. As a result, division of the cell wall is inhibited and destruction occurs.

Pharmacotherapeutics

Indications for aztreonam include infections with a wide range of gram-negative aerobic organisms, including *P. aeruginosa*. This drug is effective against most strains of *E. coli, Enterobacter, Klebsiella pneumoniae, Klebsiella oxytoca, Proteus mirabilis, Serratia marcescens, H. influenzae,* and *Citrobacter*. It's also used for complicated and uncomplicated UTIs, septicemia, and lower respiratory tract, skin and skin-structure, intra-abdominal, and gynecologic infections caused by susceptible gram-negative aerobic bacteria.

This drug is usually active against gram-negative aerobic organisms that are resistant to antibiotics hydrolyzed by beta-lactamases. (Beta-lactamase is an enzyme that makes an antibiotic ineffective.)

Aztreonam shouldn't be used alone as empiric therapy in seriously ill patients if a gram-positive or a mixed aerobic-anaerobic bacterial infection is suspected.

Interactions

✦ Probenecid increases the aztreonam level by prolonging the monobactam's tubular secretion rate in the kidneys.

✦ When aztreonam is used with an aminoglycoside, renal toxicity can occur.

✦ Cefoxitin, imipenem, or another potent inducer of beta-lactamase production may inactivate aztreonam.

✦ Use of aztreonam with clavulanic acid may produce synergistic or antagonistic effects, depending on the organism involved.

Key nursing actions
(continued)

✦ Monitor the patient for hepatic dysfunction.

✦ Watch for evidence of cholestatic hepatitis when giving erythromycin estolate or ethylsuccinate.

Features of aztreonam

✦ Is the first member of the monobactam class of drugs

✦ Inhibits cell-wall synthesis in susceptible gram-negative bacteria by binding with PBP-3

✦ Is usually active against gram-negative aerobic organisms that are resistant to antibiotics hydrolyzed by beta-lactamases

✦ Is used for wide range of gram-negative aerobic organisms, including *P. aeruginosa*

✦ Is used for complicated and uncomplicated UTIs, septicemia, and lower respiratory tract, skin and skin-structure, intra-abdominal, and gynecologic infections

Possible drug interactions

✦ Aminoglycosides
✦ Cefoxitin
✦ Clavulanic acid
✦ Imipenem
✦ Probenecid

Adverse reactions to watch for

◆ Abdominal cramps, bloating, GI bleeding, halitosis, numbness of tongue, oral ulceration, unusual taste (I.V. infusion)
◆ Anaphylaxis, erythema multiforme, exfoliative dermatitis, pruritus, urticaria
◆ *C. difficile* diarrhea
◆ Confusion, dizziness, fatigue, headache, insomnia, paresthesia, seizures, weakness
◆ Diarrhea, nausea, vomiting
◆ Discomfort, pain, swelling at I.M. injection site
◆ Hypotension
◆ Thrombophlebitis (I.V. use)
◆ Transient anemia, eosinophilia, leukocytosis, leukopenia, neutropenia, pancytopenia, thrombocytopenia, thrombocytosis
◆ Transient ECG changes, including ventricular bigeminy and premature ventricular contractions
◆ Transient increases in liver function values

Key nursing actions

◆ Monitor renal function closely if aztreonam is given with an aminoglycoside.

PATIENT TEACHING

Teaching a patient about monobactams

Whenever a monobactam is prescribed, teach the patient and his family the drug's name, dose, frequency, action, and adverse effects. Also take the following actions.
◆ Stress the importance of taking the drug for the prescribed length of time.
◆ Warn the patient who receives I.M. aztreonam that pain may occur at the injection site.
◆ Advise the patient who receives I.V. aztreonam to report pain at the infusion site.
◆ Emphasize the importance of undergoing blood tests periodically to detect adverse hematologic or hepatic reactions.
◆ Instruct the patient to notify the nurse before getting out of bed if dizziness occurs.
◆ Teach the patient how to manage mouth ulcers and perform frequent mouth care.
◆ Instruct the patient with thrombocytopenia to take bleeding precautions, such as avoiding cuts and bruises, using a soft toothbrush, and using an electric razor for shaving.
◆ Review appropriate infection-control measures with the patient and his family if leukopenia occurs.
◆ Teach the patient with anemia to stagger his activities and to rest frequently.
◆ Instruct the patient to notify the prescriber if adverse reactions occur.

Adverse reactions

The most common GI reactions to aztreonam include diarrhea, nausea, and vomiting. Less common GI reactions include GI bleeding, abdominal cramps, bloating, a transient unusual taste during or after I.V. infusion, numbness of the tongue, oral ulceration, and halitosis. *C. difficile* diarrhea may also occur.

Hematologic reactions may include transient eosinophilia, leukopenia, neutropenia, thrombocytopenia, pancytopenia, anemia, leukocytosis, and thrombocytosis.

Transient increases in AST, ALT, and alkaline phosphatase levels may occur. They return to pretreatment levels shortly after stopping the drug. Hepatitis, jaundice, and other manifestations of hepatotoxicity are rare.

Hypotension and transient electrocardiogram (ECG) changes, including ventricular bigeminy and premature ventricular contractions, may occur. Seizures, confusion, insomnia, dizziness, paresthesia, weakness, fatigue, and headache may also occur as adverse CNS reactions.

Thrombophlebitis may occur in patients receiving I.V. aztreonam. Discomfort, pain, and swelling at the injection site may also occur in patients receiving I.M. aztreonam, although the drug is generally well tolerated when given by this route.

Hypersensitivity and dermatologic reactions may include anaphylaxis, urticaria, pruritus, erythema multiforme, and exfoliative dermatitis.

Nursing considerations

◆ Obtain specimens for culture and sensitivity testing before giving the first dose of aztreonam. Notify the prescriber if results reveal organisms that are resistant to aztreonam.
◆ Monitor the patient periodically for adverse reactions and drug interactions during therapy. If any occur, notify the prescriber.
◆ Closely monitor the patient's renal function if aztreonam is used with an aminoglycoside.

◆ Monitor the patient closely for hypersensitivity reactions. If a hypersensitivity reaction occurs, withhold aztreonam, notify the prescriber, and switch the patient to a different antibiotic. Keep standard emergency equipment nearby.

◆ Maintain seizure precautions throughout therapy.

◆ If the patient experiences confusion, dizziness, or other adverse CNS reactions, take safety precautions.

◆ Monitor the patient's complete blood count (CBC) and liver function studies for abnormalities.

◆ If leukocytopenia occurs, take infection-control measures.

◆ If thrombocytopenia occurs, take bleeding precautions.

◆ If anemia occurs, stagger the patient's activities and provide frequent rest periods.

◆ If adverse hematologic or hepatic reactions occur, notify the prescriber.

◆ Teach the patient and his family about the prescribed drug. (See *Teaching a patient about monobactams*.)

NITROFURANTOIN

The antibacterial nitrofurantoin is used to treat acute and chronic UTIs. It isn't useful in the treatment of pyelonephritis or perinephric disease.

Pharmacokinetics

After oral administration, nitrofurantoin is absorbed rapidly and well from the GI tract. Taking the drug with food enhances the drug's bioavailability and lessens GI distress. Because it dissolves more slowly, the macrocrystalline form of the drug is absorbed more slowly and causes less GI distress.

The drug is 20% to 60% protein-bound. It crosses the placental barrier and appears in breast milk. It's also distributed in bile.

Nitrofurantoin is partially metabolized by the liver; 30% to 50% is excreted unchanged in urine.

Pharmacodynamics

Usually bacteriostatic, nitrofurantoin may become bactericidal. This change depends on the drug level in urine and the infecting organism's susceptibility. Although nitrofurantoin's exact mechanism of action is unknown, it appears to inhibit the formation of acetyl coenzyme A from pyruvic acid, thereby inhibiting energy production by the infecting organism. The drug may also disrupt bacterial cell-wall formation.

Pharmacotherapeutics

Because the absorbed drug concentrates in the urine, nitrofurantoin is used to treat UTIs. It has a higher antibacterial activity in acid urine. Nitrofurantoin isn't effective against systemic bacterial infections.

Interactions

◆ Probenecid and sulfinpyrazone inhibit renal excretion of nitrofurantoin, reducing its efficacy and increasing its toxic potential.

◆ A magnesium salt or antacid containing magnesium can decrease the extent and rate of nitrofurantoin absorption.

◆ Nitrofurantoin may decrease the antibacterial activity of norfloxacin or nalidixic acid.

Key nursing actions
(continued)

◆ Watch for hypersensitivity reactions.

◆ Maintain seizure precautions throughout therapy.

◆ If the patient is confused, dizzy, or has other CNS reactions, take safety precautions.

◆ Monitor CBC and liver function studies.

Features of nitrofurantoin

◆ Is usually bacteriostatic, but may be bactericidal

◆ May inhibit formation of acetyl coenzyme A from pyruvic acid, which inhibits energy production by infecting organisms

◆ May disrupt bacterial cell-wall synthesis

◆ Is used for UTIs

◆ Is ineffective against systemic bacterial infections

Possible drug interactions

◆ Antacids containing magnesium

◆ Magnesium salts

◆ Nalidixic acid

◆ Norfloxacin

◆ Probenecid

◆ Sulfinpyrazone

Detecting pneumonitis in geriatric patients

During nitrofurantoin therapy, geriatric patients are the most likely to experience acute pneumonitis. To detect this adverse reaction, monitor the patient for signs and symptoms, which typically appear in the first week of treatment. Signs and symptoms of acute pneumonitis include sudden fever, chills, cough, dyspnea, chest pain, eosinophilia, and pulmonary infiltration that may appear as consolidation or pleural effusion on X-rays.

Adverse reactions to watch for

◆ Abdominal pain, anorexia, diarrhea, Gi iritation, nausea, vomiting
◆ Acute pneumonitis, especially in older patients
◆ Anaphylaxis, arthralgia, chills, fever
◆ Angioneurotic edema; eczematous, erythematous, or maculopapular rash; pruritus; urticaria
◆ Asthmatic attacks in patients with a history of asthma
◆ Dark yellow or brown urine
◆ Hypersensitivity reactions
◆ Peripheral neuropathy

Key nursing actions

◆ Monitor the patient for hypersensitivity reactions involving the skin, lungs, liver, blood.
◆ Give nitrofurantoin with food or milk to minimize adverse GI reactions.
◆ Obtain a urine culture and sensitivity test before and during therapy to determine drug effectiveness. Continue therapy for 3 days after urine is sterile.

Adverse reactions

GI irritation is the most common adverse reaction to nitrofurantoin. Anorexia, nausea, and vomiting occur more commonly than diarrhea and abdominal pain. Some patients have experienced peripheral neuropathy, which usually begins with paresthesia and dysesthesia of the legs and can progress to a debilitating state.

Hypersensitivity reactions may occur and involve the skin, lungs, blood, and liver. Chills, fever, arthralgia (a characteristic of systemic lupus erythematosus), and anaphylaxis may also occur. Dermatologic hypersensitivity reactions include maculopapular, erythematous, or eczematous rashes; urticaria; angioneurotic edema; and pruritus.

Pulmonary reactions include asthmatic attacks in patients with a history of asthma and acute pneumonitis especially in older patients. (See *Detecting pneumonitis in geriatric patients.*)

Hematologic reactions are rare but may include leukopenia, granulocytopenia, and megaloblastic anemia. In patients with G6PD deficiency, nitrofurantoin can precipitate an acute episode of hemolytic anemia, although this is rare. Non–dose-related hepatotoxicity occurs rarely as well as chronic active hepatitis, cholestatic jaundice, and cholestatic hepatitis. Nitrofurantoin may color the urine dark yellow or brown.

Nursing considerations

◆ Don't give nitrofurantoin with probenecid, sulfinpyrazone, an antacid, nalidixic acid, and norfloxacin.
◆ Monitor the patient for adverse reactions and drug interactions during nitrofurantoin therapy. If any occur, notify the prescriber.
◆ Monitor the patient for hypersensitivity reactions that may involve the skin, lungs, blood, and liver. Keep standard emergency equipment nearby because anaphylaxis may occur.
◆ If a hypersensitivity reaction occurs, withhold the drug and notify the prescriber. Provide symptomatic relief.
◆ Give nitrofurantoin with food or milk to minimize adverse GI reactions.
◆ Obtain a urine culture and sensitivity test before and during therapy to determine drug effectiveness. Continue nitrofurantoin therapy for 3 days after urine sterility is confirmed.
◆ Teach the patient and his family about the prescribed drug. (See *Teaching a patient about nitrofurantoin.*)

PENICILLINS

Penicillins remain among the most important and useful antibacterials, despite the availability of numerous others. These antibacterials can be divided into four groups:
+ aminopenicillins, such as amoxicillin, amoxicillin and clavulanate potassium, and ampicillin.
+ extended-spectrum penicillins, such as carbenicillin, piperacillin, and ticarcillin.
+ natural penicillins, such as penicillin G benzathine, penicillin G benzathine and procaine, penicillin G potassium, penicillin G procaine, penicillin G sodium, and penicillin V potassium.
+ penicillinase-resistant penicillins, such as cloxacillin, dicloxacillin, nafcillin, and oxacillin.

Pharmacokinetics

After oral administration, penicillins are absorbed mainly in the duodenum and the upper jejunum of the small intestine. Absorption of oral penicillin varies and depends on such factors as the particular penicillin used, pH of the patient's stomach and intestine, and presence of food in the GI tract.

Most penicillins should be given 1 hour before or 2 hours after meals when the stomach is empty to enhance absorption. Amoxicillin, penicillin V, and amoxicillin and clavulanate can be given without regard to meals.

Penicillins are distributed widely to most areas of the body, including the lungs, liver, kidneys, muscle, bone, and placenta. High drug levels also appear in urine, making penicillins useful in treating UTIs.

Penicillins are metabolized to a limited extent in the liver to inactive metabolites; they're excreted 60% unchanged by the kidneys. Nafcillin and oxacillin are also excreted in bile.

Features of penicillins
+ Are among the most important and useful antibacterials
+ Belong to four groups: aminopenicillins, extended-spectrum penicillins, natural penicillins, penicillinase-resistant penicillins
+ Are usually bactericidal
+ Bind reversibly to several enzymes outside bacterial cytoplasmic membranes
+ Inhibit cell-wall synthesis, rapidly destroying bacterial cells
+ Are used for gram-positive, gram-negative, and anaerobic organisms

Possible drug interactions

+ Aminoglycosides
+ Anticoagulants
+ Chloramphenicol
+ Hormonal contraceptives
+ Methotrexate
+ Neomycin
+ Probenecid
+ Tetracycline
+ Warfarin

Adverse reactions to watch for

+ Anaphylactic reactions, drug fever, rash, serum sickness
+ Coma, seizures (with penicillin G at more than 20 million units daily in patients with decreased renal function)
+ Diarrhea, glossitis, nausea, vomiting (with oral use, most commonly with ampicillin)
+ Hepatotoxicity (with oxacillin)
+ Hypersensitivity reactions
+ Interstitial nephritis, renal impairment (with large parenteral dosages of penicillin G)
+ Positive Coombs' test
+ Prolonged bleeding time from platelet dysfunction
+ Pseudomembranous colitis (with aminopenicillins and extended-spectrum penicillins)

Pharmacodynamics

Usually, penicillins are bactericidal. They bind reversibly to several enzymes outside the bacterial cytoplasmic membrane. These enzymes are PBPs and are involved in cell-wall synthesis and cell division. Interference with these processes inhibits cell-wall synthesis, causing rapid destruction of the cell.

Pharmacotherapeutics

No other class of antibacterials provides as wide a spectrum of activity as the penicillins. As a class, they cover gram-positive, gram-negative, and anaerobic organisms. Specific penicillins have a greater activity against specific organisms.

Penicillin is given by I.M. injection when oral administration is inconvenient or a patient's compliance is questionable. Because long-acting preparations of penicillin G (penicillin G benzathine and penicillin G procaine) are relatively insoluble, give these drugs I.M.

Interactions

+ Probenecid increases the penicillin level.
+ A penicillin can reduce renal tubular secretion of methotrexate, increasing the risk of methotrexate toxicity.
+ Tetracycline or chloramphenicol can reduce penicillin's bactericidal action.
+ Neomycin decreases the absorption of penicillin V.
+ Penicillin V or ampicillin can reduce the effectiveness of a hormonal contraceptive.
+ When used with an anticoagulant, large doses of an I.V. penicillin can increase bleeding.
+ Nafcillin and dicloxacillin may inhibit warfarin activity.
+ High dosages of penicillin G or an extended-spectrum penicillin can inactivate an aminoglycoside.
+ Penicillin can reduce the effects of an aminoglycoside, especially if mixed in the same I.V. solution.

Adverse reactions

Hypersensitivity reactions are the major adverse reactions to penicillins. Anaphylactic reactions, serum sickness, drug fever, or rash may occur. Large dosages, prolonged therapy, or parenteral administration may also lead to allergic reactions.

 CLINICAL ALERT Some patients may experience an allergic reaction to tartrazine, a dye contained in certain penicillin preparations.

Carbenicillin and ticarcillin, which are given as disodium salts, can increase the sodium intake. Because of this, the drugs may pose a problem for patients with cardiac disease or decreased renal function.

Penicillins can produce adverse hematologic effects. A positive Coombs' test for hemolytic anemia can occur in patients receiving dosages of I.V. penicillin G equal to more than 10 million units per day in uremic patients or 40 million units per day in patients with normal renal function. Stopping the drug usually returns the hemoglobin to the baseline normal value. Penicillins (especially carbenicillin and ticarcillin) may induce platelet dysfunction, causing prolonged bleeding time. Platelet function returns to normal when the drug is stopped.

Occasionally, hepatotoxicity has developed during oxacillin therapy. Adverse GI reactions, such as glossitis, nausea, vomiting, and diarrhea, are usually linked to oral use; they're most common with ampicillin therapy. The aminopenicillins and extended-spectrum penicillins can produce pseudomembranous colitis.

Seizures or coma caused by direct CNS irritation can occur with penicillin G in dosages greater than 20 million units daily in patients with decreased renal function.

Renal impairment and interstitial nephritis may occur in patients receiving large parenteral dosages of penicillin G. Usually, these reactions begin within 5 to 10 days after therapy begins. Signs and symptoms may include fever, eosinophilia, hematuria, proteinuria, or pyuria.

Nursing considerations
✦ Obtain a complete patient history to assess the risk of allergic reaction whenever penicillin therapy is considered.
✦ Don't mix an aminoglycoside with an extended-spectrum penicillin or a high dose of penicillin G. Keeping them separate will prevent an inactivated aminoglycoside.
✦ Give oral penicillin 1 hour before or 2 hours after meals to ensure an optimal drug level.
✦ Give penicillin G benzathine and procaine I.M. only.
✦ Monitor the patient closely for adverse reactions and interactions during penicillin therapy. Keep in mind that the patient may become sensitized to penicillin through exposure.
✦ For a patient who also receives warfarin, closely monitor his coagulation test results at the start of warfarin therapy and for up to 3 weeks after discontinuation of nafcillin or dicloxacillin.
✦ Stop penicillin at once if the patient exhibits rapidly developing dyspnea and hypotension, which indicates anaphylactic shock. Notify the prescriber and give immediate treatment, such as epinephrine, corticosteroids, antihistamines, and other resuscitative measures.
✦ Monitor the patient's temperature for a sudden elevation that may indicate drug fever. Notify the prescriber if a fever occurs.
✦ Monitor a patient with decreased renal function who receives more than 20 million units of penicillin G daily for seizures or decreased level of consciousness. Maintain seizure precautions during therapy.
✦ In a patient receiving large parenteral dosages of penicillin G, observe for signs of renal impairment or interstitial nephritis, such as fever, eosinophilia, hematuria, proteinuria, or pyuria; these signs usually occur 5 to 10 after therapy begins. Stop the drug and give corticosteroids to improve renal function.
✦ Observe a patient receiving an aminopenicillin or extended-spectrum penicillin for signs and symptoms of pseudomembranous colitis, such as abdominal pain or diarrhea. If signs or symptoms occur, notify the prescriber before giving the next dose.
✦ Monitor for adverse GI reactions in a patient receiving an oral penicillin, especially ampicillin. If nausea, vomiting, diarrhea, or glossitis occurs, monitor his hydration and give an antiemetic or antidiarrheal as needed. If GI reactions are severe, stop the drug or replace it with a parenteral form.
✦ Monitor the patient for bleeding tendencies, such as easy bruising, bleeding gums, or blood in the urine or stool.

Key nursing actions
✦ Stop penicillin at once if the patient rapidly develops dyspnea and hypotension.
✦ Monitor the temperature; sudden elevation may indicate drug fever.
✦ Watch for seizures and decreased level of consciousness if the patient with decreased renal function receives more than 20 million units of penicillin G daily. Maintain seizure precautions.
✦ Watch for evidence of renal impairment or interstitial nephritis if the patient receives large parenteral dosages of penicillin G.
✦ Observe a patient receiving an aminopenicillin or extended-spectrum penicillin for evidence of pseudomembranous colitis.
✦ Assess the patient for adverse GI reactions during oral therapy.
✦ Monitor the patient for bleeding tendencies, such as easy bruising, bleeding gums, or blood in the urine or stool.
✦ Monitor the platelet count.

Teaching a patient about penicillins

Whenever a penicillin is prescribed, teach the patient and his family the drug's name, dose, frequency, action, and adverse effects. Also take the following actions:
+ Stress the importance of taking the drug for the prescribed length of time.
+ Advise the patient to take an oral penicillin 1 hour before or 2 hours after meals to ensure an optimal drug level.
+ Review the signs and symptoms of allergic reactions with the patient. Instruct him to withhold the drug and notify the prescriber if such a reaction occurs. If an anaphylactic reaction occurs, instruct the family to seek emergency treatment immediately.
+ Advise the patient who is allergic to penicillins to wear a medical identification necklace or bracelet.
+ Encourage the patient to have the prescribed blood or urine tests and to keep follow-up appointments.
+ Instruct the patient to notify the prescriber if the infection persists or worsens or if adverse reactions occur.
+ Describe the risks of an elevated sodium or potassium level to a patient who has cardiac disease or decreased renal function and who takes carbenicillin or ticarcillin. Teach him to recognize and report signs and symptoms of sodium or potassium imbalance.

Features of sulfonamides

+ Are bacteriostatic
+ Have a wide spectrum of activity against gram-positive and gram-negative bacteria
+ Inhibit folic acid production, which reduces the number of bacterial nucleotides
+ Are used for acute UTIs
+ May be used for recurrent or chronic UTIs based on culture and sensitivity tests
+ Are also used for infections caused by *Nocardia asteroides* and *Toxoplasma gondii*
+ Co-trimoxazole is used for various other infections, such as *Pneumocystis carinii* pneumonia, acute otitis media caused by *H. influenzae* or *S. pneumoniae*, and acute exacerbations of chronic bronchitis caused by *H. influenzae* or *S. pneumoniae*

+ Monitor the patient's platelet count during penicillin therapy. Prolonged bleeding time is most likely to occur in a patient with uremic or hepatic disease who receives carbenicillin or ticarcillin. If bleeding time is prolonged, stop the drug.
+ Advise a patient who uses a hormonal contraceptive to use a reliable alternative form of contraception during penicillin V or ampicillin therapy.
+ Teach the patient and his family about the prescribed drug. (See *Teaching a patient about penicillins.*)

SULFONAMIDES

As the first effective systemic antibacterials, sulfonamides include sulfadiazine, sulfamethoxazole and trimethoprim (co-trimoxazole), sulfasalazine, and sulfisoxazole.

Pharmacokinetics

Most sulfonamides are absorbed well and distributed widely in the body. They're metabolized in the liver to inactive metabolites and excreted by the kidneys. Because crystalluria may occur, adequate fluid intake is highly recommended.

Pharmacodynamics

Sulfonamides are bacteriostatic: they prevent the growth of microorganisms by inhibiting folic acid production. The decreased folic acid synthesis decreases the number of bacterial nucleotides and inhibits bacterial growth.

Pharmacotherapeutics

Frequently, sulfonamides are used to treat acute UTIs. With recurrent or chronic UTIs, the infecting organism may not be susceptible to sulfonamides. Therefore, the choice of therapy should be based on culture and sensitivity tests.

Sulfonamides are also used to treat infections caused by *Nocardia asteroides* and *Toxoplasma gondii.* These drugs exhibit a wide spectrum of activity against gram-positive and gram-negative bacteria.

Co-trimoxazole is also used for various other infections, such as *Pneumocystis carinii* pneumonia, acute otitis media caused by *H. influenzae* or *S. pneumoniae,* and acute exacerbations of chronic bronchitis caused by *H. influenzae* or *S. pneumoniae.*

Interactions
✦ A sulfonamide can increase the hypoglycemic effects of an oral antidiabetic, increasing the risk of a low glucose level.
✦ When taken with methenamine, a sulfonamide may lead to crystalluria.
✦ Co-trimoxazole may increase the anticoagulant effects of warfarin.
✦ Together, co-trimoxazole and cyclosporine increase the risk of renal toxicity.

Adverse reactions
Sulfonamides cause numerous adverse reactions. Renal colic, nephritis, toxic nephrosis, hematuria, proteinuria, renal calculi, and elevated BUN and creatinine levels may result from sulfonamide-induced crystalluria and tubular deposits of sulfonamide crystals. Maintaining a high urine flow rate and alkalinized urine can minimize these complications. Nausea, vomiting, and diarrhea are common.

The risk of hypersensitivity reactions appears to increase as the dosage increases. Various dermatologic reactions, including rash, pruritus, erythema nodosum, erythema multiforme of the Stevens-Johnson type, and exfoliative dermatitis, can occur. Sulfonamides can also produce photosensitivity.

Fever may develop 7 to 10 days after the initial sulfonamide dose. A reaction that resembles serum sickness may occur, producing fever, joint pain, urticarial eruptions, bronchospasm, and leukopenia. Extremely rare reactions, such as granulocytopenia, aplastic anemia, and hemolytic anemia, have been reported.

Nursing considerations
✦ Give a sulfonamide with ample amounts of fluids.
✦ Monitor the patient for adverse reactions and interactions during therapy. If they occur, notify the prescriber.
✦ Withhold the sulfonamide dose and notify the prescriber if dermatologic reactions occur. Provide skin care to relieve discomfort caused by the reaction.
✦ Monitor the patient's urine elimination pattern for such changes as an increase or decrease in the amount voided, urinary frequency, or dysuria. Notify the prescriber of such changes.

 CLINICAL ALERT **Monitor the patient's fluid intake and output. The urine output should be at least 1,500 ml per day to ensure proper hydration. Inadequate urine output can lead to crystalluria or tubular deposits of the sulfonamide.**

✦ Teach the patient and his family about the prescribed drug. (See *Teaching a patient about sulfonamides,* page 320.)

Adverse reactions to watch for
✦ Diarrhea, nausea, vomiting
✦ Elevated BUN and creatinine levels, hematuria, nephritis, proteinuria, renal calculi, renal colic, toxic nephrosis
✦ Erythema multiforme of the Stevens-Johnson type, erythema nodosum, exfoliative dermatitis, pruritus, rash
✦ Fever 7 to 10 days after the first dose
✦ Hypersensitivity reactions
✦ Photosensitivity
✦ Serum sickness–like reaction: bronchospasm, fever, joint pain, leukopenia, urticarial eruptions

Key nursing actions
✦ Give sulfonamides with ample fluids.
✦ Withhold the dose and notify the prescriber if skin reactions develop.
✦ Monitor the urine elimination pattern.
✦ Monitor the patient's fluid intake and output.

Features of tetracyclines

+ Are classified as short-acting, intermediate-acting, or long-acting
+ Are bacteriostatic
+ Penetrate bacterial cells by an energy-dependent process and inhibit protein synthesis by binding to a subunit of the ribosome
+ Have a broad-spectrum activity against gram-positive and gram-negative aerobic and anaerobic bacteria, spirochetes, mycoplasmas, rickettsiae, chlamydiae, some protozoa
+ Are used to treat Rocky Mountain spotted fever, Q fever, Lyme disease
+ Are the drugs of choice for non-gonococcal urethritis caused by *Chlamydia* and *Ureaplasma urealyticum*
+ Are used with tetracycline and streptomycin as the most effective treatment for brucellosis
+ Treat acne in low dosages because they decrease the fatty acid content of sebum

TETRACYCLINES

These broad-spectrum antibacterials may be classified as short-acting drugs (such as oxytetracycline and tetracycline), intermediate-acting drugs (such as demeclocycline) or long-acting drugs (such as doxycycline and minocycline).

Pharmacokinetics

When taken orally, tetracyclines are absorbed from the duodenum. They're distributed widely into body tissues and fluids, concentrated in bile, and excreted primarily by the kidneys. Doxycycline is also excreted in feces. Minocycline undergoes enterohepatic recirculation.

Pharmacodynamics

Because all tetracyclines are primarily bacteriostatic, they inhibit the growth or multiplication of bacteria. These drugs penetrate the bacterial cell by an energy-dependent process. In the cell, they bind primarily to a subunit of the ribosome, inhibiting the protein synthesis needed to maintain the bacterial cell.

Pharmacotherapeutics

Tetracyclines provide a broad spectrum of activity against gram-positive and gram-negative aerobic and anaerobic bacteria, spirochetes, mycoplasmas, rickettsiae, chlamydiae, and some protozoa. The long-acting compounds doxycycline and minocycline provide more action against various organisms than other tetracyclines.

Tetracyclines are used to treat Rocky Mountain spotted fever, Q fever, and Lyme disease. They're the drugs of choice for treating nongonococcal urethritis caused by *Chlamydia* and *Ureaplasma urealyticum*. Combination therapy with a tetracycline and streptomycin is the most effective treatment for brucellosis.

In low dosages, tetracyclines effectively treat acne because they can decrease the fatty acid content of sebum.

Interactions

+ A tetracycline can reduce the effectiveness of a hormonal contraceptive and may result in breakthrough bleeding.
+ A tetracycline can reduce the bactericidal action of penicillin.

LIFESPAN

Preventing tooth problems from tetracyclines

Tetracyclines can cause adverse effects on teeth and bones. To avoid these effects, take preventive measures at different stages of development. For a pregnant woman, avoid giving a tetracycline during the last half of pregnancy. For a breast-feeding woman, suggest that she stop breast-feeding during tetracycline therapy. In these women, taking tetracyclines can cause permanent tooth staining, enamel hypoplasia, and inhibited skeletal growth in their fetuses and infants.

For a child younger than age 8, avoid giving a tetracycline. Doing so helps prevent permanent tooth discoloration, enamel hypoplasia, and a decrease in the child's skeletal growth rate.

♦ An aluminum, calcium, or magnesium antacid can reduce the absorption of an oral tetracycline.
♦ An iron salt, bismuth subsalicylate, or zinc sulfate can reduce the absorption of doxycycline, oxytetracycline, or tetracycline.
♦ A barbiturate, carbamazepine, or phenytoin can increase the metabolism and reduce the antibiotic effects of doxycycline.
♦ Milk or a dairy product can bind with a tetracycline (except for doxycycline and minocycline) and prevent drug absorption.

Adverse reactions

Tetracyclines produce many of the same adverse reactions as other antibacterials, such as superinfection and GI disturbances.

Adverse GI reactions to oral tetracyclines include nausea, vomiting, abdominal distress and distention, and diarrhea. Diarrhea usually subsides when the drug is stopped; however, prolonged symptoms from pseudomembranous colitis may occur.

 CLINICAL ALERT Photosensitivity reactions, made evident by a red rash on areas exposed to sunlight, are most common in patients who receive demeclocycline or doxycycline. However, photosensitivity reactions can occur with any tetracycline.

Tetracyclines cause permanent gray-brown to yellow discoloration of the teeth when given during tooth formation. (See *Preventing tooth problems from tetracyclines.*)

Hepatotoxic reactions, which include lipid infiltration of the liver, primarily occur with I.V. tetracyclines. Nephrotoxicity can develop in patients with renal failure; the antianabolic effects of tetracyclines may increase BUN and creatinine levels. Nephrotoxicity can also occur in patients who take outdated tetracycline.

CNS toxicity, which includes vestibular disturbances, occurs primarily with minocycline. Light-headedness, loss of balance, dizziness, and tinnitus usually begin on the 2nd or 3rd day of minocycline therapy. Symptoms are reversible several days after the drug is stopped.

As with any antibiotic, superinfection commonly develops during tetracycline therapy. Overgrowth of yeast typically occurs, and oral or vaginal candidiasis requires specific therapy. Staphylococcal enterocolitis caused by tetracycline-resistant

Adverse reactions to watch for

♦ Abdominal distress and distention, diarrhea, nausea, vomiting
♦ Dizziness, light-headedness, loss of balance, tinnitus (with minocycline)
♦ Gray-brown to yellow tooth discoloration when given during tooth formation
♦ Hepatotoxic reactions (with I.V. use)
♦ Nephrotoxicity in patients with renal failure
♦ Oral or vaginal candidiasis
♦ Photosensitivity reactions
♦ Pseudomembranous colitis
♦ Staphylococcal enterocolitis
♦ Superinfection

Teaching a patient about tetracyclines

Whenever a tetracycline is prescribed, teach the patient and his family the drug's name, dose, frequency, action, and adverse effects. Also take the following actions.

✦ Stress the importance of taking the drug for the prescribed length of time.

✦ Advise the patient who experiences a hypersensitivity reaction to withhold the drug and notify the prescriber.

✦ Advise the patient not to consume milk, milk products, or drugs that contain calcium, magnesium, aluminum, or iron with the tetracycline because these products prevent tetracycline absorption.

✦ Advise the patient to take doxycycline and minocycline with food to minimize GI irritation and to take any other tetracycline on an empty stomach.

✦ Advise the patient who experiences esophageal irritation to take tetracycline with 8 oz (240 ml) of water.

✦ Warn the patient receiving oxytetracycline that the I.M. injection will be painful.

✦ Inform the patient with minocycline-induced central nervous system toxicity that the symptoms should disappear several days after the drug is stopped.

✦ Advise the patient to avoid direct sunlight, cover exposed skin, or use a sunscreen with a sun protection factor of 15 or higher during tetracycline therapy.

✦ Advise a woman who takes hormonal contraceptives to use an alternate means of contraception during tetracycline therapy and for 1 week after therapy is stopped.

✦ Instruct the patient to notify the prescriber if adverse reactions occur.

Key nursing actions

✦ Give doxycycline or minocycline with food to minimize GI distress. Give any other tetracycline 1 hour before or 2 hours after meals when the stomach is empty. Don't give drug within 3 hours of dairy products.

✦ Monitor a patient receiving I.V. oxytetracycline or tetracycline for thrombophlebitis.

✦ Monitor the patient regularly for evidence of superinfection.

✦ Inspect the patient's mouth regularly for evidence of oral candidiasis.

staphylococci can lead to severe diarrhea, dehydration, and possible circulatory collapse.

Nursing considerations

✦ Monitor the patient periodically for adverse reactions and interactions. If they occur, notify the prescriber.

✦ Give doxycycline or minocycline with food to minimize GI distress. Give any other tetracycline 1 hour before or 2 hours after meals when the stomach is empty. Don't administer drug within 3 hours of dairy products.

✦ If used with antacids that contain calcium, magnesium, or aluminum, or with iron, bismuth, or zinc, separate administration times by 2 to 3 hours.

✦ Dilute an I.V. preparation in a large volume of fluid and give by continuous slow drip.

✦ Monitor a patient receiving parenteral oxytetracycline or tetracycline for thrombophlebitis at the I.V. site.

✦ Double-check any prescription for an I.M. injection because this route usually isn't recommended. If the drug must be given I.M., inject oxytetracycline deeply into a large muscle.

✦ Monitor the patient regularly for signs of superinfection, such as oral thrush, GI disturbance, or worsening of signs and symptoms of the systemic infection.

✦ Inspect the patient's mouth regularly for signs of oral candidiasis, such as cream-colored or bluish white pseudomembranous patches on the tongue, mouth, or pharynx. Encourage a woman to report unusual vaginal discharge.

✦ Notify the prescriber if oral or vaginal candidiasis is suspected; specific therapy will be needed.

✦ For a woman who takes a hormonal contraceptive, suggest that she use a reliable alternative contraceptive during tetracycline therapy.
✦ Teach the patient and his family about the prescribed drug. (See *Teaching a patient about tetracyclines.*)

VANCOMYCIN

Vancomycin is used to treat methicillin-resistant *S. aureus,* which has become a major concern. Because of the emergence of vancomycin-resistant enterococci, however, vancomycin must be used judiciously. Generally, vancomycin shouldn't be used for any infection unless culture and sensitivity testing confirms the need for its use.

Pharmacokinetics

Because vancomycin is absorbed poorly from the GI tract, it must be given I.V. for systemic infections. The drug diffuses well into pleural, pericardial, synovial, and ascitic fluids.

The metabolism of vancomycin is unknown. About 85% of a dose is excreted unchanged in urine within 24 hours. A small amount may be eliminated through the liver and biliary tract.

Pharmacodynamics

Vancomycin inhibits bacterial cell-wall synthesis, which damages the bacterial plasma membrane. When the bacterial cell wall is damaged, the body's natural defenses can attack the organism.

Pharmacotherapeutics

Vancomycin is active against gram-positive organisms, such as *S. aureus, S. epidermidis, S. pyogenes, Enterococcus,* and *S. pneumoniae.*

I.V. vancomycin is the therapy of choice for patients with serious resistant staphylococcal infections who are hypersensitive to penicillins. Oral vancomycin is used for patients with antibiotic-induced *C. difficile* colitis who can't take metronidazole or have responded poorly to metronidazole.

When used with an aminoglycoside, vancomycin is also the treatment of choice for *E. faecalis* endocarditis in patients who are allergic to penicillin.

Interactions

✦ Vancomycin may increase the risk of toxicity when used with another drug that causes nephrotoxicity and ototoxicity, such as an aminoglycoside, amphotericin B, bacitracin, cisplatin, colistin, or polymyxin B.

Adverse reactions

Parenteral vancomycin must be given I.V. only, and care must be taken to avoid extravasation. Pain and thrombophlebitis may occur after I.V. use. I.M injection isn't recommended because it causes pain and tissue necrosis at the injection site.

Ototoxicity is the most serious reaction to parenteral vancomycin. This reaction is most likely to occur in patients with renal impairment and those receiving long-term, high-dosage I.V. therapy. Vancomycin may damage the auditory branch of cranial nerve VIII; permanent deafness can occur. Tinnitus may precede deafness and requires the drug to be stopped. Hearing loss occasionally improves after the drug is stopped, but in many cases it deteriorates further.

Features of vancomycin

✦ Inhibits bacterial cell-wall synthesis, which allows the body's natural defenses to kill organisms
✦ Is active against gram-positive organisms, such as *S. aureus, S. epidermidis, S. pyogenes, Enterococcus, S. pneumoniae*
✦ Is used for methicillin-resistant *S. aureus* but, in light of vancomycin-resistant enterococci, must be used judiciously
✦ Is used I.V. for serious resistant staphylococcal infections in patients hypersensitive to penicillins
✦ Is used for antibiotic-induced *C. difficile* colitis in patients who respond poorly to metronidazole or can't take it
✦ Is combined with an aminoglycoside for *E. faecalis* endocarditis in patients allergic to penicillin

Adverse reactions to watch for

✦ Anaphylactic reactions, drug fever, eosinophilia
✦ Azotemia, mild hematuria, proteinuria, urine casts
✦ Extravasation (with I.V. use)
✦ Hypersensitivity reactions
✦ Neutropenia
✦ Ototoxicity (tinnitus followed by possibly permanent deafness)
✦ Pain, thrombophlebitis (with I.V. use)
✦ Severe hypotensive reaction and maculopapular or erythematous rash (with rapid I.V. infusion)

Teaching a patient about vancomycin

Whenever vancomycin is prescribed, teach the patient and his family the drug's name, dose, frequency, action, and adverse effects. Also take the following actions:
✦ Stress the importance of taking the drug for the prescribed length of time.
✦ Instruct the patient to report ringing in his ears or a reduced ability to hear.
✦ Emphasize the importance of undergoing laboratory tests regularly.
✦ Instruct the patient to alert the nurse if he feels pain at the I.V. infusion site.
✦ Advise the patient to notify the prescriber if adverse reactions occur or if symptoms persist or worsen.

Occasionally, mild hematuria, proteinuria, urine casts, and azotemia may occur. The risk of nephrotoxicity increases when vancomycin is given with an aminoglycoside.

 CLINICAL ALERT Rapid I.V. infusion of vancomycin may cause a severe hypotensive reaction accompanied by a maculopapular or erythematous rash on the face, neck, chest, and arms. Known as red man syndrome, this reaction usually begins a few minutes after the infusion is started and resolves spontaneously several hours after the infusion is discontinued.

Hypersensitivity reactions occur in 5% to 10% of patients who receive vancomycin. Anaphylactic reactions, eosinophilia, and drug fever may occur. Neutropenia, which rapidly reverses after stopping the drug, may also occur.

Nursing considerations

✦ Assess the patient's renal status before therapy begins. If the patient receives another ototoxic or nephrotoxic drug, monitor the drug's peak and trough levels and the creatinine level.
✦ Don't give vancomycin I.M. because the injection is painful and can produce tissue necrosis.
✦ Don't give the drug by rapid I.V. injection. Instead, infuse it slowly in a large volume of fluid to avoid a hypotensive reaction.
✦ Don't mix it with other drugs in the same I.V. solution.
✦ Be aware that I.V. and oral forms aren't interchangeable.
✦ Monitor the patient periodically for adverse reactions and interactions during therapy. Notify the prescriber if any occur.
✦ Monitor the patient closely for signs of ototoxicity, especially if he has renal impairment or is receiving long-term, high-dosage I.V. therapy.
✦ Ask the patient about tinnitus or hearing loss during therapy. Withhold the drug and notify the prescriber if either one occurs.
✦ Teach the patient and his family about the prescribed drug. (See *Teaching a patient about vancomycin.*)

Key nursing actions

✦ Assess the patient's renal status before therapy starts.
✦ Don't give the drug by rapid I.V. infusion.
✦ Monitor the patient closely for evidence of ototoxicity.
✦ Ask the patient about tinnitus and hearing loss during therapy.

ANTIVIRALS

Antivirals are used to prevent or treat viral infections, ranging from influenza to human immunodeficiency virus (HIV) infection. Major antivirals used to treat systemic infections include amantadine and rimantadine, foscarnet, non-nucleoside reverse transcriptase inhibitors (NNRTIs), nucleoside reverse transcriptase inhibitors (NRTIs), tenofovir, protease inhibitors, ribavirin, and synthetic nucleosides.

AMANTADINE AND RIMANTADINE

Amantadine and its derivative, rimantadine, are used to prevent or treat influenza A infections.

Pharmacokinetics

After oral administration, amantadine and rimantadine are absorbed well in the GI tract and distributed widely throughout the body. Amantadine is eliminated primarily in urine; rimantadine is extensively metabolized and then excreted in urine.

Pharmacodynamics

Although amantadine's exact mechanism of action is unknown, the drug appears to inhibit an early stage of viral replication. Rimantadine inhibits viral RNA and protein synthesis.

Pharmacotherapeutics

Amantadine and rimantadine are used to prevent and treat respiratory tract infections caused by strains of the influenza A virus. They can reduce the severity and duration of fever and other symptoms in patients already infected with influenza A.

They also protect patients undergoing immunization during the 2 weeks needed for immunity to develop or patients who can't take the influenza vaccine because of hypersensitivity.

Amantadine is also used to treat parkinsonism and drug-induced extrapyramidal reactions, such as abnormal involuntary movements.

Interactions

No significant drug interactions have been documented with rimantadine.
✦ Use of an anticholinergic with amantadine increases adverse anticholinergic effects.
✦ When given with hydrochlorothiazide and triamterene, amantadine excretion decreases, which increases the amantadine level.
✦ When amantadine and trimethoprim are used together, their levels increase.

Adverse reactions

The most common adverse reactions to amantadine are nausea, anorexia, nervousness, fatigue, depression, irritability, insomnia, psychosis, anxiety, confusion, forgetfulness, and hallucinations. Other CNS reactions include headache, dizziness, lightheadedness, slurred speech, ataxia, tremor, and a sense of inebriation. Patients with seizure disorders are more prone to seizures while receiving amantadine.

Other less common adverse reactions include heart failure, orthostatic hypotension, edema, leukopenia, dermatitis, photosensitivity, dry mouth, rash, urine reten-

Features of amantadine and rimantadine

✦ Amantadine may inhibit an early stage of viral replication.
✦ Rimantadine inhibits viral RNA protein synthesis.
✦ Are used to prevent and treat respiratory tract infections caused by influenza A virus
✦ Can reduce the severity and duration of symptoms in patients already infected with influenza A
✦ Protect patients hypersensitive to influenza vaccine and patients who received vaccine but won't have immunity for 2 more weeks
✦ Amantadine is used to treat parkinsonism, drug-induced extrapyramidal reactions.

Adverse reactions to watch for

✦ Anorexia, constipation, nausea, vomiting
✦ Anxiety, confusion, depression, fatigue, forgetfulness, hallucinations, insomnia, irritability, nervousness, psychosis
✦ Ataxia, dizziness, headache, light-headedness, sense of inebriation, slurred speech, tremor
✦ Dermatitis, dry mouth, photosensitivity, rash, urine retention
✦ Edema, heart failure, orthostatic hypotension
✦ Hypersensitivity reactions
✦ Leukopenia
✦ Seizures, especially in patients with seizure disorders

Teaching a patient about amantadine and rimantadine

Whenever amantadine or rimantadine is prescribed, teach the patient and his family the drug's name, dose, frequency, action, and adverse effects. Also take the following actions.
✦ Instruct the patient to take the drug after meals for maximum absorption.
✦ Advise a geriatric patient to take the drug in two daily doses rather than a single dose to avoid adverse neurologic reactions.
✦ Instruct the patient with insomnia to take the drug several hours before bedtime.
✦ Tell the patient to stand or change positions slowly if orthostatic hypotension occurs.
✦ Instruct the patient to report adverse reactions, especially signs of central nervous system (CNS) disturbances (dizziness, depression, anxiety, and nausea) and renal impairment (change in urine or in urine elimination pattern).
✦ Caution the patient not to perform activities that require alertness or physical coordination if adverse CNS reactions occur.
✦ Teach the patient to use infection-control measures, such as staying away from crowds or people with infections, if leukopenia occurs.
✦ Advise the patient to be alert for excessive anticholinergic effects if he also takes an anticholinergic.
✦ Teach the patient how to handle such adverse reactions as dry mouth or constipation.
✦ Instruct the patient to limit salt and fluid intake if fluid retention occurs.
✦ Instruct the patient to notify the prescriber if adverse reactions or interactions occur.

tion, constipation, and vomiting. Amantadine may also cause hypersensitivity reactions.

Similar adverse reactions have been reported with rimantadine. However, they tend to be less severe.

Nursing considerations
✦ Give the drug cautiously to a patient who also receives an anticholinergic.
✦ Closely monitor the patient for excessive anticholinergic effects.
✦ Monitor the patient for adverse reactions or drug interactions during therapy. Notify the prescriber if any occur.
✦ If the patient experiences insomnia, give amantadine or rimantadine early in the day to prevent sleep loss.
✦ Take seizure precautions when giving amantadine to a patient with a history of seizures.
✦ Closely monitor the patient with a history of heart failure for exacerbation or recurrence of heart failure as evidenced by shortness of breath, tachycardia, jugular vein distention, or crackles in the lungs.
✦ Reduce the dosage for a patient with renal impairment or a history of seizures.
✦ Teach the patient and his family about the prescribed drug. (See *Teaching a patient about amantadine and rimantadine*.)

Key nursing actions
✦ Monitor the patient for excessive anticholinergic effects.
✦ If the patient develops insomnia, give the drug early in the day.
✦ Take seizure precautions if the patient has a history of seizures.
✦ If the patient has a history of heart failure, watch closely for worsening or recurrence.

FOSCARNET

The antiviral foscarnet is most commonly used to treat cytomegalovirus (CMV) retinitis in patients with acquired immunodeficiency syndrome (AIDS).

Pharmacokinetics

After I.V. infusion, foscarnet is poorly bound to plasma proteins. In patients with normal renal function, the majority of a dose is excreted unchanged in urine.

Pharmacodynamics

Foscarnet prevents viral replication by selectively inhibiting DNA polymerase, an enzyme that helps form DNA from a precursor substance that exists in DNA.

Pharmacotherapeutics

Primarily, foscarnet is used to treat CMV retinitis in patients with AIDS. If CMV retinitis progresses or relapses, patients may be retreated with foscarnet or may begin combination therapy with foscarnet and ganciclovir. Foscarnet is also used to treat acyclovir-resistant herpes simplex virus (HSV) infections in immunocompromised patients.

Interactions

◆ Together, foscarnet and pentamidine increase the risk of hypocalcemia and renal toxicity.
◆ Use of foscarnet with another drug that alters the calcium level may result in hypocalcemia.
◆ When foscarnet is used with a nephrotoxic drug, such as amphotericin B or an aminoglycoside, the risk of renal impairment increases.

Adverse reactions

With foscarnet, adverse reactions include fever, fatigue, rigors, asthenia, malaise, pain, infection, sepsis, headache, paresthesia, dizziness, involuntary muscle contractions, hypoesthesia, neuropathy, seizures, anorexia, nausea, vomiting, diarrhea, abdominal pain, anemia, granulocytopenia, leukopenia, mineral and electrolyte imbalances, depression, confusion, anxiety, coughing, dyspnea, rash, increased sweating, altered renal function, vision disturbances, and death.

Nursing considerations

◆ Don't give foscarnet by rapid I.V. or bolus infusion because high levels are linked to toxicity.
◆ Monitor the patient periodically for adverse reactions or drug interactions during foscarnet therapy. Notify the prescriber if any occur.
◆ Closely monitor the patient's renal function, especially the creatinine level, during therapy. Because foscarnet can cause renal dysfunction, adjust the dosage to changes in renal function.
◆ Because of the risk of renal toxicity, aggressively hydrate the patient with each treatment.
◆ Closely monitor the patient's electrolyte levels because transient changes may increase the risk of cardiac disturbances and seizures.
◆ Regularly monitor the patient's CBC during therapy. Notify the prescriber of any abnormalities.

Features of foscarnet

◆ Prevents viral replication by selectively inhibiting DNA polymerase
◆ Is mainly used for CMV retinitis in patients with AIDS
◆ Is also used for acyclovir-resistant HSV infections in immunocompromised patients

Adverse reactions to watch for

◆ Abdominal pain, anorexia, diarrhea, nausea, vomiting
◆ Altered renal function
◆ Anemia, granulocytopenia, leukopenia
◆ Anxiety, confusion, depression
◆ Asthenia, dizziness, fatigue, headache, hypoesthesia, involuntary muscle contractions, malaise, neuropathy, pain, paresthesia, rigors, seizures
◆ Coughing, dyspnea
◆ Fever, infection, sepsis
◆ Increased sweating, rash
◆ Mineral and electrolyte imbalances
◆ Vision disturbances

Key nursing actions

◆ Monitor renal function, especially the creatinine level.
◆ Hydrate the patient aggressively with each treatment.
◆ Monitor electrolyte levels closely.
◆ Monitor the CBC regularly.
◆ Assess the patient for evidence of infection if leukopenia develops.

Teaching a patient about foscarnet

Whenever foscarnet is prescribed, teach the patient and his family the drug's name, dose, frequency, action, and adverse effects. Also take the following actions.

✦ Instruct the patient to notify the nurse if he feels pain or discomfort at the I.V. infusion site.

✦ Inform a pregnant patient that foscarnet use during pregnancy is indicated only if the potential benefit to her justifies the potential risk to her fetus.

✦ Advise the patient to seek assistance with walking and getting out of bed if vision disturbances occur.

✦ Tell the patient to immediately report any symptoms of hypocalcemia, such as perioral tingling, numbness in the arms or legs, and paresthesia.

✦ Advise the patient that the drug doesn't cure cytomegalovirus-induced retinitis and that retinitis may progress during or after treatment.

✦ Explain the importance of adequate hydration during therapy.

✦ Instruct the patient to notify the prescriber if adverse reactions occur.

Features of NNRTIs

✦ Delavirdine and nevirapine interfere with the action of reverse transcriptase enzyme so replication can't occur

✦ Efavirenz competes for reverse transcriptase through non-competitive inhibition

✦ Are used with other antivirals to treat HIV infection

✦ Nevirapine is used for patients whose condition has begun to deteriorate

Possible drug interactions

✦ Benzodiazepines
✦ Clarithromycin
✦ Hormonal contraceptives
✦ Indinavir
✦ Protease inhibitors
✦ Rifabutin
✦ Saquinavir
✦ Warfarin

✦ Closely monitor the patient for signs and symptoms of infection, such as fever, chills, cough, and purulent drainage, if he develops leukopenia. Take infection-control measures until his white blood cell (WBC) count returns to normal.

✦ If anemia occurs, stagger the patient's activities and provide frequent rest periods.

✦ Teach the patient and his family about the prescribed drug. (See *Teaching a patient about foscarnet.*)

NON-NUCLEOSIDE REVERSE TRANSCRIPTASE INHIBITORS

NNRTIs are used with other antiretrovirals to treat HIV infection. Drugs in this class include delavirdine, efavirenz, and nevirapine.

Pharmacokinetics

After absorption and distribution, delavirdine and efavirenz are highly protein-bound; nevirapine is widely distributed throughout the body. All three drugs are metabolized by the cytochrome P450 liver enzyme system. Excretion occurs in urine and feces.

Pharmacodynamics

Delavirdine and nevirapine interfere with the action of reverse transcriptase enzyme by binding to the enzyme and preventing it from exerting an effect so replication can't occur. Efavirenz competes for the enzyme through non-competitive inhibition.

Pharmacotherapeutics

NNRTIs are used with other antiretrovirals to treat HIV infection; nevirapine is specifically indicated for patients whose condition has begun to deteriorate.

WARNING

Managing nevirapine reactions

Because nevirapine can produce a life-threatening rash, you must be prepared to detect and manage this adverse reaction and related ones by following these steps:

✦ During nevirapine therapy, be especially alert for a severe rash or a rash accompanied by fever. Most rashes occur in the first 6 weeks of therapy.

✦ Monitor the patient for related signs and symptoms, such as blistering, oral lesions, conjunctivitis, muscle or joint aches, or general malaise.

✦ Report a rash or any related signs and symptoms to the prescriber.

✦ If a rash occurs during the first 14 days of therapy, don't increase the dosage until the rash has resolved.

Interactions

✦ Delavirdine may increase the level of a benzodiazepine, clarithromycin, rifabutin, saquinavir, or warfarin.

✦ Delavirdine may significantly increase the indinavir level, which requires a decreased indinavir dosage.

✦ Efavirenz interacts with indinavir, which requires an increased indinavir dose.

✦ Nevirapine may decrease the activity of a protease inhibitor or hormonal contraceptive.

Adverse reactions

Common adverse reactions to delavirdine are fatigue, headache, asthenia, nausea, and rash. Common reactions to efavirenz include dizziness, diarrhea, and rash; to nevirapine include fever and nausea.

 CLINICAL ALERT The use of nevirapine has been linked to the development of a severe rash. In some cases, the rash may be severe enough to become life-threatening.

Nursing considerations

✦ Use an NNRTI cautiously in a patient with renal or hepatic impairment.

✦ Monitor the patient's CBC and liver function test results before starting therapy and throughout therapy.

✦ Monitor the patient periodically for adverse reactions and drug interactions during NNRTI therapy. If they occur, alert the prescriber.

✦ Monitor the patient for a rash and related reactions. (See *Managing nevirapine reactions*.)

✦ Be alert for signs of resistance, which can develop with monotherapy. For best results, combination therapy with other retrovirals is recommended.

✦ Administer efavirenz at bedtime to minimize adverse CNS effects.

 CLINICAL ALERT If nevirapine therapy is interrupted for more than 7 days, restart therapy as if the patient were receiving the drug for the first time.

✦ Teach the patient and his family about the prescribed drug. (See *Teaching a patient about NNRTIs*, page 330.)

Adverse reactions to watch for

delavirdine
✦ Asthenia
✦ Fatigue
✦ Headache
✦ Nausea
✦ Rash

efavirenz
✦ Diarrhea
✦ Dizziness
✦ Rash

nevirapine
✦ Fever
✦ Life-threatening rash
✦ Nausea

Key nursing actions

✦ Monitor the CBC and liver function tests before and during therapy.

✦ Watch for rash and related reactions.

✦ Watch for evidence of resistance if the patient receives monotherapy.

✦ If nevirapine therapy stops for more than 7 days, restart as though the patient were receiving the drug for the first time.

Teaching a patient about NNRTIs

Whenever a non-nucleoside reverse transcriptase inhibitor (NNRTI) is prescribed, teach the patient and his family the drug's name, dose, frequency, action, and adverse effects. Also take the following actions.

✦ Tell the patient to stop the drug and call the prescriber if a rash occurs.
✦ Instruct the patient to take efavirenz at bedtime.
✦ Inform the patient that these drugs don't reduce the risk of transmitting the human immunodeficiency virus to others through sexual contact or blood contamination.
✦ Stress the importance of returning regularly for blood tests.
✦ Advise a woman of childbearing age that hormonal contraceptives shouldn't be used with nevirapine.
✦ Caution the patient not to perform activities that require alertness if dizziness or other adverse central nervous system reactions occur.
✦ Instruct the patient to notify the prescriber if adverse reactions occur.

Features of NRTIs

✦ Must be converted to active metabolites to act
✦ Abacavir inhibits HIV-1 transcriptase
✦ Didanosine and zalcitabine block HIV replication
✦ Lamivudine and stavudine inhibit viral DNA replication
✦ Zidovudine prevents viral DNA from replicating

NUCLEOSIDE REVERSE TRANSCRIPTASE INHIBITORS

NRTIs are used to treat advanced HIV infections. Drugs in this class include abacavir, didanosine, lamivudine, stavudine, zalcitabine, and zidovudine. Zidovudine was the first drug approved by the Food and Drug Administration for treating AIDS and AIDS-related complex.

Pharmacokinetics

After oral administration, abacavir is rapidly and extensively absorbed. It's distributed in the extravascular space, and about 50% binds with plasma proteins. The drug is metabolized by enzymes and primarily excreted in urine with the remainder excreted in feces.

Because didanosine is degraded rapidly in gastric acid, didanosine tablets and powder contain a buffering drug to increase pH. The exact route of metabolism isn't fully understood. About half of an absorbed dose is excreted in urine.

Lamivudine and stavudine are rapidly absorbed after administration, and are excreted by the kidneys.

Oral zalcitabine is absorbed well from the GI tract when given on an empty stomach. Absorption is reduced when the drug is given with food. Zalcitabine penetrates the blood-brain barrier.

Zidovudine is absorbed well from the GI tract, distributed widely throughout the body, metabolized by the liver, and excreted by the kidneys.

Pharmacodynamics

NRTIs must undergo conversion to their active metabolites to produce their action. Abacavir is converted to an active metabolite that inhibits the activity of HIV-1 transcriptase by competing with a natural component and incorporating into viral DNA.

Didanosine and zalcitabine undergo cellular enzyme conversion to their active antiviral metabolites to block HIV replication.

Lamivudine and stavudine are converted to their active metabolites, which inhibit viral DNA replication.

EYE ON DRUG ACTION

How zidovudine works

Zidovudine can inhibit replication of human immunodeficiency virus (HIV). The first two illustrations show how HIV invades cells and then replicates itself. The bottom illustration shows how zidovudine blocks the virus from transforming.

HIV invasion and replication

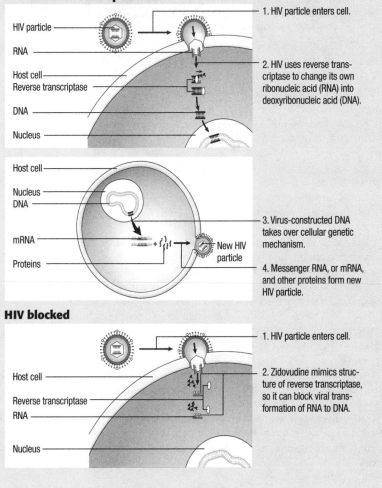

1. HIV particle enters cell.

2. HIV uses reverse transcriptase to change its own ribonucleic acid (RNA) into deoxyribonucleic acid (DNA).

3. Virus-constructed DNA takes over cellular genetic mechanism.

4. Messenger RNA, or mRNA, and other proteins form new HIV particle.

HIV blocked

1. HIV particle enters cell.

2. Zidovudine mimics structure of reverse transcriptase, so it can block viral transformation of RNA to DNA.

Uses of NRTIs

+ Are used, usually with other antivirals, to treat HIV infection and AIDS
+ I.V. zidovudine is used for hospitalized patients and those who can't take oral drugs. Also used to prevent HIV transmission from mother to fetus and to treat AIDS-related dementia
+ Oral zidovudine is used in multidrug regimen to treat HIV infection

Zidovudine is converted by cellular enzymes to an active form, zidovudine triphosphate, which prevents viral DNA from replicating. (See *How zidovudine works.*)

Pharmacotherapeutics

NRTIs are used to treat HIV and AIDS. Abacavir, lamivudine, stavudine, and zalcitabine are used with other antiretroviral to treat HIV infection. Didanosine, used with other antiretrovirals, is an alternative initial treatment of HIV infection.

Possible drug interactions

✦ Acetaminophen
✦ Acyclovir
✦ Alcohol
✦ Antacids containing aluminum or magnesium
✦ Aspirin
✦ Chloramphenicol
✦ Cimetidine
✦ Cisplatin
✦ Dapsone
✦ Delavirdine
✦ Doxorubicin
✦ Ethionamide
✦ Flucytosine
✦ Fluoroquinolones
✦ Ganciclovir
✦ Gold salts
✦ Hydralazine
✦ Indomethacin
✦ Interferon
✦ Iodoquinol
✦ Isoniazid
✦ Lorazepam
✦ Metronidazole
✦ Nitrofurantoin
✦ Pentamidine isethionate
✦ Probenecid
✦ Tetracyclines
✦ Vinblastine
✦ Vincristine

Adverse reactions to watch for

abacavir
✦ Anorexia, diarrhea, hypersensitivity reactions, nausea, vomiting

didanosine
✦ Abdominal pain, alopecia, arthritis, asthenia, CNS depression, constipation, diarrhea, dizziness, dry mouth, headache, insomnia, loss of taste, myalgia, nausea, pancreatitis, peripheral neuropathy, pruritus, rash, stomatitis, unusual taste, vomiting

WARNING

Coping with hypersensitivity reactions to abacavir

Hypersensitivity reactions to abacavir can be fatal. That's why it's important to deal with them quickly and effectively. To do that, follow these steps:
✦ Closely monitor the patient for signs and symptoms of a hypersensitivity reaction, such as fever, rash, fatigue, nausea, vomiting, diarrhea, and abdominal pain.
✦ At the first sign of hypersensitivity, stop the drug and notify the prescriber immediately.
✦ Don't restart abacavir after a hypersensitivity reaction. Otherwise, severe signs and symptoms will recur within hours and may include breathing difficulties, life-threatening hypotension, and death.

Zidovudine is given I.V. to help patients who are hospitalized and can't take oral drugs. It's also used to prevent HIV transmission from mother to fetus and to treat AIDS-related dementia. Oral zidovudine is used as part of a multidrug regimen for treating HIV infection. Doses of either form may need to be adjusted in patients with renal or hepatic disease.

Interactions

✦ Alcohol consumption can increase the abacavir level.
✦ Didanosine may reduce the absorption of delavirdine, a fluoroquinolone, or a tetracycline.
✦ Lamivudine can inhibit phosphorylation of zalcitabine.
✦ Stavudine can inhibit phosphorylation of zidovudine.
✦ Zalcitabine increases the risk of peripheral neuropathy when taken with chloramphenicol, cimetidine, cisplatin, didanosine, ethionamide, gold salts, hydralazine, iodoquinol, isoniazid, metronidazole, nitrofurantoin, or vincristine.
✦ When used together, zalcitabine and pentamidine isethionate increase the risk of pancreatitis.
✦ An antacid that contains aluminum or magnesium can reduce zalcitabine absorption.
✦ Use of zidovudine with a drug such as dapsone, doxorubicin, flucytosine, ganciclovir, interferon, pentamidine isethionate, vinblastine, or vincristine can increase the risk of cellular and renal toxicity.
✦ Use of zidovudine with acetaminophen, aspirin, cimetidine, indomethacin, probenecid, or lorazepam can increase the risk of toxicity of either drug.
✦ Together, zidovudine and acyclovir may produce profound lethargy and drowsiness.

Adverse reactions

The most common adverse reactions reported in patients taking abacavir are nausea, vomiting, diarrhea, and anorexia. Hypersensitivity reactions may also occur. (See *Coping with hypersensitivity reactions to abacavir.*)

Adverse reactions to didanosine reported in 5% or more of adults include headache, diarrhea, peripheral neuropathy, asthenia, nausea, vomiting, insomnia, rash, pruritus, abdominal pain, CNS depression, constipation, stomatitis, myalgia, arthritis, loss of taste, unusual taste in the mouth, dry mouth, pancreatitis, alopecia, and dizziness.

LIFESPAN

Reducing the dangers of lamivudine in children

Pediatric patients are unusually susceptible to lamivudine's ability to trigger pancreatitis. To reduce this danger, use the drug with extreme caution, if at all, in a child with a history of pancreatitis or other significant risk factors for pancreatitis. When the drug must be used, monitor the child for signs and symptoms of pancreatitis, such as abdominal pain, fever, anorexia, nausea, and vomiting. Also, monitor his amylase level. If you note signs or symptoms or an increased amylase level, withhold lamivudine immediately and notify the prescriber.

CLINICAL ALERT In pregnant women, combination therapy with didanosine, stavudine, and another antiretroviral has caused fatal lactic acidosis.

Typically, lamivudine causes adverse GI effects. These include nausea, diarrhea, vomiting, anorexia, decreased appetite, abdominal pain, abdominal cramps, and dyspepsia. Rarely, the drug has caused pancreatitis. It may also produce peripheral neuropathy, malaise, fatigue, headache, rash, anemia, neutropenia, pain, myalgia, arthralgia, nasal signs and symptoms, cough, and fever or chills.

Adverse reactions to stavudine include fever, asthenia, abdominal pain, diarrhea, nausea, vomiting, anorexia, arthralgia, myalgia, back pain, dyspnea, rash, diaphoresis, pruritus, and chills.

In more than 5% of patients, adverse reactions to zalcitabine include peripheral neuropathy, mouth ulcers, nausea, rash, headache, myalgia, and fatigue.

The most common adverse reactions to zidovudine are hematologic. Significant anemia occurs 4 to 6 weeks after therapy begins; granulocytopenia appears within 6 to 8 weeks. Headache has been reported in up to 50% of patients who have received zidovudine. Other CNS reactions include dizziness, agitation, restlessness, and insomnia. Nausea, vomiting, abdominal pain, diarrhea, dyspepsia, and anorexia are the most common GI reactions. Myalgia, diaphoresis, dyspnea, fever, rash, and unusual taste in the mouth may also occur.

Nursing considerations

CLINICAL ALERT Avoid monotherapy with any single drug for HIV infection. For best results, use a combination of antiretrovirals. However, don't give lamivudine with zalcitabine and don't give stavudine with zidovudine. These combinations inhibit phosphorylation.

✦ Monitor the patient periodically for adverse reactions and drug interactions during therapy. If they occur, alert the prescriber.

✦ Monitor the patient's red blood cell (RBC) and WBC counts during zalcitabine or zidovudine therapy.

✦ Monitor the patient closely for pancreatitis and peripheral neuropathy. Be aware that pancreatitis may be fatal, especially in children who receive lamivudine. (See *Reducing the dangers of lamivudine in children.*) If pancreatitis is suspected, stop the drug immediately.

✦ Give didanosine and zalcitabine on an empty stomach.

Adverse reactions to watch for
(continued)

lamivudine
✦ Abdominal cramps or pain, anemia, anorexia, arthralgia, chills, cough, diarrhea, decreased appetite, dyspepsia, fatigue, fever, headache, malaise, myalgia, nasal signs and symptoms, nausea, neutropenia, pain, pancreatitis, peripheral neuropathy, rash, vomiting

stavudine
✦ Abdominal pain, anorexia, arthralgia, asthenia, back pain, chills, diaphoresis, diarrhea, dyspnea, fever, myalgia, nausea, pruritus, rash, vomiting

zalcitabine
✦ Fatigue, headache, mouth ulcers, myalgia, nausea, peripheral neuropathy, rash

zidovudine
✦ Abdominal pain, agitation, anemia, anorexia, diaphoresis, diarrhea, dizziness, dyspepsia, dyspnea, fever, granulocytopenia, headache, insomnia, myalgia, nausea, rash, restlessness, unusual taste, vomiting

Key nursing actions
✦ Monitor RBC and WBC counts during zalcitabine or zidovudine therapy.
✦ Monitor the patient closely for pancreatitis and peripheral neuropathy. (Pancreatitis can be fatal, especially in children who receive lamivudine.)
✦ Give didanosine and zalcitabine when the patient has an empty stomach.

Teaching a patient about NRTIs

Whenever a nucleoside reverse transcriptase inhibitor (NRTI) is prescribed, teach the patient and his family the drug's name, dose, frequency, action, and adverse effects. Also take the following actions.

✦ Instruct the patient to take the NRTI as directed even if it means interrupting sleep.
✦ Inform the patient that the NRTI doesn't reduce the risk of transmitting the human immunodeficiency virus to others through sexual contact or blood contamination.
✦ Caution the patient to avoid over-the-counter drugs and to check with the prescriber, pharmacist, or nurse before taking any.
✦ Instruct the patient to take didanosine or zalcitabine on an empty stomach.
✦ Tell the patient to immediately report signs and symptoms of pancreatitis, such as abdominal pain and vomiting. Also tell him to report numbness, tingling, or pain in his hands or feet.
✦ Instruct the patient to notify the prescriber if other adverse reactions occur.
✦ Advise the patient with phenylketonuria that didanosine contains phenylalanine.
✦ Stress the importance of returning regularly for blood tests.
✦ Caution the patient not to perform activities that require alertness if dizziness or other adverse central nervous system reactions occur.

✦ Use didanosine or stavudine cautiously in a pregnant woman.
✦ Teach the patient and his family about the prescribed drug. (See *Teaching a patient about NRTIs*.)

TENOFOVIR

Tenofovir is used with other antiretrovirals in the treatment of HIV. Tenofovir is a nucleotide reverse transcriptase inhibitor (or NtRTI) and works similarly to the NRTIs.

Pharmacokinetics

Tenofovir is absorbed much better after a high-fat meal. Then it's distributed in small amounts into plasma and serum proteins. Its metabolism probably isn't mediated by cytochrome P450 liver enzymes, and the drug is excreted via the kidneys.

Pharmacodynamics

Tenofovir stops HIV by competing with substrates. It's subsequently incorporated into the DNA chain, halting HIV replication.

Pharmacotherapeutics

Along with other drugs, tenofovir is used to treat HIV infection.

Interactions

✦ A drug that's eliminated through the kidneys or that decreases renal function may increase the tenofovir level.
✦ Tenofovir may increase the didanosine level, worsening didanosine's adverse effects.

Features of tenofovir

✦ Stops HIV replication by competing with substrates and being incorporated into the DNA chain
✦ Is used with other drugs to treat HIV infection
✦ Is absorbed much better after a high-fat meal

Teaching a patient about tenofovir

Whenever tenofovir is prescribed, teach the patient and his family the drug's name, dose, frequency, action, and adverse effects. Also take the following actions.
✦ Inform the patient that the drug doesn't reduce the risk of transmitting the human immunodeficiency virus to others through sexual contact or blood contamination.
✦ Instruct the patient to take the drug with a meal to enhance its bioavailability.
✦ If the patient takes tenofovir and didanosine (buffered form), advise him to take tenofovir 2 hours before or 1 hour after didanosine.
✦ Instruct the patient to notify the prescriber if adverse reactions occur.

Adverse reactions

The most common adverse reactions to tenofovir are GI disturbances, such as nausea, diarrhea, vomiting, and flatulence. Tenofovir may be linked to bone abnormalities, such as osteomalacia and decreased bone mineral density, and renal toxicity because of increased creatinine and phosphaturia levels.

 CLINICAL ALERT Potentially fatal lactic acidosis and severe hepatomegaly with steatosis have been reported rarely in patients taking tenofovir alone or with another antiretroviral. Women and patients who are obese or who have had prior exposure to NRTIs may be at risk.

Nursing considerations

✦ Assess the patient for liver disease before tenofovir therapy begins. Use the drug with caution in a patient with preexisting liver disease. Monitor his liver function periodically, and suspend treatment if hepatotoxicity is suspected.
✦ Monitor the patient for signs and symptoms of bone abnormalities and renal toxicity.
✦ Monitor the patient periodically for adverse reactions and drug interactions during therapy. If they occur, alert the prescriber.
✦ Teach the patient and his family about the prescribed drug. (See *Teaching a patient about tenofovir*.)

PROTEASE INHIBITORS

In HIV infection, protease inhibitors act against the enzyme HIV protease and prevent it from dividing a larger viral precursor protein into the active smaller enzymes that the virus needs to fully mature. The result is an immature, noninfectious cell.

Drugs in this class include amprenavir, indinavir, lopinavir and ritonavir, nelfinavir, ritonavir, and saquinavir.

Pharmacokinetics

Amprenavir is metabolized in the liver to active and inactive metabolites, and is minimally excreted as unchanged drug in urine and feces.

Adverse reactions to watch for

✦ Bone abnormalities, such as osteomalacia and decreased bone mineral density
✦ Diarrhea, flatulence, nausea, vomiting
✦ Lactic acidosis
✦ Renal toxicity caused by increased creatinine level and phosphaturia
✦ Severe hepatomegaly with steatosis

Key nursing actions

✦ Assess the patient for liver disease before therapy starts.
✦ Monitor the patient for evidence of bone abnormalities and renal toxicity.

Features of protease inhibitors

✦ Inhibit the activity of HIV protease and prevent the cleavage of viral polyproteins
✦ Are used in combination therapy to treat HIV infection
✦ Are combined (as lopinavir and ritonavir) for their positive effects on the HIV RNA level and CD4 counts

Possible interactions

- Alpha-adrenergic blockers
- Amiodarone
- Antiarrhythmics
- Antidepressants
- Antiemetics
- Antifungals
- Antilipemics
- Antimalarials
- Antineoplastics
- Beta blockers
- Calcium channel blockers
- Carbamazepine
- Cimetidine
- Corticosteroids
- Dexamethasone
- Didanosine
- Ergot derivatives
- Erythromycin
- Immunosuppressants
- Methylphenidate
- Midazolam
- Pentoxifylline
- Phenobarbital
- Phenothiazines
- Phenytoin
- Quinidine
- Rifabutin
- Rifampin
- St. John's wort
- Triazolam
- Warfarin

Adverse reactions to watch for

amprenavir
- Diarrhea, loose stools, nausea, vomiting
- Hyperglycemia, hypertriglyceridemia
- Oral and perioral paresthesia
- Rash

Indinavir is rapidly absorbed and moderately bound to plasma proteins. It's metabolized by the liver into seven metabolites. The drug is excreted mainly through feces.

Lopinavir is extensively metabolized by the liver's cytochrome P-450 system; ritonavir inhibits lopinavir's metabolism, which increases the lopinavir level. The antiviral activity of the combination is mainly due to lopinavir.

Nelfinavir's bioavailability is unknown. Food increases its absorption. It's highly protein-bound, metabolized in the liver, and excreted primarily in feces.

Ritonavir is well absorbed, metabolized by the liver, and broken down into at least five metabolites. It's mainly excreted in feces, with some elimination through the kidneys.

Saquinavir is poorly absorbed from the GI tract. It's widely distributed, highly bound to plasma proteins, metabolized by the liver, and excreted mainly by the kidneys.

Pharmacodynamics
All of these drugs inhibit the activity of HIV protease and prevent the cleavage of viral polyproteins.

Pharmacotherapeutics
Protease inhibitors are used in combination therapy to treat HIV infection. Lopinavir is used with ritonavir because this combination has positive effects on the HIV RNA level and on CD4 counts.

Interactions
- Buffering drugs in didanosine decrease gastric absorption of indinavir.
- Indinavir can inhibit the metabolism of midazolam or triazolam, increasing the risk of potentially fatal events, such as arrhythmias.
- Rifampin significantly reduces the indinavir level.
- Indinavir or ritonavir may increase the nelfinavir level.
- Nelfinavir may greatly increase the levels of amiodarone, ergot derivatives, midazolam, quinidine, rifabutin, or triazolam.
- Carbamazepine, phenobarbital, or phenytoin may reduce nelfinavir's effectiveness.
- Ritonavir inhibits lopinavir metabolism, leading to an increased lopinavir level.
- Ritonavir may increase the effects of cimetidine, erythromycin, methylphenidate, pentoxifylline, a phenothiazine, warfarin, or an alpha-adrenergic blocker, antiarrhythmic, antidepressant, antiemetic, antifungal, antilipemic, antimalarial, antineoplastic, beta blocker, calcium channel blocker, corticosteroid, or immunosuppressant.
- Carbamazepine, dexamethasone, phenobarbital, and phenytoin may reduce saquinavir's action.
- St. John's wort may increase hepatic metabolism of a protease inhibitor, which decreases the drug's therapeutic effects.

Adverse reactions
Common adverse reactions to amprenavir are oral and perioral paresthesia, nausea, vomiting, diarrhea or loose stools, hyperglycemia, hypertriglyceridemia, and rash.

Indinavir's common adverse reactions include abdominal pain, asthenia, fatigue, flank pain, malaise, nausea, diarrhea, vomiting, acid regurgitation, anorexia,

Avoiding the risks of protease inhibitors

In certain patients, protease inhibitors pose special risks. To avoid these risks, take the following steps:
✦ Discourage breast-feeding in mothers who receive saquinavir mesylate. It's not known whether this drug appears in breast milk.
✦ Urge a mother to stop breast-feeding during indinavir sulfate therapy. This drug appears in breast milk.

dry mouth, headache, insomnia, dizziness, sleeplessness, taste perversion, and back pain.

Rash was commonly reported with the use of lopinavir and ritonavir. The most common adverse effects with ritonavir include asthenia and GI and neurologic disturbances, such as nausea, diarrhea, vomiting, anorexia, abdominal pain, taste perversion, and circumoral and peripheral paresthesia.

Most adverse reactions to saquinavir are mild. The most common ones are diarrhea, abdominal discomfort, and nausea. Less common reactions include rash, eczema, and photosensitivity. These reactions rarely occur: confusion, ataxia, weakness, acute myeloblastic leukemia, hemolytic anemia, Stevens-Johnson syndrome, seizures, severe cutaneous reaction related to increased liver function test results, isolated elevation of transaminases, thrombophlebitis, headache, thrombocytopenia, exacerbation of chronic liver disease with grade 4 elevated liver function tests, jaundice, ascites, and right and left upper quadrant abdominal pain. Because many HIV-infected patients have numerous diseases, it's not fully clear whether these effects are drug reactions or disease symptoms.

Nursing considerations
✦ Monitor the patient periodically for adverse reactions and drug interactions during protease inhibitor therapy. Notify the prescriber if any occur.
✦ Warn the patient taking saquinavir to avoid exposure to ultraviolet light, because photosensitization may occur.
✦ Use protease inhibitors cautiously in a patient with impaired liver function because the liver metabolizes all of these drugs.
✦ Caution a breast-feeding woman about protease inhibitor use. (See *Avoiding the risks of protease inhibitors.*)
✦ Don't give amprenavir with high-fat foods.
✦ For optimal absorption, give indinavir without food and with a full glass of water at least 1 hour before a meal.
✦ Separate indinavir and didanosine administration by at least 1 hour.
✦ Give ritonavir or lopinavir and ritonavir with food.
✦ Give saquinavir within 2 hours after a full meal.
✦ Teach the patient and his family about the prescribed drug. (See *Teaching a patient about protease inhibitors.* page 338.)

(See *Teaching a patient about protease inhibitors.* page 338.)

Adverse reactions to watch for
(continued)

indinavir
✦ Abdominal pain, asthenia, back pain, fatigue, flank pain, headache, malaise,
✦ Acid regurgitation, anorexia, diarrhea, dry mouth, nausea, taste perversion, vomiting
✦ Dizziness, insomnia

lopinavir and ritonavir
✦ Rash

ritonavir
✦ Abdominal pain, anorexia, diarrhea, nausea, taste perversion, vomiting
✦ Asthenia
✦ Oral and peripheral paresthesia

saquinavir
✦ Abdominal discomfort, diarrhea, nausea

Key nursing actions
✦ If patient takes saquinavir, warn about possible photosensitivity.
✦ Give these drugs cautiously to patients with impaired liver function.
✦ Caution pregnant women about protease inhibitors.

Teaching a patient about protease inhibitors

Whenever a protease inhibitor is prescribed, teach the patient and his family the drug's name, dose, frequency, action, and adverse effects. Also take the following actions.

◆ Advise the patient that no protease inhibitor has been shown to reduce the risk of transmitting the human immunodeficiency virus through sexual contact or blood contamination.
◆ Instruct the patient to avoid exposure to ultraviolet light during saquinavir mesylate therapy because photosensitization may occur.
◆ Advise the patient to take saquinavir mesylate within 2 hours after a full meal.
◆ Tell the patient to take ritonavir or ritonavir and lopinavir with food.
◆ Instruct the patient to take indinavir sulfate without food and with a full glass of water at least 1 hour before a meal.
◆ Tell the patient to take ritonavir or indinavir sulfate every day as prescribed. If a dose is missed, he should take the next dose as soon as possible. However, he shouldn't take a double dose.
◆ Suggest that the patient improve the taste of ritonavir by mixing it with chocolate milk, Ensure, or Advera up to 1 hour before taking it.
◆ Advise the patient to store moisture-sensitive indinavir capsules in the original container with the desiccant.
◆ Advise a breast-feeding woman to avoid breast-feeding while taking a protease inhibitor because the drug may appear in breast milk.
◆ Tell the patient not to take amprenavir with high-fat foods.
◆ Instruct the patient to store ritonavir in the refrigerator. Advise him that, if needed, the drug can be unrefrigerated for up to 30 days.

RIBAVIRIN

Currently, ribavirin is available to treat respiratory syncytial virus (RSV) infections in children. It's also used with interferon alfa-2b for treating chronic hepatitis C. It's given by aerosol inhalation with a small-particle aerosol generator, such as the Viratek Model 2, or by capsule for hepatitis C treatment.

Pharmacokinetics

After nasal or oral inhalation, ribavirin is absorbed well. It has a limited, specific distribution and reaches its highest levels in the respiratory tract and in RBCs. Ribavirin capsules are rapidly absorbed after administration and distributed in the plasma.

The drug is metabolized in the liver and by RBCs. It's excreted primarily by the kidneys, with some excreted in feces.

Pharmacodynamics

The mechanism of action of ribavirin isn't known completely, but the drug's metabolites inhibit viral DNA and RNA synthesis, subsequently halting viral replication.

Pharmacotherapeutics

Ribavirin therapy is used to treat severe lower respiratory tract infections caused by RSV in infants and young children. It's also used to treat chronic hepatitis C.

Features of ribavirin
◆ Has metabolites that inhibit viral DNA and RNA synthesis, halting viral replication
◆ Is used for severe RSV infections in infants and young children
◆ Is used for chronic hepatitis C

Interactions

✦ Ribavirin reduces zidovudine's antiviral activity; combined use may cause blood toxicity.

✦ Use of ribavirin with digoxin can cause digoxin toxicity, producing such effects as GI distress, CNS abnormalities, and arrhythmias.

Adverse reactions

Reactions to ribavirin include worsening of respiratory function, ventilator dependence, pneumothorax, apnea, cardiac arrest, and hypotension. Reticulosis also has been reported. Other adverse reactions include rash, conjunctivitis, and erythema of the eyelids.

Nursing considerations

✦ Give inhaled ribavirin with the Viratek SPAG-2 only. Don't use any other aerosol-generating device.

✦ For a patient who is mechanically ventilated, use heated wire connection tubing with bacterial filters in the system's expiratory limb; otherwise, ribavirin can precipitate in the ventilator and jeopardize adequate ventilation. Suction the patient every 1 to 2 hours.

✦ Monitor the patient closely for adverse reactions and drug interactions during ribavirin therapy and report them to the prescriber.

✦ Monitor the patient's cardiac status throughout ribavirin therapy. If hypotension or cardiac dysfunction occurs, notify the prescriber. Keep standard emergency equipment nearby and, if cardiac arrest occurs, be prepared to begin cardiopulmonary resuscitation.

✦ Use sterile USP water for injection, not bacteriostatic water. Water used to reconstitute this aerosol drug must not contain any antimicrobial product.

✦ Store a reconstituted solution at room temperature for up to 24 hours; discard after 24 hours.

✦ Monitor the patient for anemia during oral ribavirin therapy.

✦ Teach the patient and his family about the prescribed drug. (See *Teaching a patient about ribavirin.*)

Adverse reactions to watch for

✦ Apnea, pneumothorax, ventilator dependence, worsening of respiratory function

✦ Cardiac arrest, hypotension

✦ Conjunctivitis, erythema of the eyelids

✦ Rash

✦ Reticulosis

Key nursing actions

✦ Give inhaled ribavirin only with the Viratek SPAG-2.

✦ Monitor the patient's cardiac status throughout therapy. If hypotension or cardiac dysfunction occurs, notify the prescriber. Keep emergency equipment nearby.

✦ Assess the patient for anemia during oral therapy.

Features of synthetic nucleosides

acyclovir

+ Is useful against HSV types 1 and 2 and varicella-zoster virus with minimal toxicity to body cells
+ Must be metabolized to active form in cells infected by herpesvirus
+ Oral form is used mainly for initial and recurrent HSV type 2 infections
+ I.V. form is used for initial HSV type 2 infections in patients with normal immune systems; for initial and recurrent skin and mucous membrane HSV type 1 and 2, herpes zoster, disseminated varicella-zoster virus, and varicella infections in immunocompromised patients

famciclovir

+ Is a prodrug that changes rapidly to the active antiviral compound penciclovir; inhibits replication in HSV types 1 and 2 and varicella zoster cells
+ Is used to treat acute herpes zoster and recurrent genital herpes infections

ganciclovir

+ Potent antiviral activity against HSV and CMV
+ Converted to ganciclovir triphosphate in CMV-infected cells; may produce antiviral activity by inhibiting viral DNA synthesis
+ Used for CMV retinitis in immunocompromised patients, including those with AIDS and other CMV infections, such as encephalitis

valacyclovir

+ Is converted to acyclovir

valganciclovir

+ Is converted to famciclovir

SYNTHETIC NUCLEOSIDES

Synthetic nucleosides are used for various viral syndromes, including herpes and CMV infections, which can occur in immunocompromised patients. This drug class includes acyclovir, famciclovir, ganciclovir, valacyclovir, and valganciclovir.

Pharmacokinetics

When given orally, acyclovir has slow absorption that's only 15% to 30% complete. The drug is distributed throughout the body and metabolized primarily inside infected cells; most of the drug is excreted in urine.

Famciclovir is less than 20% bound to plasma proteins. It's extensively metabolized in the liver and excreted in urine.

Ganciclovir is given I.V. because it's absorbed poorly from the GI tract. More than 90% of ganciclovir isn't metabolized and is excreted unchanged by the kidneys.

Valacyclovir and valganciclovir are readily absorbed from the GI tract and minimally bound to plasma proteins. Both drugs are metabolized in the liver and intestinal cell walls: valacyclovir is converted to acyclovir, and valganciclovir is converted to ganciclovir. They're excreted primarily in urine.

Pharmacodynamics

Acyclovir, which is useful against herpes, is an effective antiviral that causes minimal toxicity to cells. A derivative of acyclovir, ganciclovir has potent antiviral activity against HSV and CMV. To be effective, acyclovir and ganciclovir must be metabolized to their active form in cells infected by the herpesvirus. Acyclovir enters virus-infected cells, where it's changed through a series of steps to acyclovir triphosphate. Acyclovir triphosphate inhibits virus-specific DNA polymerase, an enzyme needed for viral growth, and disrupts viral replication.

Upon entry into CMV-infected cells, ganciclovir is converted to ganciclovir triphosphate, which may produce its antiviral activity by inhibiting viral DNA synthesis. Valacyclovir is rapidly converted to acyclovir. Valganciclovir is a prodrug which is converted to famciclovir.

Famciclovir is a prodrug, or a precursor of a drug, that undergoes rapid change to the active antiviral compound penciclovir. It enters viral cells (HSV types 1 and 2 and varicella zoster), where it inhibits viral replication.

Pharmacotherapeutics

Acyclovir is used to treat infection caused by herpes viruses, including HSV types 1 and 2, and varicella-zoster virus. Oral acyclovir is used primarily to treat initial and recurrent HSV type 2 infections.

Acyclovir I.V. is used to treat severe initial HSV type 2 infections in patients with normal immune systems. In immunocompromised patients, it's used to treat initial and recurrent skin and mucous membrane HSV type 1 and 2 infections, herpes zoster infections (shingles), disseminated varicella-zoster virus infections, and varicella infections (chickenpox).

Ganciclovir is used to treat CMV retinitis in immunocompromised patients, including those with AIDS and other CMV infections, such as encephalitis. Valganciclovir is also effective against CMV retinitis.

Famciclovir is used to treat acute herpes zoster and recurrent genital herpes infections. Valacyclovir is also effective against herpes infections.

Interactions

✦ Probenecid can reduce the excretion of acyclovir, famciclovir, ganciclovir, or valganciclovir, increasing the level and risk of toxicity of the synthetic nucleoside.
✦ When used with a drug that's toxic to the kidneys, acyclovir increases the risk of kidney damage.
✦ Use of ganciclovir with a drug that damages tissue cells, such as amphotericin B, dapsone, doxorubicin, flucytosine, pentamidine isethionate, a trimethoprim and sulfa combination, vincristine, or vinblastine, inhibits the replication of rapidly dividing cells in the bone marrow, GI tract, skin, and sperm-producing cells.
✦ When taken with ganciclovir or valganciclovir, imipenem and cilastatin increases the risk of seizures.
✦ When taken with ganciclovir or valganciclovir, zidovudine increases the risk of granulocytopenia.

Adverse reactions

Reversible kidney impairment may occur with rapid I.V. injection or infusion of acyclovir. Common reactions to oral acyclovir include headache, nausea, vomiting, and diarrhea. Hypersensitivity reactions may also occur with acyclovir.

Common adverse reactions to famciclovir and valacyclovir include headache and nausea.

The most common reactions to ganciclovir are granulocytopenia and thrombocytopenia.

Adverse reactions reported to valganciclovir include diarrhea, pyrexia, nausea, neutropenia, anemia, headache, vomiting, insomnia, abdominal pain, retinal detachment, peripheral neuropathy, thrombocytopenia, and paresthesia.

Nursing considerations

✦ Adjust the dosage for a patient with decreased renal function, especially during parenteral therapy.
✦ Give I.V. infusions over 60 minutes to prevent drug crystals from precipitating in the renal tubules.
✦ Keep the patient well hydrated during parenteral therapy to ensure sufficient urine output.
✦ Monitor the patient periodically for adverse reactions and drug interactions during synthetic nucleoside therapy. Notify the prescriber if any occur.
✦ Closely monitor the patient's renal function, especially the creatinine level, during parenteral therapy.
✦ Avoid inhalation or direct skin contact when giving ganciclovir because of its carcinogenic potential.
✦ Monitor the patient's CBC regularly during therapy. Also monitor his neutrophil and platelet counts.
✦ If the patient develops leukopenia, closely monitor him for signs and symptoms of infection. Take infection-control measures until the his WBC count returns to normal.
✦ If the patient develops thrombocytopenia, closely monitor him for signs of bleeding. Test his urine, feces, and vomitus for occult blood. Take bleeding precautions until his platelet level returns to normal.
✦ If anemia occurs, stagger the patient's activities and provide frequent rest periods.
✦ Notify the prescriber of abnormalities in blood test results.

Adverse reactions to watch for

acyclovir
✦ Diarrhea, headache, nausea, vomiting
✦ Hypersensitivity reactions
✦ Reversible kidney impairment (with rapid I.V. delivery)

famciclovir and valacyclovir
✦ Headache
✦ Nausea

ganciclovir
✦ Granulocytopenia
✦ Thrombocytopenia

valganciclovir
✦ Abdominal pain, diarrhea, nausea, vomiting
✦ Anemia, neutropenia, thrombocytopenia
✦ Headache, insomnia
✦ Paresthesia, peripheral neuropathy, pyrexia
✦ Retinal detachment

Key nursing actions

✦ Keep the patient well hydrated during parenteral therapy to ensure sufficient urine output.
✦ Monitor renal function closely, especially the creatinine level, during parenteral therapy.
✦ Ganciclovir is carcinogenic; don't inhale it or let it touch your skin.
✦ Check the patient's CBC and neutrophil and platelet counts during therapy.

Teaching a patient about synthetic nucleosides

Whenever a synthetic nucleoside is prescribed, teach the patient and his family the drug's name, dose, frequency, action, and adverse effects. Also take the following actions.

✦ Instruct the patient to report pain or discomfort at the I.V. site.
✦ Advise the patient to take a mild analgesic at home for headache.
✦ Advise a woman of childbearing age to use effective contraception within 90 days because of its potential effects on the fetus.
✦ Advise a breast-feeding woman to stop breast-feeding during therapy and not to resume for at least 3 days after taking the last ganciclovir dose.
✦ Caution the patient to avoid activities that require alertness if vertigo occurs.
✦ Stress the importance of returning for regular blood tests. If leukopenia occurs, teach the patient about infection-control measures; if thrombocytopenia occurs, teach him about taking bleeding precautions.
✦ Inform the patient that the drug doesn't cure genital herpes but can decrease the duration and severity of symptoms.
✦ Teach the patient how to avoid infecting others with the herpes virus.
✦ Urge the patient to recognize and report the early signs and symptoms of herpes infection, such as tingling, itching, and pain. Explain that treatment is more effective if therapy begins within 48 hours of rash onset.
✦ Instruct the patient to notify the prescriber if adverse reactions occur.

CLINICAL ALERT Ganciclovir and valganciclovir aren't interchangeable and overdose may occur.

✦ Teach the patient and his family about the prescribed drug. (See *Teaching a patient about synthetic nucleosides.*)

Features of antituberculotics

✦ Halt the progress of mycobacterial infections; aren't always curative
✦ May need to be given over many months
✦ Are used in antituberculotic combinations to thwart bacterial resistance

ANTITUBERCULOTICS

Antituberculotics are used to treat tuberculosis (TB), which is caused by *Mycobacterium tuberculosis*. They're also effective against less common mycobacterial infections caused by *M. kansasii, M. avium-intracellulare, M. fortuitum,* and related organisms.

Not always curative, these drugs can halt the progression of a mycobacterial infection. Unlike most antibiotics, antituberculotics may need to be given over many months. This creates problems, such as patient noncompliance, the development of bacterial resistance, and drug toxicity.

Traditionally, ethambutol, isoniazid, and rifampin were the mainstays of multidrug TB therapy. Because of the emergence of drug-resistant TB strains, however, a four-drug regimen is now recommended for initial treatment: isoniazid, pyrazinamide, rifampin, and streptomycin or ethambutol. Streptomycin or ethambutol is needed only if a local resistance pattern to isoniazid isn't documented or exceeds 4%.

The antituberculotic regimen should be modified if local testing shows resistance to one or more of these drugs. For example, if a health care facility has outbreaks of TB that's resistant to isoniazid and rifampin, then patients in that facility should initially receive five-drug or six-drug regimens. (See *Using fluoroquinolones and streptomycin.*)

Pharmacokinetics

Most antituberculotics are given orally. When given orally, these drugs are absorbed well from the GI tract and distributed widely throughout the body. They're metabolized primarily in the liver and excreted by the kidneys.

Pharmacodynamics

Antituberculotics are specific for mycobacteria. At usual doses, ethambutol and isoniazid are tuberculostatic, meaning they inhibit the growth of *M. tuberculosis.* In contrast, rifampin is tuberculocidal and destroys the mycobacteria. Because bacterial resistance to isoniazid and rifampin can develop rapidly, they should always be used with other antituberculotics.

Ethambutol's exact mechanism of action remains unclear, but it may be related to inhibition of cell metabolism, arrest of multiplication, and cell death. Ethambutol acts only against replicating bacteria.

Although isoniazid's exact mechanism of action isn't known, it's thought to inhibit the synthesis of mycolic acids, important components of the mycobacterium cell wall. This inhibition disrupts the cell wall. Only replicating, not resting, bacteria appear to be inhibited.

The exact mechanism of action of pyrazinamide isn't known, but the antimycobacterial activity appears to be linked to the drug's conversion to the active metabolite pyrazinoic acid. Pyrazinoic acid, in turn, creates an acidic environment.

Actions and uses of antituberculotics

ethambutol
- Is tuberculostatic
- May inhibit cell metabolism, stop replication, and cause cell death
- Acts only against replicating bacteria
- Is used with isoniazid and rifampin for uncomplicated pulmonary TB and for infections with *M. bovis* and most strains of *M. kansasii*

isoniazid
- Is tuberculostatic
- May inhibit the synthesis of mycolic acids in cell walls of replicating cells
- Is usually used with ethambutol, rifampin, or streptomycin; bacterial resistance develops rapidly if it's used alone

pyrazinamide
- May act through conversion to pyrazinoic acid
- Is a first-line TB drug, combined with ethambutol, rifampin, and isoniazid

rifampin
- Is tuberculocidal
- Inhibits RNA synthesis in susceptible organisms mainly in replicating bacteria but also somewhat in resting bacteria
- Is a first-line drug for pulmonary TB with other antituberculotics
- Is used for asymptomatic carriers of *Neisseria meningitidis* when the risk of meningitis is high

Rifampin inhibits RNA synthesis in susceptible organisms. The drug is effective primarily for replicating bacteria but may also have some effect on resting bacteria.

Pharmacotherapeutics

Ethambutol is used with isoniazid and rifampin to treat patients with uncomplicated pulmonary TB. The drug is also used to treat infections resulting from *M. bovis* and most strains of *M. kansasii.*

Isoniazid usually is used with ethambutol, rifampin, or streptomycin. This is because combination therapy for TB and other mycobacterial infections can prevent or delay the development of resistance.

Although isoniazid is the most important drug for treating TB, bacterial resistance develops rapidly if it's used alone. However, resistance doesn't pose a problem when isoniazid is used alone to prevent TB in individuals who have been exposed to the disease, and no evidence exists of cross-resistance between isoniazid and other antituberculotics. Isoniazid is typically given orally, but may be given I.V., if needed.

Pyrazinamide is recommended as a first-line TB drug, combined with ethambutol, rifampin, and isoniazid. It's a highly specific drug that's active only against *M. tuberculosis.* Resistance to pyrazinamide may develop rapidly when the drug is used alone.

Rifampin is a first-line drug for treating pulmonary TB with other antituberculotics. It combats many gram-positive and some gram-negative bacteria but is seldom used for nonmycobacterial infections because bacterial resistance develops rapidly. It's used to treat asymptomatic carriers of *Neisseria meningitidis* when the risk of meningitis is high, but it isn't used to treat *N. meningitidis* infections because of the risk of bacterial resistance.

Interactions

◆ When used with isoniazid, cycloserine and ethionamide may produce additive CNS effects, such as drowsiness, dizziness, headache, lethargy, depression, tremor, anxiety, confusion, and tinnitus.
◆ An antacid that contains aluminum may reduce the absorption of oral isoniazid and decrease the isoniazid level.
◆ Isoniazid may increase the level of carbamazepine, diazepam, ethosuximide, phenytoin, primidone, theophylline, or warfarin.
◆ When a corticosteroid is taken with isoniazid, the effects of both drugs are decreased.
◆ Isoniazid may reduce the level of itraconazole, ketoconazole, or an oral antidiabetic.
◆ When given together, isoniazid, ethionamide, pyrazinamide, and rifampin increase the risk of hepatotoxicity.
◆ Pyrazinamide may increase the phenytoin level.
◆ Rifampin can decrease the effects of an ACE inhibitor, antiarrhythmic, anticoagulant, azole antifungal, barbiturate, benzodiazepine, beta blocker, buspirone, chloramphenicol, corticosteroid, cyclosporine, or hormonal contraceptive.

Adverse reactions

Adverse reactions to antituberculotics primarily affect the GI tract, the peripheral nervous system, and the hepatic system. Fortunately, these reactions are seldom severe enough to interrupt TB therapy.

Possible drug interactions

◆ ACE inhibitors
◆ Aluminum-containing antacids
◆ Antiarrhythmics
◆ Anticoagulants
◆ Azole antifungals
◆ Barbiturates
◆ Benzodiazepines
◆ Beta blockers
◆ Buspirone
◆ Carbamazepine
◆ Chloramphenicol
◆ Corticosteroids
◆ Cycloserine
◆ Cyclosporine
◆ Diazepam
◆ Ethionamide
◆ Ethosuximide
◆ Hormonal contraceptives
◆ Itraconazole
◆ Ketoconazole
◆ Oral antidiabetics
◆ Phenytoin
◆ Primidone
◆ Theophylline
◆ Warfarin

Spotting the long-term effects of isoniazid

During the first 6 months of isoniazid therapy, be sure to monitor the patient's liver enzyme levels because the drug has caused transient elevations in ALT, AST, and bilirubin levels in 10% to 20% of patients. Monitor the liver enzyme levels even more closely after treatment has stopped because isoniazid may cause severe, possibly fatal hepatitis many months after the drug is stopped. Also assess the patient for signs and symptoms of hepatitis, such as jaundice, hepatomegaly, abdominal pain, anorexia, and clay-colored stool.

Optic neuritis is the only significant adverse reaction to ethambutol. Signs and symptoms include decreased visual acuity, loss of red-green color discrimination, visual field constriction, and central and peripheral scotomas (areas of depressed vision in the visual field). This adverse reaction occurs in less than 1% of patients receiving 15 mg/kg, but is more common in patients who receive higher dosages or who have renal dysfunction. Stopping ethambutol usually reverses optic neuritis, but if vision impairment is severe, recovery may not be complete. Pruritus, joint pain, GI distress, malaise, headache, dizziness, and confusion have also been reported with ethambutol therapy. Occasionally, this drug increases the uric acid level and precipitates an acute gout episode.

The most common hypersensitivity reactions to ethambutol are rash and fever. Hypersensitivity reactions rarely occur with ethambutol and tend to be mild. Leukopenia, anaphylaxis, and peripheral neuritis with paresthesia of the arms and legs have been reported.

Peripheral neuritis occurs in 20% of patients receiving 6 mg/kg of isoniazid daily, and the percentage of affected patients increases with the dosage. Usually preceded by paresthesia of the feet and hands, peripheral neuritis is more likely to affect an alcoholic, diabetic, or malnourished patient or one who is predisposed to peripheral neuritis. Typically, it produces muscle twitching, dizziness, ataxia, stupor, and paresthesia. A daily dose of 10 to 50 mg of pyridoxine (vitamin B_6) may prevent this reaction. Isoniazid may also affect the liver. (See *Spotting the long-term effects of isoniazid.*)

Isoniazid may precipitate seizures in a patient with a seizure disorder. It may produce optic neuritis and atrophy, mental abnormalities (such as euphoria and memory impairment), and sedation or incoordination.

Although hypersensitivity reactions to isoniazid seldom occur, they produce fever, skin eruptions (morbilliform, maculopapular, purpuric, or exfoliative), lymphadenopathy, and vasculitis. These reactions usually appear 3 to 7 weeks after therapy begins.

Generally, pyrazinamide is well tolerated during short-course therapy. Its major limiting adverse reaction is hepatotoxicity, which appears to be dose-related and can occur anytime during therapy. Renal excretion of urates is inhibited by pyrazinamide, which can result in hyperuricemia and precipitation of gout in predisposed patients. GI disturbances, including nausea, vomiting, and anorexia, may also occur.

Adverse reactions to watch for

ethambutol
✦ Acute gout episode
✦ Confusion, dizziness
✦ Fever, rash
✦ GI distress
✦ Headache, joint pain, malaise, pruritus
✦ Optic neuritis

isoniazid
✦ Incoordination
✦ Liver effects
✦ Mental abnormalities
✦ Optic neuritis and atrophy
✦ Peripheral neuritis
✦ Sedation
✦ Seizures in a patient with a seizure disorder

pyrazinamide
✦ Anorexia, nausea, vomiting
✦ Hepatotoxicity

rifampin
✦ Abdominal cramps, anorexia, diarrhea, epigastric pain, flatulence, nausea, vomiting
✦ Elevated ALT, AST, bilirubin, and alkaline phosphatase levels
✦ Joint pain, muscle aches and cramps
✦ Transient asymptomatic jaundice and red-orange discoloration of sweat, tears, saliva, urine, and feces

Predicting rifampin's adverse reactions

Because the rate of acetylation of rifampin is genetically determined, you can roughly predict a patient's response to the drug based on his ethnic background. For example, about 50% of Blacks and Caucasians are considered slow acetylators (inactivators) of rifampin. On the other hand, most Inuits and Asians are considered rapid acetylators. Slow acetylation may lead to a higher rifampin level and an increased risk of toxic reactions.

The most common adverse reactions to rifampin include epigastric pain, nausea, vomiting, abdominal cramps, flatulence, anorexia, and diarrhea. Joint pain and muscle aches and cramps may also occur. All these reactions, which are most likely to occur during the first 2 weeks of therapy, may subside as biliary excretion of rifampin increases and its half-life decreases; interruption of therapy seldom is needed. Rifampin can elevate ALT, AST, bilirubin, and alkaline phosphatase levels, which may eventually necessitate stopping the drug. Transient asymptomatic jaundice and red-orange discoloration of sweat, tears, saliva, urine, and feces may also occur but don't require the stopping the drug. (See *Predicting rifampin's adverse reactions*.)

Intermittent doses of rifampin ranging from 900 to 1,200 mg produce hypersensitivity reactions in about 1% of patients so treated. This reaction appears as a flulike syndrome characterized by dyspnea with or without wheezing, purpura related to thrombocytopenia, leukopenia and, rarely, anaphylaxis. A patient with this reaction probably can tolerate a reduced rifampin dosage; only 3% of patients require stopping the drug.

Nursing considerations

✦ Monitor the patient for adverse reactions and drug interactions during therapy. If any occur, notify the prescriber.
✦ Assess the patient for sensory deficits when giving ethambutol or isoniazid.
✦ Monitor the patient closely for hypersensitivity reactions. Keep standard emergency equipment nearby.
✦ Monitor the patient's liver function test results during isoniazid, pyrazinamide, or rifampin therapy; uric acid level during ethambutol therapy; and WBC count during rifampin or ethambutol therapy.
✦ Monitor the patient's hydration if nausea, vomiting, anorexia, or diarrhea results from rifampin, pyrazinamide, or ethambutol therapy. Give an antiemetic or antidiarrheal as needed.
✦ If the patient experiences a headache during ethambutol therapy or joint pain or muscle aches or cramps during rifampin therapy, give an analgesic.
✦ If the patient experiences adverse CNS reactions, such as confusion or incoordination, take safety measures. For example, place the patient's bed in the lowest position, keep the bed rails raised, and supervise movement.
✦ Maintain seizure precautions when giving isoniazid to a patient with a seizure disorder.

Key nursing actions

✦ Assess the patient for sensory deficits when giving ethambutol or isoniazid.
✦ Watch closely for hypersensitivity reactions. Keep emergency equipment nearby.
✦ Monitor the patient's liver function during isoniazid, pyrazinamide, or rifampin therapy; uric acid level during ethambutol therapy; and WBC count during rifampin or ethambutol therapy.
✦ Monitor hydration if nausea, vomiting, anorexia, or diarrhea results from rifampin, pyrazinamide, or ethambutol therapy. Give an antiemetic or antidiarrheal as needed.

Teaching a patient about antituberculotics

Whenever an antituberculotic is prescribed, teach the patient and his family the drug's name, dose, frequency, action, and adverse effects. Also take the following actions.

✦ Stress the importance of taking the drug for the prescribed length of time.

✦ Teach the patient to take rifampin 1 hour before or 2 hours after a meal because food affects drug absorption.

✦ Instruct the patient to take isoniazid at least 1 hour before taking an antacid containing aluminum.

✦ Teach the patient to take pyridoxine with isoniazid to prevent peripheral neuritis.

✦ Instruct the patient taking isoniazid to consult the prescriber if signs and symptoms of hepatic dysfunction appear, such as nausea, vomiting, fatigue, weakness, and anorexia.

✦ Instruct the patient taking isoniazid or ethambutol to report vision changes immediately.

✦ Advise the patient that rifampin may produce red-orange urine, tears, sputum, sweat, and feces that stain clothes, linen, and soft contact lenses.

✦ Advise a woman who takes rifampin and uses hormonal contraceptives to use an alternate form of birth control.

✦ Reassure the patient who experiences adverse reactions early in rifampin therapy that most of them will subside with continued treatment.

✦ Teach the patient the importance of having periodic blood tests performed.

✦ Advise the patient to take a mild analgesic (unless contraindicated) for joint pain, muscle aches or cramps, or headache.

✦ Caution the patient not to perform activities that require alertness or motor coordination if adverse central nervous system reactions occur.

✦ Instruct the patient to notify the prescriber if adverse reactions occur.

Key nursing actions
(continued)

✦ If the patient has adverse CNS reactions, such as confusion or incoordination, take safety measures.

✦ Maintain seizure precautions when giving isoniazid to a patient with a seizure disorder.

✦ Assess the patient for additive CNS effects during therapy with isoniazid and cycloserine or ethionamide.

✦ Watch for treatment failure if the patient receives rifampin and another drug, such as an anticoagulant, corticosteroid, or hormon contraceptive. Adjust the dosage as indicated.

✦ Give rifampin 1 hour before or 2 hours after a meal because food affects the rate and extent of absorption.

✦ Give isoniazid at least 1 hour before giving an antacid containing aluminum to prevent an interaction.

✦ Monitor the patient for additive CNS effects during therapy with isoniazid and cycloserine or ethionamide.

✦ Monitor for treatment failure in a patient who receives rifampin and another drug, such as an anticoagulant, corticosteroid, or hormonal contraceptive. Adjust the dosage as indicated.

✦ If giving 6 mg/kg of isoniazid daily or more, monitor the patient for peripheral neuritis, which is exhibited initially by paresthesia of the hands and feet followed by muscle twitching, dizziness, ataxia, and stupor.

✦ Give pyridoxine with isoniazid to prevent peripheral neuritis.

✦ Monitor the patient for optic neuritis when giving isoniazid or 15 mg/kg or more of ethambutol.

✦ Teach the patient and his family about the prescribed drug. (See *Teaching a patient about antituberculotics.*)

ANTIFUNGALS

Used to treat fungal infections, antifungals include amphotericin B, azole antifungals, caspofungin, flucytosine, nystatin, and terbinafine.

AMPHOTERICIN B

The potency of amphotericin B has made it the most widely used drug for treating severe systemic fungal infections. It comes in several forms, including lipid-based preparations that may decrease renal or systemic toxicity.

Pharmacokinetics

After I.V. administration, amphotericin B is distributed throughout the body and excreted by the kidneys. Its metabolism isn't well defined.

Pharmacodynamics

Amphotericin B works by binding to sterol, a lipid, in the fungal cell membrane, altering cell permeability and allowing intracellular components to leak out. The drug usually inhibits fungal growth and multiplication but, if the level is high enough, the drug can destroy fungi.

Pharmacotherapeutics

Usually, amphotericin B is used to treat severe systemic fungal infections and meningitis. It's typically the drug of choice for severe infections caused by *Candida, Paracoccidioides brasiliensis, Blastomyces dermatitidis, Coccidioides immitis, Cryptococcus neoformans,* and *Sporothrix schenckii.* It's also effective against *Aspergillus fumigatus, Microsporum audouinii, Rhizopus, Candida glabrata, Trichophyton,* and *Rhodotorula.*

Because the drug is highly toxic, its use is limited to patients who have a definitive diagnosis of life-threatening infections and who are under close medical supervision.

Interactions

✦ Together, amphotericin B and flucytosine produce synergistic effects and are commonly combined in therapy for candidal or cryptococcal infections, especially cryptococcal meningitis.
✦ When amphotericin B is used with acyclovir, an aminoglycoside, or cyclosporine, the risk of renal toxicity increases.
✦ Digoxin, a corticosteroid, or an extended-spectrum penicillin may worsen hypokalemia produced by the drug, which may lead to heart problems.
✦ Amphotericin B can increase the risk of digoxin toxicity.
✦ When given with a nondepolarizing skeletal muscle relaxant, such as pancuronium bromide, amphotericin B can increase muscle relaxation.
✦ An electrolyte solution may inactivate amphotericin B when used as a diluent.

Adverse reactions

Amphotericin B probably is the most toxic antibiotic in use today. Almost all patients receiving I.V. amphotericin B experience chills, fever, nausea, vomiting, anorexia, muscle and joint pain, headache, abdominal pain, weight loss, and dyspepsia, especially at the beginning of low-dosage therapy. As therapy continues and the dosage is increased to the optimum level, these reactions usually subside. Most patients also develop normochromic or normocytic anemia that significantly decreases the hematocrit.

Up to 80% of patients receiving amphotericin B may develop some degree of nephrotoxicity, causing the kidneys to lose their concentrating ability. This promotes the loss of renal stores of potassium, bicarbonate, water, and phosphate. Nephrotoxicity usually disappears within 3 months after stopping the drug, but this toxicity sometimes leads to permanent renal impairment.

Up to 25% of patients receiving amphotericin B may develop hypokalemia, which can become severe and lead to extreme muscle weakness and ECG changes. Distal renal tubular acidosis commonly occurs, contributing to the development of hypokalemia.

Other adverse reactions to I.V. amphotericin B therapy include phlebitis and thrombophlebitis. Rarely, hypotension, hypertension, flushing, paresthesia, and seizures may occur.

Nursing considerations

✦ Refrigerate amphotericin B until it's used.

 CLINICAL ALERT Don't substitute amphotericin B preparations. Different preparations aren't interchangeable because their dosages vary. Confusing them may cause permanent damage or death.

✦ Shake the vial vigorously for at least 3 minutes before giving to properly disperse the particles.
✦ Don't give the solution if it contains precipitate.
✦ When giving I.V., use an in-line filter with a mean pore diameter of 1 micron or larger. Smaller filters will remove appreciable amounts of the drug from the solution.
✦ Infuse other antibiotics separately—not through the I.V. line used to give amphotericin B.
✦ Monitor the patient regularly for adverse reactions and drug interactions during amphotericin B therapy. Notify the prescriber if any occur.
✦ Monitor the patient's electrolyte levels, particularly watching for changes in potassium, magnesium, calcium, and phosphorus levels.
✦ During I.V. infusion, monitor the patient's vital signs. Fever may occur, but usually will subside within 4 hours after the infusion is stopped. To relieve the fever and chills caused by the infusion, give an antihistamine or antipyretic. An antiemetic may be used to relieve other reactions, such as nausea and vomiting.
✦ Check the I.V. site for phlebitis. To reduce phlebitis, rotate the site routinely and add small doses of heparin or corticosteroids to the infusion. If phlebitis becomes severe, use alternate-day therapy. The patient may receive amphotericin B via a central line, which permits greater drug dilution in the blood and decreases the severity of the phlebitis.
✦ Before beginning therapy, monitor the patient's BUN and creatinine levels every other day during initial therapy and once per week after the optimal dosage is reached. Reduce the dosage or alternate-day therapy if the patient's creatinine level approaches 3 mg/dl.
✦ Monitor the patient's fluid intake and output, and observe him for signs of nephrotoxicity.
✦ Notify the prescriber if nephrotoxicity is suspected.
✦ Teach the patient and his family about the prescribed drug. (See *Teaching a patient about amphotericin B,* page 350.)

Key nursing actions
✦ Don't interchange amphotericin B preparations.
✦ Monitor levels of electrolytes, especially potassium, magnesium, calcium, phosphorus.
✦ Check the patient's vital signs during I.V. infusions.
✦ Monitor BUN and creatinine levels before and during therapy.
✦ Document the intake and output, and assess the patient for evidence of nephrotoxicity.

Features of azole antifungals

fluconazole
+ Inhibits fungal cytochrome P450, which weakens fungal cell walls
+ Is used for mouth, throat, and esophageal candidiasis and serious systemic candidal infections, including UTIs, peritonitis, and pneumonia
+ Is also used for cryptococcal meningitis

itraconazole
+ Interferes with fungal wall synthesis by inhibiting ergosterol formation and increasing cell-wall permeability and osmotic instability
+ Is used for blastomycosis, nonmeningeal histoplasmosis, candidiasis, aspergillosis, and fungal nail disease

ketoconazole
+ Interferes with sterol synthesis in fungal cells, damaging cell membranes and increasing permeability
+ Is usually fungistatic but may be fungicidal
+ Is used for topical and systemic infections with susceptible fungi, which include dermatophytes and most other fungi

voriconazole
+ Interferes with fungal wall synthesis by inhibiting ergosterol formation and increasing cell-wall permeability and osmotic instability
+ Is used for invasive aspergillosis and serious infections caused by *Fusarium* and *Scedosporium apiospermum* in patients who can't tolerate or don't respond to other drugs

PATIENT TEACHING

Teaching a patient about amphotericin B

Whenever amphotericin B is prescribed, teach the patient and his family the drug's name, dose, frequency, action, and adverse effects. Also take the following actions.
+ Stress the importance of returning regularly for blood tests and follow-up appointments.
+ Inform the patient who receives I.V. amphotericin B that chills, fever, GI upset, muscle and joint pain, headache, abdominal pain, weight loss, and dyspepsia probably will occur. Reassure him that these reactions usually subside with continued therapy.
+ Instruct the patient to report decreased urination, cloudy or bloody urine, or other adverse reactions.

AZOLE ANTIFUNGALS

The azole class of antifungal drugs includes fluconazole, itraconazole, ketoconazole, and voriconazole. Fluconazole, itraconazole, and voriconazole are triazole derivatives; ketoconazole is an imidazole derivative. Most of these synthetic drugs offer a broad spectrum of activity.

Pharmacokinetics

After oral administration, fluconazole is about 90% absorbed. It's distributed into all body fluids, and more than 80% of a dose is excreted unchanged in urine.

Oral bioavailability is highest when itraconazole is taken with food. Voriconazole is more effective when taken 1 hour before or after a meal. Both drugs bind to plasma proteins and are extensively metabolized in the liver into a large number of metabolites. They're minimally excreted in feces.

When given orally, ketoconazole is absorbed variably and distributed widely. It undergoes extensive liver metabolism and is excreted through bile and feces.

Pharmacodynamics

Fluconazole inhibits fungal cytochrome P450, an enzyme responsible for fungal sterol synthesis, which causes fungal cell walls to weaken.

Itraconazole and voriconazole interfere with fungal wall synthesis by inhibiting the formation of ergosterol and increasing cell-wall permeability. This action makes the fungus susceptible to osmotic instability.

Within fungal cells, ketoconazole interferes with sterol synthesis, which damages the cell membrane and increases permeability. This damage leads to a loss of essential cell elements and inhibits cell growth. Ketoconazole usually produces fungistatic effects but can also produce fungicidal effects under certain conditions.

Pharmacotherapeutics

Fluconazole is used to treat mouth, throat, and esophageal candidiasis and serious systemic candidal infections, including UTIs, peritonitis, and pneumonia. The drug is also used to treat cryptococcal meningitis.

Itraconazole is effective in treating blastomycosis, nonmeningeal histoplasmosis, candidiasis, aspergillosis, and fungal nail disease.

Ketoconazole is indicated for topical and systemic infections caused by susceptible fungi, which include dermatophytes and most other fungi.

Voriconazole is used to treat invasive aspergillosis and serious infections caused by *Fusarium* and *Scedosporium apiospermum* in patients who can't tolerate or don't respond to other drugs.

Interactions

- Use of an azole antifungal with warfarin may increase the risk of bleeding.
- Fluconazole may increase cyclosporine and phenytoin levels.
- Fluconazole may increase the level of an oral antidiabetic (such as glipizide, glyburide, or tolbutamide), increasing the risk of hypoglycemia.
- Cimetidine or rifampin can enhance metabolism of fluconazole and reduce its level.
- Fluconazole may increase the activity of zidovudine.
- An antacid, H_2-receptor antagonist, phenytoin, or rifampin can lower the itraconazole level.
- Use of ketoconazole with a drug that decreases gastric acidity (such as an antacid, an anticholinergic, cimetidine, famotidine, nizatidine, or ranitidine) may decrease absorption of ketoconazole and reduce its antifungal effects.
- Use of ketoconazole with phenytoin may alter the metabolisms and levels of both drugs.
- Ketoconazole may decrease the theophylline level.
- Use of ketoconazole with another hepatotoxic drug may increase the risk of liver disease.
- Ketoconazole may increase cyclosporine and creatinine levels.
- Rifampin may decrease the ketoconazole level.
- Ketoconazole may inhibit the metabolism—and increase the levels—of carbamazepine, a protease inhibitor, quinidine, and a sulfonylurea.
- Voriconazole may inhibit the metabolism of a benzodiazepine, a calcium channel blocker, phenytoin, a sulfonylurea, and tacrolimus.
- Voriconazole may increase the levels of pimozide and quinidine, which may lead to a prolonged QT interval and torsades de pointes. This interaction prohibits use of these drugs together.

Adverse reactions

Patients receiving fluconazole may experience transient elevations in AST, ALT, alkaline phosphatase, and bilirubin levels. Less common reactions include dizziness, nausea, vomiting, abdominal pain, diarrhea, rash, and headache. Hypokalemia and increased BUN and creatinine levels have also been reported.

The most common adverse reactions to itraconazole are headache and nausea.

The most common reactions to ketoconazole are nausea and vomiting. Reactions in less than 1% of patients include pruritus, rash, dermatitis, urticaria, headache, insomnia, dizziness, vivid dreams, lethargy, paresthesia, diarrhea, flatulence, abdominal pain, and endocrine reactions, such as gynecomastia and breast pain. Hepatotoxicity, although rare, is reversible when the drug is stopped. Rarely, ketoconazole can also cause anaphylaxis, arthralgia, chills, fever, tinnitus, impotence, and photophobia.

Adverse reactions to voriconazole are uncommon. However, the drug may alter renal function. Vision changes may occur if voriconazole therapy lasts more than 28 days.

An I.V. azole antifungal may produce an infusion reaction at the start of or during the infusion.

Possible drug interactions

- Antacids
- Anticholinergics
- Benzodiazepines
- Calcium channel blockers
- Carbamazepine
- Cimetidine
- Cyclosporine
- Famotidine
- Hepatotoxic drugs
- H_2-receptor antagonists
- Nizatidine
- Oral antidiabetics
- Phenytoin
- Pimozide
- Protease inhibitors
- Quinidine
- Ranitidine
- Rifampin
- Sulfonylureas
- Tacrolimus
- Theophylline
- Warfarin
- Zidovudine

Adverse reactions to watch for

fluconazole
- Abdominal pain, diarrhea, dizziness, headache, hypokalemia, increased BUN and creatinine levels, nausea, rash, vomiting
- Transient elevations in AST, ALT, alkaline phosphatase, bilirubin levels

itraconazole
- Headache, nausea

ketoconazole
- Nausea, vomiting

voriconazole
- Altered renal function, vision changes

Avoiding fetal harm from voriconazole

When taken during pregnancy, voriconazole may harm the fetus. To avoid fetal harm, urge a woman of childbearing age to use an effective contraceptive during therapy. If voriconazole must be used during pregnancy or if the patient becomes pregnant while taking the drug, inform her of the potential hazard to the fetus.

Key nursing actions

✦ Monitor the patient's AST, ALT, alkaline phosphatase, bilirubin, BUN, and creatinine levels during fluconazole therapy.

✦ Stop fluconazole if the patient develops a rash and it continues.

✦ Monitor hydration if nausea, vomiting, or diarrhea develops. Give an antiemetic or antidiarrheal as needed.

✦ Perform baseline liver function tests and monitor results periodically if the patient receives ketoconazole, itraconazole, or voriconazole.

✦ Assess renal function during voriconazole therapy.

✦ Watch for infusion reactions.

✦ Monitor liver function tests during ketoconazole therapy.

Nursing considerations

✦ Don't give I.V. fluconazole faster than 200 mg/hour by continuous infusion.

✦ Monitor the patient periodically for adverse reactions and drug interactions. If they occur, alert the prescriber.

✦ Monitor the patient's AST, ALT, alkaline phosphatase, bilirubin, BUN, and creatinine levels during fluconazole therapy. Notify the prescriber of abnormal results.

✦ Monitor the patient who develops a rash; if it continues, stop fluconazole.

✦ Monitor the patient's hydration if nausea, vomiting, or diarrhea occurs. Give an antiemetic or antidiarrheal as needed.

✦ Use itraconazole cautiously in a patient with hypochlorhydria, which can accompany HIV infection. Such a patient may not absorb the drug readily.

✦ Caution the woman of childbearing age about the use of voriconazole. (See *Avoiding fetal harm from voriconazole.*)

✦ Obtain nail specimens for laboratory testing to diagnose onychomycosis before initiating itraconazole therapy.

✦ Perform baseline liver function tests and monitor results periodically for a patient receiving ketoconazole, itraconazole, or voriconazole. If he has baseline hepatic impairment, avoid therapy unless his condition is life-threatening. If liver dysfunction occurs during therapy, notify the prescriber immediately.

✦ Monitor the patient's renal function during voriconazole therapy. Use the I.V. form cautiously in a patient whose creatinine clearance falls below 50 ml/minute.

✦ Monitor the patient for an infusion reaction. If a reaction occurs, stop the infusion and notify the prescriber.

✦ Give ketoconazole at least 2 hours after the patient receives a drug that decreases gastric acidity.

 CLINICAL ALERT Monitor the patient's liver function tests during ketoconazole therapy. If test results show persistent elevations and the patient displays signs of hepatotoxicity, stop the drug.

✦ If phenytoin, theophylline, or cyclosporine are used with ketoconazole, monitor the levels of these drugs. The patient may need dosage adjustments or alternate therapy.

✦ Give ketoconazole on an empty stomach, if possible, to promote absorption. If the patient experiences GI distress, however, give the drug with food.

✦ Teach the patient and his family about the prescribed drug. (See *Teaching a patient about azole antifungals.*)

Teaching a patient about azole antifungals

Whenever an azole antifungal is prescribed, teach the patient and his family the drug's name, dose, frequency, action, and adverse effects. Also take the following actions.

✦ Stress the importance of taking the drug for the prescribed length of time.
✦ Inform the patient when to expect therapeutic results from the azole antifungal. For example, mucosal infections respond to ketoconazole in days, skin infections in weeks, and nail infections in months.
✦ Instruct the patient to notify the prescriber if he notices signs and symptoms of liver disease, such as dark or amber-colored urine, pale stools, abdominal pain, unusual fatigue, or yellowing of the eyes or skin.
✦ Instruct the patient to notify the prescriber if other adverse reactions occur.
✦ Teach the patient the importance of having routine blood tests while taking drugs that interact with fluconazole.
✦ Instruct the patient to take bleeding precautions if he takes warfarin during fluconazole therapy.
✦ Instruct a diabetic patient to monitor his glucose level regularly and to watch for signs and symptoms of hypoglycemia if he takes glyburide or glipizide with fluconazole.
✦ Advise the patient to report breast enlargement, breast pain, or rash during ketoconazole therapy.
✦ Caution the patient not to perform activities that require alertness if ketoconazole produces dizziness or drowsiness.
✦ Advise the patient when to take ketoconazole if he also takes other drugs that decrease gastric acidity.
✦ Teach the patient relaxation techniques if insomnia results from ketoconazole. Advise him to take a prescription sedative if insomnia persists.
✦ Advise the patient to take ketoconazole on an empty stomach or, if he experiences GI distress, to take it with food and to notify the prescriber if GI reactions persist or worsen.
✦ Instruct the patient not to substitute itraconazole capsules for oral solution; to use 10 ml of solution at a time; and to take the solution without food or to take capsules with a full meal.
✦ Tell the patient to take oral voriconazole at least 1 hour before or 1 hour after a meal.
✦ Advise the patient to avoid driving or operating machinery while taking voriconazole because vision changes may occur.
✦ Tell the patient to avoid strong, direct sunlight during voriconazole therapy.
✦ Advise a woman of childbearing age to avoid pregnancy during itraconazole or voriconazole therapy.

CASPOFUNGIN

Caspofungin belongs to a relatively new class of drugs known as *echinocandins*, or *glucan synthesis inhibitors*. Its major use is in patients who haven't responded to other antifungals, such as amphotericin B or itraconazole.

Pharmacokinetics

After I.V. administration, caspofungin is highly protein-bound, with little distribution into RBCs. The drug is metabolized slowly and excreted in urine and feces.

Pharmacodynamics

Caspofungin inhibits the synthesis of an integral component of the fungal cell wall.

Features of caspofungin

✦ Belongs to a relatively new class of drugs known as *echinocandins* or *glucan synthesis inhibitors*
✦ Inhibits the synthesis of an integral component of fungal cell walls
✦ Is used for invasive aspergillosis in patients who haven't responded to or can't tolerate other antifungals

Teaching a patient about caspofungin

Whenever caspofungin is prescribed, teach the patient and his family the drug's name, dose, frequency, action, and adverse effects. Also take the following actions.
✦ Urge the patient to tell the prescriber if he takes any other drugs because they may interact with caspofungin.
✦ Tell the patient to notify the nurse if he notices rash, facial swelling, itching, or warmth.
✦ Instruct the patient to report signs and symptoms of phlebitis, such as redness, warmth, or pain at the infusion site.
✦ Instruct the patient to notify the prescriber if other adverse reactions occur.

Adverse reactions to watch for

✦ Abdominal pain, anorexia, diarrhea, nausea, vomiting
✦ Anemia, eosinophilia, hypokalemia
✦ Chills, fever, sweating
✦ Hematuria, proteinuria
✦ Histamine-mediated symptoms, such as rash, facial swelling, pruritus, and sensation of warmth
✦ Infused vein complications, phlebitis
✦ Pain, headache, myalgia, paresthesia
✦ Tachycardia, tachypnea

Key nursing actions

✦ Plan for therapy to last no longer than 2 weeks.
✦ Inspect the I.V. site carefully for phlebitis.
✦ Observe the patient for histamine-mediated reactions.

Pharmacotherapeutics

The drug is used for invasive aspergillosis in patients who haven't responded to or can't tolerate other antifungals, but the drug hasn't been studied as an initial drug for this disorder.

Interactions

✦ Caspofungin can decrease the tacrolimus level, which may require higher doses of tacrolimus.
✦ A drug that induces drug metabolism (such as carbamazepine, efavirenz, nelfinavir, nevirapine, or phenytoin) may decrease caspofungin clearance.
✦ Cyclosporine can decrease caspofungin clearance.

 CLINICAL ALERT Use of caspofungin with cyclosporine may cause elevated liver enzyme levels, which prohibits their combined use.

Adverse reactions

Common adverse reactions to caspofungin are paresthesia, tachycardia, anorexia, anemia, pain, myalgia, tachypnea, chills, and sweating. Other adverse reactions include fever, headache, phlebitis, infused vein complications, nausea, vomiting, diarrhea, abdominal pain, proteinuria, hematuria, eosinophilia, hypokalemia, and histamine-mediated symptoms, such as rash, facial swelling, pruritus, and sensation of warmth.

Nursing considerations

 CLINICAL ALERT Never mix caspofungin in — or dilute it with — a dextrose solution.

✦ Plan for short-term therapy. Safety information on treatment longer than 2 weeks is limited.
✦ Monitor the I.V. site carefully for phlebitis.
✦ Observe the patient for histamine-mediated reactions.
✦ Monitor the patient periodically for adverse reactions and drug interactions. If they occur, alert the prescriber.

✦ Teach the patient and his family about the prescribed drug. (See *Teaching a patient about caspofungin.*)

FLUCYTOSINE

The only antimetabolite that suppresses fungal growth, flucytosine is rarely used alone. Instead, it's usually given with amphotericin B.

Pharmacokinetics

Flucytosine is absorbed well from the GI tract and distributed widely. It undergoes little metabolism and is excreted primarily by the kidneys.

Pharmacodynamics

Flucytosine penetrates fungal cells where it's converted to its active metabolite fluorouracil. Then fluorouracil is incorporated into the RNA of the fungal cells, which alters their protein synthesis and causes cell death.

Pharmacotherapeutics

Although amphotericin B is effective in treating candidal and cryptococcal meningitis alone, flucytosine is given with it to reduce the dosage and the risk of toxicity. This combination therapy is the treatment of choice for cryptococcal meningitis.

Flucytosine can be used alone to treat lower urinary tract *Candida* infections because it reaches a high level in urine. It's also used effectively to treat infections caused by *T. glabrata, Phialophora, Aspergillus,* and *Cladosporium.*

Interactions

✦ Cytarabine may antagonize flucytosine's antifungal activity, possibly by competitive inhibition.
✦ Cytosine may inactivate flucytosine.

Adverse reactions

Bone marrow suppression typically occurs when the flucytosine level exceeds 100 mcg/ml and may lead to leukopenia, thrombocytopenia, anemia, pancytopenia, or granulocytopenia.

Adverse GI reactions to flucytosine include nausea, vomiting, abdominal distention, diarrhea, and anorexia. Rarely, bowel perforation and hepatotoxicity may occur.

Azotemia, increased BUN and creatinine levels, crystalluria, and renal impairment may also occur.

Flucytosine may produce unpredictable adverse reactions, including confusion, headache, somnolence, vertigo, hallucinations, dyspnea, respiratory arrest, and rash.

Nursing considerations

✦ Monitor the patient periodically for adverse reactions and drug interactions. If they occur, notify the prescriber.
✦ Monitor the patient's hematologic and liver function test results as well as his BUN and creatinine levels. Notify the prescriber of abnormal test results.
✦ Monitor the patient's fluid intake and output. Notify the prescriber if he experiences azotemia, crystalluria, or decreased urine output, all of which may indicate renal impairment.

Features of flucytosine

✦ Penetrates fungal cells where it's converted to fluorouracil, which is incorporated into fungal RNA and alters protein synthesis
✦ Is rarely used alone; usually is given with amphotericin B
✦ Can be used alone to treat lower urinary tract *Candida* infections
✦ Is used with amphotericin B for candidal and cryptococcal meningitis, because drug allows a reduced amphotericin B dosage and risk of toxicity

Adverse reactions to watch for

✦ Abdominal distention, anorexia, diarrhea, nausea, vomiting
✦ Azotemia, increased BUN and creatinine levels, crystalluria, renal impairment
✦ Bone marrow suppression (when drug level exceeds 100 mcg/ml)
✦ Confusion, hallucinations, headache, somnolence, vertigo
✦ Dyspnea, respiratory arrest
✦ Rash

Teaching a patient about flucytosine

Whenever flucytosine is prescribed, teach the patient and his family the drug's name, dose, frequency, action, and adverse effects. Also take the following actions.
- ✦ Stress the importance of taking the drug for the prescribed length of time.
- ✦ Teach the patient the importance of returning for blood tests.
- ✦ Instruct the patient about infection-control measures or bleeding precautions as needed.
- ✦ Instruct the patient to report sore throat, fever, easy bruising, bleeding, unusual fatigue or weakness, changes in urine output, severe nausea, vomiting, or rash.
- ✦ Instruct the patient to notify the prescriber if other adverse reactions occur.
- ✦ Advise the patient to take a flucytosine dose consisting of several capsules over 15 minutes to minimize nausea or vomiting.
- ✦ Tell the patient to take a missed dose as soon as possible, but not to take a double dose. Explain that missing a dose is safer than overmedicating with a double dose.
- ✦ Caution the patient against performing activities that require alertness if dizziness or other adverse central nervous system reactions occur.

Key nursing actions

- ✦ Monitor hematologic and liver function test results and BUN and creatinine levels. Notify the prescriber of abnormal results.
- ✦ Monitor fluid intake and output.
- ✦ Inspect the patient's skin regularly for rash.
- ✦ Monitor the drug level regularly; the therapeutic level is 25 to 120 mcg/ml.
- ✦ Assess the patient for fluid volume deficit.

✦ Regularly inspect the patient's skin for a rash, which may suggest a hypersensitivity reaction to flucytosine.

✦ Regularly monitor the patient's flucytosine level during long-term therapy; the therapeutic level ranges from 25 to 120 mcg/ml.

✦ Monitor the patient for fluid volume deficit if anorexia, nausea, vomiting, or diarrhea occurs. Give an antiemetic or antidiarrheal as needed.

✦ If adverse GI reactions persist or worsen, notify the prescriber.

✦ Teach the patient and his family about the prescribed drug. (See *Teaching a patient about flucytosine*.)

NYSTATIN

This antifungal is used topically or orally for local fungal infections because it's extremely toxic when given parenterally.

Features of nystatin

- ✦ Binds to sterols in fungal cell membranes and alters membrane permeability
- ✦ May be fungicidal or fungistatic, depending on the organism present
- ✦ Is used mainly for fungal skin infections
- ✦ Topical form is used for skin or mucous membrane candidal infections, such as oral thrush, diaper rash, vaginal and vulvar candidiasis, and candidiasis between skin folds
- ✦ Oral form is used for candidal infections in the GI tract

Pharmacokinetics

Oral nystatin undergoes little or no absorption, distribution, or metabolism. It's excreted unchanged in feces. Topical nystatin isn't absorbed through the skin or mucous membranes.

Pharmacodynamics

Nystatin binds to sterols in fungal cell membranes and alters membrane permeability, which leads to loss of cell components. Nystatin can act as a fungicidal or fungistatic drug, depending on the organism present.

Pharmacotherapeutics

Nystatin is used primarily for fungal skin infections. It's effective against *Candida*. Topical nystatin is used for skin or mucous membrane candidal infections, such as

Teaching a patient about nystatin

Whenever nystatin is prescribed, teach the patient and his family the drug's name, dose, frequency, action, and adverse effects. Also take the following actions.
◆ Instruct the patient who takes the suspension form for oral candidiasis to divide the dose in half, place one-half in each side of the mouth, swish the suspension in the mouth for as long as possible, and then swallow it.
◆ Instruct the patient who takes tablets for oral candidiasis to dissolve the tablet in the mouth. Emphasize that he must not chew it or swallow it whole.
◆ Advise the patient who uses topical nystatin to report signs of a hypersensitivity reaction, such as redness or skin irritation.
◆ Teach the patient how to apply topical nystatin properly. Also stress the importance of compliance with therapy and good hygiene.
◆ Instruct the patient to insert vaginal nystatin tablets high in the vagina. Also inform her that vaginal drainage from the tablets may stain clothing.
◆ Instruct the patient to avoid using occlusive dressings during therapy with nystatin ointment or cream because they provide a favorable environment for fungal growth.
◆ Advise the patient with a foot infection to apply nystatin topical powder to shoes and socks as a preventive measure.
◆ Instruct the patient to take the drug for the length of time prescribed — usually 14 days — even though symptomatic relief may occur within the first few hours to days.
◆ Instruct the patient to notify the prescriber if adverse reactions occur.

oral thrush, diaper rash, vaginal and vulvar candidiasis, and candidiasis between skin folds. Oral nystatin is used for candidal infections in the GI tract.

Interactions
Nystatin doesn't interact significantly with other drugs.

Adverse reactions
Reactions to nystatin seldom occur, but may include diarrhea, nausea, vomiting, and abdominal pain, especially with doses higher than 5 million units. A patient may report a bitter taste. Topical nystatin may also cause skin irritation. A hypersensitivity reaction may occur with oral or topical administration.

Nursing considerations
◆ Monitor the patient periodically for adverse reactions. If any reactions occur, notify the prescriber.
◆ If the patient receives high dosages of nystatin, monitor him for diarrhea, nausea, vomiting, and abdominal pain.
◆ Inspect the patient's skin regularly for signs of irritation. If skin irritation occurs, stop the drug.
◆ Teach the patient and his family about the prescribed drug. (See *Teaching a patient about nystatin.*)

Adverse reactions to watch for
◆ Abdominal pain, diarrhea, nausea, vomiting (especially with doses larger than 5 million units)
◆ Bitter taste
◆ Hypersensitivity reaction
◆ Skin irritation (with topical form)

Key nursing actions
◆ If the patient receives large doses, watch for abdominal pain, diarrhea, nausea, vomiting.
◆ Inspect the skin regularly for irritation.

Teaching a patient about terbinafine

Whenever terbinafine is prescribed, teach the patient and his family the drug's name, dose, frequency, action, and adverse effects. Also take the following actions.
◆ Stress the importance of taking the drug for the prescribed length of time. Inform the patient that successful treatment may take 10 weeks for toenail infections and 4 weeks for fingernail infections.
◆ Tell the patient to report vision disturbances immediately because changes in the ocular lens and retina can occur.
◆ Advise the patient to immediately report signs and symptoms of liver problems, such as persistent nausea, anorexia, fatigue, vomiting, right upper quadrant pain, jaundice, dark urine, or pale stools.
◆ Instruct the patient to notify the prescriber if other adverse reactions occur.

Features of terbinafine
◆ May inhibit squalene epoxidase, which blocks the synthesis of ergosterol, an essential component of fungal cell membranes
◆ Is used to treat tinea unguium, a fungal infection of the toenail or fingernail

Adverse reactions to watch for
◆ Abdominal pain, cholestatic jaundice, diarrhea, dyspepsia, flatulence, hepatobiliary dysfunction, nausea
◆ Anaphylaxis, hypersensitivity reactions
◆ Headache
◆ Neutropenia
◆ Pruritus, rash, Stevens-Johnson syndrome, toxic epidermal necrolysis
◆ Taste or vision disturbances

TERBINAFINE

An allylamine antifungal, terbinafine inhibits fungal cell growth by inhibiting an enzyme responsible for the manufacture of ergosterol.

Pharmacokinetics

Terbinafine is well absorbed and distributed, especially if taken with food. It's extensively metabolized, and more than ⅔ of a dose is excreted in urine.

Pharmacodynamics

The drug may inhibit squalene epoxidase, which blocks the biosynthesis of ergosterol, an essential component of fungal cell membranes.

Pharmacotherapeutics

Terbinafine is used to treat tinea unguium, a fungal infection of the toenail or fingernail.

Interactions
◆ Cimetidine decreases terbinafine clearance.
◆ Rifampin increases terbinafine clearance.
◆ Terbinafine can increase caffeine and dextromethorphan levels.
◆ Terbinafine can decrease the cyclosporine level.

Adverse reactions

 CLINICAL ALERT In rare instances, terbinafine has caused hepatic impairment, even in patients with no history of liver disease.

The most common reaction to terbinafine is headache. Uncommon reactions include vision disturbances, taste disturbances, diarrhea, dyspepsia, abdominal pain, nausea, flatulence, hepatobiliary dysfunction, cholestatic jaundice, neutropenia, rash, pruritus, Stevens-Johnson syndrome, toxic epidermal necrolysis, hypersensitivity reactions, and anaphylaxis.

Nursing considerations

 CLINICAL ALERT Avoid using terbinafine if liver disease is suspected, and obtain baseline liver enzyme levels before treatment begins.

✦ Monitor the patient's CBC and liver enzyme levels during therapy that lasts longer than 6 weeks. If hepatobiliary dysfunction or cholestatic hepatitis develops, stop the drug.
✦ Avoid using terbinafine tablets in a patient with acute or chronic liver disease.
✦ Monitor the patient periodically for adverse reactions and drug interactions during terbinafine therapy. Alert the prescriber if any occur.
✦ Teach the patient and his family about the prescribed drug. (See *Teaching a patient about terbinafine*.)

DROTRECOGIN ALFA

This unique drug is a recombinant form of human activated protein C.

Pharmacokinetics
After I.V. infusion, drotrecogin alfa achieves a median steady state level in 2 hours. Information about the drug's distribution, metabolism, and excretion isn't available.

Pharmacodynamics
Although drotrecogin alfa's anti-infective action isn't known, it may work by producing dose-dependent reductions in D-dimer and interleukin-6. Activated protein C exerts an antithrombotic effect by inhibiting factors Va and VIIIa.

Pharmacotherapeutics
Drotrecogin alfa is used to treat adults who have severe sepsis, acute organ dysfunction, and a high risk of death. The drug has antithrombotic, anti-inflammatory, and fibrinolytic properties.

Interactions
✦ Drotrecogin alfa may interact with another drug that affects hemostasis, such as an anticoagulant, antiplatelet drug, or thrombolytic, possibly increasing the risk of bleeding.

Adverse reactions
Bleeding is the most common adverse reaction to drotrecogin alfa. In clinical studies, most bleeding events took the form of ecchymosis and GI bleeding.

Nursing considerations
✦ Assess the patient for conditions that contraindicate the use of drotrecogin alfa. (See *Contraindications for drotrecogin alfa*, page 360.)
✦ When preparing the infusion, use aseptic technique.

Key nursing actions
✦ Avoid terbinafine if the patient may have liver disease.
✦ Check baseline liver enzyme levels before therapy starts.
✦ Monitor the CBC and liver enzyme levels if therapy lasts more than 6 weeks.

Features of drotrecogin alfa
✦ Is a recombinant form of human activated protein C
✦ May work via dose-dependent reductions in D-dimer and interleukin-6
✦ May exert an antithrombotic effect by inhibiting factors Va and VIIIa
✦ Has antithrombotic, anti-inflammatory, and fibrinolytic properties
✦ Is used for adults with severe sepsis, acute organ dysfunction, and a high risk of death

Adverse reactions to watch for
✦ Bleeding
✦ Ecchymosis
✦ GI bleeding

Contraindications for drotrecogin alfa

This drug is contraindicated in patients who are hypersensitive to the drug or any of its components. It's also contraindicated in patients with active internal bleeding and those who have had hemorrhagic stroke in the past 3 months or intracranial or intraspinal surgery in the past 2 months. In addition, the drug is contraindicated in patients with severe head trauma, trauma with increased risk of life-threatening bleeding, an epidural catheter, an intracranial neoplasm or mass lesion, or cerebral herniation.

Key nursing actions

◆ Monitor the patient closely for bleeding.

◆ Stop the drug 2 hours before an invasive surgical procedure.

◆ Use PT to monitor coagulation status.

◆ Give drotrecogin alfa through a dedicated I.V. line or dedicated lumen of a multilumen central venous catheter.

◆ Don't expose the drug to heat or direct sunlight.

◆ Monitor the patient closely for bleeding. If clinically significant bleeding occurs, stop the infusion.

◆ Stop the drug 2 hours before an invasive surgical procedure. Restart it after hemostasis has been achieved, usually 12 hours after major invasive surgery or immediately after an uncomplicated, less invasive procedure.

◆ Because the drug has little effect on PT, use this value to monitor the patient's coagulation status.

◆ Teach the patient and his family about the prescribed drug. (See *Teaching a patient about drotrecogin alfa.*)

PATIENT TEACHING

Teaching a patient about drotrecogin alfa

Whenever drotrecogin alfa is prescribed, teach the patient and his family the drug's name, dose, frequency, action, and adverse effects. Also take the following actions.

◆ Inform the patient or his caregiver about potential adverse reactions.

◆ Instruct the patient or his caregiver to promptly report signs of bleeding, such as bleeding gums, nosebleeds, pink or reddish urine, and black or tarry stool.

◆ Advise the patient or his caregiver that bleeding may occur for up to 28 days after treatment.

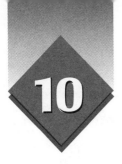

10

Antineoplastics

In the 1940s, antineoplastics, or chemotherapeutics, were developed to treat cancer. However, these drugs commonly had serious adverse effects. Today, many of these toxicities can be minimized so they aren't as devastating to the patient. With modern chemotherapy, childhood malignancies, such as acute lymphoblastic leukemia, and adult cancers, such as testicular cancer, are curable in most patients. Novel treatments, such as using monoclonal antibodies or interferons and targeting cancer-specific proteins, are improving the length of time that a patient remains in remission.

Antineoplastics may be used to cure cancer, prevent its spread, relieve cancer symptoms, or prolong survival. For a patient with a systemic cancer, such as leukemia, chemotherapy may be curative. In another patient, these drugs may be used as an adjunct based on the premise that micrometastases, although undetectable, exist. In a patient with an advanced neoplastic disorder, chemotherapy may be palliative to reduce tumor size and relieve pain and other symptoms.

Chemotherapy can include alkylating drugs, antimetabolites, antibiotic antineoplastics, aromatase inhibitors, hormonal antineoplastics, natural antineoplastics, monoclonal antibody drugs, targeted-therapy drugs, topoisomerase I inhibitors, or unclassified antineoplastics. Typically, chemotherapy is combined with other cancer treatments. For example, it may be given preoperatively to reduce tumor size and allow less radical surgery.

CELL CYCLE

To understand the pharmacodynamics of antineoplastics, you need to know about the cell cycle. All cells in the body follow a series of basic steps for division and replication. This series of steps is called the cell cycle; each step is a phase. During each phase, biochemical events that are necessary for cell division occur. (See *Understanding the cell cycle,* page 362.)

In the first phase, gap$_1$ (G$_1$), the cell manufactures the enzymes needed for deoxyribonucleic acid (DNA) synthesis. The time a cell spends in G$_1$ varies greatly but averages about 18 hours.

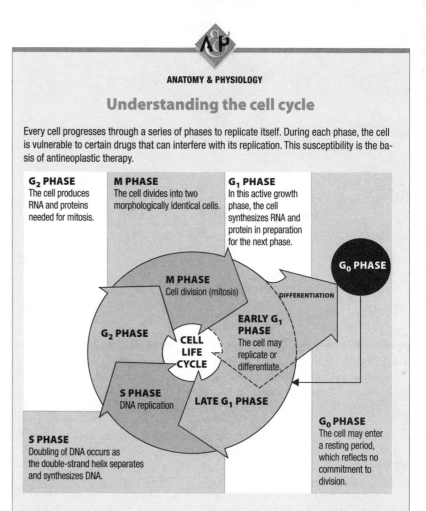

ANATOMY & PHYSIOLOGY

Understanding the cell cycle

Every cell progresses through a series of phases to replicate itself. During each phase, the cell is vulnerable to certain drugs that can interfere with its replication. This susceptibility is the basis of antineoplastic therapy.

G_2 PHASE
The cell produces RNA and proteins needed for mitosis.

M PHASE
The cell divides into two morphologically identical cells.

G_1 PHASE
In this active growth phase, the cell synthesizes RNA and protein in preparation for the next phase.

G_0 PHASE

M PHASE
Cell division (mitosis)

DIFFERENTIATION

G_2 PHASE

CELL LIFE CYCLE

EARLY G_1 PHASE
The cell may replicate or differentiate.

S PHASE
DNA replication

LATE G_1 PHASE

G_0 PHASE
The cell may enter a resting period, which reflects no commitment to division.

S PHASE
Doubling of DNA occurs as the double-strand helix separates and synthesizes DNA.

Chemotherapy and the cell cycle

✦ Cells are susceptible to different drugs in different phases of the cell cycle.

✦ Chemotherapy affects all cells in the cell cycle, especially hematopoietic and epithelial cells.

Next, the cell enters the S (synthesis) phase. In this phase, DNA replication occurs in preparation for mitosis, or cell division. This phase lasts 10 to 20 hours.

Then, the cell enters the G_2 phase, when specialized DNA proteins and ribonucleic acid (RNA) are synthesized for later mitosis. This phase lasts about 3 hours.

Finally, the cell is ready to divide and enters the M (mitosis) phase, which lasts for 1 hour. During the M phase, the cell progresses through four subphases:
✦ prophase, when the chromosomes aggregate or clump
✦ metaphase, when the chromosomes line up in the middle of the cell
✦ anaphase, when the chromosomes segregate
✦ telophase, when the cell divides, producing two morphologically identical cells.

From the M phase, the cell may follow one of three paths. It may differentiate into a functional cell, enter the resting (G_0) phase, or begin the cycle again by entering the G_1 phase. Resting cells in the G_0 phase may move on to the G_1 phase and progress through the cell cycle.

In different phases of the cycle, cells are susceptible to different drugs because the drugs interfere with specific biochemical events that occur in these phases. Chemotherapy affects all cells that are in the cell cycle, not just cancer cells. The systems of the body with high growth rates and a large percentage of cells in the cell cycle are the hematopoietic and the epithelial systems. This explains why chemotherapy has such a pronounced effect on a patient's bone marrow.

MECHANISMS OF ACTION

Although not completely understood, cancer seems to occur when one cell undergoes a malignant transformation and produces an abnormal cell. Antineoplastics interfere with cell reproduction, leading to tumor destruction.

During administration of an antineoplastic, a fixed percentage of cells die. After treatment, the remaining cells reproduce, and resting cells in the G_0 phase may return to a reproducing phase. (Cells in the G_0 phase are less sensitive to chemotherapy because they aren't synthesizing DNA actively.) Total eradication of cancer cells, therefore, depends on repeated doses of the antineoplastic. An interval between treatments permits healthy cells to recover. The optimal interval between treatments is that which allows enough time for recovery of healthy cells, yet not enough time for the tumor to totally repopulate itself.

Because cancer cells are at various phases in the cell cycle, therapy usually combines drugs that act on cells in different phases or that have different sites of action.

Although an antineoplastic kills cells as soon as they pass through a specific cell cycle, this action doesn't produce an immediate response in the patient. Most patients need at least three treatments before a response can be evaluated by physical examination, X-ray, computed tomography scanning, magnetic resonance imaging, or biological marker determination.

Tumor regression depends on several factors, such as the percentage of cells killed, the rate of regrowth, and the development of resistant cells. Evaluation of chemotherapy is difficult, however, because the cancer may be undetectable but still present. Therefore, treatment may continue for a while after the disease is no longer detectable.

TUMOR RESISTANCE

Combination drug regimens may be used for patients with tumor resistance. Tumor cell populations are heterogeneous, which means that some cells are sensitive to antineoplastics; others aren't. When an antineoplastic is given, it initially kills drug-sensitive cells. Repeated doses kill more drug-sensitive cells. Over time, however, tumor cells that aren't drug-sensitive remain and replicate, producing a drug-resistant tumor. If these resistant cells are also resistant to other drugs, they'll be even more difficult to kill. In addition, cancer cells can mutate, making drug-sensitive cells become drug resistant.

Drug resistance may develop by one or more of the following mechanisms: decreased drug entry into the tumor cells, decreased drug-activating enzymes, increased drug-deactivating enzymes, increased levels of target enzymes, decreased target enzyme affinity for the drug, increased DNA repair, or development of alternate pathways that circumvent the drug's action. In general, the greater the number of chemotherapeutics in a regimen, the less likely that drug resistance will occur.

HANDLING ANTINEOPLASTICS

Although the safe handling of antineoplastics remains controversial, most experts recommend conservative, protective methods. For maximum safety, use the following techniques when handling antineoplastics:
+ Mix antineoplastics in a class II biological safety cabinet only.

How antineoplastics work

+ Antineoplastics interfere with cell reproduction to destroy tumors.
+ During administration, a fixed percentage of cancer cells die. Afterward, the remaining cells continue reproducing.
+ Eradication of cancer cells depends on repeated antineoplastic doses. A gap between treatments permits healthy cells to recover.
+ Because cancer cells are at various phases in the cell cycle, therapy usually combines drugs that act on different cell phases or that have different sites of action.
+ Although an antineoplastic kills cells as soon as they pass through a specific cell cycle, this action doesn't produce an immediate response in the patient.

Understanding tumor resistance

+ When an antineoplastic is given, it initially kills drug-sensitive cells.
+ Over time, tumor cells that aren't drug-sensitive remain and replicate, producing a drug-resistant tumor.
+ Drug resistance may develop via a range of mechanisms.
+ In general, the greater the number of chemotherapeutics in a regimen, the less likely drug resistance is to develop.

✦ Wear powder-free, disposable, latex surgical gloves and a protective barrier garment with a closed front and long, cuffed sleeves to protect your body when mixing or giving antineoplastics. Wearing double gloves is recommended. Latex-sensitive individuals should use gloves made of an alternate material, such as nitrile.

✦ Reconstitute and give antineoplastics in syringes or I.V. sets with needleless systems.

✦ Use a closed-delivery technique when giving these drugs. Don't prime I.V. lines and syringes into a sink or waste basket; use sterile 2" × 2" gauze pads or alcohol wipes instead.

✦ After mixing and giving these drugs, dispose of any waste in a leakproof, punctureproof container labeled "hazardous waste." Such containers must be disposed of by incineration or burial at a hazardous chemical waste site.

✦ If a spill occurs, follow your facility's policy for cleaning up hazardous materials.

GIVING ANTINEOPLASTICS

Before giving an antineoplastic, reinforce the information about the benefits and risks of treatment that the patient has received. A patient who consents to investigational chemotherapy should receive additional information. Throughout the patient's therapy, continue to teach and reinforce this information to promote patient safety and compliance.

To give an antineoplastic safely, select an appropriate site and vein; consider drug compatibilities; determine the drug's vesicant, or blister-causing, potential; consider its sequencing and delivery; and prevent and treat extravasation.

For a patient who must receive several treatments with potentially damaging drugs, site and vein selection is especially important. To select an appropriate I.V. site, begin with a distal spot, such as the hand, and proceed to proximal areas, such as up the forearm.

Before giving any antineoplastic drug, consider drug compatibilities. As a rule, antineoplastics shouldn't be mixed with any other drugs. Although little research has been done to determine exact incompatibilities, the nature and toxicity of these drugs usually prohibit mixing.

To choose the proper drug sequencing and delivery technique, check the drug's vesicant potential. For intermittent drug delivery, give a vesicant drug by direct push or delivery into the side port of an infusing I.V. line. For continuous infusion, give a vesicant only via a central line or vascular access device. Give a nonvesicant drug (including an irritant) by direct I.V. push, through the side port of an infusing I.V. line, or as a continuous infusion. Some facilities require that the vesicant be given first because vein integrity decreases over time.

During the administration of any I.V. antineoplastic, the patient's safety depends on your assessment of the infusion site during drug delivery. To ensure patency of the vein, be sure to elicit a blood return before, during, and after giving the drug.

To prevent extravasation, stabilize the needle and check frequently for blood return. Although no definitive measures exist to treat extravasation of an antineoplastic, conservative measures include stopping the infusion, aspirating any residual drug from the tubing and needle, instilling an I.V. antidote if available, and removing the needle. After giving an antidote, apply heat or cold and elevate the affected limb.

How to give antineoplastics

✦ Select an appropriate site and vein. Start with a distal site, such as in the hand, and move proximally, such as up the forearm.

✦ Consider drug compatibilities. As a rule, antineoplastics shouldn't be mixed with any other drugs.

✦ Determine the drug's vesicant potential.

✦ For intermittent drug delivery, give a vesicant by direct push or delivery into the side port of an infusing I.V. line.

✦ For continuous infusion, give a vesicant only via a central line or vascular access device.

✦ Give a nonvesicant (including an irritant) by direct I.V. push, through the side port of an infusing I.V. line, or as a continuous infusion.

✦ To ensure vein patency, elicit a blood return before, during, and after giving the drug.

✦ Prevent extravasation by stabilizing the needle and checking frequently for blood return.

✦ Treat extravasation with conservative measures.

ADVERSE REACTIONS

Adverse reactions to antineoplastics result from their systemic effects. Some reactions can be life-threatening, requiring modification of the drug dosage or treatment regimen. Others are less severe, but may be stressful to the patient.

Nausea and vomiting are common adverse reactions. Chemotherapy can cause nausea and vomiting by three basic mechanisms. First, oral drugs can irritate the gastric mucosa directly, causing less severe nausea and vomiting than that caused by the other two mechanisms.

Second, other antineoplastics can stimulate the chemoreceptor trigger zone. The risk of nausea and vomiting from this mechanism depends on the drug's emetic potential.

Third, chemotherapy can cause psychogenic nausea and vomiting, which originates in the cerebral cortex. Known as anticipatory emesis, this reaction can be disabling. A patient who remembers the unpleasantness of previous chemotherapy may feel nauseated or may vomit just by thinking about future treatments. This reaction may become so severe that sights, sounds, and smells related to treatment may induce emesis, no matter how far removed the patient is from the actual treatment setting.

Chemotherapy-induced nausea and vomiting is of great concern because it can cause fluid and electrolyte imbalances, noncompliance with the treatment regimen, wound dehiscence, pathologic fractures, and Mallory-Weiss syndrome, or tears that lead to massive bleeding at the esophageal-gastric junction. It also can cause distress by limiting the patient's ability and motivation to take an active role in life.

To combat chemotherapy-induced nausea and vomiting, give an antiemetic. Usually, an antiemetic is given with other antiemetics that act by different mechanisms. A combination regimen is more effective than a single drug, especially for a strong emetic drug, such as cisplatin. To help control psychogenic factors related to nausea and vomiting, teach the patient relaxation techniques that can help minimize feelings of isolation and anxiety, encourage him to express anxieties, and help him use relaxation techniques during chemotherapy.

Adverse reactions to watch for

+ Chemotherapy-induced nausea and vomiting is of great concern because it can cause fluid and electrolyte imbalances, noncompliance, wound dehiscence, pathologic fractures, and Mallory-Weiss syndrome.
+ To combat chemotherapy-induced nausea and vomiting, most patients receive multiple antiemetics that act by differing mechanisms.

ALKYLATING DRUGS

Given alone or with other drugs, alkylating drugs effectively act against various malignant neoplasms. These drugs fall into six classes: busulfan, alkylating-like drugs, ethylenimines, nitrogen mustards, nitrosoureas, and triazenes.

All of these drugs produce their antineoplastic effects by damaging DNA. They halt the replication process of DNA by cross-linking its strands so that amino acids don't pair up correctly. Alkylating drugs are cell cycle–phase nonspecific. This means that their alkylating actions may take place at any phase of the cell cycle. (See *How alkylating drugs work,* page 366.)

BUSULFAN

Historically, the alkyl sulfonate busulfan has been used to treat chronic myelogenous leukemia, polycythemia vera, which is an increased red blood cell (RBC) mass and an increased number of white blood cells (WBCs) and platelets, and other myeloproliferative disorders, which are disorders marked by overactive bone mar-

Features of alkylating drugs

+ Halt the replication of cancer cell DNA by cross-linking its strands so that amino acids don't pair up correctly
+ Are given alone or with other drugs
+ Include six drug classes
+ Are cell cycle–phase nonspecific

How alkylating drugs work

Alkylating drugs can attack deoxyribonucleic acid (DNA) in two ways, as shown in the illustrations below.

BIFUNCTIONAL ALKYLATION

Some drugs become inserted between two base pairs in the DNA chain, forming an irreversible bond between them. This is called *bifunctional alkylation,* which causes cytotoxic effects that can destroy or poison cells.

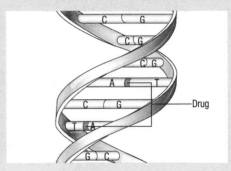

MONOFUNCTIONAL ALKYLATION

Other drugs react with just one part of a pair, separating it from its partner and eventually causing it and its attached sugar to break away from the DNA molecule. This is called *monofunctional alkylation,* which eventually may cause permanent cell damage.

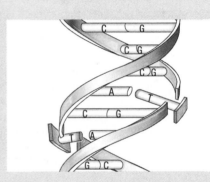

Features of busulfan

- ✦ Forms covalent bonds with DNA molecules through alkylation
- ✦ Affects mainly granulocytes and, to a lesser degree, platelets
- ✦ Is used for chronic myelogenous leukemia and in conditioning regimens for bone marrow transplantation
- ✦ Is also effective for polycythemia vera

row. In high doses, it's also used to treat leukemia during bone marrow transplantation.

Pharmacokinetics

Busulfan is absorbed rapidly and well from the GI tract. Little is known about its distribution. The drug is metabolized extensively in the liver before it's excreted in urine. Its half-life is 2 to 3 hours.

Pharmacodynamics

Through alkylation, busulfan forms covalent bonds with the DNA molecules by substituting an alkyl group for an active hydrogen atom.

Pharmacotherapeutics

Busulfan primarily affects granulocytes, which are a type of WBC, and, to a lesser degree, platelets. Because of its action on granulocytes, this drug is used for treating chronic myelogenous leukemia and in conditioning regimens for bone marrow transplantation.

Busulfan is also effective in treating polycythemia vera. However, other drugs are usually used to treat this disorder because busulfan can cause severe myelosuppression, or halting of bone marrow function.

Interactions

✦ When busulfan is used with an anticoagulant or aspirin, the risk of bleeding increases.

✦ Use of busulfan with thioguanine may cause hepatotoxicity, esophageal varices, or portal hypertension.

Adverse reactions

The major adverse reaction to busulfan is bone marrow suppression, which usually is dose-related and reversible. Bone marrow suppression produces severe leukopenia, anemia, and thrombocytopenia. Granulocytopenia occurs rarely and can progress to pancytopenia, which may be fatal.

Nausea, vomiting, and diarrhea are uncommon. Hyperuricemia may occur. With long-term therapy, an addisonian-like wasting syndrome with hyperpigmentation and weight loss sometimes occurs. Busulfan may also produce irreversible interstitial pulmonary fibrosis, which is also known as busulfan lung, after 1 to 3 years of use.

Nursing considerations

✦ Monitor the patient for adverse reactions during busulfan therapy. Alert the prescriber if any occur.

✦ Monitor the patient's complete blood count (CBC) to detect such abnormalities as leukopenia, thrombocytopenia, or anemia. If abnormalities occur, notify the prescriber before giving the next dose of busulfan.

✦ Take infection control measures and bleeding precautions. If leukopenia occurs, monitor the patient for signs of infection. If thrombocytopenia occurs, monitor the patient for signs of bleeding. Also observe for early signs and symptoms of intracranial hemorrhage. Avoid I.M. injections and venipunctures when the patient's platelet count is low. When a venipuncture must be done, apply firm pressure to the site for at least 5 minutes afterward.

✦ Use an anticoagulant cautiously during busulfan therapy and observe for signs of bleeding.

✦ Monitor the patient's uric acid level to detect hyperuricemia. If hyperuricemia occurs, give allopurinol and ensure that the patient consumes at least 2 qt (2 L) of fluid daily, unless contraindicated.

✦ Use other appropriate interventions for a patient with bone marrow suppression, nausea, or vomiting.

✦ Monitor pulmonary function test results for a patient receiving long-term busulfan therapy. Also perform respiratory assessments regularly, particularly noting changes in the quality of respirations, such as progressive dyspnea, or a persistent cough. Alert the prescriber if respiratory abnormalities occur.

✦ Teach the patient and his family about the prescribed drug. (See *Teaching a patient about busulfan,* page 368.)

Adverse reactions to watch for

✦ Addisonian-like wasting syndrome with hyperpigmentation and weight loss (with long-term therapy)
✦ Bone marrow suppression, which can cause severe leukopenia, anemia, and thrombocytopenia
✦ Diarrhea, nausea, vomiting
✦ Hyperuricemia
✦ Irreversible interstitial pulmonary fibrosis

Key nursing actions

✦ Monitor CBC.
✦ Take infection control measures and bleeding precautions.
✦ Monitor the uric acid level.
✦ Perform respiratory assessments regularly, and check pulmonary function test results if the patient is receiving long-term therapy.

ALKYLATING-LIKE DRUGS

Carboplatin, cisplatin, and oxaliplatin are heavy metal complexes that contain platinum. Because their action resembles that of a bifunctional alkylating drug, they are called alkylating-like drugs.

Pharmacokinetics

The distribution and metabolism of carboplatin aren't defined clearly. After giving carboplatin I.V., it's eliminated primarily by the kidneys. The elimination of carboplatin is biphasic. Its initial half-life is 1 to 2 hours; its terminal half-life is 2½ to 6 hours.

When given intrapleurally or intraperitoneally, cisplatin may exhibit significant systemic absorption. Highly protein-bound, cisplatin reaches a high level in the kidneys, liver, intestines, and testes but penetrates the central nervous system (CNS) poorly. The drug undergoes some liver metabolism, followed by excretion through the kidneys.

Oxaliplatin is 70% to 95% bound to plasma proteins; its binding increases over time. The drug is widely distributed into most body tissues and is eliminated in three distinct phases.

With all alkylating-like drugs, platinum is detectable in tissue for at least 4 months after the last dose.

Pharmacodynamics

Like alkylating drugs, carboplatin, cisplatin, and oxaliplatin are cell cycle–nonspecific and inhibit DNA synthesis. They act like bifunctional alkylating drugs by cross-linking strands of DNA and inhibiting DNA synthesis.

Pharmacotherapeutics

Alkylating-like drugs are used to treat several cancers. Carboplatin is used primarily for ovarian and lung cancer.

Cisplatin is prescribed to treat bladder and ovarian cancer. It's the drug of choice for testicular cancer. Its unlabeled uses include treatment of head, neck, and lung cancer.

Features of alkylating-like drugs

◆ Are heavy metal complexes that contain platinum
◆ Are cell cycle–nonspecific
◆ Inhibit DNA synthesis by cross-linking DNA strands
◆ Carboplatin is used mainly for ovarian and lung cancer
◆ Cisplatin is used for bladder and ovarian cancer and is the drug of choice for testicular cancer
◆ Oxaliplatin is used with other drugs for colorectal cancer

Oxaliplatin is used with other drugs to treat colorectal cancer.

Interactions
✦ When carboplatin, cisplatin, or oxaliplatin is used with an aminoglycoside, the risk of nephrotoxicity increases.
✦ Use of carboplatin or cisplatin with bumetanide, ethacrynic acid, or furosemide can increase the risk of ototoxicity.
✦ Cisplatin may reduce the phenytoin level.

Adverse reactions
Alkylating-like drugs produce many of the same adverse reactions as the alkylating drugs. Carboplatin can produce bone marrow suppression, especially affecting platelet formation, which may require a dosage adjustment. Cisplatin doesn't usually cause severe leukopenia or thrombocytopenia; however, it may cause anemia. Oxaliplatin commonly causes anemia, leukopenia, and thrombocytopenia.

Nephrotoxicity occurs in 28% to 36% of patients receiving cisplatin, usually after multiple courses of therapy. With long-term cisplatin therapy, neurotoxicity also can occur, producing sensory and motor peripheral neuropathies, loss of proprioception, loss of taste, and intestinal ileus. Neurotoxicity is less common with carboplatin. Carboplatin also has a lower nephrotoxic potential.

Cisplatin may produce electrolyte imbalances, especially hypomagnesemia. Up to 30% of patients receiving cisplatin report tinnitus and hearing loss, which is often permanent. These adverse reactions are much less common with carboplatin. Cisplatin also produces marked nausea and vomiting in almost all patients and requires prophylactic antiemetic therapy, usually with ondansetron or granisetron. Carboplatin usually produces less-severe nausea and vomiting that aren't as prolonged.

Other common reactions to oxaliplatin include pain, peripheral neuropathy, fatigue, headache, insomnia, fever, flushing, peripheral edema, nausea, vomiting, diarrhea, stomatitis, abdominal pain, anorexia, constipation, dyspepsia, taste perversion, back pain, arthralgia, dyspnea, cough, upper respiratory tract infection, injection site reaction, hand-foot syndrome, and allergic reaction.

Nursing considerations
✦ Monitor the patient for adverse reactions and drug interactions during therapy. Alert the prescriber if any occur.
✦ Review the patient's CBC and platelet count before giving the initial dose and with each subsequent dose.
✦ If leukopenia occurs, monitor the patient for signs and symptoms of infection. Take infection-control measures until the patient's WBC count returns to normal.
✦ If thrombocytopenia occurs, monitor the patient for signs and symptoms of bleeding. Take bleeding precautions until the platelet count returns to normal. Avoid all I.M. injections and venipunctures when the platelet count is low. When a venipuncture must be done, apply firm pressure to the site for at least 5 minutes afterward.
✦ Reconstitute cisplatin with sterile water for injection. Cisplatin remains stable for 24 hours in normal saline solution at room temperature; don't refrigerate solutions.

 CLINICAL ALERT Don't use an aluminum needle to reconstitute or give an alkylating-like drug because the drug will interact with the aluminum, forming a black precipitate that can't be injected.

Key nursing actions
- Review the CBC and platelet count before giving each dose.
- Check renal function tests before giving each dose.
- Give enough fluid to keep the patient's urine output at 100 ml/hour for 4 consecutive hours before cisplatin therapy and for 24 hours afterward.
- Give magnesium to replace any lost during cisplatin therapy.
- Give mannitol before a cisplatin infusion.

Features of thiotepa
- Is an ethylenimine derivative and multifunctional alkylating drug
- Disrupts DNA replication, RNA transcription, and nucleic acid function
- Is used to treat bladder cancer and for palliation of lymphomas and ovarian or breast carcinomas
- Can be used for intracavitary effusions, which may make drug useful for lung cancer

✦ Check the results of renal function tests before giving the initial dose and with each subsequent dose. Adjust the carboplatin dosage based on renal function or desired platelet nadir.

✦ Give sufficient fluid to maintain the patient's urine output at 100 ml/hour for 4 consecutive hours before cisplatin therapy and for 24 hours afterward. Notify the prescriber if the urine output is less than 100 ml/hour during the first 24 hours.

✦ Give magnesium to replace any that's lost during cisplatin therapy.

✦ Give mannitol before a cisplatin infusion. Also give a mannitol infusion to maintain urine output during and for 6 to 24 hours after a cisplatin infusion.

✦ Teach the patient and his family about the prescribed drug. (See *Teaching a patient about alkylating-like drugs.*)

ETHYLENIMINES
Thiotepa, an ethylenimine derivative, is a multifunctional alkylating drug.

Pharmacokinetics
After giving thiotepa I.V., it's 100% bioavailable. Significant systemic absorption may occur when thiotepa is given into pleural or peritoneal spaces to treat malignant effusions or is instilled into the bladder.

Thiotepa crosses the blood-brain barrier and is metabolized extensively in the liver. The drug and its metabolites are excreted in urine.

Pharmacodynamics
Thiotepa exerts its cytotoxic activity by interfering with DNA replication and RNA transcription. Ultimately, it disrupts nucleic acid function and causes cell death.

Pharmacotherapeutics
Thiotepa is an alkylating drug that's used to treat bladder cancer. Thiotepa is also prescribed for palliative treatment of lymphomas and ovarian or breast carcinomas.

WARNING

Spotting hematologic reactions to ethylenimines

Adverse hematologic reactions to ethylenimines include anemia, leukopenia, thrombocytopenia, and pancytopenia. Because they may be fatal, stay alert for the signs and symptoms listed in the table below.

HEMATOLOGIC REACTION	SIGNS AND SYMPTOMS
Anemia	• Fatigue • Exertional dyspnea • Dizziness • Headache • Insomnia • Pallor • Decreased red blood cell count and hemoglobin
Leukopenia	• Fever or chills • Cough or hoarseness • Lower back or side pain • Difficult or painful urination • Decreased white blood cell count
Thrombocytopenia	• Unusual bleeding or bruising • Black, tarry stools • Blood in urine • Petechiae • Decreased platelet count
Pancytopenia	• All of the above

The Food and Drug Administration (FDA) has approved thiotepa for the treatment of intracavitary effusions. This drug may also prove useful in treating lung cancer.

Interactions
✦ Use of thiotepa with aspirin or an anticoagulant may increase the risk of bleeding.
✦ Use of thiotepa with a neuromuscular blocker may prolong muscular paralysis.
✦ Use of thiotepa with another alkylating drug or with radiation therapy may intensify toxic reactions rather than enhance therapeutic ones.
✦ When used with succinylcholine, thiotepa may cause prolonged respirations and apnea, possibly by inhibiting the activity of cholinesterase, the enzyme that deactivates succinylcholine.

Adverse reactions
The major adverse reaction to thiotepa is hematologic toxicity, which is usually dose-related and cumulative. (See *Spotting hematologic reactions to ethylenimines.*)

Possible drug interactions
✦ Alkylating drugs
✦ Anticoagulants
✦ Aspirin
✦ Neuromuscular blockers
✦ Succinylcholine

Adverse reactions to watch for

+ Alopecia
+ Anorexia, nausea, vomiting
+ Exudation from S.C. lesions
+ Dizziness, headache, throat tightness
+ Febrile reactions
+ Hematologic toxicity (usually dose-related and cumulative)
+ Hives, pruritus, rash
+ Hyperuricemia
+ Injection site pain
+ Lower abdominal pain, bladder irritability, hematuria, hemorrhagic cystitis (rare)
+ Stomatitis, ulceration of intestinal mucosa

Key nursing actions

+ Monitor the CBC for hematologic abnormalities.
+ Take bleeding precautions and watch for evidence of bleeding.
+ Take safety measures if the patient is dizzy.
+ Monitor the uric acid level.
+ Watch for hematuria and dysuria, which may indicate hemorrhagic cystitis.

PATIENT TEACHING

Teaching a patient about ethylenimines

Whenever an ethylenimine is prescribed, teach the patient and his family the drug's name, dose, frequency, action, and adverse effects. Also take the following actions.
+ Inform the patient that thiotepa instillation may cause lower abdominal pain, bladder irritability (with dysuria and frequent urination), and hematuria. Reassure him that these signs and symptoms will subside.
+ Inform the patient that thiotepa may cause alopecia. Reassure him that hair loss is reversible when the treatment ends.
+ Instruct the patient to inform the prescriber immediately if hives, rash, or pruritus occurs. Any of these may indicate a hypersensitivity reaction.
+ Caution the patient not to perform activities that require alertness if dizziness occurs.
+ Inform the patient that pain may occur at the injection site during the infusion and that measures will be taken to minimize the discomfort.
+ Advise the patient to notify the prescriber if throat tightness occurs during thiotepa therapy.
+ Teach the patient to use infection control measures and bleeding precautions as needed.
+ Advise the patient with anemia to stagger activities and to rest frequently.
+ Teach the patient how to handle troublesome adverse reactions, such as GI distress and stomatitis.
+ Stress the importance of returning for follow-up visits and complete blood cell counts.
+ Instruct the patient to notify the prescriber if adverse reactions occur.

Nausea, vomiting, and anorexia are uncommon. Stomatitis and ulceration of the intestinal mucosa may occur, especially with bone marrow transplant doses.

Other adverse reactions to thiotepa include injection site pain, alopecia, headache, dizziness, and throat tightness as well as hyperuricemia, febrile reactions, and exudation from subcutaneous (S.C.) lesions.

Hypersensitivity reactions are rare, but hives, rash, and pruritus occasionally occur. In some patients, thiotepa instillation has caused lower abdominal pain, bladder irritability, hematuria and, rarely, hemorrhagic cystitis.

Nursing considerations

+ Monitor the patient for adverse reactions and drug interactions. If any occur, alert the prescriber.
+ Monitor the patient's CBC for abnormalities that indicate anemia, leukopenia, thrombocytopenia, or pancytopenia.
+ If leukopenia occurs, take infection control measures and monitor the patient for signs and symptoms of infection.
+ Take bleeding precautions and monitor the patient for signs and symptoms of bleeding.
+ Stagger the patient's activities and provide frequent rest periods if the patient experiences anemia.
+ Notify the prescriber immediately if pancytopenia occurs.
+ Take safety measures if the patient experiences dizziness. For example, place the bed in the lowest position, keep the side rails up, and supervise the patient's ambulation.
+ Monitor the patient's uric acid level; an elevation may indicate hyperuricemia.

✦ Monitor the patient for hematuria and dysuria, which may indicate hemorrhagic cystitis.

✦ Teach the patient and his family about the prescribed drug. (See *Teaching a patient about ethylenimines.*)

NITROGEN MUSTARDS

The largest group of alkylating drugs, nitrogen mustards include chlorambucil, cyclophosphamide, estramustine, ifosfamide, mechlorethamine, melphalan, and uracil mustard. Mechlorethamine was the first nitrogen mustard introduced.

Pharmacokinetics

The absorption and distribution of nitrogen mustards vary widely. However, they're all metabolized in the liver and excreted by the kidneys. Mechlorethamine undergoes such rapid metabolism that no active drug remains after a few minutes. Most nitrogen mustards possess more intermediate half-lives than mechlorethamine.

Pharmacodynamics

Through alkylation, nitrogen mustards form covalent bonds with DNA molecules. Alkylated DNA can't replicate properly, thereby resulting in cell death. Unfortunately, cells may develop resistance to the cytotoxic effects of nitrogen mustards.

Pharmacotherapeutics

Because they produce leukopenia, nitrogen mustards are effective in treating malignant neoplasms that elevate the WBC count, such as Hodgkin's disease and leukemia.

Nitrogen mustards also prove effective against non-Hodgkin's lymphoma, multiple myeloma, melanoma, and cancers of the breast, ovaries, uterus, lung, brain, testes, bladder, prostate, and stomach.

Interactions

✦ A drug or food containing calcium, such as an antacid or dairy product, can reduce estramustine absorption.

✦ Use of cyclophosphamide with a cardiotoxic drug can produce additive cardiac effects.

✦ Cyclophosphamide may reduce the digoxin level.

✦ Use of ifosfamide with allopurinol, chloral hydrate, phenytoin, or a barbiturate can increase the risk of ifosfamide toxicity.

✦ A corticosteroid can reduce the effects of ifosfamide.

✦ Melphalan may reduce the lung toxicity threshold of carmustine.

✦ Interferon alfa may reduce the melphalan level.

Adverse reactions

Bone marrow suppression, as evidenced by severe leukopenia and thrombocytopenia, is an anticipated adverse reaction to nitrogen mustards. Nausea and vomiting from CNS irritation are also common reactions. They may occur 30 minutes after the dose, as with mechlorethamine, or they may not begin for hours, as with cyclophosphamide.

Damage to rapidly proliferating cells produces stomatitis and alopecia. The swollen, inflamed mucous membranes that characterize stomatitis can lead to a nutritional problem because of the pain caused by stomatitis. Alopecia, which is

Features of nitrogen mustards

✦ Represent the largest group of alkylating drugs
✦ Form covalent bonds with DNA molecules, preventing proper replication
✦ Allow cells to become resistant to nitrogen mustards' cytotoxic effects
✦ Are used for malignant neoplasms that elevate WBC count, such as Hodgkin's disease and leukemia
✦ Are also used for non-Hodgkin's lymphoma, multiple myeloma, melanoma, and cancers of the breast, ovaries, uterus, lung, brain, testes, bladder, prostate, and stomach

Adverse reactions to watch for

✦ Alopecia
✦ Altered fertility
✦ Amenorrhea, irregular menses
✦ Bone marrow suppression (severe leukopenia, thrombocytopenia)
✦ Decreased spermatogenesis
✦ Fatigue
✦ Hemorrhagic cystitis (with cyclophosphamide, ifosfamide)
✦ Hepatotoxicity (with chlorambucil)
✦ Myelosuppression (with ifosfamide)
✦ Nausea, vomiting
✦ Stomatitis

caused by hair follicle damage, results in thinning hair 2 to 3 weeks after the first dose of a nitrogen mustard. However, hair loss isn't usually significant for two or three courses of treatment. Once treatment ends, hair growth resumes. Many patients experience fatigue during nitrogen mustard therapy.

 CLINICAL ALERT Because nitrogen mustards are powerful local vesicants, direct contact with the drugs or their vapors can cause severe reactions, especially of the skin, eyes, and respiratory tract. Mechlorethamine extravasation may cause painful inflammation and induration.

A patient may experience alterations in fertility. After several courses of nitrogen mustard treatment, women may experience amenorrhea or irregular menses. Men may have decreased spermatogenesis. Many patients, however, experience no alteration in fertility, and women treated with nitrogen mustards have conceived and given birth to normal children.

Hemorrhagic cystitis may develop within 48 hours of an I.V. dose of cyclophosphamide or after several months of oral low-dose therapy. Cyclophosphamide metabolites in the urine irritate the bladder lining, which produces this adverse reaction. Adequate hydration usually prevents hemorrhagic cystitis.

Myelosuppression and hemorrhagic cystitis are dose-limiting toxicities for ifosfamide. Giving mesna, a cystitis prophylactic, may alleviate the cystitis reaction. Ifosfamide may also cause adverse CNS reactions, such as somnolence, confusion, and hallucinations.

Chlorambucil may produce hepatotoxicity, but this reaction seldom occurs. Rarely, chlorambucil and cyclophosphamide may cause pulmonary reactions, such as interstitial pneumonitis or pulmonary fibrosis.

Like other alkylating drugs, nitrogen mustards have been implicated in producing hematologic and other malignancies, although this is rare. Anaphylaxis is another uncommon adverse reaction.

Nursing considerations

✦ Monitor the patient for adverse reactions and drug interactions. If any occur, alert the prescriber.
✦ Give the nitrogen mustard with an antiemetic to control or lessen nausea and vomiting. If fluid intake is inadequate despite antiemetic use, give I.V. fluids.
✦ If stomatitis occurs, monitor the patient's nutritional status. To relieve stomatitis, provide frequent oral care, apply a topical drug for pain relief, and provide a pureed or liquid diet.
✦ If fatigue occurs, assist the patient with activities of daily living. Limit the patient's activities and stagger those that are necessary. Provide rest periods — especially after treatment — when the patient is most likely to feel fatigued.
✦ Monitor all infusion sites for signs of extravasation, such as pain and swelling at the site. Change infusion sites according to facility protocol and as needed.
✦ Monitor the patient for signs of hemorrhagic cystitis, such as hematuria and dysuria, during cyclophosphamide or ifosfamide therapy.
✦ Increase the fluid intake of the patient receiving I.V. cyclophosphamide to at least 2 qt (2 L) daily. After treatment, instruct the patient to maintain increased fluids for 2 to 3 days.
✦ Give cyclophosphamide or ifosfamide earlier in the day rather than at bedtime to prevent prolonged contact between the drug's metabolites and the bladder.
✦ Give mesna with ifosfamide and 4 and 8 hours after treatment to help prevent hemorrhagic cystitis.

Key nursing actions
✦ Give the drug with an antiemetic.
✦ If stomatitis occurs, monitor the nutritional status.
✦ If fatigue occurs, assist with activities of daily living.
✦ Monitor all infusion sites for extravasation.
✦ Watch for evidence of hemorrhagic cystitis during cyclophosphamide or ifosfamide therapy.
✦ Increase the fluid intake of a patient receiving I.V. cyclophosphamide to at least 2 L daily.
✦ Frequently monitor blood counts, especially the CBC.

Teaching a patient about nitrogen mustards

Whenever a nitrogen mustard is prescribed, teach the patient and his family the drug's name, dose, frequency, action, and adverse effects. Also take the following actions.

✦ Inform the patient that the nitrogen mustard can produce alopecia, which can't be prevented. Explain that alopecia affects men and women and may include eyebrows, eyelashes, scalp hair, and other body hair. Reassure the patient that hair loss is reversible when the treatment ends.

✦ Instruct the patient to increase his oral fluid intake the day before cyclophosphamide or ifosfamide therapy to help prevent hemorrhagic cystitis. Advise him that fluid intake shouldn't include caffeinated beverages, such as coffee or tea.

✦ Encourage the patient to take oral cyclophosphamide earlier in the day, to maintain good fluid intake, and to void before going to bed.

✦ Discuss ways to relieve adverse reactions. For example, suggest dietary changes to relieve nausea, vomiting, or stomatitis; frequent oral care to help manage stomatitis; and activity restriction to help the patient manage fatigue.

✦ Advise the patient not to perform activities that require alertness until ifosfamide's adverse central nervous system effects are known.

✦ Teach the patient to use infection control measures and bleeding precautions during nitrogen mustard therapy.

✦ Inform the patient that fertility may be altered during nitrogen mustard therapy. Advise a woman that amenorrhea or irregular menses also may occur.

✦ Stress the importance of returning for follow-up visits and blood tests.

✦ Instruct the patient to notify the prescriber if adverse reactions occur.

✦ Advise the patient to notify the prescriber if any other symptoms appear because the nitrogen mustard may cause a secondary hematologic or other malignancy, such as leukemia.

✦ Provide written materials about the nitrogen mustard for home reference.

✦ Wear gloves and follow facility protocol when giving a nitrogen mustard, and avoid inhaling the vapors. Direct contact with the drug or its vapors can cause severe reactions, especially of the skin, eyes, and respiratory tract.

✦ Give the nitrogen mustard exactly as directed in the manufacturer's guidelines.

✦ Give mechlorethamine immediately after reconstitution because it's unstable in solution. Most other nitrogen mustards, which remain stable in solution, can be prepared a while before they're given.

✦ Reduce I.V. administration pain by altering the infusion rate, further diluting the drug if indicated, or warming the injection site to distend the vein and increase blood flow.

✦ Use appropriate interventions for a patient with bone marrow suppression, nausea, vomiting, stomatitis, or alopecia.

✦ Frequently monitor the patient's blood counts, especially his CBC.

✦ If leukopenia occurs, take infection-control measures and monitor the patient for signs of infection.

✦ Teach the patient and his family about the prescribed drug. (See *Teaching a patient about nitrogen mustards*.)

How to handle nitrogen mustards

✦ Wear gloves.
✦ Follow facility protocol.
✦ Avoid inhaling the vapors.
✦ Avoid direct contact with the drug.
✦ Give the drug exactly as directed by the manufacturer.

NITROSOUREAS

These alkylating drugs work by halting cancer cell reproduction. Nitrosoureas include carmustine, lomustine, and streptozocin.

Pharmacokinetics

When given topically to treat mycosis fungoides, a rare skin malignancy, carmustine is 5% to 28% systemically absorbed. After oral administration, lomustine is absorbed adequately, although incompletely. Because streptozocin is poorly absorbed orally, it's always given I.V.

Nitrosoureas are attracted to fat, or lipophilic, distributing to fatty tissues and cerebrospinal fluid (CSF). The drugs are metabolized extensively before they're excreted in urine.

Pharmacodynamics

During bifunctional alkylation, nitrosoureas interfere with amino acids, purines, and DNA needed for cancer cells to divide. This action halts cellular reproduction.

Pharmacotherapeutics

The nitrosoureas are highly lipid soluble, which allows them or their metabolites to easily cross the blood-brain barrier. Because of this ability, nitrosoureas are used to treat brain tumors and meningeal leukemias.

Interactions

✦ Cimetidine may increase carmustine's bone marrow toxicity.
✦ Streptozocin prolongs the elimination half-life of doxorubicin, prolonging the leukopenia and thrombocytopenia.

Adverse reactions

Carmustine and lomustine produce bone marrow suppression that begins 4 to 6 weeks after treatment and lasts for 1 to 2 weeks. The bone marrow suppression is cumulative — that is, it can become more severe and prolonged with repeated doses.

Severe nausea lasts for 2 to 6 hours after carmustine and lomustine doses. Lomustine may also cause anorexia for a few days. Severe nausea and vomiting also occur with streptozocin and may persist for more than 24 hours.

Nephrotoxicity and renal impairment may occur with the nitrosoureas. In about two-thirds of patients receiving streptozocin, renal dysfunction occurs and is dose-limiting.

High-dose carmustine may produce reversible hepatotoxicity. Carmustine may also cause pulmonary toxicity, which is characterized by pulmonary infiltrates or fibrosis. These pulmonary reactions are dose-related; their incidence is much higher in patients who receive cumulative doses of more than 1,400 mg/m². Hematologic toxicity and mild glucose intolerance are rare adverse reactions to streptozocin.

The patient may experience intense pain at the infusion site with carmustine because the drug may cause vein irritation. Streptozocin is irritating to tissues. With extravasation, the drug can cause tissue necrosis.

Nursing considerations

✦ Monitor the patient for adverse reactions and drug interactions. If any occur, alert the prescriber.
✦ Monitor the patient's CBC for abnormalities, such as delayed bone marrow suppression. Observe the patient for signs and symptoms of infection, bleeding, or

Features of nitrosoureas

✦ Interfere with amino acids, purines, and DNA needed for cancer cells to divide
✦ Are used to treat brain tumors and meningeal leukemias because high lipid solubility allows the drugs or metabolites to easily cross the blood-brain barrier

Adverse reactions to watch for

✦ Bone marrow suppression
✦ Hematologic toxicity and mild glucose intolerance (with streptozocin)
✦ Intense pain at the infusion site (with carmustine)
✦ Nephrotoxicity, renal impairment
✦ Pulmonary toxicity (with carmustine)
✦ Reversible hepatotoxicity (with carmustine)
✦ Severe nausea, vomiting
✦ Tissue irritation or, with extravasation, necrosis (with streptozocin)

anemia. Take infection control measures, bleeding precautions, or energy conservation measures as needed.

✦ Monitor the patient's urinalysis, blood urea nitrogen (BUN) level, and creatinine level for abnormalities that indicate nephrotoxicity and renal impairment. Keep in mind that mild proteinuria may be an early sign of nephrotoxicity.

✦ Monitor the patient's hepatic function test results during high-dose carmustine therapy. If abnormalities occur, lower the dosage or change to a different drug.

✦ Monitor the patient's chest X-ray results and assess his respiratory status regularly during carmustine therapy to detect signs and symptoms of pulmonary toxicity, such as the appearance of pulmonary infiltrates or fibrosis on the X-ray and shortness of breath. If pulmonary toxicity occurs, decrease the dosage or change to another drug.

✦ Inspect the patient's I.V. site for signs of tissue damage or vein irritation, such as redness, swelling, or pain on touch, before giving each dose of carmustine or streptozocin. Change I.V. sites according to facility policy and as needed.

✦ Dilute a carmustine infusion and give it over 1 to 2 hours if vein irritation occurs. Also use warmth to dilate the veins and increase blood flow to further dilute the drug.

✦ Stop the streptozocin infusion immediately and notify the prescriber if extravasation occurs. This vesicant drug can cause tissue necrosis.

✦ Teach the patient and his family about the prescribed drug. (See *Teaching a patient about nitrosoureas.*)

TRIAZENES

The triazene dacarbazine functions as an alkylating drug after the liver activates it.

Pharmacokinetics

After I.V. injection, dacarbazine is distributed throughout the body and metabolized in the liver. Within 6 hours, 30% to 46% of a dose is excreted by the kidneys (half of the dose is excreted unchanged, and half is excreted as one of the metabo-

Key nursing actions

✦ Monitor the CBC.

✦ Observe for evidence of infection, bleeding, or anemia.

✦ Monitor the patient's urinalysis and BUN and creatinine levels.

✦ Monitor hepatic function test results during high-dose carmustine therapy. If abnormalities occur, lower the dosage or change drugs.

✦ Assess the patient's chest X-ray results and respiratory status regularly during carmustine therapy to detect pulmonary toxicity.

✦ Inspect the I.V. site for tissue damage or vein irritation.

Features of dacarbazine

+ Is metabolized to an alkylating drug, which inhibits RNA and protein synthesis
+ Is cell cycle–nonspecific
+ Is used mainly for melanoma, but also with other drugs for Hodgkin's disease

Adverse reactions to watch for

+ Alopecia
+ Flulike syndrome
+ Leukopenia, thrombocytopenia
+ Nausea, vomiting
+ Pain at the infusion site
+ Phototoxicity
+ Severe tissue damage from extravasation

Key nursing actions

+ Monitor the CBC regularly.
+ Measure the patient's temperature and watch for evidence of infection.
+ Observe for evidence of bleeding.
+ Withhold food for 4 to 6 hours before giving dacarbazine; give an antiemetic.
+ Inspect the infusion site before and during administration.

lites). In patients with kidney or liver dysfunction, the drug's half-life may increase to 7 hours.

Pharmacodynamics

After dacarbazine is metabolized in the liver to an alkylating drug, it seems to inhibit RNA and protein synthesis. Like other alkylating drugs, dacarbazine is cell cycle–nonspecific.

Pharmacotherapeutics

Dacarbazine is used primarily to treat patients with melanoma, but it's also used with other drugs to treat patients with Hodgkin's disease.

Interactions

No significant interactions have been reported with dacarbazine.

Adverse reactions

Leukopenia and thrombocytopenia can result from dacarbazine use. In most patients, nausea and vomiting begin within 1 to 3 hours after the dose and may last up to 12 hours. Dacarbazine infusion typically causes pain at the infusion site, which may require further drug dilution or a slower infusion rate. If extravasation occurs, dacarbazine may cause severe tissue damage. Phototoxicity also occurs, as does a flulike syndrome and alopecia.

Nursing considerations

+ Monitor the patient for adverse reactions during therapy. If any occur, alert the prescriber.
+ Regularly monitor the patient's CBC for abnormalities that indicate leukopenia or thrombocytopenia.
+ Regularly monitor the patient's temperature, and observe for signs and symptoms of infection. If leukopenia occurs, take infection-control measures.
+ Monitor the patient for signs of bleeding. If thrombocytopenia occurs, maintain bleeding precautions. Avoid I.M. injections and venipunctures in a patient with a low platelet count. Whenever a venipuncture must be done, apply firm pressure to the site for at least 5 minutes afterward.
+ Withhold food for 4 to 6 hours before dacarbazine therapy, and give an antiemetic to decrease nausea. Nausea and vomiting usually subside after 1 or 2 days of treatment.
+ Discard refrigerated solution after 3 days; discard room temperature solution after 8 hours.
+ Inspect the patient's infusion site for signs of extravasation before and during dacarbazine administration. Drug extravasation may cause severe tissue damage.
+ If extravasation occurs, stop the infusion immediately and notify the prescriber.
+ Give dacarbazine as an I.V. infusion in 50 to 100 ml of dextrose 5% in water (D_5W) or normal saline solution over 30 minutes. If pain occurs at the infusion site, dilute the infusion up to 250 ml, slow the infusion rate, or apply warmth to the vein.
+ Teach the patient and his family about the prescribed drug. (See *Teaching a patient about triazenes.*)

Teaching a patient about triazenes

Whenever a triazene is prescribed, teach the patient and his family the drug's name, dose, frequency, action, and adverse effects. Also take the following actions.

✦ Stress the importance of returning for complete blood counts regularly.

✦ Teach the patient to recognize and report signs and symptoms of infection and bleeding. Review infection control measures and bleeding precautions that he can use as needed.

✦ Advise the patient to avoid sunlight and sunlamps for the first 2 days after treatment.

✦ Instruct the patient to withhold food for 4 to 6 hours before dacarbazine therapy to help decrease nausea.

✦ Reassure the patient that flulike syndrome may be treated with a mild antipyretic, such as acetaminophen.

✦ Inform the patient that dacarbazine may cause alopecia. Discuss ways to cope with alopecia, such as wearing a wig or scarf.

✦ Instruct the patient to notify the prescriber if adverse reactions occur.

ANTIMETABOLITES

Because antimetabolites structurally resemble DNA base pairs, these drugs can become involved in the synthesis of nucleic acids and proteins.

Antimetabolites differ sufficiently from the DNA base pairs to interfere with this synthesis. Because the antimetabolites are cell cycle–specific and primarily affect cells that actively synthesize DNA, these drugs are referred to as *S phase–specific.* These drugs affect normal cells that are reproducing actively as well as cancer cells.

Antimetabolites, which are classified by the metabolite affected, include folic acid analogues, purine analogues, and pyrimidine analogues.

FOLIC ACID ANALOGUES

Although researchers have developed many folic acid analogues, the early compound methotrexate remains the most commonly used. The drug may be used as methotrexate or methotrexate sodium.

Pharmacokinetics

Methotrexate is absorbed well and distributed throughout the body. At usual dosages, the drug doesn't readily enter the CNS. The drug can accumulate in any fluid collection, such as ascites, pleural effusion, pericardial effusion, or peripheral edema. This could result in prolonged elimination and increased toxicity, especially myelosuppression and mucositis.

Although methotrexate is metabolized partially, it's excreted primarily unchanged in urine. The drug exhibits a three-part disappearance from plasma; the rapid distributive phase is followed by a second phase, which reflects kidney clearance. The last phase, the terminal half-life, is 3 to 10 hours for a low dose and 8 to 15 hours for a high dose.

Features of antimetabolites

✦ Structurally resemble DNA base pairs but differ enough to interfere with the synthesis of nucleic acids and proteins

✦ Are cell cycle–specific

✦ Mainly affect cells that actively synthesize DNA, and so are called *S phase–specific*

✦ Affect normal cells that are reproducing actively as well as cancer cells

Actions and uses of methotrexate

+ Reversibly inhibits the enzyme dihydrofolate reductase, blocking folic acid processing and inhibiting DNA and RNA synthesis
+ Is especially useful in acute lymphoblastic leukemia, choriocarcinoma, osteogenic sarcoma, non-Hodgkin's lymphomas, and carcinomas of the head, neck, bladder, testis, and breast
+ Is prescribed in low doses for other conditions that don't respond to conventional therapy, such as severe psoriasis, graft-versus-host disease, and rheumatoid arthritis

Adverse reactions to watch for

+ Acute or chronic hepatotoxicity
+ Alopecia
+ Bone marrow suppression
+ Fatigue
+ Increased uric acid level
+ Intrathecal form: ataxia, coma, confusion, fever, headache, irritability, paralysis, paresis, seizures, somnolence, stiff neck, tremor, coma
+ Nausea, vomiting
+ Nephrotoxicity
+ Photosensitivity
+ Pulmonary toxicity
+ Stomatitis

Pharmacodynamics

Methotrexate reversibly inhibits the action of the enzyme dihydrofolate reductase, thereby blocking folic acid processing and inhibiting DNA and RNA synthesis. The result is cell death.

Pharmacotherapeutics

Methotrexate is especially useful in treating acute lymphoblastic leukemia (abnormal growth of lymphocyte precursors, the lymphoblasts), choriocarcinoma (cancer that develops from the chorionic portions of the products of conception), osteogenic sarcoma (bone cancer), non-Hodgkin's lymphomas, and carcinomas of the head, neck, bladder, testis, and breast.

The drug is also prescribed in low doses to treat other conditions—such as severe psoriasis, graft-versus-host disease, and rheumatoid arthritis—that don't respond to conventional therapy.

Interactions

+ Probenecid decreases methotrexate excretion, increasing the risk of methotrexate toxicity, including fatigue, bone marrow suppression, and stomatitis.
+ A salicylate or nonsteroidal anti-inflammatory drug, especially diclofenac, indomethacin, ketoprofen, or naproxen, can increase methotrexate toxicity.
+ Cholestyramine can reduce methotrexate absorption from the GI tract.
+ Use of alcohol with methotrexate increases the risk of liver toxicity.
+ Use of cotrimoxazole with methotrexate may produce blood cell abnormalities.
+ Penicillin decreases renal tubular secretion of methotrexate, increasing the risk of methotrexate toxicity.

Adverse reactions

Bone marrow suppression can occur with any methotrexate dosage schedule. It's greatest 10 to 14 days after a methotrexate dose. Stomatitis may develop 5 to 10 days after therapy begins. Patients receiving high-dosage methotrexate therapy are susceptible to severe stomatitis, which may result in a nutritional deficit. Fatigue may also occur.

Although rare, methotrexate can cause acute or chronic hepatotoxicity. Acute hepatotoxicity produces transient elevations in liver function tests 1 to 3 days after the drug is given. Chronic hepatotoxicity may result in cirrhosis and, less commonly, acute liver atrophy. It occurs with high-dosage, long-term methotrexate therapy and is related to the length and frequency of dosing and to a total dose of 1.5 g or more.

Pulmonary toxicity, exhibited as pneumonitis or pulmonary fibrosis, may occur. With high doses, nephrotoxicity also can occur, raising the BUN and creatinine levels. Tumor cell destruction by methotrexate may increase the uric acid concentration, which may worsen nephrotoxicity.

Photosensitivity may occur in patients despite protection from the sun. A sunburnlike rash is the primary dermatologic reaction. Alopecia occurs in about 10% of patients receiving methotrexate.

Although rare, nausea and vomiting may be the first adverse reactions to high-dose methotrexate therapy. They typically occur less than 1 hour after the dose.

CLINICAL ALERT Intrathecal methotrexate can cause severe adverse reactions, including seizures, paresis, paralysis, and death. It may also produce less severe adverse reactions, such as headache, fever, neck stiffness, confusion, and irritability. Intrathecal administration may also produce systemic toxicity marked by tremor, ataxia, somnolence, and seizures. Rarely, systemic toxicity progresses to coma and death. Because methotrexate preparations that contain preservatives may cause more adverse reactions, use only preservative-free methotrexate and diluents for intrathecal administration.

During high-dose methotrexate therapy, leucovorin may be used to minimize adverse reactions.

Nursing considerations

✦ Monitor the patient for adverse reactions and drug interactions during methotrexate therapy. Alert the prescriber if any occur.
✦ Monitor the patient's BUN and creatinine levels before each treatment to detect signs of nephrotoxicity. If the levels are abnormal, consult the prescriber about therapy modification.
✦ Encourage fluid intake and give I.V. fluids and sodium bicarbonate to increase urine alkalinity and volume and prevent nephrotoxicity in a patient receiving high-dose therapy.
✦ Accurately document the patient's fluid intake and output, and monitor his urine pH during high-dose therapy.
✦ Regularly monitor the patient's liver function test results during methotrexate therapy to detect early changes in liver function that suggest cirrhosis or acute liver atrophy.
✦ Monitor the patient for signs of liver dysfunction, such as jaundice, darkened urine, or clay-colored stools.
✦ Regularly monitor the patient's CBC and platelet count during methotrexate therapy to detect bone marrow suppression.
✦ If leukopenia occurs, monitor the patient for signs of infection. Also take infection control measures until the WBC count returns to normal.
✦ If thrombocytopenia occurs, observe the patient for signs and symptoms of bleeding. Take bleeding precautions until the platelet count returns to normal.
✦ Monitor the methotrexate level, especially during high-dose therapy.
✦ Give leucovorin with high doses of methotrexate to limit the duration of sensitive cells' exposure to methotrexate.
✦ Use only preservative-free methotrexate and diluents for intrathecal administration.
✦ Teach the patient and his family about the prescribed drug. (See *Teaching a patient about folic acid analogues,* page 382.)

Key nursing actions

✦ Check the BUN and creatinine levels before each treatment.
✦ Encourage fluid intake, and give I.V. fluids and sodium bicarbonate to increase urine alkalinity and volume and prevent nephrotoxicity.
✦ Document fluid intake and output.
✦ Check liver function test results regularly.
✦ Watch for evidence of liver dysfunction.
✦ Assess the CBC and platelet count regularly.
✦ Monitor the methotrexate level, especially during high-dose therapy.

Features of purine analogues

✦ Incorporate into DNA and RNA
✦ Inhibit DNA and RNA synthesis and other metabolic reactions required for cell growth
✦ Are cell cycle–specific, exerting effects in the S phase
✦ Are used for acute and chronic leukemias and may be useful for lymphomas
✦ Pentostatin inhibits adenosine deaminase, blocking DNA synthesis and inhibiting RNA synthesis

PURINE ANALOGUES

Purine analogues are incorporated into DNA and RNA, interfering with nucleic acid synthesis and replication. They include cladribine, fludarabine, mercaptopurine, pentostatin, and thioguanine.

Pharmacokinetics

The pharmacokinetics of purine analogues isn't clearly defined. The drugs are largely metabolized in the liver and excreted in urine.

Pharmacodynamics

Like the other antimetabolites, fludarabine, mercaptopurine, and thioguanine first must undergo conversion via phosphorylation to the nucleotide level to be active. The resulting nucleotides are then incorporated into DNA, where they may inhibit DNA and RNA synthesis and other metabolic reactions required for cell growth.

This conversion to nucleotides is the same process that pyrimidine analogues go through but, in this case, purine nucleotides are affected. Purine analogues are cell cycle–specific, exerting their effects during the S phase.

Although the exact mechanism of pentostatin's antitumor effect is unknown, the drug inhibits the enzyme adenosine deaminase, blocking DNA synthesis and inhibiting RNA synthesis.

Pharmacotherapeutics

Purine analogues are used to treat acute and chronic leukemias and may be useful in treating lymphomas.

Interactions

No significant interactions occur with cladribine or thioguanine.

✦ Use of fludarabine with pentostatin may cause severe pulmonary toxicity, which can be fatal.

✦ Allopurinol may decrease mercaptopurine metabolism, which can increase bone marrow suppression.

✦ Use of pentostatin with allopurinol may increase the risk of renal and hepatic toxicities.

✦ Pentostatin may enhance the effects of vidarabine and increase the risk of toxicity.

Adverse reactions

Purine analogues produce bone marrow suppression, which may not begin for 1 to 6 weeks after therapy is initiated. Leukopenia usually occurs first, followed by thrombocytopenia and anemia.

Nausea, vomiting, anorexia, mild diarrhea, and stomatitis occur in patients receiving purine analogues. Uric acid levels may also rise as a result of purine catabolism from cellular destruction.

Fludarabine, when used at high doses, may cause severe neurologic effects, including blindness, coma, and death. It may also cause tumor lysis syndrome, which may lead to hyperuricemia, hyperphosphatemia, hypocalcemia, metabolic acidosis, hyperkalemia, hematuria, urate crystalluria, and renal impairment. The onset of this syndrome may be signaled by flank pain and hematuria.

Many patients receiving mercaptopurine develop cholestatic jaundice after 1 to 2 months of therapy. Usually, this adverse reaction occurs with doses that exceed 2.5 mg/kg daily. The patient should report this reaction immediately because the jaundice may be reversible if the drug is stopped. If not, the reaction may be fatal. Jaundice has also been reported with thioguanine use.

The most severe adverse reactions to pentostatin involve the renal system and CNS. Use of higher-than-recommended dosages without adequate hydration may contribute to renal toxicity. Adverse CNS reactions appear to depend on the dosage schedule. Therefore, most prescribers recommend a dosage interval of 2 weeks or more.

Nursing considerations

✦ Monitor the patient for adverse reactions and drug interactions during purine analogue therapy. Alert the prescriber if any occur.

✦ Monitor the CBC weekly or as prescribed, watching for a precipitous decrease.

✦ Observe the patient for signs of bleeding and infection. Take infection control measures and bleeding precautions if bone marrow suppression occurs.

✦ Monitor the patient taking mercaptopurine or thioguanine for signs of cholestatic jaundice, such as pain in the right upper quadrant and elevated liver enzyme levels. Cholestatic jaundice may progress to hepatic necrosis, which may be reversible if the drug is stopped promptly.

✦ Monitor the patient for severe neurologic abnormalities during high-dose fludarabine therapy.

✦ Periodically monitor the patient's uric acid level.

Adverse reactions to watch for

✦ Anorexia, mild diarrhea, nausea, stomatitis, vomiting
✦ Bone marrow suppression
✦ Increased uric acid level

fludarabine
✦ Severe neurologic effects
✦ Tumor lysis syndrome

mercaptopurine
✦ Cholestatic jaundice

pentostatin
✦ CNS effects
✦ Renal effects

Key nursing actions

✦ Monitor the CBC weekly or as prescribed.
✦ Observe for evidence of bleeding and infection.
✦ Watch for evidence of cholestatic jaundice during mercaptopurine or thioguanine therapy.
✦ Monitor for severe neurologic abnormalities during high-dose fludarabine therapy.
✦ Periodically check uric acid level.
✦ Document fluid intake and output.

Teaching a patient about purine analogues

Whenever a purine analogue is prescribed, teach the patient and his family the drug's name, dose, frequency, action, and adverse effects. Also take the following actions.

✦ Stress the importance of returning regularly for follow-up blood tests.

✦ Review infection control measures, bleeding precautions, and energy-conservation measures that the patient may use as needed.

✦ Instruct the patient taking mercaptopurine or thioguanine to report any of the following to the prescriber immediately: yellowed skin or sclera, right upper quadrant pain, darkened urine, or clay-colored stools.

✦ Advise the patient taking fludarabine to report flank pain or hematuria as well as neurologic abnormalities to the prescriber immediately.

✦ Teach the patient how to manage troublesome adverse reactions, such as GI distress and stomatitis.

✦ Advise the patient to drink at least thirteen 8-oz (240-ml) glasses of fluid daily to prevent renal damage.

✦ Instruct the patient to report other adverse reactions to the prescriber.

✦ Document the patient's fluid intake and output. To minimize the effects of uric acid level elevation, encourage him to drink at least 3 qt (3 L) of fluid daily, and adjust the allopurinol dosage.

✦ Notify the prescriber if the patient's uric acid level remains elevated.

✦ Teach the patient and his family about the prescribed drug. (See *Teaching a patient about purine analogues.*)

PYRIMIDINE ANALOGUES

Pyrimidine analogues are a diverse group of drugs that inhibit the production of pyrimidine nucleotides necessary for DNA synthesis. Drugs in this class include capecitabine, cytarabine, floxuridine, fluorouracil, and gemcitabine.

Pharmacokinetics

Because pyrimidine analogues are absorbed poorly when given orally, they're usually given by other routes. With the exception of cytarabine, pyrimidine analogues are distributed well throughout the body, including CSF. They're metabolized extensively in the liver and are excreted in urine.

Pharmacodynamics

Pyrimidine analogues kill cancer cells by interfering with the natural function of pyrimidine nucleotides.

Pharmacotherapeutics

These antimetabolites may be used to treat many tumors. However, they're primarily indicated in the treatment of acute leukemias, GI tract adenocarcinomas (such as colorectal, pancreatic, esophageal, and stomach cancers), carcinomas of the breast and ovaries, and non-Hodgkin's lymphomas.

Features of pyrimidine analogues

✦ Are diverse drugs that inhibit the production of pyrimidine nucleotides needed for DNA synthesis

✦ Are used to treat many tumors

✦ Are mainly used for acute leukemias, GI tract adenocarcinomas (such as colorectal, pancreatic, esophageal, and stomach cancers), carcinomas of the breast and ovaries, and non-Hodgkin's lymphomas

Interactions

Floxuridine and gemcitabine produce no interactions that have been reported as significant.

✦ An antacid may increase capecitabine absorption.

✦ Capecitabine can increase the pharmacodynamic effects of warfarin and the risk of bleeding.

✦ Capecitabine may increase the phenytoin level.

✦ Cytarabine may decrease the absorption of digoxin, except in capsule form.

✦ Leucovorin may increase the fluorouracil level and enhance its toxicity.

Adverse reactions

Bone marrow suppression marked by neutropenia and thrombocytopenia is the major dose-limiting adverse reaction to pyrimidine analogues. This reaction is noticeable 7 to 14 days after a dose, with bone marrow recovery occurring 21 to 28 days after the drug is stopped.

Stomatitis and esophagopharyngitis may occur 5 to 10 days after therapy begins. These adverse reactions can be particularly distressing to the patient because the oral cavity ulcerations and sloughing may be extremely painful and prevent eating.

Like most antineoplastics, pyrimidine analogues can cause fatigue. Lack of energy can limit activities severely as well as the patient's involvement in therapy.

Pyrimidine analogues don't cause severe nausea and vomiting. Nausea and anorexia may occur with capecitabine, fluorouracil, or floxuridine therapy. Diarrhea may occur with fluorouracil and may be severe enough to limit or stop therapy.

Other common adverse reactions to capecitabine are fatigue, paresthesia, pyrexia, diarrhea, stomatitis, abdominal pain, constipation, anorexia, dyspepsia, neutropenia, thrombocytopenia, anemia, lymphopenia, hand-and-foot syndrome, and dermatitis.

Cytarabine may produce fever and flulike symptoms within 24 hours after therapy begins. This drug produces a rash in 4% of patients. Intrathecal cytarabine usually doesn't cause systemic toxicity. It's more likely to cause nausea, vomiting, fever, and transient headaches. High-dose cytarabine can cause severe cerebellar neurotoxicity, chemical conjunctivitis, diarrhea, fever, and hand-and-foot syndrome.

Hepatic arterial infusion of floxuridine has been linked to bile duct sclerosis and liver cirrhosis.

In most cases, fluorouracil is relatively well tolerated. However, it can produce several hypersensitivity reactions, including mild to severe skin reactions. Such reactions may take the form of pruritus on the limbs or less commonly on the trunk, photosensitivity with erythema or increased skin pigmentation, darkened veins with prolonged drug use, or a rash on the hands and feet with prolonged high-dose infusions. Other hypersensitivity reactions may include increased lacrimation, nasal discharge, or epistaxis; these reactions disappear after therapy is stopped. Alopecia commonly occurs with fluorouracil.

Nursing considerations

✦ Store fluorouracil at room temperature and protect it from light.

✦ Don't use a cloudy fluorouracil solution. If crystals form, dissolve the solution by warming it.

✦ Use plastic I.V. containers to give a continuous fluorouracil infusion because the solution is more stable in plastic I.V. bags than in glass bottles.

✦ Reconstitute floxuridine with sterile water for injection. For the actual infusion, dilute further in D_5W or normal saline solution.

Adverse reactions to watch for

✦ Anorexia, nausea (with capecitabine, fluorouracil, floxuridine)

✦ Bone marrow suppression (neutropenia, thrombocytopenia)

✦ Esophagopharyngitis

✦ Fatigue

✦ Stomatitis

capecitabine

✦ Abdominal pain, constipation, diarrhea, dyspepsia, stomatitis

✦ Anemia, lymphopenia

✦ Dermatitis

✦ Fatigue, paresthesia, pyrexia

✦ Hand-and-foot syndrome

cytarabine

✦ Fever, flulike symptoms

✦ Intrathecal use: fever, nausea, transient headache, vomiting

✦ Rash

fluorouracil

✦ Diarrhea

✦ Hypersensitivity reactions (including mild to severe skin reactions)

Teaching a patient about pyrimidine analogues

Whenever a pyrimidine analogue is prescribed, teach the patient and his family the drug's name, dose, frequency, action, and adverse effects. Also take the following actions.
◆ Stress the importance of returning for follow-up blood tests.
◆ Teach the patient how to manage stomatitis and esophagopharyngitis at home.
◆ Review energy-conservation measures that the patient can use at home if fatigue occurs.
◆ Teach the patient to use infection control measures and bleeding precautions as needed.
◆ Teach the patient how to manage troublesome adverse GI reactions.
◆ Advise the patient receiving fluorouracil that photosensitivity may occur. Instruct him to avoid sun exposure or to wear a sunscreen, hat, and sunglasses when sun exposure is unavoidable.
◆ Inform the patient that fluorouracil may cause increased lacrimation, nasal discharge, or epistaxis. Reassure him that these reactions disappear after therapy is stopped.
◆ Inform the patient that cytarabine may precipitate fever and flulike symptoms up to 24 hours after it's given. Advise him to take an antipyretic and an analgesic, as prescribed.
◆ Inform the patient that reversible alopecia may occur during fluorouracil therapy.
◆ Tell the patient to take capecitabine with water within 30 minutes after breakfast and dinner.
◆ Instruct the patient taking capecitabine to notify the prescriber if he's also taking folic acid.
◆ Instruct the patient to notify the prescriber if adverse reactions occur.

Key nursing actions
◆ Monitor the CBC to detect bone marrow suppression.
◆ Review the results of liver function tests regularly during intra-arterial floxuridine therapy.
◆ Assess for fever and flulike symptoms during cytarabine therapy.
◆ During capecitabine therapy, monitor the patient for hyperbilirubinemia, severe nausea, and evidence of hand-and-foot syndrome, such as numbness, paresthesia, swelling, erythema, desquamation, blistering, and severe pain of hands or feet.

◆ Discard refrigerated floxuridine solution after 2 weeks because it becomes unstable after this time.
◆ Use preservative-free normal saline solution for intrathecal cytarabine.
◆ Discard reconstituted cytarabine solution 48 hours after reconstitution because it becomes unstable after this time.
◆ Monitor the patient for adverse reactions. If any occur, alert the prescriber.
◆ Monitor the patient's CBC to detect bone marrow suppression. If neutropenia occurs, monitor the patient for signs of infection. Also take infection-control measures until the neutrophil count returns to normal. If thrombocytopenia occurs, monitor the patient for signs and symptoms of bleeding. Also take bleeding precautions until the thrombocyte count returns to normal. If hematologic abnormalities occur, limit the pyrimidine analogue dosage.
◆ Regularly review the results of the patient's liver function tests throughout intra-arterial floxuridine therapy.
◆ Monitor the patient for fever and flulike symptoms during cytarabine therapy. Give a mild analgesic and antipyretic to reduce the fever and ease discomfort.
◆ During capecitabine therapy, monitor the patient for hyperbilirubinemia, severe nausea, and signs and symptoms of hand-and-foot syndrome, such as numbness, paresthesia, painless or painful swelling, erythema, desquamation, blistering, and severe pain of hands or feet.
◆ Teach the patient and his family about the prescribed drug. (See *Teaching a patient about pyrimidine analogues.*)

ANTIBIOTIC ANTINEOPLASTICS

Antibiotic antineoplastics are antimicrobials that produce tumor-destroying effects by binding with DNA. They inhibit the cellular processes of normal and malignant cells.

Drugs in this class include bleomycin, dactinomycin, daunorubicin, doxorubicin, idarubicin, mitomycin, mitoxantrone, and valrubicin. Daunorubicin, doxorubicin, idarubicin, and valrubicin belong specifically to the anthracycline class of antibiotics. They have been isolated from cultures of *Streptomyces peucetius*.

Pharmacokinetics

Because antibiotic antineoplastics are usually given I.V., no absorption occurs. They're considered 100% bioavailable.

Some of these drugs are also given directly into the body cavity being treated. Bleomycin, doxorubicin, and mitomycin sometimes are given as topical bladder instillations in which significant systemic absorption doesn't occur. When bleomycin is injected into the pleural space for malignant effusions, up to one-half of the dose is absorbed.

Distribution of these antineoplastics varies as does their metabolism and elimination.

Pharmacodynamics

With the exception of mitomycin, antibiotic antineoplastics intercalate, or insert themselves, between adjacent base pairs of a DNA molecule, physically separating them.

DNA looks like a twisted ladder with the rungs made up of pairs of nitrogenous bases. These drugs insert themselves between these nitrogenous bases. Then, when the DNA chain replicates, an extra base is inserted opposite the intercalated antibiotic, resulting in a mutant DNA molecule. The overall effect is cell death.

Mitomycin is activated inside the cell to a bifunctional or trifunctional alkylating drug. The drug produces single-strand breakage of DNA. It also cross-links DNA and inhibits DNA synthesis.

Pharmacotherapeutics

Antibiotic antineoplastics act against many cancers, including:
✦ Hodgkin's disease and non-Hodgkin's lymphoma
✦ testicular carcinoma
✦ squamous cell carcinoma of the head, neck, and cervix
✦ Wilms' tumor (a malignant neoplasm of the kidney, occurring in young children)
✦ osteogenic sarcoma, and rhabdomyosarcoma (malignant neoplasm composed of striated muscle cells)
✦ Ewing's sarcoma (a malignant tumor that originates in bone marrow, typically in long bones or the pelvis) and other soft-tissue sarcomas
✦ breast, ovarian, bladder, and lung cancer
✦ melanoma
✦ carcinomas of the GI tract
✦ choriocarcinoma
✦ acute leukemia.

Features of antibiotic antineoplastics

✦ Insert themselves (except mitomycin) between adjacent base pairs of a DNA molecule, resulting in a mutant DNA molecule after replication
✦ Are used for many cancers, including acute leukemia, bladder cancer, breast cancer, carcinoma of GI tract, choriocarcinoma, Ewing's and other soft-tissue sarcomas, Hodgkin's disease, melanoma, non-Hodgkin's lymphoma, osteogenic sarcoma, ovarian cancer, rhabdomyosarcoma, squamous cell carcinoma of head-neck-cervix, testicular carcinoma, Wilms' tumor

Adverse reactions to watch for

◆ Alopecia
◆ Bone marrow suppression
◆ Cardiomyopathy
◆ Nausea, vomiting
◆ Severe tissue damage from extravasation
◆ Stomatitis

bleomycin
◆ Anaphylactic reaction
◆ Chills, fever
◆ Irreversible pulmonary fibrosis
◆ Skin toxicity

doxorubicin
◆ Potentiated effects of radiation therapy
◆ Red urine

mitoxantrone
◆ Blue-green urine

Interactions
◆ Bleomycin may decrease the digoxin or phenytoin level.
◆ Doxorubicin may reduce the digoxin level.
◆ Use of fludarabine or pentostatin with idarubicin increases the risk of fatal lung toxicity and isn't recommended.
◆ Together, mitomycin and a vinca alkaloid may cause acute respiratory distress.

Adverse reactions
Antibiotic antineoplastics produce many of the same reactions as other drugs used to treat malignant neoplasms. The primary reaction is bone marrow suppression. Except for bleomycin, all of these drugs produce moderate to severe leukopenia and thrombocytopenia. Mitomycin causes delayed myelosuppression that requires 6 to 8 weeks for the bone marrow to recover.

Bone marrow suppression, stomatitis, and alopecia result from the antineoplastics' effects on rapidly proliferating tissues. Because bone marrow, epithelial tissue, and hair follicles have faster growth rates then many other body tissues, these cells are more vulnerable to antineoplastics.

Nausea and vomiting may result from chemical irritation of the emetic center in the brain. Vomiting may also result from psychogenic factors leading to anticipatory emesis.

If extravasated, all antibiotic antineoplastics, except bleomycin, produce severe tissue damage. Extravasation can occur with even the most careful use.

Bleomycin may produce fever and chills. If these effects become intense, the patient should receive immediate treatment with antihistamines and antipyretics. Patients who develop fever and chills with bleomycin therapy must be premedicated with antihistamines and antipyretics before each bleomycin use. Bleomycin can result in irreversible pulmonary fibrosis, but this effect is rare, usually affecting patients older than age 70 who have received more than the recommended lifetime dosage. About 50% of patients who receive bleomycin develop skin toxicity after receiving 150 to 200 units. Toxicity begins with urticaria and may produce hyperpigmentation. Anaphylactic reactions have occurred in 1% of patients receiving bleomycin for lymphoma. Therefore, test doses should be given.

The anthracycline antibiotic antineoplastics may cause irreversible cardiomyopathy. These effects are cumulative, dose-related, and irreversible. Patients taking a cumulative dose of more than 550 mg/m^2 of daunorubicin or doxorubicin have a higher risk. If the patient had radiation therapy to the chest, the risk of cardiomyopathy increases as he approaches the lifetime dosage of 400 mg/m^2. Therefore, total lifetime dosages are limited to prevent these effects. These drugs may also produce acute ECG changes.

Doxorubicin may potentiate the effects of radiation therapy and cause hyperpigmentation of the irradiated area or increased stomatitis or enteritis. Doxorubicin may color the urine red; mitoxantrone may color it blue-green.

Although uncommon, mitomycin may cause renal or pulmonary toxicity.

Nursing considerations
◆ Monitor the patient for adverse reactions and drug interactions during therapy. If any occur, notify the prescriber.
◆ Monitor the patient for bone marrow suppression during treatment with any antibiotic antineoplastic except bleomycin. Expect acute complications when the absolute granulocyte count falls below 1,000/mm^3. As the count declines, encourage the patient to maintain adequate nutritional and fluid intake. During the nadir, the patient should avoid crowds and anyone with an active contagious infection.

Teaching a patient about antibiotic antineoplastics

Whenever an antibiotic antineoplastic is prescribed, teach the patient and his family the drug's name, dose, frequency, action, and adverse effects. Also take the following actions.

✦ Instruct the patient to watch for and immediately report signs and symptoms of infection, such as fever and sore throat. Emphasize this to a hospitalized patient who is at risk for contracting an infection from hospital procedures, such as venipunctures, urinary catheters, and other actions that alter skin integrity.

✦ Teach the patient to use bleeding precautions and energy conservation measures if needed.

✦ Instruct the patient to alert the nurse if pain or discomfort occurs at the infusion site during the infusion.

✦ Teach the patient how to manage troublesome adverse reactions, such as nausea, vomiting, and stomatitis.

✦ Provide information and support for the patient with alopecia. Inform him that hair loss is temporary, but that hair regrowth may be a different color or texture.

✦ Teach the patient to recognize the signs and symptoms of pulmonary fibrosis and interstitial pneumonia, such as dry, unproductive cough and dyspnea.

✦ Instruct the patient receiving bleomycin to take his temperature at home. Stress the importance of reporting fever and chills to the prescriber.

✦ Advise the patient receiving bleomycin to report urticaria or hyperpigmentation, which may signal skin toxicity.

✦ Teach the patient receiving daunorubicin, doxorubicin, idarubicin, or valrubicin to recognize and report the signs and symptoms of heart failure.

✦ Inform the patient that localized hyperpigmentation and increased stomatitis or enteritis may occur if he receives doxorubicin during radiation therapy.

✦ Stress the importance of returning for follow-up blood tests.

✦ Inform the patient that doxorubicin may color his urine red and mitoxantrone may color it blue-green temporarily.

✦ Give the patient printed information about the prescribed antibiotic antineoplastic for home reference.

✦ Instruct the patient to notify the prescriber if adverse reactions occur.

✦ Monitor the hematocrit and platelet count to detect anemia or thrombocytopenia from bone marrow suppression. Because RBCs have a longer life than WBCs and platelets, anemia doesn't usually occur unless the patient has occult or overt blood loss. When the platelet count is below 50,000/mm³, take additional safety precautions, such as avoiding I.M. injections to prevent trauma. Give supportive platelet transfusions and packed RBCs as needed.

✦ Use extreme caution when giving daunorubicin, doxorubicin, idarubicin, mitomycin, or mitoxantrone because they are powerful vesicants. To give a vesicant safely, give by I.V. push into the side port of a freely infusing I.V. line, which enables close supervision of the site throughout use.

✦ If infiltration or extravasation is suspected, stop the infusion immediately and notify the prescriber. Apply cold compresses and elevate the affected limb. To decrease tissue damage, instill hydrocortisone into the affected site via an I.V. catheter, S.C. injection, or as indicated by facility protocol.

✦ Teach the patient and his family about the prescribed drug. (See *Teaching a patient about antibiotic antineoplastics*.)

Key nursing actions

✦ Monitor for bone marrow suppression (except with bleomycin).

✦ Check the hematocrit and platelet count to detect anemia or thrombocytopenia.

✦ Use extreme caution when giving daunorubicin, doxorubicin, idarubicin, mitomycin, or mitoxantrone because they are powerful vesicants. Give them by I.V. push into the side port of a freely infusing I.V. line and closely supervise the site throughout use.

Features of aromatase inhibitors

anastrozole

+ Is a selective nonsteroidal aromatase inhibitor that lowers estradiol level
+ Binds to the heme of the CYP unit of the aromatase enzyme, which converts adrenal androgens to estrone and estradiol in peripheral tissues

exemestane

+ Is a steroidal aromatase inhibitor that reduces the estrogen level, decreasing cell growth in estrogen-dependent breast cancer
+ Is used in postmenopausal women for advanced breast cancer that has progressed after tamoxifen therapy

letrozole

+ Is a nonsteroidal competitive inhibitor of the aromatase enzyme that inhibits conversion of androgens to estrogens, leading to decreased tumor mass or slowed progress
+ Used for metastatic breast cancer that progresses after therapy with an antiestrogen, such as tamoxifen

anastrozole and letrozole

+ Are used for hormone receptor-positive or hormone receptor-unknown locally advanced or metastatic breast cancer, for advanced breast cancer with disease progression after tamoxifen therapy in postmenopausal women, and for adjunctive treatment of hormone receptor-positive early breast cancer

AROMATASE INHIBITORS

Anastrozole, exemestane, and letrozole belong to a class of antineoplastics called aromatase inhibitors. All three drugs are used to treat breast cancer in postmenopausal women.

Pharmacokinetics

After oral use, anastrozole is well absorbed into the systemic circulation. About 85% of the drug is metabolized in the liver, and 11% is excreted by the kidneys.

Oral exemestane is rapidly absorbed. It's extensively distributed, highly protein-bound, and cleared from the systemic circulation primarily by metabolism.

Letrozole is rapidly and completely absorbed from the GI tract. It's slowly metabolized to an inactive metabolite, which is excreted by the kidneys.

Pharmacodynamics

Anastrozole is a selective nonsteroidal aromatase inhibitor that significantly lowers the estradiol level. It competitively binds to the heme of the cytochrome P450 (CYP) unit of the aromatase enzyme. This inhibits the enzyme, which converts adrenal androgens to estrone and estradiol in peripheral tissues.

Exemestane is a steroidal aromatase inhibitor that reduces the estrogen level, which decreases cell growth in estrogen-dependent breast cancer. The drug acts as a false substrate for the aromatase enzyme. It's processed to an intermediate substance that binds irreversibly to the enzyme, which causes it to become inactivated.

As a nonsteroidal competitive inhibitor of the aromatase enzyme, letrozole selectively inhibits the conversion of androgens to estrogens. A decreased estrogen level leads to decreased tumor mass or delayed progression of tumor growth in some women.

Pharmacotherapeutics

In postmenopausal women, anastrozole and letrozole are used as first-line treatments for hormone receptor-positive or hormone receptor-unknown locally advanced or metastatic breast cancer. It's also used in postmenopausal women to treat advanced breast cancer with disease progression after tamoxifen therapy and as an adjunct to treatment of hormone receptor-positive early breast cancer.

LIFESPAN

Avoiding the developmental dangers of anastrozole

For a woman of childbearing age, rule out pregnancy before initiating anastrozole treatment. During treatment, urge the patient to use effective contraception and to let the prescriber know if she plans to become pregnant or suspects she may be pregnant. These actions can help prevent fetotoxicity and pregnancy loss.

For a breast-feeding woman, use anastrozole cautiously. Although it isn't known whether the drug appears in breast milk, the manufacturer recommends caution because of possible risks to the infant.

Exemestane is indicated for advanced breast cancer in postmenopausal women, which has progressed after tamoxifen treatment.

In postmenopausal women, letrozole is also used for metastatic breast cancer that progresses after therapy with an antiestrogen, such as tamoxifen.

Interactions
No significant interactions have been reported with anastrozole or letrozole.
◆ A drug that induces CYP 3A4 enzymes, such as carbamazepine, nafcillin, or phenytoin, may decrease the exemestane level.

Adverse reactions
Common adverse reactions to anastrozole include headache, asthenia, hot flashes, and nausea. Reactions to exemestane commonly include depression, insomnia, anxiety, fatigue, pain, hot flashes, nausea, and dyspnea. The most common adverse reactions to letrozole are nausea and bone, limb, and back pain.

Nursing considerations
◆ Avoid using anastrozole in a patient with hormone receptor-negative disease or who didn't respond to previous tamoxifen therapy. Such patients rarely respond to anastrozole. (See *Avoiding the developmental dangers of anastrozole.*)
◆ For a patient with advanced breast cancer, continue anastrozole therapy until the tumor progresses.
◆ Continue treatment with exemestane until tumor progression is apparent.
◆ Don't adjust the letrozole dosage for a patient with a creatinine clearance of 10 ml/minute or more.

 CLINICAL ALERT Use letrozole cautiously in a patient with severe liver impairment. Be aware that a dosage adjustment isn't needed for a patient with mild to moderate liver dysfunction.

◆ Give letrozole without regard to food because food doesn't affect its absorption.
◆ Monitor the patient for adverse reactions and drug interactions during aromatase inhibitor therapy. If any occur, alert the prescriber.
◆ Teach the patient and his family about the prescribed drug. (See *Teaching a patient about aromatase inhibitors.*)

Adverse reactions to watch for

anastrozole
◆ Asthenia
◆ Headache
◆ Hot flashes
◆ Nausea

exemestane
◆ Anxiety
◆ Depression
◆ Dyspnea
◆ Fatigue
◆ Hot flashes
◆ Insomnia
◆ Nausea
◆ Pain

letrozole
◆ Bone, limb, and back pain
◆ Nausea

Key nursing actions
◆ Avoid using anastrozole in a patient with hormone receptor-negative disease or who didn't respond to previous tamoxifen therapy. Such patients rarely respond to anastrozole.
◆ Use letrozole cautiously in a patient with severe liver impairment.

HORMONAL ANTINEOPLASTICS

Hormonal antineoplastics are prescribed to alter the growth of malignant neoplasms or to manage and treat their physiologic effects. Hormonal drugs prove effective against hormone-dependent tumors, such as cancers of the prostate, breast, and endometrium. Lymphomas and leukemias are usually treated with therapies that include corticosteroids because of their ability to affect lymphocytes.

Types of hormonal antineoplastics include androgens, antiandrogens, antiestrogens, gonadotropin-releasing hormone analogues, and progestins.

ANDROGENS

Therapeutically useful androgens are synthetic derivatives of naturally occurring testosterone. They include fluoxymesterone, methyltestosterone, testolactone, testosterone cypionate, testosterone enanthate, and testosterone propionate.

Pharmacokinetics

The pharmacokinetic properties of therapeutic androgens resemble those of naturally occurring testosterone.

Oral androgens, fluoxymesterone, methyltestosterone, and testolactone, are absorbed well. The parenteral ones, testosterone enanthate and testosterone propionate, are designed specifically for slow absorption after I.M. use.

Androgens are distributed well throughout the body, metabolized extensively in the liver, and excreted in urine. The duration of parenteral androgens is longer because the oil suspension is absorbed slowly. Parenteral androgens are given one to three times per week.

Pharmacodynamics

Androgens probably act by one or more mechanisms. These drugs may reduce the number of prolactin receptors or may bind competitively to those that are available. These drugs may inhibit estrogen synthesis or competitively bind at estrogen receptors; these actions prevent estrogen from affecting estrogen-sensitive tumors.

Pharmacotherapeutics

Androgens are indicated for the palliative treatment of advanced breast cancer, particularly in postmenopausal women with bone metastasis.

Interactions

✦ An androgen may decrease the dose requirements for insulin.
✦ An androgen may increase the effects of an oral anticoagulant.
✦ Use of an androgen with a hepatotoxic drug increases the risk of hepatotoxicity.

Adverse reactions

Dose-related nausea and vomiting are the most common adverse reactions to androgens. Fluid retention caused by sodium retention may also occur. A woman may develop masculine characteristics, including increased facial hair, acne, clitoral hypertrophy, increased libido, and a deeper voice.

Prolonged high dosages of androgens have produced jaundice, which may limit their use in patients with liver dysfunction. Also, patients with bone metastasis are at greater risk for developing hypercalcemia during prolonged androgen therapy.

Features of androgens

✦ Are synthetic derivatives of naturally occurring testosterone
✦ Prevent estrogen from affecting estrogen-sensitive tumors, possibly by reducing the number of prolactin receptors, binding competitively to those available, inhibiting estrogen synthesis, or competitively binding to estrogen receptors
✦ Are used for palliation of advanced breast cancer, particularly in postmenopausal women with bone metastasis

Adverse reactions to watch for

✦ Virilization in women
✦ Fluid and sodium retention
✦ Hypercalcemia
✦ Jaundice
✦ Nausea, vomiting

Teaching a patient about androgens

Whenever an androgen is prescribed, teach the patient and his family the drug's name, dose, frequency, action, and adverse effects. Also take the following actions.

✦ Inform the patient that systemic reactions to the androgen include fluid retention, nausea, and vomiting. Teach him to recognize signs and symptoms and to report them to the prescriber. Instruct the patient to weigh himself daily and to restrict sodium and fluid intake if fluid retention occurs. If nausea and vomiting occur, advise the patient to request an antiemetic and take it before meals as prescribed.

✦ Inform a woman well in advance about potential virilization and provide emotional support. Advise her that prolonged androgen therapy can cause hirsutism, mild scalp hair loss, a deeper voice, facial acne, clitoral enlargement, increased libido, and breast regression. If therapy is stopped at the onset of virilization, the conditions may disappear. If therapy is continued, the conditions may become irreversible.

✦ Teach the patient to recognize the signs and symptoms of jaundice, including yellowed skin or sclera, darkened urine, clay-colored stools, and pruritus, and to report any of these findings immediately to the prescriber.

✦ Teach the patient and his family to recognize and report the signs and symptoms of hypercalcemia, including anorexia, nausea, vomiting, lethargy, and polyuria. Explain that these effects may be caused by a treatable complication.

✦ Instruct the patient to notify the prescriber if adverse reactions occur.

Nursing considerations

✦ Monitor the patient for adverse reactions and drug interactions during therapy. If any occur, alert the prescriber.

✦ Monitor the patient's hydration status if nausea or vomiting occurs during androgen therapy. Give an antiemetic before meals as needed.

✦ Monitor the patient for signs and symptoms of fluid retention. Be especially alert for these signs in a patient with a history of heart failure. If fluid retention occurs, restrict the patient's fluid intake to about six 8-oz (240-ml) glasses daily and limit his sodium intake to 2 g.

✦ Monitor the results of liver function tests for a patient who receives prolonged high dosages of an androgen. Also monitor him for jaundice.

 CLINICAL ALERT Use extreme caution with I.M. injections to avoid inadvertent I.V. or S.C. injection. Because I.M. preparations are oil suspensions, a serious oil embolism can occur if an I.M. androgen is given into a vein.

✦ Use a 1" needle to inject an I.M. androgen, and inject the drug deeply into muscle tissue. If irritation or inflammation develops, apply ice for comfort.

✦ Monitor the patient's calcium level monthly to detect hypercalcemia, especially in a patient with bone metastasis who receives prolonged androgen therapy.

✦ Prevent hypercalcemia by mobilizing the patient as much as possible and maintaining adequate hydration. Limiting dietary calcium intake doesn't significantly affect the calcium level.

✦ Teach the patient and his family about the prescribed drug. (See *Teaching a patient about androgens*.)

Key nursing actions

✦ Monitor hydration if nausea or vomiting occurs. Give an antiemetic before meals as needed.

✦ Watch for evidence of fluid retention.

✦ Track the results of liver function tests during prolonged therapy with high doses of an androgen.

✦ Check the calcium level monthly.

Features of antiandrogens

+ Inhibit androgen uptake or prevent androgen binding in cell nuclei in target tissues
+ Are used with a gonadotropin-releasing hormone analogue to treat metastatic prostate cancer and prevent disease flare that occurs when a gonadotropin-releasing hormone analogue is used alone

Adverse reactions to watch for

+ Anxiety, confusion, depression, drowsiness, nervousness
+ Decreased libido, hot flashes, impotence
+ Diarrhea, nausea, vomiting
+ Elevated liver enzyme and creatinine levels
+ Gynecomastia
+ Neuromuscular dysfunction
+ Photosensitivity

Key nursing actions

+ Give the drug with a gonadotropin-releasing hormone analogue.
+ Monitor liver enzyme and creatinine levels frequently. If they exceed the safe ranges, stop the drug.
+ Monitor hydration if nausea, vomiting, or diarrhea occurs.

ANTIANDROGENS

Antiandrogens are used as an adjunct to gonadotropin-releasing hormone analogues in treating advanced prostate cancer. These drugs include bicalutamide, flutamide, and nilutamide.

Pharmacokinetics

After oral use, antiandrogens are absorbed rapidly and completely. These drugs are metabolized rapidly and extensively and excreted primarily in urine.

Pharmacodynamics

Bicalutamide, flutamide, and nilutamide exert their antiandrogenic action by inhibiting androgen uptake or preventing androgen binding in cell nuclei in target tissues.

Pharmacotherapeutics

Antiandrogens are used with a gonadotropin-releasing hormone analogue, such as leuprolide, to treat metastatic prostate cancer. This combination therapy may help prevent the disease flare that occurs when a gonadotropin-releasing hormone analogue is used alone.

Interactions

+ When used with warfarin, bicalutamide or flutamide may increase the prothrombin time.

Adverse reactions

When an antiandrogen is used with a gonadotropin-releasing hormone analogue, the most common adverse reactions are hot flashes, decreased libido, impotence, diarrhea, nausea, vomiting, and gynecomastia. Other adverse reactions include drowsiness, confusion, depression, anxiety, nervousness, photosensitivity, neuromuscular dysfunction, and elevated liver enzyme and creatinine levels.

Nursing considerations

+ Monitor the patient for adverse reactions and drug interactions during antiandrogen therapy. If any occur, alert the prescriber.
+ Give an antiandrogen with a gonadotropin-releasing hormone analogue for maximum effectiveness.
+ Monitor the patient's liver enzyme and creatinine levels frequently during antiandrogen therapy. If the levels exceed the safe ranges, stop the drug.
+ Monitor the patient's hydration status if nausea, vomiting, or diarrhea occurs. Administer an antiemetic or antidiarrheal as needed.
+ Notify the prescriber if adverse GI reactions prevent antiandrogen use.
+ Teach the patient and his family about the prescribed drug. (See *Teaching a patient about antiandrogens.*)

ANTIESTROGENS

The antiestrogen tamoxifen is a first-line treatment for advanced breast cancer with estrogen receptor–positive tumors in postmenopausal women. Tamoxifen is also used as an adjunct to treat breast cancer and reduce its occurrence in women at high risk. Other antiestrogens include fulvestrant and toremifene.

Pharmacokinetics

After I.M. injection, fulvestrant yields a peak level within 7 to 9 days and has a half-life of 40 days. After oral use, tamoxifen is absorbed well and extensively metabolized in the liver before being excreted in feces. After oral use, toremifene is well absorbed and is extensively metabolized.

Pharmacodynamics

Estrogen receptors are found in the cancer cells of 50% of premenopausal and 75% of postmenopausal women with breast cancer. These receptors respond to estrogen to induce tumor growth.

Antiestrogens bind to the estrogen receptors and inhibit estrogen-mediated tumor growth in breast tissue. The inhibition may result because of binding to receptors at the nuclear level or because the binding reduces the number of free receptors in the cytoplasm. Ultimately, DNA synthesis and cell growth are inhibited.

Tamoxifen also can retain estrogen against activity at other tissue sites, such as bone.

Pharmacotherapeutics

Antiestrogens are used to treat metastatic breast cancer that's estrogen receptor–positive or estrogen receptor–unknown. Tumors in postmenopausal women are more responsive to tamoxifen than those in premenopausal women.

Features of antiestrogens

✦ Bind to estrogen receptors and inhibit estrogen-mediated tumor growth in breast tissue; inhibition may result because of binding to receptors at the nuclear level or because binding reduces the number of free receptors in the cytoplasm

✦ Are used for metastatic breast cancer that's estrogen receptor–positive or estrogen receptor–unknown

tamoxifen

✦ Is more effective in postmenopausal women than in premenopausal women

✦ Is also used as an adjunct to surgery in postmenopausal women with axillary lymph nodes that contain cancer cells and estrogen receptor–positive tumors

Adverse reactions to watch for

fulvestrant
+ Abdominal pain, constipation, diarrhea, nausea, vomiting
+ Asthenia, headache, hot flashes
+ Back pain, bone pain, injection site pain, pelvic pain
+ Cough, dyspnea

tamoxifen
+ Hot flashes, nausea, vomiting
+ Ocular lesions, retinopathy, superficial corneal opacity (with high dosages)
+ Transient mild leukopenia or thrombocytopenia
+ Tumor flare, which may increase the number and size of lesions or increase bone pain

toremifene
+ Cataracts
+ Hypercalcemia
+ Sweating
+ Vaginal discharge

Key nursing actions
+ Monitor hydration if nausea or vomiting occurs. Give an antiemetic as needed.
+ Monitor WBC and platelet counts regularly.
+ Watch for tamoxifen-induced tumor flare.
+ Assess for decreased visual acuity.
+ Check the calcium level closely for the first weeks of toremifene therapy in a patient with bone metastases to detect hypercalcemia.

Tamoxifen is also used as an adjunct to surgery in postmenopausal women with axillary lymph nodes that contain cancer cells and estrogen receptor–positive tumors.

Interactions
No significant interactions have been reported with fulvestrant.
+ Tamoxifen or toremifene can increase the effects of warfarin, increasing the risk of bleeding.
+ Bromocriptine increases the effects of tamoxifen.
+ An antacid may affect the absorption of enteric-coated tamoxifen tablets.
+ When used with a drug that raises the calcium level, such as hydrochlorothiazide, toremifene increases the risk of hypercalcemia.
+ A drug that induces CYP 3A4 enzymes (such as carbamazepine, phenobarbital, or phenytoin) may increase toremifene metabolism.
+ A drug that inhibits CYP 3A4-6 enzymes (such as erythromycin or ketoconazole) may decrease toremifene metabolism.

Adverse reactions
Fulvestrant commonly causes asthenia, headache, hot flashes, nausea, vomiting, constipation, abdominal pain, diarrhea, bone pain, back pain, pelvic pain, dyspnea, cough, and injection site pain.

Tamoxifen is relatively nontoxic. Its most common adverse reactions include hot flashes, nausea, and vomiting. Transient mild leukopenia or thrombocytopenia occurs in about 4% of patients. In patients with bone metastasis, hypercalcemia may occur. About 1% of patients treated with tamoxifen may experience tumor flare, which may increase the number and size of lesions or increase bone pain; however, this reaction subsides quickly. Patients receiving high dosages of tamoxifen have experienced ocular lesions, retinopathy, and superficial corneal opacity, which reduce visual acuity.

Common adverse reactions with toremifene include cataracts, vaginal discharge, and sweating. Hypercalcemia may also occur.

Nursing considerations
+ Monitor the patient for adverse reactions and drug interactions during antiestrogen therapy. If any occur, alert the prescriber.
+ Monitor the patient's hydration status if nausea or vomiting occurs during antiestrogen therapy. Give an antiemetic as needed.
+ Monitor the patient's WBC and platelet counts regularly for mild leukopenia or thrombocytopenia. For a patient with bone metastasis, monitor the calcium level to detect hypercalcemia.
+ Observe the patient for signs of tamoxifen-induced tumor flare, such as increased number and size of lesions or increased bone pain. Give additional analgesics.
+ Store tamoxifen tablets at room temperature and protect them from light.
+ Monitor the patient for decreased visual acuity. High dosages of tamoxifen may produce ocular lesions, retinopathy, and superficial corneal opacity.
+ Schedule the patient for regular eye examinations by an ophthalmologist during tamoxifen therapy.
+ Report vision changes to the prescriber because tamoxifen may need to be stopped.
+ Schedule the patient for yearly gynecologic examinations and Papanicolaou tests.

Teaching a patient about antiestrogens

Whenever an antiestrogen is prescribed, teach the patient and his family the drug's name, dose, frequency, action, and adverse effects. Also take the following actions.

✦ Inform the patient that hot flashes, nausea, and occasional vomiting are the most common adverse reactions to tamoxifen, and describe how to manage them at home. Explain that tolerance to these symptoms usually develops rapidly.

✦ Instruct the patient to immediately report to the prescriber decreased visual acuity; it may be irreversible. Emphasize the need for routine eye examinations by an ophthalmologist who knows he's taking tamoxifen.

✦ Assure the patient and his family that tumor flare is an expected adverse reaction that will subside. Advise the patient to request increased analgesics in the meantime.

✦ Instruct the patient to store tamoxifen at room temperature and protect it from light.

✦ Stress the importance of returning for follow-up blood tests.

✦ Caution a woman of childbearing age to avoid pregnancy and to report suspected pregnancy immediately.

✦ Instruct the patient to take the drug exactly as prescribed.

✦ Advise the patient to take toremifene without regard to meals.

✦ Warn the patient not to stop therapy without consulting the prescriber.

✦ Inform the patient about vaginal bleeding and other adverse reactions to toremifene; tell her to notify the prescriber if bleeding occurs.

✦ Instruct the patient to inform the prescriber if adverse reactions occur.

✦ Closely monitor the calcium level during the first weeks of toremifene treatment in a patient with bone metastases because of the increased risk of hypercalcemia.

✦ Because fulvestrant is given I.M., don't use it in a patient who has bleeding diathesis or thrombocytopenia or who takes an anticoagulant.

✦ Teach the patient and his family about the prescribed drug. (See *Teaching a patient about antiestrogens.*)

GONADOTROPIN-RELEASING HORMONE ANALOGUES

Gonadotropin-releasing hormone analogues are used to treat advanced prostate cancer. They include goserelin, leuprolide, and triptorelin.

Pharmacokinetics

Goserelin is absorbed slowly for the first 8 days of therapy and rapidly and continuously thereafter. After S.C. injection, leuprolide is absorbed well. Triptorelin reaches a peak level within 1 week of I.M. injection and produces a detectable level for 4 weeks.

The distribution, metabolism, and excretion of gonadotropin-releasing hormone analogues aren't clearly defined.

Features of gonadotropin-releasing hormone analogues

✦ Act on a man's pituitary gland to increase LH secretion, which stimulates testosterone production; however, with long-term use, they inhibit LH release from the pituitary and testosterone release from the testicles.

Features of gonadotropin-releasing hormone analogues
(continued)

✦ Reduces the testosterone level, which inhibits tumor growth
✦ Are used for palliation of metastatic prostate cancer

Pharmacodynamics

Gonadotropin-releasing hormone analogues act on a man's pituitary gland to increase luteinizing hormone (LH) secretion, which stimulates testosterone production. The peak testosterone level is reached about 72 hours after daily administration.

With long-term use, however, these drugs inhibit LH release from the pituitary and subsequently inhibit testicular release of testosterone. Because prostate tumor cells are stimulated by testosterone, the reduced testosterone level inhibits tumor growth.

Pharmacotherapeutics

Gonadotropin-releasing hormone analogues are used for palliative treatment of metastatic prostate cancer. The drugs lower the testosterone level without the adverse psychological effects of castration or the adverse cardiovascular effects of diethylstilbestrol.

Interactions

No drug interactions have been identified with goserelin or leuprolide.
✦ Use of triptorelin with a hyperprolactinemic drug may decrease gonadotropin-releasing hormone receptors in the pituitary gland.

Adverse reactions to watch for

✦ Anorexia, constipation, nausea, vomiting
✦ Hot flashes
✦ Impotence
✦ Increased pain or symptoms for the first 2 weeks of treatment
✦ Peripheral edema
✦ Reduced libido

Adverse reactions

Hot flashes are the most common reactions to gonadotropin-releasing hormone analogues. Impotence and decreased libido also often occur. Disease symptoms and pain may worsen or flare during the first 2 weeks of therapy. (See *Dealing with disease flare.*)

Peripheral edema occurs in about 8% of patients. Nausea, vomiting, constipation, and anorexia occur in about 2% of patients. Thromboembolic complications are uncommon; gynecomastia and breast tenderness are rare.

Nursing considerations

✦ Monitor the patient for adverse reactions and drug interactions during therapy. If any occur, alert the prescriber.

◆ Monitor the patient for signs and symptoms of thromboembolic complications. If any occur, notify the prescriber immediately and provide emergency treatment.

 CLINICAL ALERT Monitor the patient for disease flare, which is characterized by an increase in disease symptoms and pain during the first 2 weeks of therapy with a gonadotropin-releasing hormone analogue.

◆ Increase the analgesic dosage to control pain as indicated.
◆ Monitor the patient's testosterone and prostate-specific antigen levels.
◆ Don't give triptorelin with a hyperprolactinemic drug.
◆ Teach the patient and his family about the prescribed drug. (See *Teaching a patient about gonadotropin-releasing hormone analogues.*)

PROGESTINS

Progestins are hormones used to treat various forms of cancer and include medroxyprogesterone and megestrol.

Pharmacokinetics

After I.M. injection in an aqueous or oil suspension, medroxyprogesterone is absorbed slowly from its deposit sites. When taken orally, megestrol is absorbed well.

These drugs are distributed well throughout the body and may sequester in fatty tissue. Progestins are metabolized in the liver and excreted as metabolites in urine.

Pharmacodynamics

The mechanism of action of progestins in treating tumors isn't completely understood. The drugs may bind to a specific receptor to act on hormonally sensitive cells.

Key nursing actions
◆ Watch for evidence of thromboembolic complications.
◆ Monitor the patient for disease flare.
◆ Check the testosterone and prostate-specific antigen levels.

Features of progestins
◆ May bind to a specific receptor to act on hormonally sensitive cells
◆ Are cytostatic
◆ Are used (especially megesterol) for palliation of advanced endometrial, breast, and renal cancers

Because progestins don't exhibit a cytotoxic activity, they're considered cytostatic. In other words, they prevent cells from multiplying.

Pharmacotherapeutics

Progestins are used for the palliative treatment of advanced endometrial, breast, and renal cancers. Of these drugs, megestrol is used most often.

Interactions

No drug interactions have been identified for megestrol. Medroxyprogesterone has significant drug interactions.

✦ Medroxyprogesterone may interfere with bromocriptine's effects, causing menstruation to stop.

✦ Aminoglutethimide or rifampin may reduce the progestin effects of medroxyprogesterone.

Adverse reactions

Mild fluid retention and related weight gain are probably the most common reactions to progestins. Thromboemboli can develop with the use of progestins and may cause stroke, pulmonary dysfunction, blocked blood flow to a limb, and local, superficial tenderness or swelling. Breakthrough bleeding, spotting, changes in menstrual flow, and breast tenderness may also occur with progestins. In addition, liver function abnormalities may occur.

 CLINICAL ALERT Oil in an injectable progestin can cause oil embolus if the drug is inadvertently injected into a vein. At high doses, injectable progestins can produce gluteal abscesses. Patients who are hypersensitive to the oil carrier used for injection (usually sesame or castor oil) may have a local or systemic hypersensitivity reaction.

Nursing considerations

 CLINICAL ALERT Don't give an injectable progestin I.V. The oil in the drug's formulation can cause an oil embolus when it enters the circulation.

✦ Avoid local adverse reactions to I.M. progestin by injecting the drug deeply and applying pressure and ice afterward to lessen pain and irritation.

✦ Regularly inspect the gluteal injection sites of a parenteral progestin for signs and symptoms of abscess, such as swelling, a fluid-filled sac, and localized pain. If an abscess occurs, avoid injecting the drug into the area, provide such symptomatic relief as frequent application of warm compresses, and encourage the patient not to put pressure on the site.

✦ Monitor the patient for adverse reactions and drug interactions during progestin therapy. If any occur, alert the prescriber.

✦ Regularly monitor the patient's liver function test results and observe him for signs and symptoms of hepatotoxicity.

✦ Monitor the patient for signs and symptoms of thromboembolism. If you suspect thromboembolism, notify the prescriber immediately and prepare for emergency treatment and anticoagulation therapy.

✦ Regularly monitor the patient for local and systemic hypersensitivity reactions. Keep standard emergency equipment nearby. Notify the prescriber immediately if such reactions occur.

✦ Teach the patient and his family about the prescribed drug. (See *Teaching a patient about progestins.*)

NATURAL ANTINEOPLASTICS

This subclass of antineoplastics includes podophyllotoxins and vinca alkaloids.

PODOPHYLLOTOXINS

As semisynthetic glycosides, podophyllotoxins are cell cycle–specific and act during the G_2 and late S phases of the cell cycle. These drugs include etoposide and teniposide.

Pharmacokinetics

When taken orally, podophyllotoxins are only moderately absorbed. Although the drugs are distributed widely throughout the body, they achieve a poor CSF level.

Podophyllotoxins undergo liver metabolism and are excreted primarily in urine.

Pharmacodynamics

Although their mechanism of action isn't completely understood, podophyllotoxins produce several biochemical changes in tumor cells. At low levels, these drugs block cells at the late S or G_2 phase. At higher levels, they arrest cells in the G_2 phase.

Podophyllotoxins also can break one of the strands of the DNA molecule. In addition, they can inhibit nucleotide transport and incorporation into nucleic acids.

Pharmacotherapeutics

Etoposide is used to treat testicular cancer and small-cell lung cancer. It may also be used to treat lymphomas and leukemias, although the FDA hasn't approved these indications yet.

Teniposide is used to treat acute lymphoblastic leukemia. The drug has demonstrated some activity in treating Hodgkin's disease, lymphomas, and brain tumors.

Features of podophyllotoxins

✦ Low levels block cells at the late S or G_2 phase
✦ Higher levels arrest cells in the G_2 phase
✦ Can also break one strand of a DNA molecule and can inhibit nucleotide transport and incorporation into nucleic acids

etoposide
✦ Is used for testicular cancer and small-cell lung cancer
✦ Is used off-label for lymphoma, leukemia

teniposide
✦ Is used for acute lymphoblastic leukemia
✦ Has some activity in Hodgkin's disease, lymphomas, and brain tumors

Interactions

◆ When used with warfarin, etoposide may increase the risk of bleeding.
◆ Teniposide may increase the clearance and intracellular level of methotrexate.

Adverse reactions

Podophyllotoxins suppress bone marrow, producing nadirs in 7 to 14 days. These drugs can cause leukopenia and, less commonly, thrombocytopenia; leukopenia resolves in about 3 weeks. About 90% of patients receiving podophyllotoxins experience alopecia, which may resolve as treatment continues.

About one-third of patients receiving podophyllotoxins develop nausea and vomiting, which last 2 to 6 hours. Anorexia is another common reaction. Stomatitis occurs in 5% of patients.

Acute hypotension may result if a podophyllotoxin is infused too rapidly. Pain and burning at the injection site also have been reported.

Several rare reactions also can occur during podophyllotoxin therapy. They may take the form of acute hypersensitivity (with chills, fever, generalized erythema, pruritus, wheezing, bronchospasm, or tachycardia); transient liver function abnormalities; an elevated alkaline phosphatase level, which indicates impending hepatotoxicity; or peripheral neuropathy.

Nursing considerations

◆ Give I.V. etoposide or teniposide over 30 to 60 minutes to prevent hypotension. Monitor the patient's blood pressure before and during the infusion.
◆ Frequently monitor the patient's WBC and platelet counts during therapy, especially during the expected nadir, which occurs in days 7 to 14 for the WBC count and days 9 to 16 for the platelet count. At the nadir, the patient is at the greatest risk for problems related to leukopenia and thrombocytopenia. Acute complications occur when the absolute granulocyte count is less than 1,000/mm³ and the platelet count is less than 20,000/mm³.
◆ Monitor the patient with leukopenia for signs and symptoms of infection. Take infection control measures until the WBC count returns to normal.
◆ Monitor the patient with thrombocytopenia for signs and symptoms of bleeding. Take bleeding precautions until the platelet count has returned to normal.
◆ Give an antiemetic before podophyllotoxin use and every 2 to 4 hours thereafter, as needed, to prevent or control nausea and vomiting.
◆ Monitor the patient for signs and symptoms of acute hypersensitivity. If a hypersensitivity reaction occurs, stop the infusion and notify the prescriber immediately. During podophyllotoxin therapy, keep standard emergency equipment, diphenhydramine hydrochloride, and epinephrine nearby.
◆ Monitor the patient's liver function test results and alkaline phosphatase level. Abnormalities may indicate impending hepatotoxicity.
◆ Inspect the patient's mouth regularly for signs of stomatitis, which is temporary. Provide prophylactic mouth care before chemotherapy to help decrease stomatitis severity and increase patient comfort. Provide therapeutic mouth care, including topical antibiotics and analgesics, if required by the degree of stomatitis.
◆ Notify the prescriber if stomatitis persists or worsens.
◆ Teach the patient and his family about the prescribed drug. (See *Teaching a patient about podophyllotoxins.*)

Teaching a patient about podophyllotoxins

Whenever a podophyllotoxin is prescribed, teach the patient and his family the drug's name, dose, frequency, action, and adverse effects. Also take the following actions.

✦ Inform the patient that he may feel burning or pain at the infusion site during podophyllotoxin administration.

✦ Advise the patient to avoid people with active contagious infections, to watch for signs of infection, and to report them immediately to the prescriber.

✦ Explain that acute hypersensitivity reactions may occur with podophyllotoxin therapy. Instruct the patient to report signs or symptoms promptly.

✦ Prepare the patient for possible alopecia by explaining the timing and speed of hair loss and noting that it may affect the scalp, eyebrows, eyelashes, or other body hair.

✦ Teach the patient how to manage troublesome adverse reactions, such as nausea and stomatitis, at home.

✦ Give the patient written materials about the possible effects of the podophyllotoxin for home reference.

✦ Instruct the patient to notify the prescriber if adverse reactions persist or worsen.

VINCA ALKALOIDS

Vinca alkaloids are nitrogenous bases derived from the periwinkle plant. These drugs, which are cell cycle–specific for the M phase, include vinblastine, vincristine, and vinorelbine.

Pharmacokinetics

After I.V. use, vinca alkaloids are distributed well throughout the body. They undergo moderate liver metabolism before being eliminated through different phases, primarily in feces with a small percentage eliminated in urine.

Pharmacodynamics

Vinca alkaloids may disrupt the normal function of the microtubules (cell structures responsible for DNA movement) by binding to the protein tubulin in the microtubules.

When the microtubules can't separate chromosomes properly, the chromosomes are dispersed throughout the cytoplasm or arranged in unusual groupings. As a result, formation of the mitotic spindle is prevented, and the cells can't complete mitosis.

Cell division is arrested in metaphase, causing cell death. Therefore, vinca alkaloids are cell cycle–specific to the M phase. Interruption of microtubule function may also impair some types of cellular movement, phagocytosis (engulfing and destroying microorganisms and cellular debris), and CNS functions.

Pharmacotherapeutics

Vinblastine is used to treat metastatic testicular carcinoma, lymphomas, Kaposi's sarcoma (the most common acquired immunodeficiency syndrome [AIDS]-related cancer), neuroblastoma (a highly malignant tumor originating in the sympathetic nervous system), breast carcinoma, and choriocarcinoma.

Features of vinca alkaloids

✦ May disrupt the function of microtubules (responsible for DNA movement) by binding to tubulin in the microtubules

✦ Cell cycle–specific to the M phase

✦ Vinblastine is used for metastatic testicular carcinoma, lymphomas, Kaposi's sarcoma, neuroblastoma, breast carcinoma, choriocarcinoma.

✦ Vincristine is used in combination therapy for Hodgkin's disease, non-Hodgkin's lymphoma, Wilms' tumor, rhabdomyosarcoma, acute lymphocytic leukemia.

✦ Vinorelbine is used for non–small-cell lung cancer, metastatic breast carcinoma, cisplatin-resistant ovarian carcinoma, Hodgkin's disease.

Vincristine is helpful in combination therapy to treat Hodgkin's disease, non-Hodgkin's lymphoma, Wilms' tumor, rhabdomyosarcoma, and acute lymphocytic leukemia.

Vinorelbine is used to treat non–small-cell lung cancer. It may also be used in treating metastatic breast carcinoma, cisplatin-resistant ovarian carcinoma, and Hodgkin's disease.

Interactions

✦ Erythromycin may increase the toxicity of vinblastine.
✦ Vinblastine can decrease the phenytoin level.
✦ Vincristine can reduce the effects of digoxin.
✦ Asparaginase can decrease metabolism of vincristine and increase its risk of toxicity.
✦ A calcium channel blocker can enhance vincristine accumulation, increasing the risk of toxicity.

Adverse reactions

Minor differences in the chemical structure of the vinca alkaloids cause significant differences in toxicity. Vinblastine and vinorelbine toxicities occur primarily as bone marrow suppression, which is manifested by leukopenia and slight thrombocytopenia. Leukopenia increases the patient's risk of infection, especially if the absolute granulocyte count is less than 1,000/mm³. Dose adjustments may be needed based on the degree of neutropenia.

During vinorelbine monotherapy, interstitial pulmonary changes and acute respiratory distress syndrome have been reported and, in many patients, have been fatal. The onset of pulmonary changes occurred 3 to 8 days after treatment began.

Alopecia occurs in up to 50% of patients receiving vinca alkaloids, although hair loss is more likely with vincristine than vinblastine. Many patients experience partial alopecia; others, total. Men are equally as affected as women by alopecia of the scalp, eyebrows, eyelashes, and body. Alopecia is reversible when the drugs are stopped, and hair may begin to regrow during therapy.

Neuromuscular abnormalities occur frequently with vincristine and vinorelbine therapy and occasionally with vinblastine therapy. Peripheral neuropathies, which usually limit the dose for vincristine and vinorelbine, may include loss of deep tendon reflexes, paresthesia, numbness, pain, and tingling. Other vincristine-induced neurotoxicities include encephalopathies and cranial nerve dysfunction, such as vocal cord paralysis, ptosis (upper eyelid drooping), and jaw pain. Constipation is common with vinorelbine because it causes neuropathy.

Vinca alkaloids, which are vesicants, may cause severe local necrosis if extravasation occurs. They also may increase the uric acid level if rapid cell lysis occurs.

Stomatitis may result from vinca alkaloid use. Nausea and vomiting that may occur can be controlled with antiemetics. Prophylactic laxative use may prevent constipation caused by vincristine.

Vinblastine may produce tumor pain described as intense stinging or burning in the tumor bed, with an abrupt onset 1 to 3 minutes after giving the drug. The pain usually lasts 20 minutes to 3 hours. Vincristine may induce syndrome of inappropriate antidiuretic hormone.

Nursing considerations

✦ Monitor the patient regularly for adverse reactions and drug interactions during vinca alkaloid therapy. If any occur, alert the prescriber.

Adverse reactions to watch for

✦ Alopecia (more likely with vincristine than vinblastine)
✦ Bone marrow suppression (with vinblastine and vinorelbine)
✦ Constipation (with vinorelbine)
✦ Increased uric acid level
✦ Intense stinging or burning tumor pain (with vinblastine)
✦ Interstitial pulmonary changes and acute respiratory distress syndrome (with vinorelbine)
✦ Nausea, vomiting
✦ Neuromuscular abnormalities (with vincristine, vinorelbine, and occasionally vinblastine)
✦ Neurotoxicities involving encephalopathies and cranial nerve dysfunction, such as vocal cord paralysis, ptosis, and jaw pain (with vincristine)
✦ Peripheral neuropathies, such as loss of deep tendon reflexes, paresthesia, numbness, pain, and tingling (with vincristine and vinorelbine)
✦ Severe local necrosis from extravasation
✦ Stomatitis
✦ Syndrome of inappropriate antidiuretic hormone (with vincristine)

✦ Monitor the patient's CBC and platelet count regularly. Note the CBC nadir when caring for a patient with bone marrow suppression. At the nadir, which usually occurs 4 to 10 days after giving the drug, the patient is at the greatest risk for problems related to leukopenia and thrombocytopenia.

✦ Monitor the patient for signs and symptoms of infection if leukopenia occurs. Take infection control measures until the WBC count returns to normal.

✦ Monitor the patient with leukopenia for thrombocytopenia because the two occur sequentially. When the platelet count is under 50,000/mm³, he's at risk for bleeding. When the count drops below 20,000/mm³, he's at severe risk and probably will need a platelet transfusion. Monitor the patient with thrombocytopenia for bleeding. Take bleeding precautions until the platelet count returns to normal. Avoid rectal temperatures and I.M. injections in a patient with thrombocytopenia or leukopenia.

✦ Monitor the patient's laboratory test results to detect anemia. A patient who is dehydrated from nausea, vomiting, or anorexia may have a normal hematocrit. Once the patient is rehydrated, the hematocrit will fall, thus revealing anemia.

✦ Periodically monitor the patient's uric acid level throughout therapy to detect rapid cell lysis. If the level becomes elevated, give allopurinol. This drug prevents the rapid accumulation of uric acid.

✦ Monitor the patient for neuromuscular abnormalities during vinblastine or vincristine therapy. To detect peripheral neuropathies, assess deep tendon reflexes and ask about paresthesia, numbness, pain, and tingling. During vincristine therapy, observe for signs and symptoms of other neurotoxicities, such as encephalopathy (drowsiness or decreased level of consciousness) and cranial nerve dysfunction (vocal cord paralysis, jaw pain, or ptosis). Notify the prescriber if neuromuscular abnormalities occur.

✦ Examine the I.V. infusion site for evidence of extravasation, such as redness, swelling, or pain on touch, before giving a vinca alkaloid. If extravasation is suspected, change the infusion site to prevent severe local necrosis.

✦ Consider when the drug is given to encourage compliance. Some patients prefer treatments in the evening; patients who are employed may prefer treatments on their days off.

✦ Handle vinca alkaloids carefully. Give the prescribed drug directly into the vein or into the injection port in the tubing of a freely infusing I.V. solution. These methods allow direct observation of the injection site.

 CLINICAL ALERT Monitor the patient for intense stinging or burning in the tumor bed that begins abruptly 1 to 3 minutes after vinblastine use. Relieve pain with an analgesic as needed, because the pain may last up to 3 hours.

✦ Avoid splashing vinorelbine solution in the eyes. Severe eye irritation will result.

✦ During vinorelbine therapy, observe for signs and symptoms of interstitial pulmonary changes, such as shortness of breath, cough, or hypoxia.

✦ Give a stimulant laxative, if needed, during vincristine therapy.

✦ Teach the patient and his family about the prescribed drug. (See *Teaching a patient about vinca alkaloids,* page 406.)

Key nursing actions

✦ Monitor the CBC and platelet count.

✦ Assess the patient with leukopenia for thrombocytopenia.

✦ Check laboratory test results for anemia.

✦ Monitor the uric acid level periodically during therapy.

✦ Watch for neuromuscular abnormalities during vinblastine or vincristine therapy.

✦ Look for evidence of interstitial pulmonary changes (cough, shortness of breath, hypoxia) during vinorelbine therapy.

PATIENT TEACHING

Teaching a patient about vinca alkaloids

Whenever a vinca alkaloid is prescribed, teach the patient and his family the drug's name, dose, frequency, action, and adverse effects. Also take the following actions.

✦ Prepare the patient for alopecia by explaining when hair loss usually begins and noting that it occurs gradually and is reversible once treatment ends.

✦ Explain that burning or stinging pain commonly occurs at the tumor site after I.V. vinblastine administration. Reassure the patient that this pain isn't caused by a worsening of the tumor, but by cellular destruction that causes tissue swelling.

✦ Teach the patient and family the signs and symptoms of neurotoxicity.

✦ Plan an effective teaching program about bone marrow suppression that includes the patient's blood counts, potential sites of infection, and personal habits.

✦ Advise the patient with leukopenia to maintain proper hygiene and report signs and symptoms of infection, including fever, cough, sore throat, and a burning sensation during urination.

✦ Instruct the patient at risk for leukopenia and thrombocytopenia to avoid cuts and bruises and to use a sponge toothbrush and an electric razor.

✦ Instruct the patient to report a sudden headache, which may indicate life-threatening intracranial bleeding.

✦ Prevent colonic irritation and bleeding that result from vincristine-induced constipation by recommending a bowel program that includes prophylactic stool softeners as prescribed.

✦ Stress the importance of returning for follow-up blood tests.

✦ Caution the patient not to engage in activities that require alertness if neurotoxicity occurs.

✦ Teach the patient how to manage troublesome adverse GI reactions.

✦ Advise the patient to speak up immediately if discomfort occurs at the infusion site during administration.

✦ Instruct the patient to report other adverse reactions to the prescriber.

✦ Give the patient written materials about the prescribed vinca alkaloid for home reference.

Features of monoclonal antibodies

✦ Bind to target receptors on cancer cells and may induce programmed cell death or recruit other immune system elements to attack cancer cells

✦ Are used for solid tumors and hematologic malignancies, such as non-Hodgkin's lymphoma, chronic lymphocytic leukemia, acute myeloid leukemia

gemtuzumab
✦ May deliver a toxic chemotherapeutic dose to the tumor

MONOCLONAL ANTIBODIES

Recombinant DNA technology has produced monoclonal antibodies that are directed at targets on cancer cells. These drugs include alemtuzumab, gemtuzumab, ibritumomab, rituximab, and trastuzumab.

Pharmacokinetics
Because of their large protein molecules, monoclonal antibodies aren't absorbed orally. They have a limited volume of distribution and a long half-life, sometimes measured in weeks.

Pharmacodynamics
Monoclonal antibodies bind to target receptors on cancer cells and may cause tumor death by inducing programmed cell death or recruiting other elements of the immune system to attack cancer cells. Gemtuzumab may also cause tumor death by delivering a toxic chemotherapeutic dose to the tumor. Ibritumomab produces similar effects by delivering a radiation dose to the tumor.

Pharmacotherapeutics

These antineoplastics are active against solid tumors and hematologic malignancies, such as:

✦ non-Hodgkin's lymphoma (ibritumomab and rituximab target CD20 on malignant B-lymphocytes)
✦ chronic lymphocytic leukemia (alemtuzumab targets CD52 antigen on B-cells)
✦ acute myeloid leukemia (gemtuzumab targets CD33 antigen on myeloid leukemic cells).

Trastuzumab is used to treat metastatic breast cancer in patients whose tumors overexpress human epidermal growth factor receptor 2 (HER2) protein and who have received one or more chemotherapeutics for metastatic disease. It's also used with paclitaxel for metastatic breast cancer in patients whose tumors overexpress HER2 protein and who haven't received chemotherapy for metastatic disease.

Interactions

✦ Trastuzumab can increase the cardiac toxicity of an anthracycline.

Adverse reactions

All monoclonal antibodies can cause infusion-related toxicities, such as fever, chills, shortness of breath, hypotension, and anaphylaxis. Fatalities have been reported.

Alemtuzumab is linked to myelosuppression and an increased risk of opportunistic infections, such as *Pneumocystis* pneumonia and fungal and viral infections.

Gemtuzumab therapy may lead to tumor lysis syndrome and hyperuricemia.

 CLINICAL ALERT Severe myelosuppression may occur in any patient who receives the recommended dose of gemtuzumab. Fatal hepatic veno-occlusive disease may result from treatment with gemtuzumab and subsequent chemotherapy.

A drug regimen using ibritumomab and rituximab may cause severe, life-threatening infusion reactions, which typically begin 30 to 120 minutes after the first rituximab infusion. Signs and symptoms include hypotension, angioedema, hypoxia, or bronchospasm; interruption of treatment may be required.

Severe mucocutaneous reactions (including toxic epidermal necrolysis, Stevens-Johnson syndrome, paraneoplastic pemphigus, and lichenoid or vesiculobullous dermatitis) have occurred in patients receiving rituximab.

Use of trastuzumab may result in ventricular dysfunction and heart failure.

Nursing considerations

✦ Before trastuzumab therapy, perform a thorough baseline cardiac assessment. Obtain a complete history, perform a physical examination, and schedule diagnostic tests to identify the patient's risk of cardiotoxicity.
✦ Premedicate the patient with acetaminophen or diphenhydrinate before drug use to help reduce infusion-related reactions.
✦ Withhold alemtuzumab if the patient has a systemic infection at the time of the scheduled dose.
✦ Monitor the patient's blood pressure and assess for hypotensive symptoms during monoclonal antibody use.
✦ Monitor the patient regularly for adverse reactions and drug interactions during monoclonal antibody therapy. If any occur, alert the prescriber.
✦ Keep drugs available to treat hypersensitivity reactions to the drug.

Features of monoclonal antibodies

(continued)

ibritumomab
✦ Delivers radiation to the tumor

trastuzumab
✦ Is used for metastatic breast cancer in patients whose tumors overexpress a protein and who have received one or more drugs for metastatic disease
✦ Is used with paclitaxel for metastatic breast cancer in patients whose tumors overexpress a protein and who haven't received chemotherapy for metastatic disease

Adverse reactions to watch for

✦ Heart failure, ventricular dysfunction (with trastuzumab)
✦ Hyperuricemia, tumor lysis syndrome, severe myelosuppression (with gemtuzumab)
✦ Infusion-related toxicities (fever, chills, shortness of breath, hypotension, anaphylaxis)
✦ Myelosuppression, opportunistic infections (with alemtuzumab)
✦ Severe mucocutaneous reactions (with rituximab)

Key nursing actions
- Perform a thorough baseline cardiac assessment before trastuzumab therapy.
- Monitor the blood pressure, and assess for hypotensive symptoms.
- Obtain CBC and platelet counts weekly during therapy, more often if anemia, neutropenia, or thrombocytopenia worsens.
- Monitor liver function test results during gemtuzumab therapy.
- Review the CD4+ count after treatment with alemtuzumab until it is 200 cells/mm^3 or higher.
- Stay alert for rituximab infusion reactions and mucocutaneous reactions.

Features of targeted-therapy drugs

bortezomib
- Inhibits proteasomes involved in cell cycle functions that promote tumor growth
- Is used for relapsed multiple myeloma

◆ Obtain the patient's CBC and platelet counts weekly during therapy and more frequently if anemia, neutropenia, or thrombocytopenia worsens. Be especially alert for abnormalities during gemtuzumab therapy because this drug can cause severe myelosuppression.

◆ Monitor the results of liver function studies to detect elevations during gemtuzumab therapy.

◆ Review the patient's CD4+ counts after treatment with alemtuzumab until CD4+ count is 200 cells/mm^3 or higher.

◆ If tumor lysis syndrome occurs during gemtuzumab therapy, provide adequate hydration and allopurinol to prevent hyperuricemia.

 CLINICAL ALERT Stay alert for infusion reactions to rituximab, including hypotension, angioedema, hypoxia, and bronchospasm. If any are detected, stop treatment immediately and notify the prescriber.

◆ Assess the patient for mucocutaneous reactions to rituximab. If you detect any, avoid further infusions and treat the reaction promptly.

◆ Teach the patient and his family about the prescribed drug. (See *Teaching a patient about monoclonal antibodies.*)

TARGETED-THERAPY DRUGS

A groundbreaking approach to cancer treatment is to target the proteins linked to the growth of a specific type of cancer. Drugs in this new class include bortezomib, gefitinib, and imatinib.

Pharmacokinetics
Because bortezomib isn't absorbed orally, it must be given I.V. It's extensively distributed into body tissues and metabolized in the liver.

After oral use of gefitinib, about half of the drug is absorbed. It's widely distributed in tissues, undergoes hepatic metabolism, and is excreted mainly in feces.

When given orally, imatinib is almost completely absorbed. It's 95% bound to plasma proteins and extensively metabolized by the liver. Its half-life is about 15 hours.

Pharmacodynamics

Bortezomib inhibits the proteasomes involved in cell cycle functions that promote tumor growth.

Gefitinib inhibits epidermal growth factor receptor-1, which is overexpressed with certain cancers, such as non–small-cell lung cancer. This blocks the pathways for cancer growth, survival, and metastasis.

Imatinib binds to the adenosine triphosphate (ATP) binding area on BCR-ABL proteins. In chronic myeloid leukemia, BCR-ABL proteins stimulate other tyrosine kinase proteins and lead to abnormally high production of WBCs. The binding of imatinib effectively halts abnormal WBC production.

Pharmacotherapeutics

Bortezomib is indicated in the treatment of multiple myeloma that has relapsed after standard chemotherapy.

Gefitinib is used as a single drug in patients with non-small cell lung cancer that haven't responded to two standard chemotherapy regimens.

Imatinib is prescribed to treat chronic myeloid leukemia, acute lymphoid leukemia, and GI stromal tumors.

Interactions

No known interactions exist with bortezomib.

✦ A drug that inhibits CYP 3A4 enzymes, such as clarithromycin, erythromycin, itraconazole, or ketoconazole, can decrease gefitinib or imatinib metabolism and increase the targeted-therapy drug level.

✦ A drug that induces CYP 3A4 enzymes, such as rifampin or phenytoin, can increase gefitinib or imatinib metabolism and decrease the targeted-therapy drug level.

✦ A histamine$_2$ (H$_2$)-receptor antagonist may reduce the gefitinib level.

Adverse reactions

Bortezomib may cause asthenia, nausea, decreased appetite, constipation, thrombocytopenia, pyrexia, vomiting, anemia, peripheral neuropathy, headache, hypotension, diarrhea, and hepatotoxicity.

In clinical trials, the most frequent drug-related adverse reactions to gefitinib were diarrhea, rash, acne, dry skin, nausea, and vomiting. Other reactions include pruritus, anorexia, asthenia, and weight loss. Abnormal eyelash growth has also been reported. Interstitial lung disease has been reported in about 1% of patients taking gefitinib.

Common adverse reactions to imatinib include headache, fatigue, weakness, pyrexia, edema, cerebral hemorrhage, epistaxis, anorexia, nausea, diarrhea, abdominal pain, constipation, GI hemorrhage, neutropenia, thrombocytopenia, anemia, hypokalemia, myalgia, muscle cramps, musculoskeletal pain, arthralgia, cough, dyspnea, pneumonia, rash, petechiae, and night sweats.

Nursing considerations

✦ Use bortezomib cautiously in a patient with hepatic impairment.
✦ Monitor the patient's weight daily.
✦ Closely monitor the patient for fluid retention, which can be severe during imatinib therapy.
✦ Monitor the patient's CBC weekly for the first month of therapy with bortezomib or imatinib, then biweekly for the second month and periodically thereafter.

Features of targeted-therapy drugs
(continued)

gefitinib
✦ Inhibits epidermal growth factor receptor-1, which is overexpressed with certain cancers
✦ Is used alone for non–small-cell lung cancer that hasn't responded to two standard chemotherapy regimens

imatinib
✦ Binds to ATP binding area on BCR-ABL proteins, which halts abnormal WBC production
✦ Is used for chronic myeloid leukemia, acute lymphoid leukemia, and GI stromal tumors

Adverse reactions to watch for

bortezomib
✦ Anemia, asthenia, constipation, decreased appetite, diarrhea, headache, hepatotoxicity, hypotension, nausea, peripheral neuropathy, pyrexia, thrombocytopenia, vomiting

gefitinib
✦ Abnormal eyelash growth, acne, anorexia, asthenia, diarrhea, dry skin, interstitial lung disease, nausea, pruritus, rash, vomiting, weight loss

imatinib
✦ Abdominal pain, anemia, anorexia, arthralgia, cerebral hemorrhage, constipation, cough, diarrhea, dyspnea, edema, epistaxis, fatigue, GI hemorrhage, headache, hypokalemia, muscle cramps, musculoskeletal pain, myalgia, nausea, neutropenia, night sweats, petechiae, pneumonia, pyrexia, rash, thrombocytopenia, weakness

Teaching a patient about targeted-therapy drugs

Whenever a targeted-therapy drug is prescribed, teach the patient and his family the drug's name, dose, frequency, action, and adverse effects. Also take the following actions.

✦ Stress the importance of returning for blood tests during therapy to monitor for adverse reactions.
✦ Instruct the patient to take imatinib with food and a large glass of water and to take gefitinib without regard to food.
✦ Advise the patient not to drive or operate machinery until bortezomib's adverse central nervous system effects are known.
✦ Teach the patient how to avoid dehydration during bortezomib therapy.
✦ Instruct a woman of childbearing age to avoid pregnancy while receiving a targeted-therapy drug.
✦ Teach the patient to recognize adverse reactions and report them to the prescriber.

Key nursing actions

✦ Weigh the patient daily.
✦ Monitor closely for fluid retention, especially during imatinib therapy.
✦ Check the CBC weekly for the first month of therapy with bortezomib or imatinib, biweekly for the second month, and periodically thereafter.
✦ Monitor liver function test results carefully during bortezomib therapy.

✦ Give imatinib with food to minimize GI irritation, which commonly occurs with this drug.

 CLINICAL ALERT Carefully monitor the patient's liver function test results because bortezomib can produce hepatotoxicity, which may be severe. Decrease the dosage as needed.

✦ Consider increasing the imatinib dosage only if the patient has no severe adverse reactions or severe non–leukemia-related neutropenia or thrombocytopenia and if he displays disease progression at any time, fails to achieve a satisfactory hematologic response after at least 3 months of treatment, or loses a previously achieved hematologic response.
✦ Reconstitute bortezomib with normal saline solution and give the drug within 8 hours of preparation.
✦ Teach the patient and his family about the prescribed drug. (See *Teaching a patient about targeted-therapy drugs.*)

TOPOISOMERASE I INHIBITORS

Topoisomerase I inhibitors inhibit the enzyme topoisomerase enzyme I. They're derived from camptothecin, a naturally occurring alkaloid from the Chinese tree *Camptotheca acuminata.* Currently available drugs include irinotecan and topotecan.

Pharmacokinetics

Irinotecan and topotecan are minimally absorbed and must be given I.V. Irinotecan is a prodrug for the active metabolite SN-38. The half-life of SN-38 is about 10 hours, and it's eliminated via biliary excretion.

Topotecan undergoes pH-dependent hydrolysis. It's metabolized in the liver and excreted in significant amounts by the kidneys.

Pharmacodynamics

These drugs exert their cytotoxic effect by inhibiting the topoisomerase I enzyme, which mediates the relaxation of supercoiled DNA. Topoisomerase I inhibitors bind to the DNA-topoisomerase I complex and prevent resealing. This causes DNA strands to break, resulting in impaired DNA synthesis.

Pharmacotherapeutics

Topoisomerase I inhibitors are active against solid tumors and hematologic malignancies. Irinotecan is used to treat colorectal cancer and small-cell lung cancer. Topotecan is prescribed for treating ovarian cancer, small-cell lung cancer, and acute myeloid leukemia.

Interactions

✦ Ketoconazole significantly increases the SN-38 level, which increases the risk of irinotecan toxicity.
✦ Use of a diuretic may exacerbate the dehydration caused by irinotecan-induced diarrhea.
✦ Use of a laxative with irinotecan can induce diarrhea.
✦ Prochlorperazine can increase the risk of extrapyramidal toxicities caused by irinotecan.
✦ When used with fluorouracil and leucovorin, irinotecan may cause a thrombo-embolic event, such as myocardial infarction or stroke.

Adverse reactions

Diarrhea commonly results from irinotecan therapy. It can occur acutely during therapy; this form is cholinergically mediated and can be reversed with atropine. Or diarrhea can occur several days after chemotherapy and may persist for up to 1 week. For this form of diarrhea, the treatment of choice is loperamide given every 2 hours until stools become formed.

Irinotecan's other adverse reactions include insomnia, dizziness, asthenia, headache, fever, pain, vasodilation, edema, rhinitis, nausea, vomiting, anorexia, stomatitis, constipation, flatulence, dyspepsia, abdominal cramping and enlargement, anemia, weight loss, dehydration, back pain, dyspnea, increased cough, alopecia, sweating, rash, chills, and infection.

Topotecan can cause significant myelosuppression. It may also produce fatigue, asthenia, headache, fever, nausea, vomiting, diarrhea, constipation, abdominal pain, stomatitis, anorexia, neutropenia, leukopenia, thrombocytopenia, anemia, back and skeletal pain, dyspnea, cough, and alopecia.

Nursing considerations

✦ Irinotecan comes in a plastic blister package to prevent accidental breakage and leakage. Inspect the vial for damage and signs of leakage before removing it from the blister package. Store the vial at 59° to 86° F (15° to 30° C) and protect it from light.
✦ Withhold a diuretic during irinotecan therapy and periods of active vomiting or diarrhea to decrease the risk of dehydration.

 CLINICAL ALERT Before giving the first dose of topotecan, make sure that the patient's baseline neutrophil count exceeds 1,500/mm³ and his platelet count exceeds 100,000/mm³.

PATIENT TEACHING

Teaching a patient about topoisomerase I inhibitors

Whenever a topoisomerase I inhibitor is prescribed, teach the patient and his family the drug's name, dose, frequency, action, and adverse effects. Also take the following actions.

✦ Stress the importance of returning for blood tests during therapy to monitor for adverse reactions.

✦ Urge the patient to promptly report sore throat, fever, chills, or unusual bleeding or bruising.

✦ Caution a woman of childbearing age to avoid pregnancy and breast-feeding during therapy.

✦ Inform the patient about the risk of irinotecan-induced diarrhea and methods to treat it. Tell him to avoid laxatives.

✦ Warn the patient that hair loss may occur.

✦ Teach the patient to recognize adverse reactions and report them to the prescriber.

Key nursing actions

✦ Before giving the first dose of topotecan, make sure the baseline neutrophil count exceeds 1,500/mm³ and platelet count exceeds 100,000/mm³.

✦ Review the WBC count and CBC with differential before each dose of irinotecan.

✦ Assess the patient for diarrhea during irinotecan therapy.

✦ Temporarily stop irinotecan if neutropenic fever occurs or the absolute neutrophil count falls below 500/mm³.

✦ Be alert for evidence of bone marrow suppression.

✦ Frequently monitor peripheral blood cell counts.

✦ Review the patient's WBC count and CBC with differential before each dose of irinotecan.

 CLINICAL ALERT Monitor for diarrhea during irinotecan therapy. Watch for diaphoresis and abdominal cramping, which may precede diarrhea that occurs within 24 hours of giving the drug. Give I.V. atropine, unless contraindicated, to treat this type of diarrhea.

If diarrhea occurs more than 24 hours after giving the drug, watch for signs and symptoms of dehydration and electrolyte imbalances. Because this form of diarrhea may be life-threatening, treat it with loperamide and closely monitor the patient's fluid intake and output and electrolyte levels.

✦ Temporarily stop irinotecan if neutropenic fever occurs or if the patient's absolute neutrophil count falls below 500/mm³. Reduce the dosage if his WBC count is below 2,000/mm³, neutrophil count is below 1,000/mm³, hemoglobin is below 8 g/dl, or platelet count is below 100,000/mm³.

✦ Be alert for signs and symptoms of bone marrow suppression (especially neutropenia), which indicates a toxic topotecan level. The nadir occurs about 11 days after giving the drug. Neutropenia isn't cumulative over time.

✦ Frequently monitor the patient's peripheral blood cell counts. Don't give topotecan until his neutrophil count recovers to more than 1,000/mm³, platelet count recovers to more than 100,000/mm³, and hemoglobin recovers to more than 9 mg/dl (with transfusion, if needed).

✦ Give WBC colony-stimulating factor to promote cell growth and decrease the patient's risk of infection.

✦ Teach the patient and his family about the prescribed drug. (See *Teaching a patient about topoisomerase I inhibitors.*)

UNCLASSIFIABLE ANTINEOPLASTICS

Many other antineoplastics don't fit into existing classifications. These drugs include aldesleukin, altretamine, arsenic, asparaginases, hydroxyurea, interferons, procarbazine, and taxanes.

ALDESLEUKIN

Aldesleukin is a human recombinant interleukin-2 derivative that's used to treat metastatic renal cell carcinoma.

Pharmacokinetics

After I.V. use of aldesleukin, about 30% is absorbed into the plasma and about 70% is absorbed rapidly by the liver, kidneys, and lungs. The drug is excreted primarily by the kidneys.

Pharmacodynamics

The exact antitumor mechanism of action of aldesleukin is unknown. The drug may stimulate an immunologic reaction against the tumor.

Pharmacotherapeutics

Aldesleukin is used to treat metastatic renal cell carcinoma. It may also be prescribed to treat Kaposi's sarcoma and metastatic melanoma.

Interactions

+ Use of aldesleukin with a psychotropic drug (such as an analgesic, antiemetic, narcotic, sedative, or tranquilizer) may produce additive CNS effects.
+ A glucocorticoid may reduce aldesleukin's antitumor effects.
+ An antihypertensive may potentiate aldesleukin's hypotensive effects.
+ Use of aldesleukin with a drug that's toxic to the kidneys (such as an aminoglycoside), bone marrow (such as a cytotoxic drug), heart (such as doxorubicin), or liver (such as methotrexate or asparaginase) may increase toxicity in these organs.

Adverse reactions

During clinical trials, more than 15% of patients developed these adverse reactions to aldesleukin: pulmonary congestion, dyspnea, anemia, thrombocytopenia, leukopenia, hypomagnesemia, acidosis, oliguria, anuria, stomatitis, nausea, vomiting, pruritus, erythema, rash, dry skin, fever, chills, fatigue, malaise, weakness, edema, infection, pain, weight gain, and elevated bilirubin, transaminase, alkaline phosphatase, and creatinine levels.

Nursing considerations

+ Monitor the patient regularly for adverse reactions and drug interactions during aldesleukin therapy. If any occur, alert the prescriber.
+ Verify that the patient's cardiac, pulmonary, hepatic, and CNS functions are normal before therapy begins. Obtain the results of hematologic tests, pulmonary and cardiac function tests, blood chemistries, and chest X-rays before therapy starts and then daily during therapy.
+ Monitor the patient's CBC and platelet count for evidence of leukopenia, thrombocytopenia, or anemia. Because RBCs have a longer life than WBCs and platelets,

Features of aldesleukin

+ May stimulate an immunologic reaction against the tumor
+ Is used for metastatic renal cell carcinoma, Kaposi's sarcoma, and metastatic melanoma

Adverse reactions to watch for

+ Acidosis, hypomagnesemia
+ Anemia, leukopenia, thrombocytopenia
+ Anuria, oliguria
+ Chills, fever
+ Dry skin, erythema, pruritus, rash
+ Dyspnea, pulmonary congestion
+ Edema, weight gain
+ Elevated bilirubin, transaminase, alkaline phosphatase, and creatinine levels
+ Fatigue, malaise, weakness
+ Infection, pain
+ Nausea, stomatitis, vomiting

Key nursing actions

+ Verify that cardiac, pulmonary, hepatic, and CNS functions are normal before therapy begins.
+ Monitor the CBC and platelet count for evidence of leukopenia, thrombocytopenia, or anemia.
+ Take bleeding precautions when the platelet count falls below 50,000/mm³.
+ Monitor the patient for flulike syndrome.

anemia is less of a problem than thrombocytopenia or leukopenia unless the patient has occult or overt blood loss.
+ Monitor the patient with leukopenia for signs and symptoms of infection, such as fever, sore throat, chills, and malaise. Also take infection control measures until the patient's WBC count returns to normal.
+ Take bleeding precautions whenever the patient's platelet count falls below 50,000/mm³. Give platelet transfusions and packed RBCs during times of severe bleeding.
+ Take energy conservation measures for a patient with anemia. For example, stagger his activities, help with tasks, and arrange for frequent rest periods.
+ Monitor the patient for flulike syndrome, characterized by fever, chills, malaise, and myalgia. Give a mild antipyretic and analgesic as needed.
+ Teach the patient and his family about the prescribed drug. (See *Teaching a patient about aldesleukin.*)

ALTRETAMINE

This synthetic cytotoxic antineoplastic is used as palliative treatment for patients with ovarian cancer.

Pharmacokinetics

After oral use, altretamine is absorbed well. It's metabolized extensively in the liver and excreted by the liver and kidneys. The parent compound is poorly bound to plasma proteins.

Pharmacodynamics

The exact mechanism of action of altretamine is unknown. However, its metabolites are alkylating drugs.

Pharmacotherapeutics

Altretamine is used as palliative treatment of persistent or recurring ovarian cancer after first-line therapy with cisplatin or an alkylating drug combination.

Interactions

✦ Cimetidine may increase altretamine's half-life and its risk of toxicity.

 CLINICAL ALERT Keep in mind that the use of altretamine with a monoamine oxidase (MAO) inhibitor may cause severe orthostatic hypotension.

Adverse reactions

More than 10% of patients in clinical trials exhibited these adverse reactions to altretamine: nausea, vomiting, neurotoxicity, peripheral neuropathy, and anemia. Bone marrow suppression is common and can cause leukopenia, thrombocytopenia, and anemia.

Nursing considerations

✦ Monitor the patient regularly for adverse reactions and drug interactions during altretamine therapy. If any occur, alert the prescriber.

✦ Monitor the patient's CBC and platelet count for evidence of leukopenia, thrombocytopenia, or anemia. Typically, the nadir of bone marrow suppression occurs about 4 weeks after therapy begins; recovery, at 6 weeks. Because RBCs have a longer life than WBCs and platelets, anemia is less of a problem than thrombocytopenia or leukopenia unless the patient has occult or overt blood loss.

✦ Monitor the patient with leukopenia for signs and symptoms of infection. Also take infection control measures until his WBC count returns to normal.

✦ Take bleeding precautions whenever the patient's platelet count falls below 50,000/mm³. Give platelet transfusions and packed RBCs during times of severe bleeding.

✦ Stop the drug for at least 14 days if the patient develops GI reactions that don't respond to conventional treatments or progressive neurotoxicity or if his WBC count is less than 2,000/mm³, granulocyte count is less than 1,000/mm³, or platelet count is less than 75,000/mm³. Restart therapy with a reduced dosage. If neurologic symptoms persist despite the dosage reduction, stop the drug.

✦ Take energy conservation measures for a patient with anemia. For example, stagger his activities, help with tasks, and arrange for frequent rest periods.

✦ Monitor the patient for signs and symptoms of neurotoxicity and peripheral neuropathy. Perform a neurologic examination before each course of therapy. Immediately report signs and symptoms to the prescriber.

✦ Monitor the patient for signs and symptoms of orthostatic hypotension, such as light-headedness or dizziness upon arising, if he also receives an MAO inhibitor. Advise him to avoid sudden position changes.

✦ Teach the patient and his family about the prescribed drug. (See *Teaching a patient about altretamine,* page 416.)

Features of altretamine

✦ Has metabolites that are alkylating drugs
✦ Is used as palliative treatment for persistent or recurring ovarian cancer after first-line therapy with cisplatin or an alkylating drug combination

Adverse reactions to watch for

✦ Anemia
✦ Bone marrow suppression that can cause leukopenia, thrombocytopenia, and anemia
✦ Nausea, vomiting
✦ Neurotoxicity, peripheral neuropathy

Key nursing actions

✦ Monitor the CBC and platelet count to detect leukopenia, thrombocytopenia, or anemia.
✦ Take bleeding precautions when the platelet count falls below 50,000/mm³.
✦ Stop the drug for at least 14 days if the patient develops GI reactions unresponsive to usual treatments, progressive neurotoxicity, a WBC count less than 2,000/mm³, a granulocyte count less than 1,000/mm³, or a platelet count less than 75,000/mm³.
✦ Watch for evidence of neurotoxicity and peripheral neuropathy.
✦ Watch for evidence of orthostatic hypotension.

Features of arsenic
+ Causes damage and DNA fragmentation similar to programmed cell death in the proteins and DNA of acute promyelocytic leukemia
+ Is used for promyelocytic leukemia that has relapsed after, or been refractory to, standard chemotherapy
+ Is being investigated for treating multiple myeloma

ARSENIC

Arsenic is used to treat patients with promyelocytic leukemia (a rare form of acute myeloid leukemia) who have relapsed after standard therapy or haven't responded to it.

Pharmacokinetics

Because arsenic is inadequately absorbed orally, it must be given I.V. The drug is distributed to the heart, liver, kidneys, lungs, hair, and nails. It's metabolized through reduction by arsenate reductase and then through methylation to inactive metabolites, which are excreted in urine.

Pharmacodynamics

In the proteins and DNA of acute promyelocytic leukemia, arsenic causes damage and DNA fragmentation similar to programmed cell death.

Pharmacotherapeutics

Arsenic is used for treating promyelocytic leukemia that has relapsed after standard chemotherapy or has been refractory to it. It's being investigated for treatment of multiple myeloma.

Interactions

+ Use of arsenic with another drug that prolongs the QT interval may increase the risk of arrhythmias.

WARNING

Preventing the fatal effects of arsenic

Arsenic trioxide has been linked to acute promyelocytic leukemia (APL) differentiation syndrome. To prevent its life-threatening effects, follow these guidelines:
✦ Monitor the patient for signs and symptoms of APL differentiation syndrome, such as fever, dyspnea, weight gain, pulmonary infiltrates, and pleural or pericardial effusion, with or without leukocytosis.
✦ If you detect any of these signs or symptoms, notify the prescriber immediately.
✦ Expect to treat the syndrome with high doses of corticosteroids.

✦ Use of arsenic with a diuretic or amphotericin B may increase the risk of electrolyte imbalances.

Adverse reactions
Arsenic can cause ECG abnormalities that may progress to life-threatening arrhythmias. It also can induce a unique toxicity called acute promyelocytic leukemia (APL) differentiation syndrome. (See *Preventing the fatal effects of arsenic.*)

Adverse neurologic reactions to arsenic may include headache, insomnia, anxiety, dizziness, and tremor. Other reactions are rash, nausea, vomiting, hypokalemia, liver damage, and muscle and bone aches.

Nursing considerations
✦ Use arsenic cautiously in patients with heart failure, renal failure, prolonged QT interval, conditions that result in hypokalemia or hypomagnesemia, or a history of torsades de pointes.
✦ Before starting the drug, obtain an ECG tracing; review the patient's potassium, calcium, magnesium, and creatinine levels; and correct electrolyte imbalances.
✦ Monitor the patient's electrolyte levels and hematologic and coagulation test results at least twice weekly during treatment. Keep his potassium above 4 mEq/dl and his magnesium level above 1.8 mg/dl.
✦ Monitor the patient for syncope and rapid or irregular heart rate. If these occur, stop the drug, hospitalize him, and monitor his electrolyte levels and QTc interval. Restart the drug as indicated when electrolyte imbalances have been corrected and the QTc interval falls below 460 msec.
✦ Monitor the patient's ECG tracing at least weekly during therapy. A prolonged QTc interval commonly occurs 1 to 5 weeks after the infusion, and returns to baseline about 8 weeks after the infusion. If the QTc interval is higher than 500 msec at any time during therapy, assess the patient closely and consider stopping the drug.
✦ Teach the patient and his family about the prescribed drug. (See *Teaching a patient about arsenic,* page 418.)

Adverse reactions to watch for
✦ Anxiety, dizziness, headache, insomnia, tremor
✦ APL differentiation syndrome
✦ ECG abnormalities that may progress to life-threatening arrhythmias
✦ Hypokalemia
✦ Liver damage, nausea, vomiting
✦ Muscle and bone aches
✦ Rash

Key nursing actions
✦ Before starting the drug, obtain an ECG tracing; review potassium, calcium, magnesium, and creatinine levels; and correct electrolyte imbalances.
✦ Monitor electrolyte levels and hematologic and coagulation test results at least twice weekly during treatment.
✦ Monitor the patient for syncope and rapid or irregular heart rate.
✦ Review the ECG tracing at least weekly during therapy.

ASPARAGINASES

Asparaginases are cell cycle–specific drugs that act during the G_1 phase. They include asparaginase and pegaspargase.

Pharmacokinetics

After parenteral use, asparaginase is 100% bioavailable when given I.V. and about 50% bioavailable when given I.M. Asparaginase remains inside the blood vessels, with minimal distribution elsewhere. Its metabolism is unknown; only trace amounts appear in urine.

No information is available about the pharmacokinetics of pegaspargase.

Pharmacodynamics

Asparaginase and pegaspargase capitalize on the biochemical differences between normal cells and tumor cells. Most normal cells can synthesize asparagine, but some tumor cells depend on other sources of asparagine for survival. The asparaginases help degrade asparagine to aspartic acid and ammonia. Then, deprived of their supply of asparagine, the tumor cells die.

Pharmacotherapeutics

Asparaginase is used primarily with standard chemotherapy to induce remission in patients with acute lymphocytic leukemia. Pegaspargase is used to treat acute lymphocytic leukemia in patients who are hypersensitive to asparaginase.

Interactions

♦ Asparaginase or pegaspargase may reduce the effectiveness of methotrexate.
♦ Use of asparaginase with prednisone may lead to hyperglycemia.
♦ Use of asparaginase with vincristine can cause increased neuropathy.

Adverse reactions

Asparaginase and pegaspargase can cause several potentially serious toxicities. (See *Risks of asparaginases.*) Anaphylaxis, the most serious reaction, is more likely to occur with intermittent I.V. dosing than with daily I.V. dosing or I.M. injections.

Features of asparaginases

♦ Help degrade asparagine to aspartic acid and ammonia and, by depriving tumor cells of asparagine, kill them
♦ Asparaginase is used mainly with standard chemotherapy to induce remission in acute lymphocytic leukemia
♦ Pegaspargase is used for acute lymphocytic leukemia in patients hypersensitive to asparaginase

LIFESPAN

Risks of asparaginases

Adverse reactions to asparaginases vary with the patient's age and developmental status. For example, reactions to asparaginase in children tend to be less severe than in adults. The safety and efficacy of pegaspargase haven't been studied in children younger than age 1. However, the drug has a lower risk of adverse reactions (except hypersensitivity reactions) in older children than in adults. Neither drug is recommended for use during pregnancy or breast-feeding.

In many patients, nausea and vomiting occur shortly after asparaginase or pegaspargase use. Fever, headache, and abdominal pain may also occur. Hepatotoxicity commonly develops and is manifested by transient and mild liver enzyme elevations, which peak in the second week of therapy.

Hypersensitivity reactions occur in 20% to 35% of patients receiving asparaginase or pegaspargase. Anaphylaxis also occurs, and the risk of a reaction rises with each successive treatment. Pancreatitis, evidenced by epigastric pain, vomiting, and a high amylase level, has appeared in 5% of patients receiving asparaginase. Patients may also become hyperglycemic due to decreased insulin production. CNS toxicity may also occur in 25% of patients, producing personality changes, seizures, and abnormal electroencephalogram (EEG) tracings. Renal impairment and coagulation abnormalities, such as hypofibrinogenemia and depression of other coagulation factors, may also occur.

Nursing considerations
✦ Handle I.V. preparations of asparaginase and pegaspargase cautiously.
✦ Refrigerate reconstituted asparaginase if the preparation isn't used immediately. Use the solution only if it's clear.
✦ Give asparaginase or pegaspargase with the prescriber present because of the risk of anaphylaxis. Keep available drugs and equipment needed to treat cardiac arrest.
✦ Monitor the patient's vital signs before and during asparaginase use.
✦ Stop the asparaginase or pegaspargase infusion immediately if a hypersensitivity reaction occurs and begin emergency treatment. Keep in mind that the risk of anaphylaxis increases with each successive treatment and is more likely to occur with intermittent therapy.
✦ Monitor the patient regularly for adverse reactions and drug interactions during therapy. Alert the prescriber if any occur.
✦ Give an antiemetic as needed because nausea and vomiting are particularly noxious adverse reactions to asparaginase and pegaspargase therapy. If an antiemetic isn't prescribed, consult the prescriber and use other nursing interventions for a patient with nausea or vomiting.
✦ Monitor the patient's liver and renal function test results and amylase and glucose levels. Notify the prescriber of abnormal results.
✦ Take seizure precautions during asparaginase therapy. Stop the infusion immediately and notify the prescriber if seizures occur.
✦ Report personality changes to the prescriber. Such changes may indicate CNS toxicity from asparaginase.

Adverse reactions to watch for
✦ Abdominal pain, nausea, vomiting
✦ Anaphylaxis, hypersensitivity reactions
✦ CNS toxicity (such as personality changes, seizures, abnormal EEG tracings)
✦ Coagulation abnormalities
✦ Fever, headache
✦ Hepatotoxicity
✦ Hyperglycemia
✦ Pancreatitis
✦ Renal impairment

Key nursing actions
✦ Give asparaginase or pegaspargase with the prescriber present because of the risk of anaphylaxis. Keep emergency equipment nearby.
✦ Monitor vital signs before and during asparaginase use.
✦ Give an antiemetic as needed.
✦ Monitor liver and renal function test results and amylase and glucose levels.
✦ Take seizure precautions during asparaginase therapy.
✦ Report personality changes to the prescriber.
✦ Monitor coagulation factor levels.

Teaching a patient about asparaginases

Whenever an asparaginase is prescribed, teach the patient and his family the drug's name, dose, frequency, action, and adverse effects. Also take the following actions.

◆ Inform the patient of the risk of cardiac arrest, and provide support and reassurance.

◆ Instruct the patient to immediately report signs or symptoms of hypersensitivity, including restlessness, wheezing, facial flushing or edema, urticaria, pruritus, tachycardia, hypotension, fever, and dyspnea.

◆ Teach the patient to recognize the signs and symptoms of central nervous system (CNS) toxicity (such as personality changes and seizures) and of pancreatitis (such as abdominal tenderness, midepigastric pain, and vomiting). The CNS changes usually disappear when asparaginase is stopped but may persist. Inform the patient that CNS toxicity or pancreatitis may require the drug to be stopped.

◆ Teach the patient to recognize and report the signs and symptoms of liver damage, such as yellowed skin or sclera, dark-colored urine, clay-colored stools, and pruritus.

◆ Advise the patient to take a mild antipyretic and analgesic if a fever or headache occurs with asparaginase use.

◆ Teach the patient to take bleeding precautions if coagulation abnormalities occur.

◆ Give the patient written materials about the possible effects of asparaginase for his home reference.

◆ Instruct the patient to notify the prescriber if adverse reactions persist or worsen.

◆ Note asparaginase treatment on EEG request slips because the drug can cause abnormal EEG tracings.

◆ Pegaspargase is often given with other chemotherapeutics, such as cytarabine, daunorubicin, doxorubicin, methotrexate, and vincristine. Be alert for the adverse effects of these drugs, too.

◆ Monitor the patient's coagulation factor levels. Withhold asparaginase and give fresh frozen plasma, as indicated. Take bleeding precautions until the patient's coagulation factor levels return to normal.

◆ Teach the patient and his family about the prescribed drug. (See *Teaching a patient about asparaginases.*)

HYDROXYUREA

Usually, hydroxyurea is used to treat chronic myelogenous leukemia. However, it's also used for solid tumors and head and neck cancer.

Pharmacokinetics

After oral use, hydroxyurea is absorbed readily and distributed well into the CSF. It reaches a peak level 2 hours after use. About half of a dose is metabolized by the liver to carbon dioxide, which is excreted by the lungs, or to urea, which is excreted by the kidneys. The other half is excreted unchanged in urine.

Features of hydroxyurea

◆ Inhibits ribonucleotide reductase, which is required for DNA synthesis

◆ Kills cells in the S phase and holds other cells in the G_1 phase, where they're most susceptible to radiation

Pharmacodynamics

Hydroxyurea exerts its effect by inhibiting the enzyme ribonucleotide reductase, which is required for DNA synthesis. The drug kills cells in the S phase of the cell cycle and holds other cells in the G_1 phase, where they're most susceptible to radiation.

Pharmacotherapeutics

Hydroxyurea is used to treat selected myeloproliferative disorders. It may produce temporary remissions in some patients with metastatic malignant melanomas as well. In addition, the drug is used with radiation to treat carcinomas of the head, neck, and lung.

Interactions

✦ A cytotoxic drug or radiation therapy can enhance the toxicity of hydroxyurea.

Adverse reactions

Hydroxyurea causes dose-related bone marrow suppression characterized primarily by leukopenia. It may also produce drowsiness, headache, nausea, vomiting, and anorexia. These adverse reactions are usually dose-related. Mild dermatologic reactions may include pruritus, facial erythema, and a maculopapular rash.

Rarely, a patient receiving radiation will experience exacerbated radiation erythema when taking hydroxyurea. Stomatitis and alopecia may also occur but are rare. Patients taking hydroxyurea may need to take allopurinol to prevent uric acid nephropathy and the resulting renal damage.

Nursing considerations

✦ Give oral hydroxyurea on a daily or every-third-day schedule, using a large single dose rather than divided doses to attain a higher drug level. If the patient has trouble swallowing capsules, dissolve the capsule contents in water and give immediately.
✦ Monitor the patient regularly for adverse reactions and drug interactions during hydroxyurea therapy. Alert the prescriber if any occur.
✦ Regularly monitor the patient's WBC count for leukopenia. If leukopenia occurs, monitor him for signs and symptoms of infection. Also take infection control measures until the WBC count returns to normal.
✦ Use other appropriate nursing interventions for a patient with leukopenia, nausea, vomiting, stomatitis, or alopecia.
✦ Monitor the patient's uric acid, BUN, and creatinine levels during therapy to detect signs of uric acid nephropathy, such as rising uric acid, BUN, and creatinine levels.
✦ Encourage the patient with signs of nephropathy to drink at least eight 8-oz (240-ml) glasses of fluid daily. Also give allopurinol.
✦ Notify the prescriber if uric acid nephropathy occurs.
✦ Teach the patient and his family about the prescribed drug. (See *Teaching a patient about hydroxyurea,* page 422.)

Features of hydroxyurea
(continued)

✦ Is used to treat selected myeloproliferative disorders
✦ May produce temporary remission in some patients with metastatic malignant melanoma
✦ Is used with radiation for carcinomas of head, neck, and lung

Adverse reactions to watch for

✦ Anorexia, nausea, vomiting
✦ Bone marrow suppression
✦ Drowsiness, headache
✦ Facial erythema, maculopapular rash, pruritus
✦ Uric acid nephropathy

Key nursing actions

✦ Monitor the WBC count regularly for leukopenia.
✦ Review uric acid, BUN, and creatinine levels during therapy to detect uric acid nephropathy.
✦ Urge the patient with signs of nephropathy to drink at least eight 8-oz glasses of fluid daily. Also give allopurinol.

Teaching a patient about hydroxyurea

Whenever hydroxyurea is prescribed, teach the patient and his family the drug's name, dose, frequency, action, and adverse effects. Also take the following actions.

+ Stress the importance of returning for follow-up blood tests.
+ Instruct the patient to watch for signs and symptoms of infection and to report them immediately to the prescriber.
+ Advise the patient to avoid people with contagious infections.
+ Teach the patient about using an oral or suppository antiemetic if nausea and vomiting occur during hydroxyurea therapy.
+ Explain that mild, reversible dermatologic reactions, such as pruritus, maculopapular rash, and facial erythema, may occur. Instruct the patient to keep previously irradiated skin clean, dry, and protected from sunlight. Also instruct him to report exacerbation of erythema at an irradiated site to the prescriber.
+ Caution the patient to avoid activities that require alertness if drowsiness occurs.
+ Teach the patient how to manage stomatitis at home.
+ Prepare the patient for possible alopecia by explaining the timing and speed of hair loss and noting that it may affect the scalp, eyebrows, eyelashes, or other body hair.
+ Stress the importance of taking hydroxyurea exactly as prescribed to maximize therapeutic effects and minimize adverse ones.
+ Instruct the patient to drink at least eight 8-oz (240-ml) glasses of fluid daily during hydroxyurea therapy.
+ Give the patient written materials about hydroxyurea therapy for home reference.
+ Instruct the patient to notify the prescriber if other adverse reactions occur.

Features of interferons

+ Are so named for their ability to interfere with viral replication
+ Are active against cancer and condylomata acuminata
+ Come in three types: alfa, beta, and gamma

alfa interferons

+ Appear to bind to specific receptors on cell membranes, where they prompt intracellular events that include enzyme induction
+ Are used for blood malignancies, especially hairy cell leukemia
+ Are also used for AIDS-related Kaposi's sarcoma, condylomata acuminata, chronic myelogenous leukemia, non-Hodgkin's lymphoma, multiple myeloma, melanoma, and renal cell carcinoma

INTERFERONS

A family of naturally occurring glycoproteins, interferons are so named because of their ability to interfere with viral replication. These drugs have anticancer activity as well as activity against condylomata acuminata (soft, wartlike growths on the skin and mucous membrane of the genitalia caused by a virus). The three types of interferons are:

+ alfa interferons derived from WBCs
+ beta interferons derived from fibroblasts (connective tissue cells)
+ gamma interferons derived from fibroblasts and lymphocytes.

Currently, only alfa interferons (alfa-2a, alfa-2b, and alfa-n3) are available commercially. Beta and gamma interferons are limited to investigational use.

Pharmacokinetics

After I.M. or S.C. use, alfa interferons are usually absorbed well. Information about their distribution is unavailable. Alfa interferons are filtered by the kidneys, where they're degraded. Hepatic metabolism and biliary excretion of interferons are negligible.

Pharmacodynamics

Although their exact mechanism of action is unknown, alfa interferons appear to bind to specific receptors on cell membranes. When bound, they initiate intracellular events that include the induction of certain enzymes.

This process may account for their ability to inhibit viral replication, suppress cell proliferation, enhance macrophage activity (engulfing and destroying microorganisms and other debris), and increase the cytotoxicity of lymphocytes for target cells.

Pharmacotherapeutics

Alfa interferons have shown their most promising activity in treating blood malignancies, especially hairy cell leukemia. Their approved indications currently include hairy cell leukemia, AIDS-related Kaposi's sarcoma, and condylomata acuminata.

Alfa interferons also demonstrate some activity against chronic myelogenous leukemia, non-Hodgkin's lymphoma, multiple myeloma, melanoma, and renal cell carcinoma.

Interactions

◆ When used with a CNS depressant, an interferon may enhance CNS depression.
◆ An interferon can substantially increase the half-life of a methylxanthine, such as aminophylline or theophylline.
◆ Use of an interferon with a live virus vaccine may potentiate viral replication, increasing the vaccine's adverse effects and decreasing the body's antibody response.
◆ When used with radiation therapy or a drug that causes blood abnormalities or bone marrow suppression, an interferon may increase bone marrow suppression.
◆ When used with interleukin-2, an alfa interferon can increase the risk of renal failure.

Adverse reactions

The most common adverse reaction to alfa interferons is a flulike syndrome that may produce fever, fatigue, myalgia, headache, chills, and arthralgia.

Hematologic toxicity occurs in up to 50% of patients and may cause leukopenia, neutropenia, thrombocytopenia, and anemia. Adverse GI reactions, such as anorexia, nausea, and diarrhea, occur in 30% to 50% of patients receiving an alfa interferon. CNS disturbances, which occur in 10% to 20% of patients, may include dizziness, confusion, paresthesia, numbness, lethargy, and depression.

Cough and dyspnea can result from interferon therapy, as can hypotension, edema, chest pain, and heart failure. Adverse dermatologic reactions may include alopecia, rash, and dry skin. Interferons may also cause an elevated liver transaminase level and abnormalities in renal function tests.

Nursing considerations

◆ Monitor the patient regularly for adverse reactions and drug interactions during interferon therapy. If any occur, alert the prescriber.
◆ Monitor the patient's blood pressure to detect hypotension. Regularly inquire about chest pain. Monitor for signs and symptoms of heart failure. Notify the prescriber if assessments reveal hypotension or signs of heart failure.
◆ Monitor the patient's CBC and platelet count for evidence of leukopenia, neutropenia, thrombocytopenia, or anemia. Observe the patient with leukopenia for signs and symptoms of infection. Take infection control measures until his WBC count returns to normal. Observe the patient with thrombocytopenia for signs of bleeding. Also take bleeding precautions until his platelet count returns to normal. If anemia occurs, encourage him to take energy conservation measures until his RBC count returns to normal.

Adverse reactions to watch for

◆ Abnormal renal function tests
◆ Alopecia, dry skin, rash
◆ Anorexia, diarrhea, nausea
◆ Chest pain, edema, heart failure, hypotension
◆ Confusion, depression, dizziness, lethargy, numbness, paresthesia
◆ Cough, dyspnea
◆ Elevated liver transaminase level
◆ Flulike syndrome including arthralgia, chills, fatigue, fever, headache, myalgia
◆ Hematologic toxicity

Key nursing actions

+ Monitor the blood pressure to detect hypotension.
+ Assess the CBC and platelet count for evidence of leukopenia, neutropenia, thrombocytopenia, or anemia.
+ Check the liver transaminase level and renal function test results.
+ Assess the patient for flulike symptoms, such as fever, headache, fatigue, myalgia, chills, and arthralgia.
+ Monitor for CNS disturbances, including dizziness, confusion, paresthesia, numbness, lethargy, and depression.

PATIENT TEACHING

Teaching a patient about interferons

Whenever an interferon is prescribed, teach the patient and his family the drug's name, dose, frequency, action, and adverse effects. Also take the following actions.
+ Inform the patient about the likelihood and management of flulike symptoms. Reassure him that most people develop a tolerance to these symptoms, which tend to diminish with continued therapy.
+ Teach the patient or a family member how to give the drug properly.
+ Teach the patient how to manage troublesome GI reactions.
+ Caution the patient not to perform activities that require alertness if central nervous system disturbances occur.
+ Instruct the patient to report cough, dyspnea, chest pain, light-headedness, and ankle swelling because these signs and symptoms may suggest heart failure, hypotension, or a respiratory disturbance.
+ Teach the patient to use infection control measures, bleeding precautions, and energy conservation measures as needed.
+ Stress the importance of returning for follow-up blood tests.
+ Give the patient written materials about the possible effects of interferons for his home reference.
+ Instruct the patient to recognize other adverse reactions and report them to the prescriber.

+ Monitor the patient's liver transaminase level and renal function test results. If abnormal results occur, reduce the dosage.
+ Monitor the patient for flulike symptoms, such as fever, headache, fatigue, myalgia, chills, and arthralgia.
+ Give the interferon in the evening to minimize troublesome flulike symptoms during the day.
+ Monitor the patient for CNS disturbances, including dizziness, confusion, paresthesia, numbness, lethargy, and depression. Notify the prescriber immediately if these symptoms occur.
+ Consult the prescriber about premedicating the patient with acetaminophen to help relieve flulike symptoms.
+ Teach the patient and his family about the prescribed drug. (See *Teaching a patient about interferons.*)

PROCARBAZINE

Procarbazine, a methylhydrazine derivative with MAO inhibiting properties, is used to treat Hodgkin's disease and primary and metastatic brain tumors. It's cell cycle–phase specific and acts on the S phase.

Pharmacokinetics

After oral use, procarbazine is absorbed well. It readily crosses the blood-brain barrier and is well distributed into CSF.

Procarbazine is metabolized rapidly in the liver and is activated by microsomal enzymes. It's excreted in urine, primarily as metabolites. Respiratory excretion of the drug occurs as methane and carbon dioxide gas.

Pharmacodynamics

An inert drug, procarbazine must be activated metabolically in the liver before it can produce various cell changes. It can cause chromosomal damage, suppress mitosis, and inhibit DNA, RNA, and protein synthesis. Cancer cells can develop resistance to procarbazine quickly.

Pharmacotherapeutics

Used with other antineoplastics, procarbazine is prescribed to treat Hodgkin's disease. It's also used to treat primary and metastatic brain tumors. In addition, the drug may be useful against small-cell lung cancer, non-Hodgkin's lymphoma, myeloma, melanoma, and CNS tumors.

Interactions

✦ When given with a CNS depressant, procarbazine produces additive CNS depression.

 CLINICAL ALERT **Keep in mind that, when taken with meperidine (Demerol, an opioid analgesic), procarbazine may result in severe hypotension and lead to death.**

✦ Use of procarbazine with an antidepressant, sympathomimetic, or tyramine-rich food can produce hypertensive reactions.

Adverse reactions

Late-onset bone marrow suppression is the most common dose-limiting reaction to procarbazine. The platelet count nadir occurs after about 4 weeks of therapy, followed by the leukocyte count nadir. Complete recovery occurs at about 6 weeks.

Nausea and vomiting occur in 50% of patients. Stomatitis and diarrhea may also occur. Initially, procarbazine therapy may induce a flulike syndrome, including fever, chills, sweating, lethargy, and myalgia. High-dose procarbazine therapy can cause azoospermia or cessation of menses. Procarbazine may be teratogenic.

Adverse dermatologic reactions have occurred in about 3% of patients. These reactions include pruritus, acneiform rash, and hyperpigmentation.

Procarbazine may produce CNS toxicity marked by such reactions as confusion, depression, psychosis, neuropathies, fingertip paresthesia, footdrop, and lack of muscle coordination. Interstitial pneumonitis and pulmonary fibrosis may occur. Orthostatic hypotension occurs rarely.

Nursing considerations

✦ Minimize procarbazine-induced nausea and vomiting by giving the drug in divided doses and at bedtime.
✦ Place the patient on a low-tyramine diet because procarbazine's MAO inhibition can interact with tyramine, producing hypertension.
✦ Reevaluate the patient's compliance with the low-tyramine diet if he experiences hypertensive crisis.
✦ Monitor the patient regularly for adverse reactions and drug interactions during procarbazine therapy. Alert the prescriber if any occur.
✦ Monitor the patient's CBC and platelet count for evidence of leukopenia, thrombocytopenia, or anemia. Typically, the nadir of bone marrow suppression occurs about 4 weeks after therapy begins; recovery, 6 weeks. Because RBCs have a longer life than WBCs and platelets, anemia is less of a problem than thrombocytopenia or leukopenia unless the patient has occult or overt blood loss.

Features of procarbazine

✦ Is an inert drug
✦ Must be activated metabolically in the liver
✦ Can cause chromosomal damage, suppress mitosis, and inhibit DNA, RNA, and protein synthesis
✦ Allows cancer cells to develop resistance to it quickly
✦ Is used with other antineoplastics for Hodgkin's disease, primary and metastatic brain tumors, small-cell lung cancer, non-Hodgkin's lymphoma, myeloma, melanoma, and CNS tumors

Adverse reactions to watch for

✦ Acneiform rash, hyperpigmentation, pruritus
✦ Azoospermia, cessation of menses
✦ Confusion, depression, psychosis
✦ Diarrhea, nausea, stomatitis, vomiting
✦ Flulike syndrome
✦ Interstitial pneumonitis, pulmonary fibrosis
✦ Late-onset bone marrow suppression
✦ Orthostatic hypotension
✦ Neuropathies, fingertip paresthesia, footdrop, lack of muscle coordination
✦ Teratogenic effects

Teaching a patient about procarbazine

Whenever procarbazine is prescribed, teach the patient and his family the drug's name, dose, frequency, action, and adverse effects. Also take the following actions.

✦ Stress the importance of returning for follow-up blood tests.

✦ Teach the patient to consume a low-tyramine diet to help prevent a drug-food interaction. The patient should avoid such foods as pickled herring, chicken or beef liver, ripe or aged cheeses, beer, Chianti, chocolate, coffee, and cola drinks.

✦ Instruct the patient to consult the pharmacist or prescriber before using an over-the-counter drug. Such a drug may contain alcohol or a central nervous system (CNS) depressant, which can interact with procarbazine.

✦ Advise the patient to stagger his activities and to rest frequently if anemia occurs.

✦ Advise the patient with leukopenia to avoid people with active contagious infections, to watch for signs and symptoms of infection, and to report them immediately to the prescriber.

✦ Teach the patient with thrombocytopenia to take bleeding precautions.

✦ Inform the patient and his family about the risk of CNS toxicity.

✦ Advise a woman to avoid pregnancy during procarbazine therapy because the drug may be teratogenic. This is particularly important because procarbazine is commonly used to treat Hodgkin's disease, which predominantly affects young adults.

✦ Inform a woman receiving high dosages of procarbazine that cessation of menses may occur and is drug-related.

✦ Instruct the patient to avoid activities that require alertness if adverse CNS reactions occur.

✦ Teach the patient how to manage troublesome adverse reactions, such as GI distress, stomatitis, and flulike syndrome.

✦ Give the patient written materials about the possible effects of procarbazine for his home reference.

✦ Instruct the patient to notify the prescriber if other adverse reactions occur.

Key nursing actions

✦ Place the patient on a low-tyramine diet to prevent tyramine interactions and hypertension.

✦ Monitor the CBC and platelet count for evidence of leukopenia, thrombocytopenia, or anemia.

✦ Take bleeding precautions when the platelet count falls below 50,000/mm³.

✦ Watch for evidence of CNS toxicity, such as fingertip paresthesia, footdrop, lack of muscle coordination, confusion, and depression.

✦ Monitor the blood pressure regularly to detect impending acute hypertensive episode.

✦ Monitor the patient with leukopenia for signs and symptoms of infection. Also take infection control measures until his WBC count returns to normal.

✦ Take bleeding precautions whenever the patient's platelet count falls below 50,000/mm³. Give platelet transfusions and packed RBCs during times of severe bleeding.

✦ Monitor the patient for signs of CNS toxicity, such as fingertip paresthesia, footdrop, lack of muscle coordination, confusion, and depression. Immediately report these signs and symptoms to the prescriber.

✦ Monitor the patient's blood pressure regularly during procarbazine therapy to detect an impending acute hypertensive episode. If the patient displays a sudden elevation in blood pressure, stop the infusion and notify the prescriber. Keep standard emergency equipment nearby and begin emergency measures to manage hypertensive crisis.

✦ Teach the patient and his family about the prescribed drug. (See *Teaching a patient about procarbazine.*)

TAXANES

Taxane antineoplastics include docetaxel and paclitaxel. These drugs are used to treat metastatic ovarian and breast carcinoma after other chemotherapy has failed.

Pharmacokinetics

After I.V. use, docetaxel has a rapid onset of action. It's excreted primarily through feces.

When given I.V., paclitaxel is highly bound to plasma proteins. It's metabolized primarily in the liver; a small amount is excreted unchanged in urine.

Pharmacodynamics

Docetaxel and paclitaxel exert their chemotherapeutic effects by disrupting the microtubule network essential for mitosis and other vital cellular functions.

Pharmacotherapeutics

Paclitaxel is used when first-line or subsequent chemotherapy has failed in treating metastatic ovarian carcinoma as well as metastatic breast cancer. Both taxanes may also be used to treat head and neck cancer, prostate cancer, and non–small-cell lung cancer.

Interactions

✦ Use of paclitaxel along with carboplatin or cisplatin may cause additive myelosuppression.
✦ Cyclosporine, erythromycin, ketoconazole, or troleandomycin may alter docetaxel metabolism.
✦ Phenytoin may decrease the paclitaxel level and reduce its efficacy.
✦ Dalfopristin or quinupristin may increase the paclitaxel level and the risk of toxicity.

Adverse reactions

Hypersensitivity reactions occur in 30% of patients who receive docetaxel. Other reactions to this drug include fluid retention, leukopenia, neutropenia, thrombocytopenia, alopecia, stomatitis, paresthesia, pain, fatigue, and weakness.

During clinical trials, 25% or more patients experienced these adverse reactions to paclitaxel: bone marrow suppression resulting in neutropenia, leukopenia, thrombocytopenia, or anemia; hypersensitivity reactions; abnormal EEG tracings; peripheral neuropathy; myalgia; arthralgia; nausea, vomiting, and diarrhea; mucositis; and alopecia.

Nursing considerations

✦ Give I.V. paclitaxel through an in-line filter. Prepare and store the drug in glass containers.
✦ Premedicate a patient with corticosteroids, diphenhydramine, or H_2-receptor antagonists to reduce the risk of severe hypersensitivity reactions and fluid retention.
✦ Give an antiemetic to a patient with nausea or vomiting.
✦ Note paclitaxel treatment on EEG request slips because the drug can cause abnormal EEG tracings. If the patient experiences significant cardiac conduction abnormalities while receiving paclitaxel, give appropriate therapy and perform continuous cardiac monitoring during subsequent infusions.
✦ Monitor the patient regularly for adverse reactions and drug interactions during taxane therapy. If any occur, alert the prescriber.
✦ Monitor the patient's CBC and platelet counts for evidence of leukopenia, thrombocytopenia, or anemia. Typically, the nadir of bone marrow suppression occurs about 4 weeks after therapy begins; recovery, at 6 weeks. Because RBCs have a

Features of taxanes
✦ Disrupt the microtubule network essential for mitosis and other vital cell functions
✦ Used to treat head and neck cancer, prostate cancer, and non–small-cell lung cancer
✦ Paclitaxel is used when other chemotherapy has failed to treat metastatic ovarian carcinoma or metastatic breast cancer.

Adverse reactions to watch for

docetaxel
✦ Alopecia
✦ Fatigue, pain, paresthesia, weakness
✦ Fluid retention
✦ Hypersensitivity reactions
✦ Leukopenia, neutropenia, thrombocytopenia
✦ Stomatitis

paclitaxel
✦ Abnormal EEG tracings, peripheral neuropathy
✦ Alopecia
✦ Arthralgia, myalgia
✦ Bone marrow suppression leading to anemia, leukopenia, neutropenia, thrombocytopenia
✦ Diarrhea, mucositis, nausea, vomiting
✦ Hypersensitivity reactions

Teaching a patient about taxanes

Whenever a taxane is prescribed, teach the patient and his family the drug's name, dose, frequency, action, and adverse effects. Also take the following actions.

✦ Stress the importance of returning for follow-up blood tests.

✦ Advise the patient to stagger his activities and take frequent rests if anemia occurs.

✦ Advise the patient with leukopenia to avoid people with active contagious infections, to watch for signs and symptoms of infection, and to report them immediately to the prescriber.

✦ Teach the patient with thrombocytopenia to take bleeding precautions.

✦ Teach the patient how to manage troublesome adverse reactions, such as GI distress.

✦ Give the patient written materials about the possible effects of the taxane for his home reference.

✦ Instruct the patient to notify the prescriber if other adverse reactions occur.

✦ Prepare the patient for alopecia by explaining the timing and speed of hair loss and noting that it may affect the scalp, eyebrows, eyelashes, or other body hair.

✦ Stress the importance of taking premedication before taking the drug to minimize noxious adverse effects.

Key nursing actions

✦ Monitor the CBC and platelet counts for evidence of leukopenia, thrombocytopenia, or anemia.

✦ Take bleeding precautions when the platelet count falls below 50,000/mm³.

longer life than WBCs and platelets, anemia is less of a problem than thrombocytopenia or leukopenia unless the patient has occult or overt blood loss.

✦ Monitor the patient with leukopenia for signs and symptoms of infection, such as fever, sore throat, chills, and malaise. Also take infection control measures until his WBC count returns to normal.

✦ Take bleeding precautions whenever the patient's platelet count falls below 50,000/mm³. Give platelet transfusions and packed RBCs during times of severe bleeding.

✦ Take energy conservation measures for a patient with anemia. For example, stagger his activities, help with tasks, and arrange for frequent rest periods.

✦ Teach the patient and his family about the prescribed drug. (See *Teaching a patient about taxanes.*)

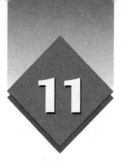

Hematologic drugs

Three types of drugs are used to treat hematologic disorders: hematinics, anticoagulants, and thrombolytics. Hematinics provide essential building blocks for red blood cell (RBC) production. Anticoagulants alter the coagulant properties of the blood. Thrombolytic drugs dissolve *thrombi*, or blood clots.

To comprehend how these drugs produce their effects, you need a clear understanding of hematologic structures and functions.

HEMATOLOGIC SYSTEM

The hematologic system includes *plasma*, the liquid component of blood, and blood cells, including RBCs, white blood cells (WBCs), and platelets. RBCs, or erythrocytes, transport oxygen to tissues. WBCs, or leukocytes, defend the body against invading organisms. Platelets aid in *hemostasis*, or stopping bleeding.

ERYTHROPOIESIS

Through erythropoiesis, RBCs are produced. RBCs are small—about 7 microns in diameter. Shaped like a biconcave disk, the RBC has a large surface area relative to its volume. It can change shape as it moves through narrow blood vessels and can withstand the turbulence in small capillaries. RBCs are the most numerous of the blood's formed elements. Normally, the RBC count is about 5,500,000/mm^3 of blood.

RBCs carry oxygen to cells and exchange it for carbon dioxide. They carry most of these gases in combination with hemoglobin. Each RBC contains 200 to 300 million molecules of hemoglobin. One hemoglobin molecule contains four iron atoms, enabling it to combine with four oxygen molecules to form oxyhemoglobin. The globin is the protein part of the hemoglobin molecule and combines with carbon dioxide to form carbaminohemoglobin.

Drugs used to treat hematologic disorders
◆ Hematinics provide building blocks for RBC production.
◆ Anticoagulants alter the coagulant properties of blood.
◆ Thrombolytic drugs dissolve thrombi.

Reviewing erythropoiesis

✦ Erythropoiesis produces RBCs at variable rates, depending on how many RBCs the body needs.

✦ RBCs are the most numerous of the formed elements in blood.

✦ Shaped like biconcave disks, RBCs carry oxygen to cells and exchange it for carbon dioxide.

✦ Each RBC carries 200 to 300 million hemoglobin molecules.

✦ RBCs are formed from stem cells in the bone marrow and live 105 to 120 days.

✦ To produce RBCs, the bone marrow needs adequate iron, vitamin B_{12}, amino acids, copper, and cobalt.

✦ Anemia results from a significant decrease in RBCs and hemoglobin.

✦ Phagocytes in the spleen and bone marrow destroy RBC fragments through phagocytosis.

✦ During phagocytosis, hemoglobin releases iron, and bilirubin is formed; both are transported to the liver, where iron is stored and bilirubin is excreted in bile.

✦ The bone marrow reuses stored iron to make new RBCs.

RBC maturation occurs in the bone marrow and involves nucleated cells called hemocytoblasts, or stem cells. The stem cells divide by mitosis and evolve through several stages to mature erythrocytes. When an RBC leaves the bone marrow and enters the blood, the cell contains hemoglobin.

The life span of an RBC is 105 to 120 days. After that, it breaks down, usually in the capillaries and in the reticuloendothelial cells in the lining of the hepatic blood vessels. Phagocytes in the spleen and bone marrow envelop and destroy RBC fragments, a process known as *phagocytosis.* During phagocytosis, hemoglobin releases its iron and the pigment bilirubin is formed. The iron and bilirubin are transported to the liver, where the iron is stored and the bilirubin is excreted in bile. Then the bone marrow reuses the stored iron to produce new RBCs. In healthy individuals, the number of RBCs remains constant, with RBCs being produced as they're destroyed.

Erythropoiesis becomes more rapid when more RBCs are needed. For example, cell production increases when RBCs are lost in hemorrhage and when tissue hypoxia occurs. Hemorrhage and hypoxia stimulate the kidneys to produce the hormone erythropoietin, which accelerates RBC production in the bone marrow.

The bone marrow requires adequate supplies of iron, vitamin B_{12}, amino acids, copper, and cobalt to produce RBCs.

Anemia represents a significant decrease in RBC count and hemoglobin. Although many types of anemia exist, the two major types are microcytic anemia, from iron deficiency, and macrocytic anemia, from vitamin B_{12} or folic acid deficiency.

BLOOD COAGULATION

The pathways involved in blood coagulation include the intrinsic (intravascular) and the extrinsic (extravascular) pathways. (See *Understanding coagulation pathways.*) The intrinsic pathway is activated by injury to the endothelial layer of the blood vessel, which disrupts blood flow. This disruption initiates a chain of events that forms a blood clot. Atherosclerotic plaque formation is a condition that activates this type of clotting.

The extrinsic pathway is activated by injury to tissues and vessels, such as surgical wounds or burns, releasing tissue thromboplastin into the circulation. Thromboplastin, a powerful procoagulant, stimulates a chain of events that forms a thrombus.

The body also produces blood clots to repair blood vessel damage caused by normal wear and tear. Platelets adhere to the damaged area and release adenosine diphosphate (ADP), which makes platelets sticky and helps a clot to form. Vasoconstriction in the damaged blood vessel reduces blood flow and produces blood stasis, allowing time for the clot to form.

The body maintains a delicate balance between clot formation (coagulation) and clot destruction (fibrinolysis). Coagulation is inhibited by:

✦ the liver and reticuloendothelial system, which remove clotting factors from the blood

✦ antithrombins, which neutralize thrombin

✦ adequate blood flow, which dilutes clotting factors

✦ the fibrinolytic system, which interferes with the action of thrombin on fibrinogen.

Certain diseases are characterized by abnormal coagulation. Thrombus formation can occur in the venous system, causing venothrombosis (such as a pulmonary

ANATOMY & PHYSIOLOGY

Understanding coagulation pathways

Various factors can affect coagulation through the intrinsic and extrinsic pathways, as illustrated here. A naturally occurring protein, antithrombin III neutralizes thrombin. Heparin increases the thrombin-neutralizing action of antithrombin III, so its effect on coagulation is multiplied. Oral anticoagulants diminish the action of vitamin K, responsible for the formation of factors II, VII, IX, and X in the liver.

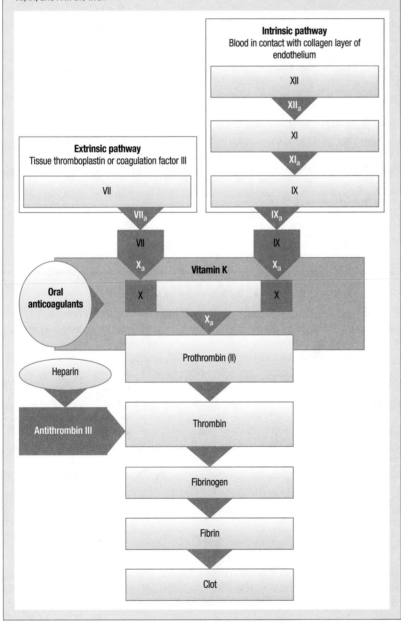

Reviewing coagulation

✦ Blood coagulation occurs via two pathways: intrinsic (intravascular) and extrinsic (extravascular).

✦ The intrinsic pathway is activated by injury to the endothelial layer of a blood vessel.

✦ The extrinsic pathway is activated by injury to tissues and vessels.

✦ The body produces blood clots to repair damage to blood vessels.

✦ A clot forms when platelets adhere to the injured area. They release adenosine phosphate, which increases their tendency to stick together in the clot.

✦ Vasoconstriction at the injured area helps to reduce blood flow, allowing time for the clot to stabilize.

✦ The body maintains a delicate balance between coagulation (clot formation) and fibrinolysis (clot destruction).

✦ Coagulation is inhibited by the liver and reticuloendothelial system, antithrombins, normal blood flow, and the fibrinolytic system.

embolus), or in the arterial system, causing arterial thrombosis (such as a cerebrovascular thrombosis from a diseased mitral valve).

Anticoagulants and antiplatelet drugs are used to treat or prevent thrombotic disorders. These drugs act by inhibiting the formation of thrombin and of factors II, VII, IX, and X (oral anticoagulants) and II, Xa, XIa, and XII (heparin) in the liver or by interfering with platelet aggregation.

FIBRINOLYSIS

Conditions such as blood stagnation or blood vessel damage trigger the coagulation mechanism and activate the fibrinolytic system. The fibrinolytic system restricts clot propagation in the circulation, breaks down blood clots, and removes the fibrin networks as the injured area heals.

When the fibrinolytic system is activated, tissue plasminogen activator (tPA) is released from storage areas in the endothelium. tPA is released during stress reactions, vigorous exercise, hypoglycemia, and anabolic steroid use. tPA binds to fibrin and converts inactive circulating plasminogen to plasmin, the proteolytic enzyme that digests fibrin threads, fibrinogen, prothrombin, and factors V, VIII, and XII. Then plasmin causes clot lysis.

Normally, plasmin is inactivated in the circulation by alpha$_2$ antiplasmin, a physiologic inhibitor that prevents too much circulating plasmin, which can cause blood hypocoagulability. However, plasmin bound to fibrin is resistant to alpha$_2$ antiplasmin. Usually, fibrinolysis is restricted to a thrombus area, which prevents generalized fibrinolysis and bleeding.

Fibrinolysis of a thrombus produces fibrin degradation products (FDPs). FDPs, which normally aren't present in blood, interfere with platelet aggregation and produce an anticoagulant effect.

HEMATINICS

Used to treat anemias, hematinics provide the essential building blocks for RBC production. These drugs do this by increasing hemoglobin, the necessary element for oxygen transportation.

This class of drugs includes iron, vitamin B$_{12}$, folic acid, epoetin alfa, and darbepoetin alfa. Iron, vitamin B$_{12}$, and folic acid are used to treat microcytic (iron-deficient) and macrocytic (megaloblastic) anemia. Microcytic anemia is characterized by small, incompletely hemoglobinated RBCs and results from inadequate dietary intake of iron or excessive blood loss, which may occur with slow, insidious GI bleeding or heavy menstrual bleeding. Macrocytic anemia is characterized by abnormally large RBCs and results from inadequate intake or insufficient GI absorption of vitamin B$_{12}$ or folic acid.

Epoetin alfa and darbepoetin alfa are used to treat normocytic anemia, which is characterized by a decreased number of RBCs and stems from erythropoietin deficiency.

IRON

Oral and parenteral iron supplements are used to treat the most common form of anemia—iron deficiency anemia. They include ferrous fumarate, ferrous gluconate, ferrous sulfate, iron dextran, iron sorbitol, iron sucrose, polysaccharide iron complex, and sodium ferric gluconate complex.

Pharmacokinetics

Iron is absorbed primarily from the duodenum and upper jejunum of the intestine by active transport. The ferrous form is absorbed three times faster than the ferric form. The ferrous salts don't vary in absorption, but do vary in the amount of elemental iron supplied.

The amount of iron absorbed depends partially on the body stores of iron. When body stores are low or RBC production is accelerated, iron absorption may increase by 20% to 30%. On the other hand, when total iron stores are large, only about 5% to 10% of iron is absorbed. Also, enteric-coated preparations decrease iron absorption because they don't release iron until after it leaves the duodenum.

Iron is transported by the blood and bound to transferrin, its carrier plasma protein. About 30% of the iron is stored primarily as hemosiderin or ferritin in the reticuloendothelial cells of the liver, spleen, and bone marrow. About two-thirds of the total body iron is contained in hemoglobin. Iron is excreted in urine, stool, sweat, and through intestinal cell sloughing. It also appears in breast milk.

Pharmacodynamics

Although iron has other roles, its most important role is the production of hemoglobin. About 80% of iron in the plasma goes to the bone marrow, where it's used for erythropoiesis.

Pharmacotherapeutics

Oral iron therapy is used to prevent or treat iron deficiency anemia. It's also used to prevent anemias in children ages 6 months to 2 years because this is a period of rapid growth and development. Pregnant women may need iron supplements to replace the iron used by the developing fetus. Treatment for iron-deficient anemia usually lasts for 6 months.

Parenteral iron therapy is used for patients who can't absorb oral preparations, don't comply with oral therapy, or have bowel disorders (such as ulcerative colitis). Patients who have end-stage renal disease and receive hemodialysis may receive parenteral iron at the end of their dialysis session. Parenteral iron therapy corrects the iron store deficiency quickly; however, the anemia isn't corrected any faster. Two parenteral iron products are available. Iron dextran may be given by I.M. injection or slow continuous I.V. infusion. Iron sucrose, which is indicated for use in hemodialysis patients, is given by I.V. infusion.

Interactions

+ Antacids, cholestyramine, cimetidine, colestipol, or magnesium trisilicate can reduce oral iron absorption.
+ Coffee, tea, eggs, and milk can reduce oral iron absorption.
+ Oral iron may reduce absorption of levothyroxine, methyldopa, penicillamine, quinolones (ciprofloxacin, gatifloxacin, levofloxacin, lomefloxacin, norfloxacin, ofloxacin, moxifloxacin, and sparfloxacin), or tetracyclines (demeclocycline, doxycycline, minocycline, oxytetracycline, and tetracycline).

Adverse reactions

The most common adverse reactions to iron are GI irritation, such as heartburn, anorexia, nausea, vomiting, and constipation or diarrhea. The patient's stools may also appear darker. Liquid oral iron preparations may stain the patient's teeth.

Parenteral forms may cause hypersensitivity reactions. (See *Testing for parenteral iron sensitivity,* page 434.) They may also produce hypotension, seizures, recurrence of arthritis, leukocytosis, headache, backache, dizziness, malaise, transitory paresthesia, and shivering.

Features of iron

+ Is available as oral and parenteral supplements
+ Is used to increase hemoglobin production in iron deficiency anemia
+ Is used mainly for erythropoiesis in bone marrow

Oral therapy

+ Is used to prevent or treat iron deficiency anemia and to prevent anemia in pregnant women and children ages 6 months to 2 years

Parenteral therapy

+ Is used for patients who can't absorb oral forms, don't comply with oral therapy, or have bowel disorders
+ Corrects deficient iron stores quickly, but doesn't correct anemia faster than oral therapy

Adverse reactions to watch for

Oral forms

+ Anorexia, constipation, dark stools, diarrhea, heartburn, nausea, vomiting
+ Stained teeth (with liquid forms)

Parenteral forms

+ Arthritis recurrence
+ Backache, headache
+ Dizziness, hypotension
+ Hypersensitivity reactions
+ Leukocytosis
+ Malaise
+ Seizures, shivering, transitory paresthesia

Key nursing actions

✦ Monitor the patient's iron level regularly and CBC with differential to evaluate the drug's effects.
✦ Watch for acute hypersensitivity reactions, which can be fatal, during parenteral therapy. Keep emergency equipment nearby.
✦ Urge the patient to drink at least eight 8-ounce (240-ml) glasses of fluid daily (unless contraindicated), increase his dietary fiber intake, and exercise regularly to prevent constipation. If constipation occurs, give a laxative.

WARNING

Testing for parenteral iron sensitivity

Parenteral iron can cause acute hypersensitivity reactions, including anaphylaxis, dyspnea, urticaria, other rashes, pruritus, arthralgia, myalgia, fever, sweating, and allergic purpura. To test for drug sensitivity and prevent serious reactions, always give a test dose of iron dextran before beginning therapy.

Carefully assess the patient's response to the test dose. If no adverse reactions occur within 1 hour, give the total dose. If adverse reactions occur, notify the prescriber immediately. To treat anaphylaxis, keep epinephrine and standard emergency equipment readily available.

Nursing considerations

✦ Monitor the patient closely for adverse reactions and drug interactions. Notify the prescriber if any occur.
✦ Regularly monitor the patient's iron level and complete blood count (CBC) with differential to evaluate the drug's effectiveness. Increased iron level and hemoglobin indicate effective therapy; a decreased WBC count indicates leukocytosis, an adverse reaction.

PATIENT TEACHING

Teaching a patient about iron

Whenever an iron preparation is prescribed, teach the patient and his family the drug's name, dose, frequency, action, and adverse effects. Also take the following actions.
✦ Inform the patient of his daily iron requirement.
✦ Help the patient explore possible causes of anemia, such as inadequate diet or excessive menstrual bleeding, to prevent recurrence.
✦ Advise the patient to include iron-rich foods in his diet.
✦ Teach the patient how to prevent accidental iron poisoning in small children.
✦ Teach the patient to take liquid preparations with a straw to prevent tooth stains.
✦ Inform the patient that iron preparations normally darken the stool. However, he should notify the prescriber if bloody stool or abdominal cramping or pain occurs.
✦ Inform the patient receiving I.M. iron that soreness, inflammation, and skin discoloration may occur at the injection site.
✦ Advise the patient not to perform activities that require alertness if dizziness or malaise develops.
✦ Instruct the patient to take an oral iron preparation between meals and 2 hours before or after taking a prescribed antacid.
✦ Tell the patient how to prevent or relieve constipation.
✦ Instruct the patient who develops seizures to withhold the next iron dose and notify the prescriber.
✦ Advise the patient to check with the prescriber before taking any new prescription or over-the-counter drugs.
✦ Instruct the patient to notify the prescriber if adverse reactions occur.

✦ Give oral iron supplements between meals and within at least 2 hours of antacids.

 CLINICAL ALERT **Closely monitor the patient for an acute hypersensitivity reaction to parenteral iron, which can be fatal. Keep standard emergency equipment nearby.**

✦ Infuse I.V. iron at 1 ml/minute. More rapid infusion may cause phlebitis and vessel reddening, or flushing, at the infusion site. Use only single-dose vials for I.V. therapy. Multi-dose vials contain the preservative phenol, which can cause serious adverse reactions.
✦ Administer I.M. iron by the Z-track method to avoid leakage into subcutaneous tissue and to prevent skin discoloration at the injection site. Inject the drug into a muscle mass on the upper outer buttock.
✦ Encourage the patient to drink at least eight 8-ounce (240-ml) glasses of fluid daily (unless contraindicated), increase his fiber intake, and exercise regularly to prevent constipation. If constipation occurs, give a laxative.
✦ Give iron to a patient who refuses transfusions but needs elective surgery.
✦ Teach the patient and his family about the prescribed drug. (See *Teaching a patient about iron*.)

VITAMIN B$_{12}$

Used to treat vitamin B$_{12}$ deficiencies and pernicious anemia, the most common forms of vitamin B$_{12}$ supplements are cyanocobalamin and hydroxocobalamin.

Pharmacokinetics

Vitamin B$_{12}$ is available in oral and injectable forms. A substance called intrinsic factor, secreted by the gastric mucosa, is needed for vitamin B$_{12}$ absorption. Patients with a deficiency of intrinsic factor develop vitamin B$_{12}$-deficiency pernicious anemia. Because patients with this disorder can't absorb vitamin B$_{12}$, an injectable form of the drug is used to treat this type of anemia.

After I.M. or S.C. injection, cyanocobalamin is absorbed and binds to transcobalamin II for transport to the tissues. Then it's transported in the bloodstream to the liver, where 90% of the body's supply of vitamin B$_{12}$ is stored. Although hydroxocobalamin is absorbed more slowly from the injection site, its uptake in the liver may be greater than that of cyanocobalamin.

With either drug, the liver slowly releases vitamin B$_{12}$ as needed by the body. About 3 to 8 mcg of vitamin B$_{12}$ are excreted in bile each day and then reabsorbed in the ileum. Within 48 hours after a vitamin B$_{12}$ injection, 50% to 95% of the dose appears in urine, with the major portion excreted in the first 8 hours. Vitamin B$_{12}$ also appears in breast milk.

Pharmacodynamics

When vitamin B$_{12}$ is given, it replaces vitamin B$_{12}$ that the body normally would absorb from the diet. This vitamin is essential for cell growth and replication and for the maintenance of myelin (nerve coverings) throughout the nervous system. Vitamin B$_{12}$ may also be involved in lipid and carbohydrate metabolism.

Pharmacotherapeutics

Cyanocobalamin and hydroxocobalamin are used to treat pernicious anemia, a megaloblastic anemia characterized by decreased gastric production of hydrochloric acid and the deficiency of *intrinsic factor*, a substance normally secreted by the

Features of vitamin B$_{12}$

✦ Is essential for cell growth and replication and for myelin maintenance throughout the nervous system
✦ May be involved in lipid and carbohydrate metabolism
✦ Is commonly used as cyanocobalamin and hydroxocobalamin supplements
✦ Replaces vitamin B$_{12}$ that normally would be supplied by diet
✦ Is used to treat pernicious anemia, a megaloblastic anemia marked by decreased gastric hydrochloric acid production and deficient intrinsic factor, which is secreted by parietal cells of the gastric mucosa and is essential for vitamin B$_{12}$ absorption

Teaching a patient about vitamin B₁₂

Whenever a vitamin B_{12} preparation is prescribed, teach the patient and his family the drug's name, dose, frequency, action, and adverse effects. Also take the following actions.
- Explain that the patient should start to feel better 24 hours after therapy begins.
- Teach the patient and his family how to give vitamin B_{12} subcutaneously or intramuscularly if long-term therapy is needed.
- Teach the patient how to store the drug properly.
- Stress the importance of regular laboratory testing to monitor the effectiveness of therapy or to detect adverse hematologic reactions.
- Emphasize the importance of compliance with the drug regimen.
- Teach the patient that a well-balanced diet can eliminate vitamin deficiencies.
- Instruct the patient to eat vitamin B_{12}-rich foods, such as meat, seafood, milk, eggs, liver, and legumes.
- Reassure the patient with exanthema that it's transient.
- Reassure the patient with diarrhea that it usually remains mild. Tell him to ask the prescriber for a prescription for an antidiarrheal if needed.
- Instruct the patient to notify the prescriber if adverse reactions occur.

Adverse reactions to watch for

Parenteral therapy
- Heart failure, peripheral vascular thrombosis, pulmonary edema
- Hypersensitivity reactions that could result in anaphylaxis
- Hypokalemia
- Mild diarrhea
- Optic nerve atrophy in patients with hereditary optic nerve atrophy
- Polycythemia vera
- Pruritus, transient exanthema, urticaria
- Swollen feeling throughout the body

Key nursing actions
- Monitor the patient's hematocrit, reticulocyte count, and folate level to determine treatment effectiveness.
- Keep emergency equipment nearby during parenteral therapy in case anaphylaxis develops.

parietal cells of the gastric mucosa that is essential for vitamin B_{12} absorption. Intrinsic factor deficiencies are common in patients who have had total or partial gastrectomies or total ileal resection.

Interactions
- Alcohol, aminosalicylic acid, chloramphenicol, colchicine, or neomycin may decrease oral cyanocobalamin absorption.

Adverse reactions
No dose-related adverse reactions occur with vitamin B_{12} therapy. However, rare reactions may occur when vitamin B_{12} is given parenterally. These include hypersensitivity reactions that could result in anaphylaxis and death; cardiovascular reactions (pulmonary edema, heart failure, and peripheral vascular thrombosis); hematologic reactions (polycythemia vera); hypokalemia; dermatologic reactions (pruritus, transient exanthema, and urticaria); and GI reactions (mild diarrhea). Severe, swift optic nerve atrophy has been reported in patients with hereditary optic nerve atrophy. Some patients report a feeling of swelling throughout the entire body.

Nursing considerations
- Monitor the patient's hematocrit, reticulocyte count, and folate level to determine the effectiveness of therapy. Also, monitor his potassium level to detect hypokalemia.

 CLINICAL ALERT Keep standard emergency equipment readily available during parenteral iron therapy because of the risk that the patient could develop anaphylaxis.

✦ Give I.V. vitamin B_{12} to a patient who can't take vitamin B_{12} orally. Give a higher dosage of cyanocobalamin to a critically ill patient with a neurologic or infectious disease or hyperthyroidism. Because cobalt is an essential element of vitamin B_{12}, give an intradermal test dose to a patient with cobalt hypersensitivity.

✦ Store the parenteral drug in a light-resistant container at room temperature.

✦ Encourage the patient to eat foods rich in vitamin B_{12}, such as meat, seafood, milk, eggs, and liver.

✦ Monitor the patient for adverse reactions or drug interactions. If any occur, notify the prescriber.

✦ Monitor the patient's compliance by reviewing the results of laboratory tests, especially during lifelong therapy.

✦ Stress the importance of monthly B_{12} injections for the patient with pernicious anemia.

✦ If the patient receives long-term therapy with I.M. injections, emphasize the need for treatment because neurologic damage (such as degenerative spinal cord lesions) can occur as early as 3 months after a vitamin B_{12} deficiency develops.

✦ Teach the patient and his family about the prescribed drug. (See *Teaching a patient about vitamin B_{12}.*)

FOLIC ACID

Also known as *folate*, folic acid is used to treat megaloblastic anemia that's caused by folic acid deficiency. Usually, this type of anemia is seen in tropical or nontropical sprue, anemia due to poor nutritional intake, pregnancy, infancy, or childhood.

Pharmacokinetics

After oral or parenteral administration, folic acid is rapidly absorbed in the first third of the small intestine and distributed to all body tissues. Synthetic folic acid is readily absorbed even in patients with malabsorption syndromes. Folic acid is metabolized in the liver. Excess folic acid is primarily excreted unchanged in urine and a small amount is excreted in feces. It also appears in breast milk.

Pharmacodynamics

Folic acid is an essential component for normal RBC production and growth and is required for nucleoprotein synthesis. A folic acid deficiency results in pernicious anemia and low serum and RBC folate levels.

Pharmacotherapeutics

Folic acid is used to treat folic acid deficiency. Pregnant women and patients undergoing treatment for liver disease, hemolytic anemia, alcohol abuse, skin disease, or renal impairment typically need preventive folic acid therapy.

Interactions

✦ Folic acid in large doses may counteract the effectiveness of an anticonvulsant (such as phenytoin), which may lead to seizures.

✦ Aspirin, methotrexate, pentamidine, sulfasalazine, triamterene, or trimethoprim may reduce the effectiveness of folic acid.

✦ Cycloserine, glutethimide, hormonal contraceptives, or isoniazid can interfere with folic acid absorption.

Adverse reactions to watch for

+ Altered sleep patterns, difficulty concentrating, irritability, over-activity
+ Anorexia, nausea

Key nursing actions

+ Assess the effect of therapy, especially in the first 2 weeks.
+ If a patient receives large folic acid doses and an anticonvulsant, take seizure precautions.
+ Watch for recurring megaloblastic anemia if the patient takes a drug that disrupts folic acid absorption.

Features of epoetin alfa and darbepoetin alfa

+ May be given S.C. or I.V.
+ Replace erythropoietin, which forms in the kidneys from hypoxia or anemia, prompts RBC production in bone marrow, and is deficient in normocytic anemia

epoetin alfa
+ Is used for normocytic anemia from chronic renal impairment, for anemia from chemotherapy or zidovudine therapy in patients with human immunodeficiency virus infection, and for anemia before surgery (to reduce the need for blood transfusions)

PATIENT TEACHING

Teaching a patient about folic acid

Whenever a folic acid preparation is prescribed, teach the patient and his family the drug's name, dose, frequency, action, and adverse effects. Also take the following actions.
+ Teach the patient the dietary sources of folate. Instruct him not to overcook vegetables because this may destroy folic acid compounds.
+ Teach the patient to inform all prescribers about folic acid therapy to prevent drug interactions.
+ Advise the patient to notify the prescriber if adverse reactions occur or if signs of megaloblastic anemia recur.

Adverse reactions

Allergic reactions from folic acid are rare, but may include rash, pruritus, and erythema. Folic acid may also cause anorexia, nausea, altered sleep patterns, difficulty with concentration, irritability, and overactivity.

Nursing considerations

+ Monitor the patient closely for adverse reactions and drug interactions. If any occur, notify the prescriber.
+ Monitor the effectiveness of folic acid therapy, particularly during the first 2 weeks.
+ If a patient receives large doses of folic acid during anticonvulsant therapy, take seizure precautions.
+ Monitor the patient closely for recurrence of megaloblastic anemia if he also takes a drug that interferes with folic acid absorption, such as cycloserine, glutethimide, a hormonal contraceptive, or isoniazid.
+ Teach the patient and his family about the prescribed drug. (See *Teaching a patient about folic acid.*)

EPOETIN ALFA AND DARBEPOETIN ALFA

The glycoproteins epoetin alfa and darbepoetin alfa stimulate erythropoiesis. They're used to treat normocytic anemia.

Pharmacokinetics

Epoetin alfa and darbepoetin alfa may be given S.C. or I.V. After S.C. administration, the peak epoetin alfa level occurs in 5 to 24 hours, and the peak darbepoetin alfa level occurs in 24 to 72 hours. The circulating half-life of epoetin alfa is 4 to 13 hours; of darbepoetin alfa, 49 hours. The therapeutic effects of these drugs last for several days after administration.

Pharmacodynamics

Epoetin alfa and darbepoetin alfa are used to replace the endogenous hormone erythropoietin. Normally, erythropoietin is formed in the kidneys in response to hypoxia and anemia and it stimulates RBC production in the bone marrow. Patients with disorders that decrease erythropoietin production develop chronic normocytic anemia, which requires administration of exogenous erythropoietin.

Pharmacotherapeutics

Epoetin alfa is used to treat normocytic anemia (characterized by a decrease in hemoglobin, RBC count, and packed RBC volume) caused by chronic renal impairment. It's also prescribed to treat anemia caused by chemotherapy or by zidovudine therapy in patients with human immunodeficiency virus infection. In addition, it's indicated to reduce the need for blood transfusions in anemic patients who are scheduled to have surgery.

Darbepoetin alfa is used to treat anemia caused by chronic renal impairment or by chemotherapy in patients with non-myeloid malignancies.

Interactions

No interactions have been reported with either drug.

Adverse reactions

Hypertension is the most common adverse reaction to epoetin alfa and darbepoetin alfa. It may occur even in previously hypotensive patients. Other adverse reactions may include seizures, headache, arthralgia, nausea, edema, fatigue, diarrhea, vomiting, chest pain, skin reactions at the administration site, asthenia, and dizziness.

 CLINICAL ALERT Darbepoetin alfa may cause arrhythmias, cardiac arrest, and death. Assess the patient closely during therapy, and keep emergency equipment readily available.

Nursing considerations

✦ Check the patient's blood pressure regularly to detect hypertension. Monitor him closely for other adverse reactions during therapy.
✦ Take seizure precautions and closely monitor the patient's neurologic status because of the risk of seizures, especially during the first 90 days of therapy.
✦ If the patient experiences headache, arthralgia, or chest pain, notify the prescriber. Obtain a prescription, as needed, to relieve the discomfort. If chest pain occurs, obtain an ECG tracing immediately.
✦ Evaluate the patient's hematocrit and hemoglobin regularly to monitor the effectiveness of therapy.
✦ Decrease the dosage when the hematocrit reaches the target range or rises above 4 points in 2 weeks. If the hematocrit doesn't increase by 5 to 6 points after 8 weeks of therapy and remains below the target range of 30% to 33% of blood volume, increase the dosage.
✦ Don't shake the solution. Shaking may inactivate the drug.
✦ If the solution is discolored or contains particles, don't give it.
✦ Give only one dose from the single-use vial. Don't mix the solution with other drugs because it doesn't contain preservatives.
✦ If adverse reactions occur or if therapy is ineffective, notify the prescriber.
✦ Teach the patient and his family about the prescribed drug. (See *Teaching a patient about epoetin alfa and darbepoetin alfa,* page 440.)

(See *Teaching a patient about epoetin alfa and darbepoetin alfa,* page 440.)

Features of epoetin alfa and darbepoetin alfa
(continued)

darbepoetin alfa
✦ Is used for anemia from chronic renal impairment or chemotherapy in patients with non-myeloid malignancies

Adverse reactions to watch for
✦ Arrhythmias, cardiac arrest, chest pain, edema, hypertension
✦ Arthralgia, fatigue
✦ Asthenia, dizziness, headache, seizures
✦ Diarrhea, nausea, vomiting
✦ Skin reactions at the administration site

Key nursing actions
✦ Check the patient's blood pressure regularly to detect hypertension.
✦ Take seizure precautions and closely monitor neurologic status because of the risk of seizures, especially during the first 90 days of therapy.
✦ Evaluate hematocrit and hemoglobin regularly to monitor treatment effectiveness.
✦ Decrease the dosage when hematocrit reaches the target range or rises more than 4 points in 2 weeks. If hematocrit doesn't increase by 5 to 6 points after 8 weeks of therapy and remains below the target range of 30% to 33% of blood volume, increase the dosage.

Teaching a patient about epoetin alfa and darbepoetin alfa

Whenever epoetin alfa or darbepoetin alfa is prescribed, teach the patient and his family the drug's name, dose, frequency, action, and adverse effects. Also take the following actions.
+ Stress the importance of having blood tests to assess the effectiveness of therapy.
+ Inform the patient and his family that seizures may occur, especially during the first 90 days of therapy.
+ Caution the patient not to perform activities that require alertness if dizziness occurs.
+ Advise the patient to have his blood pressure checked regularly.
+ Instruct the patient to notify the prescriber immediately or go to the nearest emergency department if chest pain occurs.
+ Instruct the patient to notify the prescriber if any other adverse reactions occur.

ANTICOAGULANTS

Anticoagulants reduce blood clotting. Major classes of anticoagulants include heparin, low–molecular-weight heparins, oral anticoagulants, oral antiplatelets, I.V. antiplatelets, direct thrombin inhibitors, and factor Xa inhibitors.

HEPARIN

Prepared from animal tissue, heparin is used to prevent clot formation. Because this drug doesn't affect the synthesis of clotting factors, it can't dissolve already-formed clots.

Pharmacokinetics

Because heparin isn't absorbed well from the GI tract, this drug must be given parenterally. Distribution is immediate after I.V. administration, but it isn't as predictable with S.C. injection. The drug is metabolized in the liver, and its metabolites are excreted in urine.

Pharmacodynamics

Heparin prevents the formation of new thrombi. First, it inhibits the formation of thrombin and fibrin by activating antithrombin III. Then antithrombin III inactivates factors IXa, Xa, XIa, and XIIa in the intrinsic and common pathways. This results in prevention of a stable fibrin clot.

In low doses, heparin increases the activity of antithrombin III against factor Xa and thrombin and inhibits clot formation. Much larger doses are needed to inhibit fibrin formation after a clot has been formed. This relationship between dose and effect is the rationale for using low-dose heparin to prevent clotting.

Whole blood clotting time, prothrombin time (PT), and partial thromboplastin time (PTT) are prolonged during heparin therapy. However, these times may be only slightly prolonged with low or ultra-low preventive doses.

Features of heparin

+ Is prepared from animal tissue
+ Doesn't dissolve existing clots because it doesn't affect the synthesis of clotting factors
+ Prevents clot formation by activating antithrombin III, which inactivates factors IXa, Xa, XIa, and XIIa in the intrinsic and common pathways, thus inhibiting formation of thrombin and fibrin
+ Is used for venous thromboemboli caused by inappropriate or excessive intravascular activation of blood clotting, disseminated intravascular coagulation, arterial clotting and embolus formation in patients with atrial fibrillation or flutter, acute myocardial infarction, intra-abdominal surgery or total hip or knee replacement, arterial and cardiac surgery, blood transfusions, extracorporeal circulation, and hemodialysis

Pharmacotherapeutics

Heparin may be used in various clinical situations to prevent the formation of new clots or the extension of existing clots. These situations include:

✦ preventing or treating venous thromboemboli, characterized by inappropriate or excessive intravascular activation of blood clotting

✦ treating disseminated intravascular coagulation, a complication of other diseases that results in accelerated clotting

✦ treating arterial clotting and preventing embolus formation in patients with atrial fibrillation or atrial flutter, arrhythmias in which ineffective atrial contractions cause blood to pool in the atria, increasing the risk of clot formation

✦ inhibiting thrombus formation and promoting cardiac circulation in an acute myocardial infarction (MI) by preventing further clot formation at the site of the already-formed clot

✦ preventing thrombus formation in patients undergoing intra-abdominal surgery or total hip or knee replacement

✦ preventing clot formation in arterial and cardiac surgery, blood transfusions, extracorporeal circulation, and hemodialysis.

Interactions

✦ When used with oral anticoagulants, heparin increases the risk of bleeding and may prolong the PT and International Normalized Ratio (INR), which are used to monitor the effects of oral anticoagulants.

✦ When used with aspirin, clopidogrel, cilostazol, dipyridamole, and nonsteroidal anti-inflammatory drugs (NSAIDs), heparin increases the risk of bleeding.

✦ Antihistamines, cephalosporins, digoxin, neomycin, nicotine, nitroglycerin, penicillins, quinidine, phenothiazines, and tetracyclines may antagonize the effects of heparin.

Adverse reactions

One advantage of heparin is that it produces relatively few adverse reactions, which usually can be prevented if the patient's PTT is maintained within the therapeutic range or 1½ to 2½ times the control. Bleeding, the most common adverse reaction, may lead to more serious consequences if it occurs in the brain (subdural hematoma), at arterial puncture sites, or in or behind the peritoneum (intraperitoneal or retroperitoneal hemorrhage). The effects of heparin can be reversed easily by giving protamine sulfate, which has a specific affinity for heparin and forms a stable salt with it.

Depending on the type of heparin used, the drug may depress the platelet count, resulting in thrombocytopenia. Bovine heparin has a greater tendency than porcine heparin to produce thrombocytopenia.

Because heparin is procured from animal sources, it can produce hypersensitivity reactions. These reactions can produce such signs and symptoms as chills, fever, urticaria, rash, and anaphylaxis, which are reversible with drug stoppage.

If therapy lasts for more than 6 months, alopecia may occur. Long-term therapy may also cause osteoporosis and spontaneous fractures.

Nursing considerations

✦ Monitor the patient closely for bleeding and other adverse reactions or drug interactions.

Possible drug interactions

✦ Antihistamines
✦ Aspirin
✦ Cephalosporins
✦ Cilostazol
✦ Clopidogrel
✦ Digoxin
✦ Dipyridamole
✦ Neomycin
✦ Nicotine
✦ Nitroglycerin
✦ Oral anticoagulants
✦ Penicillins
✦ Quinidine
✦ Tetracyclines

Adverse reactions to watch for

✦ Alopecia (with therapy that lasts more than 6 months)
✦ Bleeding, depressed platelet count, thrombocytopenia
✦ Hypersensitivity reactions (anaphylaxis, chills, fever, rash, urticaria)
✦ Osteoporosis and spontaneous fractures (with long-term therapy)

PATIENT TEACHING

Teaching a patient about heparin

Whenever heparin is prescribed, teach the patient and his family the drug's name, dose, frequency, action, and adverse effects. Also take these actions.

✦ Teach the patient and his family about home care, including how to give the drug properly and detect signs of bleeding.

✦ Help the home care patient schedule necessary partial thromboplastin time (PTT) tests. Keep in mind, however, that these tests may not be needed if the PTT is maintained at the low end of the therapeutic range (1½ times the control).

✦ Advise the patient that he may perform all normal activities of daily living if his platelet count is normal.

✦ Encourage the patient to use an electric razor and a soft toothbrush to avoid the risk of bleeding from cuts or irritated gums.

✦ Advise the patient to avoid all over-the-counter drugs, including aspirin preparations and antihistamines, unless he consults the prescriber or pharmacist first.

✦ Teach the hospitalized patient the signs and symptoms of bleeding and precautions to take after venipuncture.

✦ Reassure the patient with alopecia that hair loss is reversible.

✦ Instruct the patient and family to notify the prescriber immediately if bleeding or other adverse reactions occur.

Key nursing actions

✦ Monitor the patient's partial thromboplastin time.

✦ Observe the patient's vital signs, hemoglobin, and hematocrit for signs of bleeding.

✦ Frequently assess wounds, drainage tubes, and I.V. sites for signs of bleeding. Also observe for purpura.

✦ Check the patient's urine, stool, and vomit for occult blood.

✦ Monitor the patient's PTT. Notify the prescriber if the patient's PTT level exceeds the therapeutic range. Check the PTT and platelet count daily. Porcine heparin lowers the risk of heparin-induced thrombocytopenia.

✦ Observe the patient's vital signs, hemoglobin, and hematocrit for signs of bleeding.

✦ Frequently assess wounds, drainage tubes, and I.V. sites for signs of bleeding. Also observe for purpura, a sign of S.C. bleeding.

✦ Check the patient's urine, stool, and vomit for occult blood.

✦ If the patient develops neurologic dysfunction, a sign of intracranial bleeding, notify the prescriber immediately. Withhold the dose to reduce the severity of intracranial bleeding, bleeding at arterial puncture sites, or bleeding in or behind the peritoneum.

✦ Give S.C. into the anterior abdominal wall fold above the iliac crest and 2″ (5 cm) or more from the umbilicus to avoid the risk of bleeding. To minimize the risk of bleeding, don't aspirate or massage the injection site after giving. Apply gentle pressure to the site for 5 to 10 seconds after the injection.

 CLINICAL ALERT Don't give I.M., and avoid other I.M. injections, if possible. Check the label carefully before administration because the drug is available in different strengths. Keep in mind that it's prescribed in units rather than in milligrams.

✦ Give a trial dose of 1,000 units to a patient with a history of allergies. During the trial, observe the patient for signs of hypersensitivity.

✦ To prevent a drug interaction, check with the pharmacist before mixing any other drug with an infusion.

✦ Don't freeze or refrigerate; the drug is stable at room temperature.

✦ Inspect all vials for particles or discoloration. If either is present, discard the vial.

✦ Keep the antidote protamine sulfate readily available in case severe bleeding occurs.

✦ Teach the patient and his family about the prescribed drug. (See *Teaching a patient about heparin.*)

LOW–MOLECULAR-WEIGHT HEPARINS

Like heparin, low–molecular-weight heparins are used to treat and prevent clot formation. These drugs are obtained by depolymerization of unfractionated heparin. Their advantages are that they can be given S.C. and that they require limited monitoring.

Low–molecular-weight heparins available in the United States include dalteparin, enoxaparin, and tinzaparin.

Pharmacokinetics

After S.C. administration, dalteparin is about 90% available. It's excreted in urine. Enoxaparin is absorbed rapidly and almost completely and is nearly 90% bioavailable. It's metabolized in the liver and excreted primarily by the kidneys. Tinzaparin's volume of distribution is similar to that of blood volume, which suggests that its distribution is limited to the central compartment. Tinzaparin is partially metabolized and is eliminated by the kidneys.

Because low–molecular-weight heparins have a prolonged half-life, they can be given once or twice daily by S.C. injection.

Pharmacodynamics

Dalteparin works by enhancing the inhibition of factor Xa and thrombin by antithrombin.

Enoxaparin accelerates the formation of antithrombin III-thrombin complex and deactivates thrombin, preventing the conversion of fibrinogen to fibrin. It has a higher antifactor Xa-to-antifactor IIa activity ratio.

Tinzaparin inhibits reactions that lead to blood clotting, including the formation of fibrin clots. It also acts as a potent coinhibitor of several activated coagulation factors, especially factors Xa and IIa (thrombin). The drug binds with antithrombin, which increases its ability to inactivate the coagulation enzymes factor Xa and thrombin. It also induces the release of tissue factor pathway inhibitor, which may contribute to its antithrombotic effect.

Pharmacotherapeutics

Dalteparin is used to prevent ischemic complications in unstable angina and non–Q wave MI. It's also indicated for the prevention of deep vein thrombosis (DVT) and pulmonary embolism in patients undergoing hip replacement surgery or patients undergoing abdominal surgery who are at risk for thromboembolic complications.

Indications for enoxaparin include the prevention of pulmonary embolism and DVT after hip or knee replacement or abdominal surgery, prevention of ischemic complications of unstable angina and non–Q-wave MI, and reduction of the risk of embolism because of decreased mobility in patients with acute illness. It's also used to treat acute DVT with or without pulmonary embolism.

Tinzaparin is used to treat symptomatic DVT with or without pulmonary embolism.

WARNING

Precautions for low–molecular-weight heparins

Use low–molecular-weight heparins with extreme caution in patients who have had epidural spinal anesthesia or spinal puncture. These patients are at risk for developing epidural or spinal hematoma that can result in long-term paralysis. This risk increases with the use of epidural catheters, drugs that affect hemostasis, and traumatic or repeated epidural or spinal punctures. For such patients, frequently monitor for signs and symptoms of neurologic impairment. If you detect any, notify the prescriber and provide immediate treatment.

Also use low–molecular-weight heparins with extreme caution in patients with a history of heparin-induced thrombocytopenia, aneurysms, cerebrovascular hemorrhage, spinal or epidural punctures (as with anesthesia), uncontrolled hypertension, or threatened abortion.

Use these drugs cautiously in geriatric patients and in those with conditions that place them at increased risk for hemorrhage, such as bacterial endocarditis, congenital or acquired bleeding disorders, ulcer disease, angiodysplastic GI disease, hemorrhagic stroke, or recent spinal, eye, or brain surgery. Also use them cautiously in patients with regional or lumbar block anesthesia, blood dyscrasias, recent childbirth, pericarditis or pericardial effusion, renal insufficiency, or severe central nervous system trauma.

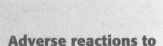

Adverse reactions to watch for

+ Anemia, fever, nausea (with enoxaparin)
+ Injection site hematoma (with dalteparin and tinzaparin)

Key nursing actions

+ Don't interchange a low-molecular-weight heparin with unfractionated heparin or another low–molecular-weight heparin. Units and dosages differ greatly.
+ Have the patient assume a sitting or supine position for dalteparin administration.
+ Obtain routine CBC and fecal occult blood tests periodically during therapy. Dalteparin or enoxaparin therapy doesn't require regular PT or PTT monitoring.
+ Monitor the patient closely for evidence of thrombocytopenia.
+ Be alert for allergic reactions to tinzaparin.

Interactions

+ When used with antiplatelets, oral anticoagulants, or thrombolytics, a low–molecular-weight heparin increases the risk of bleeding.

Adverse reactions

With low–molecular-weight heparins, the risk of bleeding complications is low. The most common adverse reaction to dalteparin and tinzaparin is injection site hematoma. Common reactions to enoxaparin are fever, nausea, and anemia.

Nursing considerations

+ Take an accurate patient history because certain conditions require cautious drug use. (See *Precautions for low–molecular-weight heparins*.)

 CLINICAL ALERT Don't interchange a low–molecular-weight heparin with unfractionated heparin or another low–molecular-weight heparin. Their units and dosages differ significantly.

+ Have the patient assume a sitting or supine position for dalteparin administration. Give the S.C. injection deeply into the U-shaped area around the navel, upper outer side of the thigh, or upper outer quadrangle of a buttock. Rotate sites daily. When injecting into the area around the navel or thigh, use your thumb and forefinger to lift up a skin fold. Insert the entire length of needle at a 45- to 90-degree angle.
+ Never give these drugs I.M.
+ Don't mix the drug with other injections or infusions unless specific compatibility data support such mixing.
+ Obtain routine CBC and fecal occult blood tests periodically during therapy. A patient who takes dalteparin or enoxaparin doesn't need regular PT or PTT monitoring.

+ Monitor the patient closely for signs and symptoms of thrombocytopenia.
+ If a thromboembolic event occurs despite prophylaxis, stop the drug.
+ Avoid using enoxaparin to prevent thrombi in a patient with prosthetic heart valves because he may be at higher risk for thromboembolism.
+ For a patient who also receives warfarin, draw blood for PT and INR just before the next scheduled tinzaparin dose because this drug can affect those values.

 CLINICAL ALERT Be alert for allergic reactions to tinzaparin. This low–molecular-weight heparin contains sodium metabisulfite, which may cause allergic reactions in susceptible people.

+ Teach the patient and his family about the prescribed drug. (See *Teaching a patient about low–molecular-weight heparins.*)

ORAL ANTICOAGULANTS

In the United States, the main oral anticoagulant used is warfarin.

Pharmacokinetics

After oral administration, warfarin is absorbed rapidly and almost completely. It's extensively bound to plasma proteins, mainly albumin. It's metabolized in the liver and excreted in urine. Although warfarin is absorbed quickly, it takes about 48 hours to produce effects and may take 3 to 4 days to achieve its full effect. This is because warfarin antagonizes the production of vitamin K-dependent clotting factors. Before warfarin can exhibit its full effect, the circulating vitamin K clotting factors must be exhausted.

Pharmacodynamics

Oral anticoagulants alter the liver's ability to synthesize vitamin K-dependent clotting factors, including prothrombin and factors VII, IX, and X. However, clotting factors already in the bloodstream continue to coagulate blood until they're depleted, so anticoagulation doesn't begin immediately.

Key nursing actions (*continued*)

+ Monitor the patient closely for evidence of thrombocytopenia.
+ Be alert for allergic reactions to tinzaparin.

Features of warfarin

+ Alters the liver's ability to synthesize vitamin K-dependent clotting factors, including prothrombin and factors VII, IX, and X
+ Produces anticoagulation after 2 to 4 days because existing clotting factors keep coagulating blood until they're depleted
+ Is the drug of choice to prevent DVT and clot formation in patients with prosthetic heart valves or diseased mitral valves
+ Is usually started for thromboembolism while the patient is receiving heparin (except outpatients at high risk for thromboembolism)
+ Is sometimes used with antiplatelet drugs, such as aspirin or clopidogrel

Pharmacotherapeutics

When prescribed to treat thromboembolism, oral anticoagulants usually are started while the patient is still receiving heparin. Warfarin, however, may be started without heparin in outpatients at high risk for thromboembolism.

Warfarin is the drug of choice to prevent DVT and clot formation in patients with prosthetic heart valves or diseased mitral valves. In some instances, warfarin is used with antiplatelet drugs, such as aspirin or clopidogrel.

Interactions

Because warfarin is highly plasma protein-bound and metabolized by the liver, the use of other drugs may alter the amount of warfarin in the body. This may increase the risk of bleeding or clotting, depending on which drug is used.

✦ A diet that's high in vitamin K reduces the effectiveness of oral anticoagulants.

✦ Use of phenytoin with oral anticoagulants may increase or decrease the effects of oral anticoagulants and can increase the risk of phenytoin toxicity.

✦ Together, chronic alcohol abuse and oral anticoagulant use increase the risk of clotting.

✦ Together, acute alcohol intoxication and oral anticoagulant use increase the risk of bleeding.

✦ When taken with oral anticoagulants, the following drugs can increase the risk of bleeding: allopurinol, an anabolic or androgenic steroid, chloral hydrate, chloramphenicol, cimetidine, clofibrate, cotrimoxazole, dextrothyroxine, disulfiram, erythromycin, gemfibrozil, heparin, indomethacin, influenza vaccine, meclofenamate, mefenamic acid, metronidazole, miconazole, nalidixic acid, phenylbutazone, piroxicam, salicylates, sulfinpyrazone, sulindac, and thyroid hormones.

✦ When taken with oral anticoagulants, these drugs can increase the risk of blood clotting, including aminoglutethimide, barbiturates, carbamazepine, cholestyramine, colestipol, corticotropin, glutethimide, mercaptopurine, methimazole, propylthiouracil, rifampin, spironolactone, or vitamin K.

Adverse reactions

The primary adverse reaction to warfarin is minor bleeding. Severe bleeding, however, may occur in the GI tract, urinary tract, or uterus. It can also occur as intraperitoneal hemorrhage from a ruptured corpus luteum, retroperitoneal hemorrhage, hemopericardium, intracranial hemorrhage, or adrenal hemorrhage. Ecchymoses and hematomas may form at arterial puncture sites (for example, after a blood gas sample is drawn).

Red-orange urine, nausea, vomiting, diarrhea, abdominal cramping, priapism, mouth ulcers, and nephropathy rarely may occur. Other rare adverse reactions to oral anticoagulants include alopecia, urticaria, dermatitis, skin necrosis, hepatitis, jaundice, fever, hypersensitivity reactions, agranulocytosis, leukopenia, and eosinophilia.

The effects of oral anticoagulants can be reversed with adequate doses of phytonadione (vitamin K_1).

Nursing considerations

✦ Closely monitor the patient — especially a geriatric patient — for bleeding and other adverse reactions. If any occur, notify the prescriber.

✦ Monitor an inpatient's PT daily or outpatient's PT every 1 to 4 weeks. Be aware that bleeding can occur even when a patient's PT falls within the therapeutic range.

Adverse reactions to watch for

✦ Abdominal cramping, diarrhea, mouth ulcers, nausea, vomiting
✦ Adrenal, intracranial, intraperitoneal, or retroperitoneal hemorrhage
✦ Agranulocytosis, eosinophilia, leukopenia
✦ Alopecia, dermatitis, skin necrosis, urticaria
✦ Ecchymoses, hematomas at arterial puncture sites
✦ Fever, hypersensitivity reactions
✦ Hemopericardium
✦ Hepatitis, jaundice
✦ Minor bleeding
✦ Nephropathy, red-orange urine
✦ Priapism
✦ Severe bleeding in the GI tract, urinary tract, or uterus

A patient with prosthetic heart valves, recurrent embolism, or rheumatic mitral valve disease will have an elevated PT ratio of 1.5 to 2.
✦ Reevaluate the patient's PT to detect interactions whenever a drug is added to or removed from the therapeutic regimen. Notify the prescriber if interactions occur. A patient who takes oral anticoagulants may receive other drugs, which can lead to serious interactions.
✦ Check and record the PT results before giving an oral anticoagulant dose. When a patient is switched from heparin to warfarin therapy, continue heparin therapy for several days until warfarin produces its therapeutic effects.
✦ If the patient's PT or INR exceeds the therapeutic range, notify the prescriber immediately and withhold the next dose.
✦ Monitor the patient's vital signs frequently to detect indications of severe internal bleeding.
✦ Treat minor bleeding by omitting one or more doses until the PT or INR returns to the therapeutic range. If minor bleeding continues, give vitamin K_1 (phytonadione).
✦ Give fresh frozen plasma or give commercial factor IX complex, if severe bleeding occurs.
✦ Teach the patient and his family about the prescribed drug. (See *Teaching a patient about oral anticoagulants.*)

Key nursing actions
✦ Closely monitor the patient — especially a geriatric patient — for bleeding and other adverse reactions.
✦ Monitor an inpatient's PT daily or an outpatient's PT every 1 to 4 weeks.
✦ Reevaluate PT whenever a drug is added to or removed from the regimen.
✦ Document PT results before giving a dose.
✦ Check vital signs frequently to detect severe internal bleeding.
✦ Treat minor bleeding by omitting one or more doses until PT or INR returns to the therapeutic range. If minor bleeding continues, give vitamin K_1.
✦ Give fresh frozen plasma or commercial factor IX complex if severe bleeding occurs.

ORAL ANTIPLATELET DRUGS

Antiplatelet drugs are used to prevent arterial thromboembolism, particularly in patients at risk for MI, stroke, and arteriosclerosis (hardening of the arteries).

Aspirin, clopidogrel, dipyridamole, sulfinpyrazone, and ticlopidine are examples of oral antiplatelet drugs.

Pharmacokinetics

After oral administration, antiplatelet drugs are absorbed very quickly, and reach peak concentration in 1 to 2 hours. They're distributed widely into most body tissues and fluids and metabolized in the liver. Aspirin and sulfinpyrazone are excreted in urine. Clopidogrel and ticlopidine are excreted in urine and feces. Dipyridamole is primarily eliminated via biliary excretion and to a lesser degree by fecal and urinary excretion.

Aspirin maintains its antiplatelet effects for about 10 days, or as long as platelets normally survive. The effects of clopidogrel generally last for about 5 days. Sulfinpyrazone may require several days of administration.

Pharmacodynamics

Antiplatelet drugs interfere with platelet activity in drug-specific and dose-related ways. In low dosages, aspirin appears to inhibit clot formation by blocking the synthesis of prostaglandin. This, in turn, prevents formation of the platelet-aggregating substance thromboxane A_2.

Clopidogrel works by inhibiting the ADP-induced platelet-fibrinogen binding and, therefore, platelet aggregation.

Dipyridamole may inhibit platelet aggregation.

Sulfinpyrazone appears to inhibit several platelet functions. At dosages of 400 to 800 mg daily, it lengthens platelet survival; dosages of more than 600 mg daily prolong the patency of arteriovenous shunts used for hemodialysis. A single dose rapidly inhibits platelet aggregation.

Ticlopidine inhibits the binding of fibrinogen to platelets during the first stage of the clotting cascade.

Pharmacotherapeutics

Antiplatelet drugs have many different uses. Aspirin is used in patients with a previous MI or unstable angina to reduce the risk of death, and to reduce the risk of transient ischemic attacks (TIAs), which temporarily reduce circulation to the brain.

Clopidogrel is used to reduce the risk of an ischemic stroke or vascular death in patients with a history of a recent MI, stroke, or established peripheral artery disease. This drug is also used to treat acute coronary syndromes, especially in patients who undergo percutaneous transluminal coronary angioplasty (PTCA) or coronary artery bypass graft (CABG) surgery.

Dipyridamole is used with warfarin or another coumarin compound to prevent thrombus formation after cardiac valve replacement. Dipyridamole may be used with aspirin to prevent thromboembolic disorders in patients who have CABG surgery or prosthetic heart valves.

After an MI, sulfinpyrazone may be used to decrease the risk of sudden cardiac death. In patients with mitral stenosis caused by rheumatic fever, it may decrease the risk of systemic embolism.

Ticlopidine is used to reduce the risk of thrombotic stroke in high-risk patients (including those with a history of frequent TIAs) and in patients who have already had a thrombotic stroke.

Interactions

✦ When used with heparin, dipyridamole, and oral anticoagulants, aspirin increases the risk of bleeding.
✦ Aspirin increases the risk of toxicity of methotrexate and valproic acid.
✦ Aspirin and ticlopidine may reduce sulfinpyrazone's effectiveness in relieving the signs and symptoms of gout.
✦ When used with aspirin and NSAIDs, clopidogrel may increase the risk of GI bleeding.
✦ When used with aspirin and oral anticoagulants, sulfinpyrazone increases the risk of bleeding.
✦ An antacid may reduce the ticlopidine level.
✦ Cimetidine can increase the risk of ticlopidine toxicity and bleeding.

Adverse reactions

In the dosage prescribed to prevent arterial clotting, aspirin most commonly produces adverse GI reactions, such as stomach pain, heartburn, nausea, constipation, hematemesis, melena, and slight gastric blood loss. Rarely, it may cause significant GI bleeding or peptic ulcer disease.

Clopidogrel may produce headache, skin ulceration, arthralgia, flulike symptoms, and upper respiratory tract infection.

Although usually well tolerated, dipyridamole can produce minimal adverse reactions that may include headache, dizziness, nausea, flushing, weakness, syncope, and mild GI distress. These disappear when the drug is stopped.

The major adverse reaction to sulfinpyrazone is epigastric discomfort, which may aggravate or reactivate peptic ulcer disease. Taking the drug with food, milk, or antacids usually reduces this discomfort.

During clinical trials with ticlopidine, 5% or more of adults displayed these adverse reactions: diarrhea, nausea, dyspepsia, rash, and elevated alkaline phosphatase and transaminase levels on liver function tests. About 2.4% of patients experiences neutropenia.

 CLINICAL ALERT With antiplatelet drugs, hypersensitivity reactions — particularly anaphylaxis — can occur. The most common reaction is bronchospasm with asthmalike symptoms. Dipyridamole may cause a rash. Other reactions to sulfinpyrazone may include rash, blood dyscrasias (anemia, leukopenia, agranulocytosis, thrombocytopenia, or aplastic anemia), and bronchoconstriction. Some patients have experienced renal dysfunction during sulfinpyrazone therapy, which disappears when the drug is stopped.

Nursing considerations

✦ Monitor the patient closely for adverse reactions and drug interactions throughout antiplatelet therapy.
✦ Monitor the patient for signs and symptoms of GI distress, such as stomach pain, heartburn, nausea, constipation, hematemesis, melena, and gastric blood loss (with aspirin); nausea (with dipyridamole); epigastric distress (with sulfinpyrazone); and diarrhea, nausea, and dyspepsia (with ticlopidine).
✦ Give aspirin and sulfinpyrazone with milk, food, or an antacid to minimize GI distress. If distress persists during aspirin therapy, use enteric-coated tablets.

Teaching a patient about oral antiplatelet drugs

Whenever an oral antiplatelet drug is prescribed, teach the patient and his family the drug's name, dose, frequency, action, and adverse effects. Also take the following actions.

✦ Instruct the patient taking aspirin or sulfinpyrazone to take it with milk, food, or an antacid and to report any severe gastric pain to the prescriber. Also tell the patient to take enteric-coated tablets as prescribed.

✦ Instruct the patient not to take aspirin if it has a strong vinegar-like odor but to purchase new tablets.

✦ Advise the patient to take dipyridamole 1 hour before meals with 8 oz (240 ml) of water.

✦ Instruct the patient to take ticlopidine with food or immediately after eating but never to take it with an antacid.

✦ Teach the patient taking ticlopidine to report any signs of infection, such as fever, chills, and sore throat, as well as severe or persistent diarrhea, yellow skin or sclera, dark urine, or light-colored stools.

✦ Stress the importance of returning for laboratory tests to monitor the effectiveness of therapy or to detect adverse reactions.

✦ Teach the patient and his family to recognize the signs and symptoms of bleeding and to report them to the prescriber.

✦ Instruct the patient taking aspirin to consult the prescriber before taking additional over-the-counter products that contain aspirin.

✦ Teach the patient to avoid participating in sports that pose a high risk of injury, which could lead to bleeding.

✦ Instruct the patient taking large doses of aspirin to recognize and report signs of salicylism (aspirin toxicity), such as ringing in the ears, nausea, and vomiting.

✦ Advise the patient not to perform activities that require alertness if dizziness, weakness, or syncope occurs.

✦ Instruct the patient to notify the prescriber immediately if adverse reactions occur.

Key nursing actions

✦ Monitor for evidence of GI distress, such as stomach pain, heartburn, nausea, constipation, hematemesis, melena, and gastric blood loss (with aspirin); nausea (with dipyridamole); epigastric distress (with sulfinpyrazone); and diarrhea, nausea, and dyspepsia (with ticlopidine).

✦ Give aspirin and sulfinpyrazone with milk, food, or an antacid to minimize GI distress.

✦ Monitor bleeding time and platelet aggregation to assess antiplatelet therapy effectiveness.

✦ Obtain a CBC with differential every 2 weeks from the second week of ticlopidine therapy through the end of the third month.

✦ Regularly auscultate breath sounds and assess respiratory rate and pattern.

✦ Watch for bronchospasm, asthmalike symptoms, or bronchoconstriction in a patient receiving aspirin or dipyridamole.

✦ Don't give aspirin if it has a strong vinegar-like odor, which indicates drug deterioration.

✦ Give dipyridamole 1 hour before meals with 8 oz (240 ml) of water.

✦ Give ticlopidine with food or immediately after eating to minimize adverse GI reactions. Don't give the drug with an antacid because it can reduce the ticlopidine level.

✦ Because guidelines haven't been established for using ticlopidine with heparin, oral anticoagulants, aspirin, or fibrinolytics, stop these drugs before ticlopidine therapy begins.

✦ Monitor the patient's bleeding time and platelet aggregation test results to assess the effectiveness of antiplatelet therapy.

✦ Obtain a CBC with differential every 2 weeks from the second week of ticlopidine therapy through the end of the third month.

✦ Auscultate the patient's breath sounds regularly, and assess for changes in his respiratory rate or pattern.

✦ Observe for bronchospasm, asthmalike symptoms, or bronchoconstriction in a patient receiving aspirin or dipyridamole. If breathing difficulty occurs, place the patient in a high Fowler's position to maximize breathing effectiveness. Give oxygen and drugs to relieve the respiratory symptoms of a hypersensitivity reaction.

✦ If adverse reactions or drug interactions occur or if antiplatelet therapy is ineffective, notify the prescriber.
✦ Teach the patient and his family about the prescribed drug. (See *Teaching a patient about oral antiplatelet drugs.*)

I.V. ANTIPLATELET DRUGS

I.V. antiplatelet drugs include abciximab, eptifibatide, and tirofiban.

Pharmacokinetics

After I.V. administration, abciximab, eptifibatide, and tirofiban are quickly distributed throughout the body. They're minimally metabolized and excreted unchanged in urine. These drugs immediately produce effects that last for about 48 hours for abciximab, or 4 to 6 hours for eptifibatide and tirofiban.

Geriatric patients and patients with renal impairment may have decreased clearance of these drugs, which prolongs the antiplatelet effects.

Pharmacodynamics

These drugs block platelet function by inhibiting the glycoprotein IIa/IIIb receptor, which is the major receptor involved in platelet aggregation.

Pharmacotherapeutics

Abciximab is used as an adjunct to PTCA or atherectomy for preventing acute cardiac ischemic complications in patients at high risk for abrupt closure of the treated coronary vessel. It's also used to treat unstable angina that doesn't respond to conventional drugs in patients scheduled for percutaneous coronary intervention within 24 hours.

Eptifibatide is indicated to treat acute coronary syndrome and to reduce ischemic complications in patients undergoing percutaneous coronary intervention.

Tirofiban is prescribed to treat acute coronary syndrome.

Interactions

✦ Use of I.V. antiplatelet drugs with heparin, NSAIDs, oral anticoagulants, other antiplatelet drugs, and thrombolytics increases the risk of bleeding.
✦ Levothyroxine and omeprazole can increase tirofiban clearance.

Adverse reactions

All I.V. antiplatelet drugs can cause serious bleeding and thrombocytopenia. They also may cause anaphylaxis in some patients. Abciximab can also produce hypotension.

Nursing considerations

✦ Use I.V. antiplatelet drugs with caution in a patient at increased risk for bleeding.
✦ Review and monitor the use of other drugs with antiplatelet drugs, which are intended for use with aspirin and heparin.

 CLINICAL ALERT For a patient receiving I.V. antiplatelet drugs, keep epinephrine, dopamine, theophylline, antihistamines, and corticosteroids readily available in case anaphylaxis occurs.

Features of I.V. antiplatelet drugs

✦ Block platelet function by inhibiting the glycoprotein IIa/IIIb receptor (the major receptor involved in platelet aggregation)

abciximab
✦ Is used as an adjunct to percutaneous transluminal coronary angioplasty or atherectomy to prevent acute cardiac ischemic complications in patients at high risk for abrupt closure of the treated coronary vessel
✦ Is also used to treat unstable angina that doesn't respond to conventional drugs in patients scheduled for percutaneous coronary intervention within 24 hours

eptifibatide
✦ Is used to treat acute coronary syndrome and to reduce ischemic complications in patients undergoing percutaneous coronary intervention

tirofiban
✦ Is used to treat acute coronary syndrome

Adverse reactions to watch for

✦ Anaphylaxis
✦ Hypotension (with abciximab)
✦ Serious bleeding
✦ Thrombocytopenia

Key nursing actions

+ Closely monitor for bleeding at the arterial access site used for cardiac catheterization and for GI tract, genitourinary tract, or retroperitoneal bleeding.
+ Take bleeding precautions.
+ Monitor platelet count, hemoglobin, and hematocrit.
+ Stop the drug and give platelets to manage severe bleeding or thrombocytopenia.

Features of direct thrombin inhibitors

argatroban
+ Reversibly binds to a thrombin-active site and inhibits thrombin-catalyzed or thrombin-induced reactions, including fibrin formation; coagulation factor V, VIII, and XIII activation; protein C activation; and platelet aggregation
+ Can inhibit the action of free and clot-related thrombin
+ Is used to prevent or treat thrombosis in patients with heparin-induced thrombocytopenia
+ Is also used for anticoagulation in patients with or at risk for heparin-induced thrombocytopenia during percutaneous coronary intervention

bivalirudin
+ Binds specifically and rapidly to thrombin to produce anticoagulant effects
+ Is used to treat unstable angina in patients undergoing PTCA

+ Closely monitor the patient for bleeding at the arterial access site used for cardiac catheterization and for internal bleeding in the GI or genitourinary tract or retroperitoneal area.
+ Take bleeding precautions. Keep the patient on bed rest for 6 to 8 hours after sheath removal or completion of the drug infusion, whichever is later. Minimize or avoid arterial and venous punctures; I.M. injections; use of urinary catheters, nasogastric tubes, or automatic blood pressure cuffs; and nasotracheal intubation.
+ Monitor the patient's platelet count, hemoglobin, and hematocrit.
+ Stop the drug and give platelets to manage severe bleeding or thrombocytopenia.
+ Teach the patient and his family about the prescribed drug. (See *Teaching a patient about I.V. antiplatelet drugs.*)

DIRECT THROMBIN INHIBITORS

Direct thrombin inhibitors include the drugs argatroban and bivalirudin.

Pharmacokinetics

After I.V. infusion, argatroban is distributed mainly in the extracellular fluid and excreted primarily in feces. Bivalirudin is cleared from the plasma by renal mechanisms and proteolytic cleavage.

Pharmacodynamics

Argatroban reversibly binds to the thrombin-active site and inhibits thrombin-catalyzed or thrombin-induced reactions, including fibrin formation; coagulation factor V, VIII, and XIII activation; protein C activation; and platelet aggregation. Argatroban can inhibit the action of free and clot-related thrombin.

Bivalirudin binds specifically and rapidly to thrombin to produce its anticoagulant effects.

Pharmacotherapeutics

Argatroban is used to prevent or treat thrombosis in patients with heparin-induced thrombocytopenia. It's also indicated for anticoagulation in patients with or at risk for heparin-induced thrombocytopenia during percutaneous coronary intervention.

Bivalirudin is prescribed to treat unstable angina in patients undergoing PTCA.

Interactions
✦ When used with antiplatelet drugs, oral anticoagulants, heparin, and thrombolytics, a direct thrombin inhibitor can increase the risk of bleeding.

Adverse reactions
Bleeding is a rare but serious reaction to direct thrombin inhibitors. Bivalirudin may also cause headache, pain, or back pain.

Nursing considerations
✦ Use direct thrombin inhibitors cautiously in patients at risk for bleeding and those with hepatic disease or a condition that increases the risk of hemorrhage, such as severe hypertension.
✦ Stop all parenteral anticoagulants before giving a direct thrombin inhibitor. Giving argatroban or bivalirudin with antiplatelet drugs, oral anticoagulants, heparin, and thrombolytics may increase the risk of bleeding.
✦ Obtain the results of coagulation tests, platelet count, hemoglobin, and hematocrit before therapy begins. Report any abnormalities to the prescriber.
✦ Teach the patient and his family about the prescribed drug. (See *Teaching a patient about direct thrombin inhibitors.*)

FACTOR XA INHIBITORS
Factor Xa inhibitors are used to prevent DVT in patients undergoing total hip and knee replacement surgery or hip fracture surgery. In the United States, the only available drug in this class is fondaparinux.

Adverse reactions to watch for
✦ Back pain, headache, pain (with bivalirudin)
✦ Bleeding

Key nursing actions
✦ Use direct thrombin inhibitors cautiously in patients at risk for bleeding and those with hepatic disease or a condition that increases the risk of hemorrhage, such as severe hypertension.
✦ Review coagulation tests, platelet count, hemoglobin, and hematocrit before therapy begins. Report abnormalities to the prescriber.

Features of fondaparinux

+ Binds to antithrombin III and potentiates, by about 300 times, the natural neutralization of factor Xa by antithrombin III
+ Interrupts the coagulation cascade, which inhibits formation of thrombin and blood clots
+ Is used only to prevent DVT in patients undergoing total hip and knee replacement surgery and surgery for hip fracture

Adverse reactions to watch for

+ Anemia, bleeding
+ Constipation, nausea
+ Edema
+ Fever
+ Rash

Key nursing actions

+ To avoid drug loss, don't expel any air bubble from the prefilled syringe.
+ Periodically monitor the patient's renal function.
+ Routinely assess for evidence of bleeding. Regularly monitor CBC, platelet count, creatinine level, and fecal occult blood test results.
+ Be aware that anticoagulant effects may last for 2 to 4 days after stopping the drug in a patient with normal renal function.

Pharmacokinetics

With S.C. administration, fondaparinux is absorbed rapidly and completely. It's distributed mainly in blood and excreted primarily unchanged in urine. Within 2 hours of administration, the drug produces its peak effect, which lasts for 17 to 24 hours.

Pharmacodynamics

Fondaparinux binds to antithrombin III and potentiates , by about 300 times, the natural neutralization of factor Xa by antithrombin III. Neutralization of factor Xa interrupts the coagulation cascade, which inhibits formation of thrombin and blood clots.

Pharmacotherapeutics

Currently, fondaparinux is indicated only in the prophylaxis of DVT in patients undergoing total hip and knee replacement surgery and surgery for hip fracture.

Interactions

+ When used with drugs that can cause bleeding, fondaparinux may increase the risk of bleeding.

Adverse reactions

Bleeding, nausea, anemia, fever, rash, constipation, and edema are the most common adverse reactions to fondaparinux.

Nursing considerations

 CLINICAL ALERT Use fondaparinux cautiously in patients who have had epidural or spinal anesthesia or spinal puncture; they're at increased risk for developing an epidural or spinal hematoma, which may cause paralysis. Use the drug with extreme caution in patients who also receive platelet inhibitors and in those at increased risk of bleeding.

+ To avoid loss of fondaparinux, don't expel any air bubble from the prefilled syringe.
+ Inspect the single-dose, prefilled syringe before giving the drug. If you see particles or discoloration, don't give it.
+ Give fondaparinux S.C. only — never I.M.
+ Don't mix fondaparinux with other injections or infusions.
+ Don't use the drug interchangeably with heparin or low–molecular-weight heparins.
+ Give S.C. into fatty tissue; rotate injection sites.
+ Periodically monitor the patient's renal function. If he experiences unstable renal function or severe renal impairment during therapy, stop the drug.
+ Routinely assess the patient for signs and symptoms of bleeding. Regularly monitor his CBC, platelet count, creatinine level, and fecal occult blood test results. If the platelet count falls below 100,000/mm^3, withhold the drug.
+ Be aware that anticoagulant effects may last for 2 to 4 days after stopping the drug in a patient with normal renal function.
+ Don't rely on the PT or PTT to measure fondaparinux activity. If coagulation parameters show unexpected changes or if major bleeding occurs, stop the drug.
+ Teach the patient and his family about the prescribed drug. (See *Teaching a patient about factor Xa inhibitors.*)

Teaching a patient about factor Xa inhibitors

Whenever a factor Xa inhibitor is prescribed, teach the patient and his family the drug's name, dose, frequency, action, and adverse effects. Also take the following actions.

✦ Explain the importance of undergoing laboratory tests to monitor the effectiveness of therapy and detect adverse reactions.

✦ Teach the patient and his family to recognize the signs and symptoms of bleeding and report them to the prescriber.

✦ Advise the patient to avoid activities that pose a risk of injury and to use a soft toothbrush and an electric razor during fondaparinux therapy.

✦ Instruct the patient to avoid over-the-counter products that contain aspirin or other salicylates.

✦ Teach the patient how to give himself the subcutaneous drug properly.

✦ Instruct the patient to notify the prescriber immediately if adverse reactions occur.

THROMBOLYTICS

Thrombolytics are used to dissolve a preexisting clot or thrombus, often in an acute or emergency situation. Currently used drugs in this class include alteplase, reteplase, streptokinase, tenecteplase, and urokinase.

Pharmacokinetics

After I.V. or intracoronary administration, thrombolytics are distributed immediately throughout the circulation, quickly activating plasminogen (a precursor to plasmin, which dissolves fibrin clots).

Alteplase, reteplase, tenecteplase, and urokinase are cleared rapidly from circulating plasma, primarily by the liver. Streptokinase is removed rapidly from circulation by antibodies and the reticuloendothelial system. These drugs don't appear to cross the placental barrier.

Pharmacodynamics

Thrombolytics convert plasminogen to plasmin, which *lyses,* or dissolves, thrombi, fibrinogen, and other plasma proteins. (See *How thrombolytics help restore circulation,* page 456.)

Pharmacotherapeutics

Each thrombolytic has specific indications. Alteplase is used to treat acute MI, pulmonary embolism, acute ischemic stroke, and peripheral artery occlusion. It's also prescribed to restore patency to clotted grafts and I.V. access devices. Reteplase and tenecteplase are used to treat acute MI. Streptokinase is prescribed to treat acute MI, pulmonary embolism, and DVT. Urokinase is preferred for pulmonary embolism, coronary artery thrombosis, and catheter clearance.

Features of thrombolytics

✦ Convert plasminogen to plasmin, which lyses thrombi, fibrinogen, and other plasma proteins

alteplase

✦ Is used to treat acute MI, pulmonary embolism, acute ischemic stroke, and peripheral artery occlusion

✦ Is also used to restore patency to clotted grafts and I.V. access devices

reteplase and tenecteplase

✦ Are used to treat acute MI

streptokinase

✦ Is used to treat acute MI, pulmonary embolism, and DVT

urokinase

✦ Is used for pulmonary embolism, coronary artery thrombosis, and catheter clearance

EYE ON DRUG ACTION

How thrombolytics help restore circulation

When a thrombus forms in an artery, the clot obstructs the blood supply, which causes ischemia and necrosis. Thrombolytics can dissolve a thrombus in a coronary or pulmonary artery, restoring the blood supply to the area beyond the blockage.

OBSTRUCTED ARTERY
A thrombus blocks blood flow through the artery and causes distal ischemia.

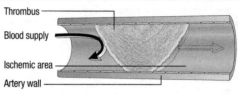

INSIDE THE THROMBUS
The thrombolytic enters the thrombus, which consists of plasminogen bound to fibrin. The drug binds to the fibrin-plasminogen complex, converting the inactive plasminogen into active plasmin. This active plasmin digests the fibrin, which dissolves the thrombus. As the thrombus dissolves, blood flow resumes.

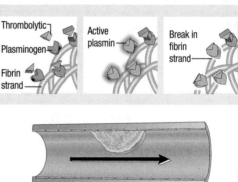

Adverse reactions to watch for

- ✦ Allergic responses (especially with streptokinase)
- ✦ Bleeding at a sutured wound or puncture site
- ✦ Flushing, headache, itching, musculoskeletal pain, nausea, urticaria (with urokinase)
- ✦ Hemorrhage in the cranium, GI or urinary tract, vagina, or behind the peritoneum
- ✦ Hemorrhagic infarct at the site of myocardial necrosis (with streptokinase)
- ✦ Hypotension unrelated to bleeding or anaphylaxis
- ✦ Major bleeding
- ✦ Reperfusion arrhythmias (with streptokinase)
- ✦ Temperature elevation (average 1.5° F [0.56° C], especially with streptokinase)

Thrombolytics are most effective when given immediately after thrombosis. They have been shown to be effective if given within 6 hours of the onset of symptoms.

Interactions
✦ When used with antiplatelet drugs, heparin, NSAIDs, and oral anticoagulants, thrombolytics can increase the risk of bleeding.
✦ Aminocaproic acid inhibits streptokinase and can be used to reverse its fibrinolytic effects.

Adverse reactions
The major reactions to thrombolytics are bleeding and allergic responses, especially with streptokinase. Thrombolytics dissolve fibrin deposits at all sites, not just at the arterial thrombus obstructing coronary or pulmonary circulation. They can cause bleeding at a sutured wound or any puncture site, such as an arterial line or central line catheter site. Major bleeding may occur in some patients, resulting from a systemic bleeding disturbance. Hemorrhaging may occur in the cranium, the GI or urinary tract, the vagina, or behind the peritoneum.

Allergic reactions to streptokinase are common because most patients possess circulating streptococcal antibodies. Urokinase has also caused allergic reactions, with such findings as urticaria, itching, flushing, nausea, headache, and musculoskeletal pain.

Streptokinase can produce hemorrhagic infarct at the site of myocardial necrosis as well as reperfusion arrhythmias. These arrhythmias usually are premature ventricular contractions that require no treatment. (After I.V. administration, alteplase may also cause reperfusion arrhythmias.) Occasionally, more serious arrhythmias, such as complex or grouped premature ventricular contractions, ventricular tachycardia, and fibrillation, may occur. Hypotension unrelated to bleeding or anaphylaxis may also occur.

Some patients experience an average temperature elevation of 1.5° F [0.56° C] after receiving a dose, particularly after receiving streptokinase. The cause of this response hasn't been established.

Nursing considerations

✦ Closely monitor the patient for bleeding and other adverse reactions, especially if he also receives heparin. Also monitor him for drug interactions.

✦ Monitor the patient's coagulation studies. Coagulation studies are recommended immediately before and 4 hours after the systemic administration of thrombolytics.

✦ Monitor the patient's vital signs frequently to assess for signs of internal bleeding and to detect hypotension, significant pulse or respiratory changes, or fever.

✦ Treat severe bleeding complications by stopping the thrombolytic infusion and infusing fresh whole blood, packed RBCs, or fresh frozen plasma. Give aminocaproic acid as an antidote.

✦ Continue to assess the patient for bleeding complications for 24 hours after thrombolytic therapy is stopped.

✦ Assess the patient's chest pain if the intracoronary route of administration is used; decreased pain may signal myocardial reperfusion. Also monitor his ECG tracings, especially noting the ST segment, and watch for reperfusion or ventricular arrhythmias or conduction disorders.

✦ Keep antiarrhythmics and a defibrillator readily accessible at all times.

✦ Observe the patient for signs of an allergic reaction.

✦ Leave the femoral venous and arterial sheaths in place for 24 hours after intracoronary thrombolytic therapy. Immobilize the patient's entire leg for 24 hours to prevent bleeding. If bleeding occurs at the femoral insertion site, apply direct pressure with a pressure dressing or aminocaproic acid–soaked sponges. Monitor the patient's color, temperature, and femoral, popliteal, and dorsalis pedis pulses every 15 minutes for 1 hour, then every 30 minutes for 8 hours, and then once each shift.

✦ Monitor the patient's neurologic status during the infusion. If the patient reports sudden severe headache or develops neurologic deficits during the infusion, stop the infusion and notify the prescriber. The patient may have developed intracranial bleeding.

✦ Reposition the patient carefully during and after the infusion to minimize bruising.

✦ Don't give the drug I.M. or insert new arterial lines during thrombolytic therapy or for 24 hours after it's ended.

✦ Give other drugs through existing I.V. sites, orally, or by nasogastric tube.

✦ Give acetaminophen rather than aspirin for fever to decrease the patient's risk of bleeding.

Key nursing actions

✦ Monitor coagulation studies.

✦ Monitor vital signs frequently to detect internal bleeding, hypotension, significant pulse or respiratory changes, or fever.

✦ Continue assessing for bleeding complications for 24 hours after thrombolytic therapy ends.

✦ Assess the patient's chest pain if the intracoronary administration route is used.

✦ Keep antiarrhythmics and a defibrillator readily accessible.

✦ Observe for evidence of an allergic reaction.

✦ Monitor neurologic status during the infusion.

✦ Reposition the patient carefully during and after the infusion to minimize bruising.

PATIENT TEACHING

Teaching a patient about thrombolytics

Whenever a thrombolytic is prescribed, teach the patient and his family the drug's name, dose, frequency, action, and adverse effects. Also take the following actions.
✦ Encourage the patient and his family to ask questions about the drug regimen.
✦ Instruct the patient to inform the nurse if adverse reactions occur or if initial symptoms, such as chest pain, improve or worsen.
✦ Teach the patient the signs and symptoms of internal bleeding and tell him to report them to the nurse or prescriber immediately.
✦ Teach the patient about proper dental care and advise him to avoid vigorous brushing, which can produce gum trauma.

✦ Notify the prescriber immediately if adverse reactions or drug interactions occur.
✦ Teach the patient and his family about the prescribed drug. (See *Teaching a patient about thrombolytics.*)

12

Endocrine drugs

Together with the central nervous system (CNS), the endocrine system regulates and integrates the body's metabolic activities and maintains homeostasis. Drugs that treat endocrine disorders include natural hormones and their synthetic analogues, hormonelike substances, and drugs that stimulate or suppress hormone secretion. These drugs belong to four major groups: antidiabetics and glucagon, thyroid and antithyroid drugs, pituitary drugs, and estrogens.

To understand endocrine pharmacology, you need to know about the endocrine system and its hormones.

ENDOCRINE SYSTEM

The endocrine system consists of glands, which are specialized cell clusters, and hormones, which are chemical transmitters secreted by the glands in response to stimulation. (See *Understanding the endocrine system,* page 460.)

PANCREATIC HORMONES

The pancreas performs exocrine and endocrine functions. Its exocrine functions include the production of enzymes needed for protein, carbohydrate, and fat digestion. Its endocrine functions arise from the islets of Langerhans in the pancreas. The islet cells consist of three specialized cell types: alpha, beta, and delta. Alpha cells produce glucagon. Beta cells produce insulin. Delta cells produce somatostatin.

During normal carbohydrate metabolism, insulin promotes glucose uptake, storage, and metabolism. It also increases protein synthesis, inhibits protein breakdown, stimulates triglyceride synthesis, and inhibits lipolysis (fat breakdown). Without insulin, the body can't metabolize glucose and must break down protein and fat for fuel.

Understanding the endocrine system

Endocrine glands secrete hormones directly into the bloodstream to regulate body function. This illustration shows the location of the endocrine glands and other organs that have endocrine functions.

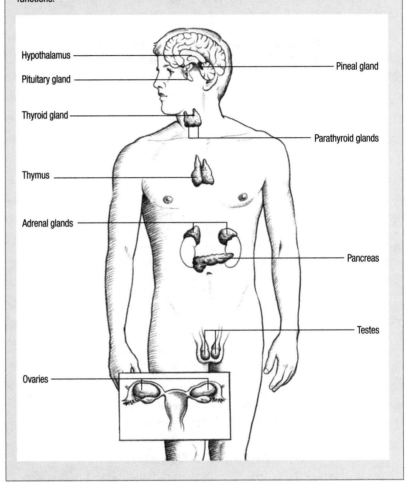

Reviewing pancreatic function
(continued)

✦ Endocrine functions arise from the islets of Langerhans, which contain three specialized cell types. Alpha cells produce glucagon. Beta cells produce insulin. Delta cells produce somatostatin.

Glucagon opposes the actions of insulin. It stimulates *glycogenolysis* (the conversion of glycogen to glucose) and *gluconeogenesis* (the production of glucose from protein breakdown), increases lipolysis, and inhibits triglyceride storage.

The glucose level primarily controls insulin and glucagon secretion. At a normal fasting glucose level of 70 to 110 mg/dl, little insulin is secreted. When the glucose level rises above 110 mg/dl, insulin secretion rapidly increases. When it falls below 70 mg/dl, glucagon secretion increases, rapidly boosting hepatic glucose production. Thus, glucagon prevents hypoglycemia and insulin prevents hyperglycemia.

Somatostatin inhibits the release of glucagon and insulin and prolongs nutrient absorption into the bloodstream. Through continual feedback and interaction, somatostatin, insulin, and glucagon maintain a normal blood glucose level.

THYROID HORMONES

The thyroid gland secretes triiodothyronine (T_3) and thyroxine (T_4), which influence the body's metabolic rate, and calcitonin, which helps regulate calcium metabolism. Secretion of these thyroid hormones is controlled primarily by thyroid-stimulating hormone (TSH), which is secreted by the anterior pituitary gland.

The thyroid gland secretes more T_4 than T_3. Although the hormones function the same physiologically, they differ in onset and intensity of action. T_3 is about four times as potent as T_4 and produces effects much more rapidly. Both hormones increase protein synthesis, stimulate cellular enzyme activity, promote growth, and enhance carbohydrate and fat metabolism. They also increase cardiac output and heart rate, respiratory rate and depth, and GI motility.

Calcitonin is secreted primarily by the thyroid gland. When the calcium level is high, calcitonin secretion increases. Calcitonin reduces the calcium level by inhibiting bone resorption, reducing osteoclast activity (bone absorption and removal), and increasing renal excretion of calcium.

PARATHYROID HORMONES

The calcium level primarily regulates parathyroid hormone secretion by the parathyroid glands. Any physiologic or pathologic alteration that increases the calcium level will suppress parathyroid gland secretion. Any decrease in the calcium level will increase parathyroid gland secretion.

Parathyroid hormones stimulate calcium and phosphate absorption from bone. These hormones also increase GI absorption and decrease renal excretion of calcium.

ANTERIOR PITUITARY HORMONES

The anterior pituitary gland secretes various hormones that help control metabolic processes in the body: growth hormone (GH), corticotropin, TSH, prolactin, follicle-stimulating hormone (FSH), and luteinizing hormone (LH).

Also called somatotropic hormone or somatotropin, GH promotes growth by increasing protein synthesis, decreasing carbohydrate use, and increasing fat mobilization and use for energy.

Corticotropin, also called adrenocorticotropin, controls cortisol secretion and enhances androgen production by the adrenal glands. This hormone also influences aldosterone secretion.

TSH, or thyrotropin, stimulates the thyroid gland to increase T_3 and T_4 production and secretion. Normally, the thyroid hormone levels remain fairly constant because of an effective feedback mechanism. Increased thyroid hormone levels inhibit TSH secretion from the pituitary gland; decreased levels stimulate TSH secretion. A hypothalamic hormone, thyrotropin-releasing hormone, regulates the increase in TSH secretion.

Prolactin promotes mammary gland development and milk production. Prolactin secretion is predominantly under the negative control of the hypothalamus, which normally synthesizes a hormone that suppresses prolactin's secretion from the pituitary gland. During lactation, however, formation of this prolactin-inhibit-

---

Reviewing thyroid hormones

+ The thyroid gland secretes T_3 and T_4, which influence the body's metabolic rate, and calcitonin, which helps regulate calcium metabolism.

+ T_3 and T_4 increase protein synthesis, stimulate cellular enzyme activity, promote growth, enhance carbohydrate and fat metabolism, and increase cardiac output, heart rate, respiratory rate and depth, GI motility.

+ Calcitonin reduces the calcium level by inhibiting bone resorption, reducing osteoclast activity, and increasing renal excretion of calcium.

Reviewing anterior pituitary hormones

+ The anterior pituitary gland secretes hormones that help control metabolic processes.

+ GH promotes growth by increasing protein synthesis, decreasing carbohydrate use, and increasing fat mobilization and use for energy.

+ Corticotropin controls cortisol secretion, enhances androgen production, and influences aldosterone secretion.

+ TSH stimulates T_3 and T_4 production and secretion.

+ Prolactin promotes mammary gland development and milk production.

+ FSH and LH are secreted in response to hypothalamic-releasing hormone and regulated by estrogen and progesterone.

ing hormone is suppressed, and sucking or breast manipulation stimulates prolactin secretion.

FSH and LH are gonadotropic hormones secreted in response to hypothalamic-releasing hormone and regulated by estrogen and progesterone levels. During each female reproductive cycle, FSH and LH levels increase and decrease. During the first phase of the cycle, increased hormone secretion stimulates new follicle growth in the ovaries. Eventually, one follicle becomes more highly developed than the others and begins to secrete large amounts of estrogen, which triggers a feedback mechanism that inhibits FSH secretion by the anterior pituitary gland. This makes the other follicles stop growing and involute. The one large follicle continues to grow through the self-stimulating effect of the secreted estrogen. Shortly before ovulation, LH and FSH secretion by the anterior pituitary gland increases markedly, producing rapid swelling of the follicle that leads to ovulation.

FSH and LH also affect men. FSH stimulates the testes to produce sperm. LH stimulates the interstitial cells in the testes to develop and produce testosterone.

POSTERIOR PITUITARY HORMONES

The posterior pituitary gland secretes antidiuretic hormone (ADH) and oxytocin. Nerve impulses from the hypothalamus regulate the secretion of these hormones.

ADH, or vasopressin, increases water reabsorption in the collecting ducts of the nephrons. Its production is regulated by osmotic receptors and volume receptors. Concentration of body fluids stimulates the osmotic receptors in the hypothalamus, increasing the impulses transmitted to the posterior pituitary to stimulate ADH secretion. This increases the water permeability of the collecting ducts.

Blood loss stimulates the volume receptors (atrial stretch receptors and baroreceptors in the carotid, aortic, and pulmonary arteries). This precipitates a marked increase in ADH secretion. ADH also exerts a potent pressor effect to maintain arterial blood pressure.

Oxytocin produces uterine contractions and milk release from the breast alveoli into the milk ducts. At the end of pregnancy, cervical stretching or irritation transmits a neurogenic reflex to the posterior pituitary gland, which stimulates increased oxytocin secretion and, subsequently, uterine contraction.

GONADAL HORMONES

The testes secrete testosterone, the major male gonadal hormone, and other male sex hormones, or androgens. These hormones produce androgenic, or masculinizing, effects, but also exert some anabolic, or building, effects. The adrenal gland also secretes androgens, but they're much less potent and don't produce significant androgenic effects.

The ovaries secrete estrogens and progesterone in response to FSH and LH. Estrogens stimulate the cellular proliferation and growth of female sex organs and related reproductive tissues. They also affect skeletal growth, fat deposition, skin vascularity, and various intracellular functions. Progesterone promotes secretory changes in the endometrium to prepare the uterus for implantation of the fertilized ovum. This hormone also evokes secretory changes in the fallopian tubes and breasts.

Estrogen or progesterone can inhibit ovulation by a negative feedback effect on the hypothalamus, which suppresses FSH and LH release.

Reviewing posterior pituitary hormones

♦ The posterior pituitary gland secretes ADH and oxytocin in response to nerve impulses from the hypothalamus.

♦ ADH increases water reabsorption in the collecting ducts of the nephrons and has a potent pressor effect.

♦ Oxytocin produces uterine contractions and the release of milk into the milk ducts.

Reviewing gonadal hormines

♦ The testes secrete testosterone (the major male gonadal hormone) and other male sex hormones, or androgens.

♦ These hormones produce androgenic, or masculinizing, effects, but also exert some anabolic, or building, effects.

♦ The ovaries secrete estrogens and progesterone in response to FSH and LH.

♦ Estrogens stimulate the growth of female sex organs and reproductive tissues. They also affect skeletal growth, fat deposition, skin vascularity, and intracellular functions.

♦ Progesterone promotes secretory changes in the endometrium to prepare the uterus for implantation of a fertilized ovum. It also evokes secretory changes in the fallopian tubes and breasts.

ANTIDIABETICS AND GLUCAGON

Insulin, a pancreatic hormone, and oral antidiabetics are hypoglycemics because they lower the glucose level. Glucagon, another pancreatic hormone, is a hyperglycemic because it raises the glucose level.

All of these drugs are used to manage diabetes mellitus, a chronic disease of insulin deficiency or resistance. Diabetes is characterized by disturbances in carbohydrate, protein, and fat metabolism. This elevates the glucose level in the body. The disease comes in two primary forms. Type 1 was formerly known as insulin-dependent diabetes mellitus. Type 2 was formerly known as non–insulin-dependent diabetes mellitus.

INSULIN

Patients with type 1 diabetes require an external source of insulin to control their glucose levels. Patients with type 2 diabetes may also need insulin at times. Insulin may be rapid-acting, short-acting, intermediate-acting, long-acting, or a combination of these forms. It may be human insulin, derived from pork, or purified (made from highly purified pancreas extracts). Insulin is measured in units.

Pharmacokinetics

Insulin isn't effective when taken orally because the GI tract breaks down its protein molecules before they reach the bloodstream.

All insulins may be given by subcutaneous (S.C.) injection. Absorption of S.C. insulin varies with the injection site, the blood supply, and degree of tissue hypertrophy at the injection site.

Regular insulin may also be given I.V. or in dialysate fluid infused into the peritoneal cavity for patients receiving peritoneal dialysis.

Upon absorption, insulin is distributed throughout the body. Insulin-responsive tissues are located in the liver, adipose tissue, and muscle. Insulin is metabolized primarily in the liver and, to a lesser extent, in the kidneys and muscle. The drug is excreted in feces and urine.

Pharmacodynamics

Insulin is an anabolic hormone that promotes the storage of glucose as glycogen. (See *How insulin aids glucose uptake*, page 464.) It also increases protein and fat synthesis; slows glycogen, protein, and fat breakdown; and promotes fluid and electrolyte balance.

Although insulin has no antidiuretic effect, this drug can correct the *polyuria* (excessive urination) and *polydipsia* (excessive thirst) caused by the osmotic diuresis from hyperglycemia by decreasing the glucose level. Insulin also facilitates potassium movement from the extracellular fluid into cells.

Pharmacotherapeutics

Insulin is indicated for type 1 diabetes. It's also prescribed for type 2 diabetes when other methods of controlling the glucose level have failed or are contraindicated, when the glucose level is elevated during periods of emotional or physical stress (such as infection and surgery), or when oral antidiabetics are contraindicated because of pregnancy or hypersensitivity.

Features of insulin

+ Is an anabolic hormone secreted by the pancreas that promotes storage of glucose as glycogen
+ Increases protein and fat synthesis; slows glycogen, protein, and fat breakdown; and promotes fluid and electrolyte balance
+ May be rapid-acting, short-acting, intermediate-acting, long-acting, or a combination
+ May be human insulin, derived from pork, or purified (made from highly purified pancreas extracts)
+ Is measured in units

Uses of insulin

+ Is used for type 1 diabetes and for type 2 diabetes when other glucose-control methods have failed or are contraindicated, when the glucose level is elevated during emotional or physical stress, or when oral antidiabetics are contraindicated because of pregnancy or hypersensitivity

EYE ON DRUG ACTION

How insulin aids glucose uptake

These illustrations show how insulin allows a cell to use glucose for energy.

1. Glucose can't enter the cell without the aid of insulin.

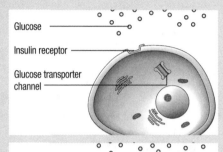

2. Normally produced by beta cells in the pancreas, insulin binds to receptors on the surface of target cells. Insulin and its receptor first move to the inside of the cell, which activates glucose transporter channels to move to the surface of the cell.

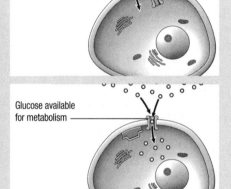

3. These channels allow glucose to enter the cell. Then the cell can use the glucose for metabolism.

Uses of insulin
(continued)

✦ Is also used to treat diabetic ketoacidosis, hyperosmolar hyperglycemic nonketotic syndrome, and severe hyperkalemia in patients with diabetes

Insulin is also used to treat two complications of diabetes: diabetic ketoacidosis, which is more common with type 1 diabetes, and hyperosmolar hyperglycemic nonketotic syndrome, which is more common with type 2 diabetes.

In patients with diabetes, insulin is also used to treat severe hyperkalemia. That's because potassium moves with glucose from the bloodstream into the cell, which lowers the potassium level.

Interactions

Some drugs interact with insulin, altering its ability to decrease the glucose level; other drugs directly affect the glucose level.

✦ Alcohol, an anabolic steroid, a monoamine oxidase (MAO) inhibitor, or a salicylate may increase the hypoglycemic effects of insulin.

✦ A corticosteroid, dextrothyroxine sodium, a sympathomimetic drug, or a thiazide diuretic may reduce insulin's effects, resulting in hyperglycemia.

✦ A beta blocker may prolong the hypoglycemic effects of insulin and may mask the signs and symptoms of hypoglycemia.

Adverse reactions

Hypoglycemia is a relatively common adverse reaction to insulin. Specific signs and symptoms vary, but may include nervousness, shakiness, diaphoresis, weakness, light-headedness, confusion, paresthesia, irritability, headache, hunger, tachycardia, and changes in speech, hearing, or vision.

 CLINICAL ALERT If untreated, hypoglycemia may progress to unconsciousness, seizures, coma, and death. Keep a source of glucose or glucagon readily available.

The Somogyi phenomenon occurs when hypoglycemia is followed by compensatory rebound hyperglycemia as the body increases glucose production to correct the problem. Typically, the phenomenon occurs late at night or early in the morning when the patient is asleep. During this time, insulin continues to be absorbed from the S.C. injection site, although insufficient glucose may be present for insulin to act. As a result, the glucose level drops rapidly. In response, the body secretes glucagon, norepinephrine, and corticosteroids to correct the hypoglycemia. An overshoot phenomenon occurs, resulting in hyperglycemia. Although the patient awakens with signs and symptoms of hyperglycemia, hypoglycemia is the problem.

The dawn phenomenon (an early morning rise in the glucose level) may result from uneven therapy. Unlike the Somogyi phenomenon, the dawn phenomenon isn't preceded by hypoglycemia. It may result from nocturnal secretion of GH, which causes insulin resistance.

A patient can experience local or systemic hypersensitivity reactions to any type of insulin, but such reactions to purified and human insulin are unlikely. Local reactions are characterized by redness, itching, or burning at the injection site. These symptoms usually disappear after 1 to 2 months of continued insulin use. Systemic hypersensitivity reactions are characterized by generalized urticaria, angioedema, dyspnea, tachycardia and, possibly, anaphylactic shock. Systemic reactions rarely occur.

Two kinds of *lipodystrophy,* or disturbance in fat metabolism, can occur with insulin injections. *Lipoatrophy,* or loss of fat tissue at the injection site, and *lipohypertrophy,* or thickening of subcutaneous fat tissue, can be prevented by rotating insulin injection sites.

Patients can develop a resistance to insulin. Although anti-insulin antibodies may play a role, insulin resistance usually results from a decreased number of insulin receptors, a postreceptor defect in insulin action, or an excess of hormones that antagonize insulin. Insulin antibodies seem more likely to develop during episodic insulin therapy for type 2 diabetes. Human insulin is preferred for episodic insulin therapy because it's the least antigenic.

Nursing considerations

✦ Frequently monitor the patient for adverse reactions, especially hypoglycemia. Also monitor for drug interactions.
✦ Monitor the patient's glucose level regularly and more frequently after the insulin dosage is increased. Check the glucose level during the night and in the early morning if you suspect the Somogyi or dawn phenomenon.
✦ Avoid delays in the patient's mealtimes to prevent hypoglycemia.

Adverse reactions to watch for

✦ Dawn phenomenon (early morning rise in the glucose level)
✦ Hypoglycemia (confusion, diaphoresis, headache, hunger, irritability, light-headedness, paresthesia, tachycardia, nervousness, shakiness, weakness, and changes in speech, hearing, or vision)
✦ Insulin resistance
✦ Lipoatrophy, lipohypertrophy
✦ Local hypersensitivity reactions (burning, itching, or redness at the injection site)
✦ Somogyi phenomenon (hypoglycemia followed by compensatory rebound hyperglycemia)
✦ Systemic hypersensitivity reactions (anaphylactic shock, angioedema, dyspnea, tachycardia, urticaria)

Key nursing actions

✦ Monitor glucose level regularly, more often after the insulin dosage is increased.
✦ Check the glucose level during the night and early in the morning if you suspect the Somogyi or dawn phenomenon.
✦ Avoid delays in the patient's mealtimes to prevent hypoglycemia.

Key nursing actions
(continued)

- ✦ Monitor the patient's calorie intake to ensure that daily requirements are met.
- ✦ Keep glucose or glucagon readily available to treat hypoglycemia. Afterward, provide a complex carbohydrate snack.
- ✦ Measure U-100 insulin in a U-100 insulin syringe.
- ✦ Prepare a U-500 dose with extreme caution. A small overdose could be fatal.
- ✦ Mix insulins in the same order every time, and give them within 5 minutes after mixing.
- ✦ Give insulin S.C. for most patients.
- ✦ Rotate and document insulin injection sites.
- ✦ Observe S.C. or I.M. injection sites for evidence of local hypersensitivity reactions (redness, itching, or burning at the site).
- ✦ Observe the patient during initial or episodic insulin therapy, particularly noting systemic hypersensitivity reactions.
- ✦ Observe for evidence of hyperglycemia, such as polyuria, polydipsia, polyphagia, weight loss, and fatigue.

PATIENT TEACHING

Teaching a patient about insulin

Whenever an insulin preparation is prescribed, teach the patient and his family the drug's name, dose, frequency, action, and adverse effects. Also take the following actions.

- ✦ Teach the patient and his family how to draw up and administer the prescribed insulin.
- ✦ Instruct the patient to rotate vials of intermediate- and long-acting insulin gently before withdrawing the dose. This ensures proper dispersion of the suspension.
- ✦ Advise the patient to use a U-100 syringe for U-100 insulin.
- ✦ Inform the patient with impaired vision of the many aids available to help withdraw the correct amount of insulin into a syringe.
- ✦ Tell the patient who must mix insulins always to follow the same order when drawing the insulins into the syringe.
- ✦ Instruct the patient to withdraw a mixture and administer it within 5 minutes or to store the mixture in the refrigerator and administer it after the binding period of 15 minutes for regular insulin with NPH insulin and 24 hours for regular insulin with lente insulin.
- ✦ Advise the patient that proper rotation of subcutaneous injection sites helps prevent lipodystrophy.
- ✦ Instruct the patient to let insulin reach room temperature before injection to minimize pain on administration.
- ✦ Instruct the patient to store insulin at a temperature below 80° F (27° C) and above 36° F (2° C). Explain that he can store an unopened vial in the refrigerator, but should never freeze insulin or leave it in direct sunlight.
- ✦ Teach the patient how to care for an insulin pump if used.
- ✦ Instruct the patient not to change the manufacturer, type, purity, species, or dosage of insulin unless instructed to do so by the prescriber.
- ✦ Teach the patient the signs and symptoms of hypoglycemia and hyperglycemia and what to do if they occur.
- ✦ Teach the patient how to monitor his glucose level. Glucose monitoring is especially important for a patient who needs rigid control of his glucose level or requires sliding-scale insulin coverage in which the dose varies with the body's need. Instruct the patient to monitor his glucose level frequently during times of stress or infection because his insulin requirement may increase. A patient may monitor his urine glucose level rather than the blood glucose level; however, this method typically provides less accurate and less reliable information.
- ✦ Teach the patient how to monitor his urine ketone level to detect ketosis, especially during illness or stress.
- ✦ Review all aspects of diabetic care that may affect insulin therapy and predispose the patient to hypoglycemia or hyperglycemia, such as diet, exercise, and stress.
- ✦ Review sick-day rules to follow during insulin therapy. For example, instruct the patient to contact the prescriber for insulin dosage adjustments and to test his blood glucose level more frequently when illness occurs.
- ✦ Instruct the patient receiving insulin to wear medical identification and to have ready access to a source of glucose, such as hard candy.
- ✦ Advise the patient to notify the prescriber if hyperglycemia or other adverse reactions occur.

✦ Monitor the patient's calorie intake to ensure that daily requirements are met. Count the calories in I.V. solutions in his daily caloric intake.

✦ Keep a source of glucose or glucagon readily available to treat a hypoglycemic reaction. After such a reaction, provide a complex carbohydrate snack.

CLINICAL ALERT Avoid dosage errors by measuring U-100 insulin in a U-100 insulin syringe. Prepare a U-500 dose with extreme caution. A small, inadvertent overdose of U-500 insulin could cause death.

✦ Don't shake insulin because the resulting froth prevents withdrawal of an accurate dose and may damage the protein molecules.

✦ Mix insulins in the same order every time and give mixed insulins within 5 minutes after mixing.

✦ Don't administer regular insulin that appears cloudy or any insulin solution that contains particles.

✦ Give insulin S.C. for most patients. Give regular insulin by I.V. or I.M., or mix it with dialysate fluid and infuse it into the peritoneal cavity for peritoneal dialysis.

✦ Give a once-daily morning dosage of insulin 30 minutes before breakfast, or a split morning and evening dosage 30 minutes before breakfast and 30 minutes before dinner, unless otherwise prescribed.

✦ Rotate and document insulin injection sites.

✦ Observe S.C. or I.M. injection sites for signs and symptoms of local hypersensitivity reactions, such as redness, itching, or burning at the site. If the reaction persists for more than 2 months or becomes worse in a patient who is taking standard insulin, switch him to human or purified insulin.

✦ Observe the patient during initial or episodic insulin therapy, particularly noting systemic hypersensitivity reactions. Keep standard emergency equipment nearby. If such a reaction occurs, switch the patient to an insulin from another source. Begin desensitization therapy.

✦ Observe the patient for signs and symptoms of hyperglycemia, such as polyuria, polydipsia, polyphagia, weight loss, and fatigue. These reactions suggest a need to change the insulin regimen.

✦ Teach the patient and his family about the prescribed drug. (See *Teaching a patient about insulin.*)

ORAL ANTIDIABETICS

Types of oral antidiabetics include:

✦ first-generation sulfonylureas, such as acetohexamide, chlorpropamide, tolazamide, and tolbutamide

✦ second-generation sulfonylureas, such as glimepiride, glipizide, and glyburide

✦ thiazolidinediones, such as pioglitazone and rosiglitazone

✦ the biguanide drug, metformin

✦ alpha-glucosidase inhibitors, such as acarbose and miglitol

✦ meglitinides, such as nateglinide and repaglinide

✦ combination therapies, such as glipizide-metformin, glyburide-metformin, and rosiglitazone-metformin.

Pharmacokinetics

Oral antidiabetics are absorbed well from the GI tract and distributed via the bloodstream throughout the body. These drugs are metabolized primarily in the liver and are excreted mostly in urine, with some excreted in bile. Glyburide is excreted equally in urine and feces; pioglitazone and rosiglitazone are largely excreted in both.

Features of oral antidiabetics

✦ Act inside and outside the pancreas to regulate glucose level

✦ May stimulate beta cells to release insulin if the pancreas is minimally functional

✦ Control glucose level by decreasing gluconeogenesis in the liver and increasing the number of insulin receptors in peripheral tissues

✦ Are used for patients with type 2 diabetes if diet and exercise don't control the glucose level

✦ Are ineffective in type 1 diabetes because beta cells aren't functioning

Pharmacodynamics

Researchers believe that oral antidiabetics produce actions inside and outside the pancreas to regulate the glucose level.

These drugs probably stimulate pancreatic beta cells to release insulin in a patient with a minimally functioning pancreas. A few weeks to a few months after a patient starts taking a sulfonylurea, his pancreatic insulin secretion drops to the pretreatment level, but his glucose level remains normal or near-normal. Most likely, the drug's actions outside the pancreas maintain this glucose control.

Oral antidiabetics also provide several actions outside of the pancreas to decrease and control the glucose level. They can go to work in the liver and decrease gluconeogenesis there. Also, by increasing the number of insulin receptors in peripheral tissues, they provide more opportunities for cells to bind sufficiently with insulin, initiating the process of glucose metabolism.

Other oral antidiabetics produce specific actions. Acarbose and miglitol inhibit enzymes, which delays glucose absorption. Metformin decreases hepatic production of glucose and intestinal absorption of glucose and improves insulin sensitivity. Nateglinide and repaglinide increase insulin secretion. Pioglitazone and rosiglitazone improve insulin sensitivity.

Pharmacotherapeutics

Oral antidiabetics are indicated for patients with type 2 diabetes if diet and exercise can't control the glucose level. These drugs aren't effective in type 1 diabetes because the pancreatic beta cells aren't functioning at a minimal level.

Combination therapy of multiple oral antidiabetics or one oral antidiabetic with insulin may be used for patients who don't respond to either drug alone.

Interactions

Hypoglycemia and hyperglycemia are the main risks when oral antidiabetics interact with other drugs.

✦ When taken with alcohol, anabolic steroids, chloramphenicol, cimetidine, clofibrate, fluconazole, gemfibrozil, MAO inhibitors, phenylbutazone, ranitidine, salicylates, sulfonamides, and warfarin, sulfonylureas can cause hypoglycemia.

✦ When used with cimetidine, nifedipine, procainamide, ranitidine, and vancomycin, metformin can cause hypoglycemia.

✦ When taken with corticosteroids, dextrothyroxine, rifampin, sympathomimetics, or thiazide diuretics, sulfonylureas can cause hyperglycemia.

✦ Together, I.V. contrast dyes and metformin may cause lactic acidosis and lead to acute renal impairment.

Adverse reactions

Hypoglycemia, the major adverse reaction to oral antidiabetics, typically results from too little food or too much drug. This reaction can also occur after an incorrect dose or, more likely, from drug or metabolite accumulation in the body.

Other common adverse reactions vary with the type of drug. Sulfonylureas can produce nausea, epigastric fullness, blood abnormalities (such as leukopenia, thrombocytopenia, and aplastic anemia), water retention, rash, hyponatremia, and photosensitivity. Metformin may cause metallic taste, nausea, vomiting, and abdominal discomfort. Acarbose and miglitol can result in abdominal pain, diarrhea,

---

Adverse reactions to watch for

✦ Hypoglycemia

acarbose and miglitol
✦ Abdominal pain, diarrhea, gas

meglitinides
✦ Upper respiratory tract infection

metformin
✦ Abdominal discomfort, metallic taste, nausea, vomiting

sulfonylureas
✦ Aplastic anemia, leukopenia, thrombocytopenia
✦ Epigastric fullness, nausea
✦ Hyponatremia, water retention
✦ Photosensitivity, rash

thiazolidinediones
✦ Swelling, weight gain

Adjusting oral antidiabetic therapy

A patient's age and developmental status can affect his oral antidiabetic drug therapy, sometimes requiring dosage adjustments or other changes in the regimen.

For example, in a child, don't use a sulfonylurea. None of these drugs are effective in type 1 (juvenile-onset) diabetes, and type 2 diabetes doesn't occur as frequently in children. Also, the safety and efficacy of these drugs haven't been established for patients in this age group.

In a pregnant woman, switch from an oral antidiabetic to insulin. This change keeps her glucose level as close to normal as possible, which helps ensure the safety of her fetus.

For a breast-feeding woman, remember that oral antidiabetics appear in breast milk, increasing the risk of hypoglycemia in the infant. If diet can't control the breast-feeding patient's blood glucose level, consider using insulin instead of an oral antidiabetic.

When caring for a geriatric patient, plan to use metformin with caution because it's substantially excreted by the kidneys. Such a patient is more likely to have age-related renal impairment, which may require the dosage to be adjusted or the drug to be stopped.

and gas. Thiazolidinediones may lead to weight gain and swelling. Meglitinides are linked to upper respiratory tract infection.

Nursing considerations

✦ Determine the patient's age and developmental status. (See *Adjusting oral antidiabetic therapy*.)
✦ Monitor the patient for adverse reactions, especially hypoglycemia.
✦ Monitor the patient's glucose level regularly and more frequently with dosage adjustments.
✦ Avoid delays in mealtimes to prevent glucose level alterations.
✦ Monitor the patient's calorie intake to ensure that daily requirements are met. Count the calories in I.V. solutions.

 CLINICAL ALERT Keep a source of glucose or glucagon readily available to treat a hypoglycemic reaction. After such a reaction, provide a complex carbohydrate snack.

✦ Give a meglitinide before meals because this type of drug has a quick onset but relatively short duration. If a meal is skipped, withhold the dose as well.
✦ Give acarbose or miglitol with the first bite of a meal.
✦ Give other oral antidiabetics 30 minutes before breakfast. If the daily dosage is divided, give the second dose 30 minutes before dinner. Give the drug on a regular schedule to minimize wide fluctuations in the patient's glucose level.
✦ Teach the patient and his family about the prescribed drug. (See *Teaching a patient about oral antidiabetics,* page 470.)

Key nursing actions

✦ Monitor for adverse reactions, especially hypoglycemia.
✦ Monitor glucose level regularly, more often with dosage adjustments.
✦ Avoid delays in mealtimes to prevent glucose level alterations.
✦ Monitor calorie intake to ensure that daily requirements are met.
✦ Keep glucose or glucagon readily available to treat a hypoglycemic reaction.

Features of glucagon

✦ Regulates the rate of glucose production by stimulating glycogenolysis (the liver conversion of glycogen back into glucose), gluconeogenesis (glucose is formed from free fatty acids and proteins), lipolysis (adipose tissue release of fatty acids, which are converted to glucose)

✦ Is used for emergency treatment of severe hypoglycemia

✦ Is also used to reduce GI motility during X-rays of the GI tract

GLUCAGON

This hyperglycemic drug, which raises the glucose level, is a hormone normally produced by alpha cells in the islets of Langerhans in the pancreas. (See *How glucagon raises the glucose level.*)

Pharmacokinetics

After S.C., I.M., or I.V. injection, glucagon is absorbed rapidly. The drug is distributed throughout the body, although its effects occur primarily in the liver. It's degraded extensively by the liver, kidneys, and plasma, and by receptor sites in plasma membranes. It's removed from the body by the liver and kidneys.

Pharmacodynamics

Glucagon regulates the rate of glucose production by stimulating glycogenolysis, gluconeogenesis, and lipolysis. In glycogenolysis, the liver converts glycogen back into glucose. In gluconeogenesis, glucose is formed from free fatty acids and proteins. In lipolysis, adipose tissue releases fatty acids, which are converted to glucose.

Pharmacotherapeutics

Glucagon is used for emergency treatment of severe hypoglycemia. The drug is also used during X-rays of the GI tract to reduce GI motility.

Interactions

✦ When used with oral anticoagulants, glucagon increases the risk of bleeding.

EYE ON DRUG ACTION

How glucagon raises the glucose level

When adequate stores of glycogen are present, glucagon can raise the glucose level in a patient with severe hypoglycemia in the following way:

◆ Initially, glucagon stimulates the formation of adenylate cyclase in liver cells.

◆ Then adenylate cyclase converts adenosine triphosphate (ATP) to cyclic adenosine monophosphate (cAMP).

◆ This product triggers a series of reactions that result in an active phosphorylated glucose molecule.

◆ In this phosphorylated form, the large glucose molecule can't pass through the cell membrane.

◆ Through glycogenolysis (the breakdown of glycogen, the stored form of glucose), the liver removes the phosphate group and allows the glucose to enter the bloodstream. This raises the glucose level for short-term energy needs.

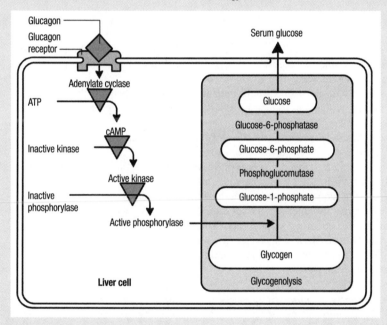

Adverse reactions

Adverse reactions to glucagon are rare. Nausea and vomiting may occur occasionally. Because of glucagon's short half-life, overdose is unlikely. No evidence of drug toxicity exists. With large dosages or prolonged treatment, hypokalemia can result. Because glucagon is a protein, an allergy to it may develop, but this reaction is rare. The body can also develop antibodies to glucagon, although the effect of such antibodies remains unknown.

Nursing considerations

◆ Monitor the patient for signs and symptoms of hypokalemia during high-dosage or long-term glucagon therapy.

Adverse reactions to watch for

◆ Hypokalemia (with large doses or prolonged treatment)
◆ Nausea, vomiting

Key nursing actions

✦ Monitor the patient for evidence of bleeding if he also receives an oral anticoagulant.

✦ After giving glucagon, give a patient with type 1 diabetes a complex carbohydrate snack as soon as possible to restore the liver glycogen level and prevent secondary hypoglycemia.

✦ If the patient is in a deep coma or doesn't wake from the coma after glucagon administration, give I.V. glucose with glucagon.

✦ Monitor the patient for signs and symptoms of bleeding if he also receives an oral anticoagulant. If bleeding occurs, notify the prescriber and decrease the oral anticoagulant dosage.

✦ After giving glucagon, give the patient with type 1 diabetes mellitus a complex carbohydrate snack as soon as possible to restore the liver glycogen level and prevent secondary hypoglycemia.

✦ Contact the prescriber immediately to obtain a prescription for I.V. glucose if the patient doesn't respond to glucagon.

✦ If the patient is in a deep coma or doesn't wake from the coma after glucagon administration, give I.V. glucose with glucagon.

✦ Mix glucagon powder only with the diluent provided.

✦ Don't give I.V. glucagon in a solution that contains calcium, potassium, or sodium chloride because precipitation can occur.

✦ Notify the prescriber if adverse reactions or drug interactions occur.

✦ Teach the patient and his family about the prescribed drug. (See *Teaching a patient about glucagon.*)

THYROID AND ANTITHYROID DRUGS

Thyroid drugs work to correct hypothyroidism. In contrast, antithyroid drugs act to correct hyperthyroidism.

THYROID DRUGS

Thyroid drugs can be natural or synthetic hormones and may contain T_3, T_4, or both. Natural thyroid drugs are made from animal thyroid and include thyroid USP (desiccated) and thyroglobulin. Both of these drugs contain T_3 and T_4.

Synthetic thyroid drugs are sodium salts of the hormones' L-isomers. These synthetic drugs include levothyroxine, which contains T_4; liothyronine, which contains T_3; and liotrix, which contains T_3 and T_4.

Pharmacokinetics

Thyroid drugs are absorbed variably from the GI tract, distributed in plasma, and bound to proteins. They're metabolized through deiodination, primarily in the liver, and excreted unchanged in feces.

Pharmacodynamics

The principal pharmacologic effect is an increased metabolic rate in body tissues. Thyroid hormones affect protein and carbohydrate metabolism and stimulate protein synthesis. They promote gluconeogenesis and increase the use of glycogen stores.

Thyroid hormones increase the heart rate and cardiac output. They may even increase the heart's sensitivity to catecholamines and increase the number of beta-adrenergic receptors in the heart. (Beta-receptor stimulation increases the heart rate and contractility).

In hypothyroid patients, these drugs may increase blood flow to the kidneys and increase the glomerular filtration rate, which produces diuresis.

Pharmacotherapeutics

Thyroid drugs act as replacement or substitute hormones to treat hypothyroidism. They're also used to treat papillary or follicular thyroid carcinoma. In addition, they're prescribed with antithyroid drugs to prevent goiter formation and hypothyroidism. In diagnostic testing, they're used to differentiate between primary and secondary hypothyroidism.

Levothyroxine is the drug of choice for thyroid hormone replacement and TSH suppression therapy.

Interactions

✦ When used with oral anticoagulants, thyroid drugs can increase the risk of bleeding.
✦ Cholestyramine or colestipol can reduce thyroid drug absorption.
✦ Phenytoin may displace thyroxine from plasma binding sites, temporarily increasing the free thyroxine level.
✦ Thyroid drugs may reduce the digoxin level, which increases the risk of arrhythmias or heart failure.
✦ Carbamazepine, phenytoin, phenobarbital, or rifampin can increase the metabolism of thyroid drugs, reducing their effectiveness.
✦ A thyroid drug may increase the theophylline level.

Adverse reactions

Most adverse reactions to thyroid drugs result from toxicity, which can be reversed by stopping the drug. Common GI signs and symptoms of thyroid toxicity include diarrhea, abdominal cramps, weight loss, and increased appetite. Cardiovascular signs and symptoms, including palpitations, diaphoresis, tachycardia, increased blood pressure, angina pectoris, and arrhythmias, may also occur, especially in older patients. (See *Using thyroid drugs safely in geriatric patients*, page 474.) Other manifestations of toxicity may include headache, tremor, insomnia, nervousness, fever, heat intolerance, and menstrual irregularities.

A patient with adrenal insufficiency should receive a corticosteroid to correct the insufficiency before thyroid therapy begins. Because thyroid drugs increase the

Features of thyroid drugs

✦ May be natural or synthetic hormones and may contain T_3, T_4, or both
✦ Natural forms are made from animal thyroid.
✦ Synthetic forms are sodium salts of the hormones' L-isomers.
✦ Increase the metabolic rate in body tissues
✦ Also affect protein and carbohydrate metabolism, stimulate protein synthesis, promote gluconeogenesis, increase the use of glycogen stores, increase the heart rate and cardiac output
✦ Are used as replacement or substitute hormones in hypothyroidism
✦ Are used to treat papillary or follicular thyroid carcinoma
✦ Are used with antithyroid drugs to prevent goiter and hypothyroidism
✦ Are used in diagnostic tests to differentiate between primary and secondary hypothyroidism

Adverse reactions to watch for

✦ Abdominal cramps, diarrhea, increased appetite, weight loss
✦ Angina, arrhythmias, diaphoresis, increased blood pressure, palpitations, tachycardia
✦ Fever, heat intolerance, headache, insomnia, nervousness, tremor
✦ Menstrual irregularities

Using thyroid drugs safely in geriatric patients

Geriatric patients are more sensitive to the effects of thyroid drugs and more likely to have other disorders that place them at risk for adverse reactions. To make thyroid therapy safer for a geriatric patient, expect to use a relatively low dosage when initiating therapy. Also closely monitor him for the drug's cardiostimulatory effects, which can lead to angina pectoris or a myocardial infarction if he has coronary artery disease. During therapy, individualize the dosage as needed.

tissue demand for adrenal hormones, thyroid therapy could precipitate an acute adrenal crisis in a patient with adrenal insufficiency.

Some thyroid preparations contain tartrazine yellow dye, which may produce bronchial asthma and other hypersensitivity reactions in a susceptible individual. Although rare, these reactions are more likely to occur in an aspirin-sensitive patient. A lactose-sensitive patient may need to avoid levothyroxine because it contains lactose. A patient who is sensitive to pork may experience GI distress when taking thyroid USP or thyroglobulin.

Nursing considerations

✦ Monitor the patient for toxicity and other adverse reactions during thyroid drug therapy. If toxicity occurs, notify the prescriber. Also, stop the drug temporarily and decrease the dosage when therapy begins again.

✦ Assess the patient for a history of pork sensitivity before giving thyroid USP or thyroglobulin, for lactose sensitivity before administering levothyroxine, and for aspirin sensitivity before giving Synthroid (levothyroxine) tablets. If the patient has a history of hypersensitivity to one thyroid drug, consult the prescriber about using another.

✦ Regularly evaluate the patient's response to therapy. Treatment should restore normal levels of T_3 and T_4. With thyroid USP or levothyroxine, expect to see a change in the patient's physical appearance and well-being in 1 to 3 weeks. With liothyronine, expect a change in 1 to 3 days.

✦ Reconstitute levothyroxine for injection immediately before use. Don't add this drug to other I.V. fluids. Discard any unused portions.

✦ Make sure that a patient with adrenal insufficiency receives corticosteroid therapy before beginning thyroid therapy.

 CLINICAL ALERT Don't withdraw a thyroid drug abruptly in a patient with myxedema, a condition that's linked to primary hypothyroidism, because doing so may precipitate myxedema coma.

✦ Watch for cardiac problems in a geriatric patient or a patient with a history of cardiac disease because T_4 may aggravate angina pectoris and lead to myocardial infarction.

✦ If the patient reports chest pain during thyroid drug therapy, notify the prescriber immediately. Give nitroglycerin to relieve pain. Obtain an ECG tracing.

Key nursing actions

✦ Monitor for toxicity and other adverse reactions during thyroid drug therapy.

✦ Assess for a history of pork sensitivity before giving thyroid USP or thyroglobulin, for lactose sensitivity before giving levothyroxine, and for aspirin sensitivity before giving Synthroid tablets.

✦ Regularly evaluate the patient's response to therapy.

✦ Watch for cardiac problems in a geriatric patient or a patient with a history of cardiac disease because T_4 may aggravate angina and lead to myocardial infarction.

Teaching a patient about thyroid drugs

Whenever a thyroid drug is prescribed, teach the patient and his family the drug's name, dose, frequency, action, and adverse effects. Also take the following actions.

✦ Teach the patient to recognize and report the signs and symptoms of hyperthyroidism, such as fatigue, breathlessness, and heat intolerance. Also instruct him to report headaches, palpitations, or nervousness, which are symptoms of thyroid hormone overdose.

✦ Remind the patient to take levothyroxine on an empty stomach to promote regular absorption and to take it in the morning to help prevent insomnia and to mimic normal hormone release.

✦ Remind the patient to store the thyroid drug in a tightly capped, light-resistant container at 59° to 86° F (15° to 30° C) to prevent deterioration.

✦ Teach the patient that different brands of thyroid drugs may vary slightly in concentration. Instruct him to check that the prescriber orders the drug by brand name and that the pharmacist doesn't substitute a different brand.

✦ Stress the importance of returning for routine thyroid tests to assess the drug's effectiveness and to detect drug toxicity.

✦ Instruct the patient to notify the prescriber if adverse reactions occur.

✦ Teach the patient and his family about the prescribed drug. (See *Teaching a patient about thyroid drugs.*)

ANTITHYROID DRUGS

Also known as *thyroid antagonists,* antithyroid drugs are used for patients with hyperthyroidism, or thyrotoxicosis. These drugs include thioamides, such as methimazole and propylthiouracil; and iodides, such as potassium iodide, stable iodine (strong iodine), and radioactive iodine (^{131}I).

Pharmacokinetics

Thioamides and iodides are absorbed through the GI tract, concentrated in the thyroid, metabolized by conjugation, and excreted in urine.

Pharmacodynamics

Drugs used to treat hyperthyroidism work in different ways. Thioamides block iodine's ability to combine with tyrosine, which prevents thyroid hormone synthesis.

Stable iodine inhibits hormone synthesis through the Wolff-Chaikoff effect, in which excess iodine decreases the formation and release of thyroid hormone.

Radioactive iodine reduces hormone secretion by destroying thyroid tissue. It does this through induction of acute radiation thyroiditis and chronic gradual thyroid atrophy. Acute radiation thyroiditis usually occurs 3 to 10 days after administering radioactive iodine. Chronic thyroid atrophy may take several years to appear.

Pharmacotherapeutics

Antithyroid drugs are commonly used to treat hyperthyroidism, especially in the form of Graves' disease (hyperthyroidism caused by autoimmunity), which accounts for 85% of all cases.

Features of antithyroid drugs

✦ Are used to treat hyperthyroidism, especially Graves' disease, which accounts for 85% of all cases

methimazole
✦ Blocks thyroid hormone formation for a longer time than propylthiouracil and is better suited for once-a-day use in mild to moderate hyperthyroidism

propylthiouracil
✦ Lowers the T_3 level faster than methimazole and usually is used for rapid improvement of severe hyperthyroidism

radioactive iodine
✦ Reduces hormone secretion by destroying thyroid tissue
✦ May be used to treat thyroid cancer

stable iodine
✦ Inhibits hormone synthesis through the Wolff-Chaikoff effect, in which excess iodine decreases thyroid hormone
✦ Is used to prepare the gland for surgical removal by firming it and decreasing its vascularity
✦ Is used after radioactive iodine therapy to control symptoms of hyperthyroidism while radiation takes effect

thioamides
✦ Block iodine's ability to combine with tyrosine, which prevents thyroid hormone synthesis

Adverse reactions to watch for

iodides

✦ Feeling of fullness in the neck, increased risk of birth defects, leukemia, metallic taste (with radioactive iodine)

✦ Iodism (chronic, dosage-dependent toxicity causing unpleasant brassy taste, burning sensation in the mouth, and increased salivation and swelling of the parotid and submaxillary glands)

✦ Tooth discoloration (with potassium iodide)

thioamides

✦ Fever, sore throat

✦ Hypersensitivity reactions (pruritus, rash, or fever in the first 3 weeks of treatment)

✦ Leukopenia, thrombocytopenia

✦ Potentially fatal granulocytopenia

Propylthiouracil, which lowers the T_3 level faster than methimazole, is usually used for rapid improvement of severe hyperthyroidism. It's also preferred for developmental reasons. (See *Reducing the risks of antithyroid drugs.*)

Because methimazole blocks thyroid hormone formation for a longer time, it's better suited for administration once per day to patients with mild to moderate hyperthyroidism. Therapy may continue for 12 to 24 months before remission occurs.

To treat hyperthyroidism, the thyroid gland may be removed by surgery or destroyed by radiation using radioactive iodine. Before surgery, stable iodine is used to prepare the gland for surgical removal by firming it and decreasing its vascularity. Radioactive iodine may also be used to treat thyroid cancer.

Stable iodine is also used after radioactive iodine therapy to control symptoms of hyperthyroidism while the radiation takes effect.

Interactions

✦ Iodides may react synergistically with lithium, which may cause hypothyroidism.

Adverse reactions

The most serious adverse reaction to thioamide therapy is potentially fatal granulocytopenia. It typically appears 4 to 8 weeks after treatment begins and usually produces a precipitous drop in white blood cell count. Thionamides may also cause thrombocytopenia and leukopenia. The patient may develop a sore throat or fever.

Hypersensitivity reactions to thioamides commonly produce pruritus, rash, or fever in the first 3 weeks of treatment.

Iodides can cause *iodism,* or chronic toxicity from iodine therapy, which is dosage-dependent. Iodism can produce an unpleasant brassy taste and burning sensation in the mouth and increased salivation and swelling of the parotid and submaxillary glands. Other signs and symptoms may include headache, rhinitis, conjunctivitis, gastric irritation, bloody diarrhea, anorexia, and depression. These reactions should disappear a few days after iodine therapy is stopped.

Potassium iodide can cause tooth discoloration. Radioactive iodine can produce a feeling of fullness in the neck and a metallic taste and can increase the risk of birth defects and leukemia.

CLINICAL ALERT Rarely, I.V. iodine administration can cause an acute hypersensitivity reaction characterized by angioedema, hemorrhagic skin lesions, and serum sickness. Radioactive iodine can also cause a rare — but acute — reaction 3 to 14 days after administration. During this time, thyroglobulin pours out of damaged follicles and can lead to acute exacerbation of hyperthyroidism and thyroid crisis. Thyroid crisis may also occur after propylthiouracil withdrawal or after giving iodine or iodinated contrast dye.

Nursing considerations
✦ Monitor the patient for adverse reactions and drug interactions during antithyroid drug therapy.
✦ Monitor the patient's complete blood count periodically to detect impending granulocytopenia, leukopenia, and thrombocytopenia. If any of these conditions exists, notify the prescriber. If laboratory results reveal fewer than 1,500 granulocytes/mm^3, stop the drug and give an antibiotic.
✦ Monitor the patient receiving an iodide for signs and symptoms of iodism, such as increased salivation and swelling of the parotid and submaxillary glands, rhinitis, GI distress, and depression. Stop iodide therapy if iodism occurs.
✦ Observe the patient for hypersensitivity reactions to the antithyroid drug.
✦ Monitor the patient for signs and symptoms of thyroid crisis after giving iodine, iodinated contrast dye, or radioactive iodine or after stopping propylthiouracil. Give emergency treatment as needed.
✦ Evaluate the patient's response to treatment. With propylthiouracil, his T$_4$ level should return to normal 14 to 60 days after therapy begins. The average time to reach a euthyroid state is 42 to 49 days, but this can vary with the drug dosage.
✦ Monitor the patient for signs and symptoms of toxicity, such as thyroid gland enlargement, and of hypothyroidism, such as depression, cold intolerance, and nonpitting edema.

CLINICAL ALERT
✦ Take full radiation precautions for 24 hours after a patient receives a dose of radioactive iodine for hyperthyroidism. The patient will have slightly radioactive urine and saliva for 24 hours, and highly radioactive vomitus for 6 to 8 hours after taking the dose.
✦ Isolate a patient who receives a dose of radioactive iodine for thyroid cancer because the patient will have radioactive urine, saliva, and perspiration for 3 days. Also take these precautions: ensure that pregnant women don't take care of the patient, provide disposable eating utensils and linens, and have the patient save all urine for 24 to 48 hours in a lead container so that the laboratory can measure the amount of radioactive material excreted. Have him drink as much fluid as possible for 48 hours after drug administration to promote excretion. Limit contact with the patient to 30 minutes per person per shift on the first day and 1 hour on the second day.

✦ Notify the prescriber if adverse reactions or drug interactions occur.
✦ Teach the patient and his family about the prescribed drug. (See *Teaching a patient about antithyroid drugs,* page 478.)

Key nursing actions
✦ Monitor CBC periodically to detect granulocytopenia, leukopenia, and thrombocytopenia.
✦ Monitor the patient receiving an iodide for evidence of iodism, such as increased salivation, swelling of the parotid and submaxillary glands, rhinitis, GI distress, and depression. Stop iodide therapy if iodism occurs.
✦ Monitor for evidence of thyroid crisis after giving iodine, iodinated contrast dye, or radioactive iodine or after stopping propylthiouracil. Give emergency treatment as needed.
✦ Evaluate the patient's response to treatment.
✦ Monitor for evidence of toxicity, such as thyroid gland enlargement. Also, watch for evidence of hypothyroidism, such as depression, cold intolerance, and nonpitting edema.
✦ Take full radiation precautions for 24 hours after a patient receives a dose of radioactive iodine for hyperthyroidism.
✦ Isolate a patient who receives radioactive iodine for thyroid cancer because he will have radioactive urine, saliva, and perspiration for 3 days.

Teaching a patient about antithyroid drugs

Whenever an antithyroid drug is prescribed, teach the patient and his family the drug's name, dose, frequency, action, and adverse effects. Also take the following actions.

◆ Instruct the patient receiving a thioamide to call the prescriber immediately if he experiences a sore throat and fever. Explain that the patient may need blood tests and a throat culture if these problems appear. Inform him that they're most likely to occur 4 to 8 weeks after drug therapy begins.

◆ Teach the patient to recognize and report the signs and symptoms of iodism during iodide therapy.

◆ If a patient is discharged fewer than 7 days after receiving radioactive iodine for thyroid cancer, advise him to avoid close prolonged contact with small children. Also instruct him not to sleep in the same room with anyone else for 7 days after treatment because of the risk of thyroid cancer for people exposed to radioactive iodine. Inform him that using the same bathroom as the rest of the family is safe.

◆ Review radiation precautions with the patient who receives radioactive iodine for hyperthyroidism or thyroid cancer.

◆ Teach the patient to recognize the signs and symptoms of hypersensitivity reactions, such as pruritus and rash. Explain that these reactions may occur during the first 3 weeks of therapy, and if they do, the prescriber may order a different drug or treat the reaction with an antihistamine.

◆ Teach the patient to recognize the signs and symptoms of hypothyroidism, which may occur after radioactive iodine therapy.

◆ Advise a pregnant patient that she shouldn't receive radiation therapy. Counsel a woman to wait several months after therapy before becoming pregnant. Advise a man not to father a child for several months after therapy.

◆ Teach the patient to keep the antithyroid drug in a light-resistant container.

◆ Advise the patient to take the antithyroid drug with meals to prevent adverse GI reactions. Radioactive iodine, however, requires overnight fasting before administration.

◆ Instruct the patient to dilute potassium iodide with water, milk, or fruit juice to mask the salty taste and to drink it through a straw to avoid tooth discoloration.

◆ Advise the patient to consult the prescriber before eating iodized salt and iodine-rich foods, such as shellfish, during antithyroid drug therapy. Also tell him to consult the prescriber before using any over-the-counter cough medicines because they may contain iodine.

◆ Instruct the patient to notify the prescriber if adverse reactions occur.

Features of pituitary drugs

◆ These drugs mimic pituitary hormones.
◆ Anterior pituitary drugs control other endocrine glands.
◆ Posterior pituitary drugs regulate fluid volume and stimulate smooth muscle contraction.

PITUITARY DRUGS

Pituitary drugs are natural or synthetic hormones that mimic the hormones produced by the pituitary gland. These drugs consist of two groups. Anterior pituitary drugs may be used diagnostically or therapeutically to control the function of other endocrine glands, such as the thyroid gland, adrenal glands, ovaries, and testes. Posterior pituitary drugs may be used to regulate fluid volume and stimulate smooth-muscle contraction in selected clinical situations.

ANTERIOR PITUITARY DRUGS

Protein hormones produced in the anterior pituitary gland regulate growth, development, and sexual characteristics by stimulating the actions of other endocrine glands. Anterior pituitary drugs include:

✦ adrenocorticotropics, such as corticotropin, cosyntropin, and repository corticotropin

✦ growth hormones, such as somatrem and somatropin

✦ gonadotropics, such as chorionic gonadotropin and menotropins

✦ thyrotropics, such as protirelin and TSH (or thyrotropin).

Pharmacokinetics

Anterior pituitary drugs aren't given orally because they're destroyed in the GI tract. Some of them can be given topically, but most require injection.

Usually, natural hormones are absorbed, distributed, and metabolized rapidly. Some analogues are absorbed and metabolized more slowly. Anterior pituitary drugs are metabolized at receptor sites and in the liver and kidneys. They're excreted primarily in urine.

Pharmacodynamics

Anterior pituitary drugs exert a profound effect on the body's growth and development. The hypothalamus controls pituitary gland secretions. In turn, the pituitary gland secretes hormones that regulate the secretions or functions of other glands.

Hormone levels in the blood help determine hormone production rates. Increased hormone levels inhibit hormone production; decreased levels raise production and secretion.

Pharmacotherapeutics

Clinical indications for anterior pituitary drugs are diagnostic and therapeutic. Corticotropin and cosyntropin are used diagnostically to differentiate between primary and secondary failure of the adrenal cortex. Corticotropin is also used to treat adrenal insufficiency.

Somatrem and somatropin are used for long-term treatment of growth failure in children with inadequate GH secretion. Somatropin can also be prescribed to treat growth failure caused by chronic renal insufficiency, short stature related to Turner's syndrome, growth failure in children with Prader-Willi syndrome. It may also be used to replace endogenous GH in adults with GH deficiency.

Chorionic gonadotropin is used to diagnose and treat cryptorchidism and to treat infertility. Menotropins is used to treat anovulation and infertility. Human TSH is used as an adjunct in diagnosing thyroid cancer.

Interactions

✦ When given with corticotropin, immunizations can increase the risk of neurologic complications and may reduce the antibody response.

✦ Corticotropin can reduce the salicylate level.

✦ When used with corticotropin, diuretics can enhance potassium loss.

✦ Barbiturates, phenytoin, and rifampin can increase corticotropin metabolism, reducing its effects.

Features of anterior pituitary drugs

corticotropin and cosyntropin

✦ Are used diagnostically to differentiate between primary and secondary failure of the adrenal cortex

corticotropin

✦ Is used to treat adrenal insufficiency

somatrem and somatropin

✦ Are used for long-term treatment of growth failure in children with inadequate GH secretion

somatropin

✦ Is used to treat growth failure from chronic renal insufficiency, short stature related to Turner's syndrome, growth failure in children with Prader-Willi syndrome

✦ Is used to replace endogenous GH in adults with GH deficiency

chorionic gonadotropin

✦ Is used to diagnose and treat cryptorchidism and to treat infertility

menotropins

✦ Is used to treat anovulation and infertility

human TSH

✦ Is used as an adjunct in diagnosing thyroid cancer

WARNING

Spotting the signs of ovarian hyperstimulation

During gonadotropic drug therapy, monitor the patient for signs and symptoms of ovarian hyperstimulation syndrome. This dangerous adverse reaction may progress rapidly to a dramatic increase in vascular permeability, which causes rapid accumulation of fluid in the peritoneal cavity, thorax, and pericardium. To detect ovarian hyperstimulation syndrome, watch for:

✦ hypovolemia
✦ hemoconcentration
✦ electrolyte imbalance

✦ ascites
✦ hemoperitoneum
✦ pleural effusion

✦ hydrothorax
✦ thromboembolism.

Adverse reactions to watch for

✦ Hypersensitivity reactions

chorionic gonadotropins and menotropins
✦ Gynecomastia
✦ Headache
✦ Injection site pain
✦ Ovarian hyperstimulation syndrome

corticotropin
✦ Dizziness, euphoria, seizures
✦ Iatrogenic Cushing's syndrome (with long-term use)
✦ Impaired wound healing
✦ Sodium and water retention

cosyntropin
✦ Flushing
✦ Pruritus

somatrem
✦ Glucose intolerance
✦ Hypothyroidism

TSH
✦ Facial flushing
✦ Headache
✦ Nausea, stomach discomfort, vomiting
✦ Urinary frequency

✦ Estrogen can increase corticotropin's effects.
✦ Use of cosyntropin with an amphetamine, an estrogen, or lithium can alter the results of adrenal function tests.
✦ Use of amphetamines or androgens with somatrem may promote epiphyseal closure.
✦ Corticosteroids can inhibit somatrem's growth-promoting action.

Adverse reactions

Because of the polypeptide nature of all pituitary drugs, the major adverse reactions are hypersensitivity reactions. Short-term, intensive drug therapy with hormones derived from animal sources increases the risk of hypersensitivity reactions. Therapy with synthetic hormones is less likely to produce these reactions.

Because the dosage must vary, the number and types of adverse reactions also vary. The most common dose-related reactions from corticotropin include sodium and water retention, impaired wound healing, dizziness, seizures, and euphoria. Less common dose-related reactions include hypokalemia, hypertension, ketosis, immunosuppression, skin hyperpigmentation, and mood elevation. Long-term use of corticotropin can cause iatrogenic Cushing's syndrome that's indistinguishable from the naturally occurring condition.

Cosyntropin administration may cause pruritus and flushing.

Somatrem may cause glucose intolerance and hypothyroidism. A large percentage of patients treated with somatrem develop antibodies to it. However, the antibodies usually don't interfere with the drug's effectiveness. Adverse reactions to somatropin are uncommon, but may include weakness, hypothyroidism, and injection site pain.

Chorionic gonadotropin and menotropins can produce ovarian hyperstimulation syndrome. (See *Spotting the signs of ovarian hyperstimulation.*) They may also cause gynecomastia, headache, and injection site pain.

TSH may cause facial flushing, urinary frequency, headache, nausea, vomiting, and stomach discomfort.

Nursing considerations

✦ Perform a hypersensitivity skin test before giving an anterior pituitary drug. After the test, document the result. If it's normal, begin therapy as indicated. If it's abnormal, notify the prescriber.

✦ Keep epinephrine 1:1,000 readily available for emergency treatment of a hypersensitivity reaction.

✦ Observe the patient for hypersensitivity reactions during the first 15 minutes of I.V. administration or immediately after I.M. or S.C. injection.

✦ Observe the patient for signs of hypersensitivity, such as urticaria, tachycardia, and pruritus, after the cosyntropin test.

✦ Monitor the patient for signs and symptoms of electrolyte imbalances and other adverse reactions during therapy with an anterior pituitary drug. Also monitor for drug interactions.

✦ Monitor the patient's thyroid function and glucose, blood urea nitrogen, and electrolyte levels during somatrem therapy.

✦ Check the urine and plasma corticosteroid levels to measure the adrenal response before and after administering corticotropin to test adrenocortical function.

✦ Place the patient on a high-potassium diet as needed to offset corticotropin-induced loss of potassium.

✦ Use caution when matching the type of preparation to the administration method. I.V. infusions of corticotropin require aqueous solutions; I.M. and S.C. injections require suspension and gelatin solutions.

✦ Give repository corticotropin and corticotropin zinc hydroxide I.M. only. Shake these drugs before injecting them into the gluteal muscle.

✦ Taper off doses of corticotropin during high-dosage therapy rather than suddenly stopping the drug because withdrawal usually causes 2 to 5 days of hypofunction.

✦ Protect corticotropin solutions from heat, temperatures below freezing, and agitation to avoid denaturing the drug's protein molecules.

✦ Refrigerate an anterior pituitary drug for storage but avoid freezing. Use the contents of reconstituted vials within 1 week.

✦ If adverse reactions or drug interactions occur, notify the prescriber.

✦ Monitor the patient for signs of fluid retention (such as ankle swelling, jugular vein distention, and crackles in the lungs upon auscultation) during corticotropin therapy.

✦ Provide a low-sodium diet and restrict fluids throughout corticotropin therapy if needed.

✦ During corticotropin therapy, weigh the patient daily, particularly noting a sudden increase of 2 lb (1 kg) or more.

✦ During corticotropin therapy, monitor the patient's blood pressure regularly to detect hypertension. Also monitor his fluid intake and output to identify electrolyte imbalances.

 CLINICAL ALERT Watch for signs and symptoms of ovarian hyperstimulation syndrome in a patient who receives chorionic gonadotropin or menotropins.

✦ Teach the patient and his family about the prescribed drug. (See *Teaching a patient about anterior pituitary drugs,* page 482.)

(See *Teaching a patient about anterior pituitary drugs,* page 482.)

Key nursing actions

✦ Perform a hypersensitivity skin test before giving the drug.

✦ Keep epinephrine 1:1,000 readily available in case of hypersensitivity reaction.

✦ Watch for evidence of electrolyte imbalances and other adverse reactions during therapy.

✦ Watch for urticaria, tachycardia, and pruritus after the cosyntropin test.

✦ Monitor thyroid function and glucose, blood urea nitrogen, and electrolyte levels during somatrem therapy.

✦ Watch for ovarian hyperstimulation syndrome in a patient who receives chorionic gonadotropin or menotropins.

corticotropin

✦ Check urine and plasma corticosteroid levels to measure the adrenal response before and after giving corticotropin to test adrenocortical function.

✦ Provide a high-potassium diet as needed to offset corticotropin-induced loss of potassium.

✦ Watch for evidence of fluid retention during therapy.

✦ Provide a low-sodium diet and restrict fluids if needed. Weigh the patient daily, noting a sudden increase of 2 lb (1 kg) or more.

✦ Monitor the patient's blood pressure and fluid intake and output.

Actions of posterior pituitary drugs

ADH

◆ Increases cyclic adenosine monophosphate, which increases the permeability of renal tubules, promoting water reabsorption

◆ Stimulates blood vessel contraction, increasing blood pressure

desmopressin

◆ Reduces diuresis and promotes clotting by increasing the factor VIII (antihemophilic factor) level

oxytocin

◆ Stimulates uterine contractions in pregnant women by increasing the permeability of uterine cell membranes to sodium ions

POSTERIOR PITUITARY DRUGS

Posterior pituitary hormones are synthesized in the hypothalamus and stored in the posterior pituitary gland. Then the posterior pituitary secretes the hormones into the blood. Posterior pituitary drugs include all forms of ADH, such as desmopressin and vasopressin, as well as the oxytocic drug, oxytocin.

Pharmacokinetics

Because enzymes in the GI tract can destroy all protein hormones, these drugs can't be given orally. Posterior pituitary drugs may be given by injection or intranasal spray.

Like other posterior pituitary drugs, oxytocin is usually absorbed, distributed, metabolized rapidly, and excreted in urine. With parenteral administration, oxytocin is absorbed rapidly; with intranasal use, absorption is erratic.

Pharmacodynamics

Under neural control, posterior pituitary hormones affect smooth-muscle contraction in the uterus, bladder, and GI tract. They also affect fluid balance through kidney reabsorption of water, and influence blood pressure through stimulation of the arterial wall muscles.

All forms of ADH increase cyclic adenosine monophosphate. This increases the permeability of the renal tubules, promoting water reabsorption. In high dosages, ADH stimulates blood vessel contraction, increasing the blood pressure.

In addition, desmopressin reduces diuresis and promotes clotting by increasing the factor VIII (antihemophilic factor) level.

In pregnant women, oxytocin may stimulate uterine contractions by increasing the permeability of uterine cell membranes to sodium ions. It can also stimulate lactation through its effect on the mammary glands.

Pharmacotherapeutics

ADH is prescribed for hormone replacement therapy in patients with *neurogenic diabetes insipidus,* or excessive loss of urine caused by a brain lesion or injury that interferes with ADH synthesis or release. However, it doesn't effectively treat nephrogenic diabetes insipidus (caused by renal tubular resistance to ADH).

Desmopressin is the drug of choice for chronic ADH deficiency. In addition, desmopressin is indicated to treat primary nocturnal enuresis. Given intranasally, this drug has a relatively long duration and a relative lack of adverse effects.

Short-term ADH treatment is indicated for patients with transient diabetes insipidus after head injury or surgery; therapy may be lifelong for patients with idiopathic hormone deficiencies. Used for short-term therapy, vasopressin elevates blood pressure in patients with hypotension caused by lack of vascular tone. It also relieves postoperative gaseous distention.

Oxytocin is used to induce labor, to complete incomplete abortions, and to treat preeclampsia, eclampsia, and premature rupture of membranes. After delivery, it's used to control bleeding and uterine relaxation, hasten uterine shrinking, and stimulate lactation.

Interactions

✦ Alcohol, demeclocycline, or lithium may decrease the ADH activity of desmopressin or vasopressin.
✦ Carbamazepine, chlorpropamide, clofibrate, or cyclophosphamide can increase ADH activity.
✦ When barbiturates or cyclopropane anesthetics are used with ADH, synergistic effects may occur and lead to coronary insufficiency or arrhythmias.
✦ Cyclophosphamide may increase the oxytocic effects of oxytocin.
✦ When used with vasopressors (such as anesthetics, ephedrine, or methoxamine), oxytocin can increase the risk of hypertensive crisis and postpartum rupture of cerebral blood vessels.

Adverse reactions

Hypersensitivity reactions are the most common adverse reactions to ADH drugs and oxytocics. These reactions occur more commonly with natural hormone extracts than with synthetic drug preparations. Large dosages of an ADH drug can cause GI distress and cardiovascular problems.

Common dose-related reactions to natural ADH drugs include circumoral and facial pallor, increased GI motility, and abdominal and uterine cramps. Other adverse reactions include tinnitus, anxiety, hyponatremia, albuminuria, eclamptic attacks, mydriasis, and transient edema. Nasal preparations can cause irritation, rhinorrhea, and nasal passage ulceration. Accidental deep inhalation of the powder preparation into the bronchial passages may cause substernal tightness, coughing,

Uses of posterior pituitary drugs

ADH
✦ Is used for hormone replacement in patients with neurogenic diabetes insipidus or idiopathic hormone deficiency

desmopressin
✦ Is the drug of choice for chronic ADH deficiency
✦ Is used to treat primary nocturnal enuresis

oxytocin
✦ Is used to induce labor, to complete incomplete abortions, and to treat preeclampsia, eclampsia, and premature rupture of membranes
✦ Is used after delivery to control bleeding and uterine relaxation, hasten uterine shrinking, and stimulate lactation

vasopressin
✦ Is used to raise blood pressure in hypotension caused by lack of vascular tone
✦ is used to relieve postoperative gaseous distention

Adverse reactions to watch for

- ✦ Cardiovascular problems, GI distress (with large doses)
- ✦ Hypersensitivity reactions (more common with natural than synthetic extracts)

Natural ADH drugs

- ✦ Abdominal cramps, increased GI motility
- ✦ Albuminurea, hyponatremia
- ✦ Anxiety
- ✦ Circumoral and facial pallor
- ✦ Eclamptic attacks
- ✦ Irritation or ulceration of nasal passage, rhinorrhea (with nasal form)
- ✦ Mydriasis
- ✦ Tinnitus
- ✦ Transient edema
- ✦ Uterine cramps

Synthetic oxytocin

- ✦ Diaphoresis, dizziness, headache, tinnitus
- ✦ GI disturbances
- ✦ Postpartum hemorrhage
- ✦ Severe water intoxication (with infusion over 24 hours)

and transient dyspnea. Large dosages may increase blood pressure. Anaphylaxis may occur after injection.

Adverse reactions to synthetic ADH drugs are rare, although high dosages can cause transient headaches, nausea, nasal congestion, rhinitis, flushing, mild abdominal cramps, and vulvar pain. Decreasing the dosage usually reduces these reactions.

Synthetic extracts have replaced natural oxytocics. Synthetic oxytocin, however, can cause adverse reactions, such as postpartum hemorrhage, GI disturbances, diaphoresis, headache, dizziness, and tinnitus. Severe water intoxication has been linked to slow oxytocin infusion over 24 hours.

 CLINICAL ALERT Excessive dosages or drug hypersensitivity may result in uterine hypertonicity, tetany, or uterine rupture. Uterine hypertonicity can produce fetal asphyxia, which may lead to fetal bradycardia and neonatal jaundice, arrhythmias, or death.

Nursing considerations

- ✦ Monitor the patient for adverse reactions and drug interactions during therapy with a posterior pituitary drug.
- ✦ Monitor the patient for hypersensitivity reactions to the posterior pituitary drug, and be prepared to deliver emergency treatment.
- ✦ If GI distress occurs, monitor the patient's hydration status. Give an antiemetic or antidiarrheal as needed.
- ✦ Frequently assess the patient's cardiovascular function. Particularly note vital sign abnormalities, such as irregular heartbeat or increased blood pressure, as well as such signs and symptoms as chest discomfort, shortness of breath, or skin color changes. Notify the prescriber if abnormalities occur.
- ✦ Monitor the patient's urine output to assess the effectiveness of antidiuretic therapy used to treat diabetes insipidus.
- ✦ Inspect the patient's nasal passages frequently when a natural ADH drug is given nasally. Be alert for nasal irritation, nasal ulcerations, or rhinorrhea.
- ✦ Assess the patient for bowel sounds, flatus passage, and resumption of bowel movements during ADH drug therapy used to improve peristalsis in the GI tract.
- ✦ Check the expiration date on the desmopressin label before use. Nasal solutions expire 1 year after the date of manufacture.
- ✦ Store parenteral and nasal desmopressin in a refrigerator at 39° F (4° C). Discard any cloudy or discolored solution.
- ✦ Ensure that a prescriber is present during I.V. or I.M. administration of oxytocin.
- ✦ Keep magnesium sulfate available during I.M. administration of oxytocin to produce endometrial relaxation, if needed.
- ✦ Assess uterine contractions and the fetal heart rate during oxytocin administration. If contractions become more frequent than every 2 minutes and last longer than 60 seconds without uterine relaxation, if contractions become excessively strong or exceed 50 mm Hg as measured on a monitor, or if the fetal heart rate indicates bradycardia, tachycardia, or irregular rhythm as measured on a monitor, stop the I.V. infusion immediately, administer oxygen, and notify the prescriber.
- ✦ Keep the plastic nasal tube for oxytocin administration clean and dry. Measure the nasal oxytocin dosage exactly because the drug is potent.

Teaching a patient about posterior pituitary drugs

Whenever a posterior pituitary drug is prescribed, teach the patient and his family the drug's name, dose, frequency, action, and adverse effects. Also take the following actions.

◆ Teach the patient how to give himself the drug. Instruct the patient to clear his nasal passages before administering a nasal preparation, to hold the squeeze bottle upright, and to spray into the nostril while sitting with the head vertical. Advise him not to administer a nasal preparation while lying down or with his head tilted back.

◆ Teach the patient how to measure his fluid intake and output and how to interpret 24-hour fluid measurement during antidiuretic hormone therapy.

◆ Instruct the patient to never increase the number of vasopressin sprays without consulting the prescriber.

◆ Explain the purpose of I.V. oxytocin to the patient and describe the expected outcome. Advise her that I.V. oxytocin is always given under a prescriber's supervision.

◆ Advise the patient to notify the prescriber if adverse reactions occur.

◆ If adverse reactions or drug interactions occur or if the drug is ineffective, notify the prescriber.

◆ Monitor the patient for early signs of water intoxication when giving oxytocin. Document the patient's fluid intake and output.

◆ Notify the prescriber if the patient displays signs or symptoms of water intoxication.

◆ Teach the patient and his family about the prescribed drug. (See *Teaching a patient about posterior pituitary drugs.*)

ESTROGENS

Estrogens mimic the physiologic effects of natural female sex hormones. They're used to correct estrogen-deficient states and, along with hormonal contraceptives, to prevent pregnancy.

Estrogens that treat endocrine system disorders include natural hormones (such as conjugated estrogens, estradiol, and estropipate) and synthetic versions (such as esterified estrogens, estradiol, estradiol cypionate, estradiol valerate, and ethinyl estradiol).

Pharmacokinetics

Estrogens are absorbed well and distributed throughout the body. Metabolism occurs in the liver, and the metabolites are excreted primarily by the kidneys.

Pharmacodynamics

The exact mechanism of action of estrogens isn't clearly understood, but they may increase the synthesis of deoxyribonucleic acid, ribonucleic acid, and protein in estrogen-responsive tissues in female breasts, urinary tract, and genital organs.

Key nursing actions

◆ Watch for hypersensitivity reactions.

◆ If GI distress occurs, monitor the patient's hydration.

◆ Assess cardiovascular function frequently.

◆ Monitor urine output if the patient has diabetes insipidus.

◆ Inspect the nasal passages if giving a nasal drug form.

◆ Check for bowel sounds, flatus passage, and resumption of bowel movements if therapy is intended to improve peristalsis.

◆ Assess uterine contractions and the fetal heart rate during oxytocin administration.

◆ Check for early evidence of water intoxication when giving oxytocin. Document fluid intake and output.

Features of estrogens

◆ Mimic the physiologic effects of natural female sex hormones

◆ May increase synthesis of DNA, RNA, and protein in estrogen-responsive tissues in female breasts, urinary tract, and genital organs

◆ Are used for hormone replacement in postmenopausal women to relieve signs and symptoms of decreased ovarian function

◆ Are used for hormone replacement therapy in women with primary ovarian failure or female hypogonadism and in patients who have undergone surgical castration

Applying the findings of the Women's Health Initiative

In 2003, the Women's Health Initiative reported increased risks of myocardial infarction, stroke, breast cancer, pulmonary emboli, and deep vein thrombosis in women who received 0.625 mg conjugated equine estrogens and 2.5 mg medroxyprogesterone acetate for 5 years, compared to women who received placebo. Although researchers didn't study other doses, the risks are assumed to be similar.

Based on these findings, adapt care appropriately:

✦ Use estrogens (with or without progesterone) at the lowest effective dose and for the shortest duration possible. This use is recommended by the American College of Obstetrics and Gynecology and the Food and Drug Administration for women who want hormone replacement therapy to relieve menopausal symptoms.

✦ Avoid the use of estrogens and progestins to prevent chronic disease, as recommended by the United States Preventive Task Force.

✦ Inform the patient that the long-term safety of short-term therapy hasn't been studied yet.

Features of estrogens
(continued)

✦ Are used for palliation in advanced, inoperable breast cancer in postmenopausal women and prostate cancer in men

Adverse reactions to watch for

✦ Acne, hypersensitivity reactions, melasma, rash, urticaria

✦ Altered libido, depression, dizziness, migraine headaches

✦ Altered menstrual flow, amenorrhea, breakthrough bleeding, dysmenorrhea, spotting, vaginal candidiasis

✦ Altered thyroid and liver function test results, cholestatic jaundice, decreased glucose tolerance

✦ Breast tenderness, enlargement, and secretions

Pharmacotherapeutics

Estrogens are prescribed primarily for hormone replacement therapy in postmenopausal women to relieve signs and symptoms of decreased ovarian function. (See *Applying the findings of the Women's Health Initiative.*)

Less commonly, estrogens are used as hormonal replacement therapy in women with primary ovarian failure or female hypogonadism and in patients who have undergone surgical castration. They're also used palliatively to treat advanced, inoperable breast cancer in postmenopausal women and prostate cancer in men.

Interactions

✦ Estrogens may decrease the effects of anticoagulants, which increases the risk of blood clots.

✦ Antibiotics, barbiturates, carbamazepine, phenytoin, primidone, and rifampin can reduce estrogen effectiveness.

✦ Estrogens can interfere with folic acid absorption from food, which may lead to folic acid deficiency.

Adverse reactions

Most adverse reactions to estrogens are mild and don't have serious or long-term consequences. However, endometrial and breast cancer may be more likely to occur in women taking estrogens. The risk of endometrial cancer increases fourfold to eightfold in women taking estrogens. Most of the risk appears to be dose-related — higher dosages over longer periods increase the risk.

Long-term estrogen use may cause increased blood pressure (sometimes in the hypertensive range) and thromboembolic disease, such as deep vein thrombosis and pulmonary embolism. The risk of thromboembolic disease increases markedly with cigarette smoking, especially in women older than age 35.

Teaching a patient about estrogens

Whenever an estrogen is prescribed, teach the patient and his family the drug's name, dose, frequency, action, and adverse effects. Also take the following actions.

◆ Advise the patient to read the estrogen package insert. Explain and reinforce this information as needed.

◆ Instruct the patient to report signs and symptoms of disorders linked to estrogen use, such as abdominal pain, abdominal mass, severe headache, slurred speech, vomiting, dizziness, faintness, weakness, numbness, heaviness in the chest, shortness of breath, blurred vision, blind spots, breast lumps, yellow skin or sclera, dark urine, or light-colored stools.

◆ Counsel a woman of childbearing age to use effective contraception because estrogens can cause congenital birth defects.

◆ Inform the patient that corneal curvature may change, causing vision disturbances or intolerance of hard or rigid gas-permeable contact lenses.

◆ Explain to the patient on cyclic therapy for postmenopausal symptoms that withdrawal bleeding may occur but doesn't indicate fertility restoration.

◆ Instruct the patient with diabetes to monitor his glucose level regularly and adjust the insulin or oral antidiabetic dosage as prescribed if estrogen causes hyperglycemia.

◆ Instruct the patient to avoid activities that require alertness if dizziness occurs.

◆ Stress the importance of returning for follow-up examinations and laboratory tests to detect adverse reactions.

◆ Teach a woman how to perform breast self-examination.

◆ Instruct the patient to notify the prescriber if adverse reactions occur.

Adverse reactions to watch for
(continued)

◆ Decreased absorption of dietary folic acid, increased lipoprotein levels

◆ Fluid retention, increased blood pressure

◆ Increased risk of breast cancer, endometrial cancer, gallbladder disease

◆ Intolerance of hard or rigid contact lenses, vision disturbances

◆ Thromboembolic disease (with long-term use)

The risk of gallbladder disease increases with estrogen use. Adverse metabolic reactions may include decreased glucose tolerance, altered thyroid and liver function test results, increased lipoprotein levels, fluid retention, decreased absorption of dietary folic acid, and cholestatic jaundice.

Adverse genitourinary reactions may include breakthrough bleeding, spotting, altered menstrual flow, dysmenorrhea, amenorrhea, and increased risk of vaginal candidiasis. Breast tenderness, enlargement, and secretions can also occur.

Adverse CNS reactions may include depression, migraine headaches, dizziness, and altered libido. Changed corneal curvature may cause vision disturbances or intolerance of hard or rigid gas-permeable contact lenses. Adverse skin reactions include melasma and acne. Urticaria, skin rashes, and rarely, hypersensitivity reactions may occur.

Nursing considerations

◆ Teach the patient and his family about the prescribed drug. (See *Teaching a patient about estrogens.*)

◆ Monitor the patient for adverse reactions and drug interactions during estrogen therapy.

◆ Perform a complete health history and physical examination before estrogen therapy begins and every 6 to 12 months thereafter.

◆ Before estrogen administration, determine if the patient is hypersensitive to natural oils, such as sesame, peanut, or castor oil. Some I.M. estrogen injections are dispersed in such oils.

Key nursing actions

✦ Perform a complete health history before therapy starts and every 6 to 12 months afterward.
✦ Monitor blood pressure often.
✦ Monitor glucose level regularly.
✦ Assess for evidence of folic acid deficiency.
✦ Monitor these results: metyrapone test, platelet count, thyroid and liver function tests, prothrombin time, and folate, triglyceride, and phospholipid levels.
✦ Check for evidence of fluid retention.

 CLINICAL ALERT Observe the patient for signs and symptoms of a thromboembolic disorder, such as deep vein thrombosis (producing calf tenderness, redness, and warmth) or pulmonary embolism (causing the sudden onset of shortness of breath, chest pain, and anxiety). Notify the prescriber immediately if they occur. Be prepared to administer treatment as needed.

✦ Monitor the patient's blood pressure frequently to detect estrogen-induced hypertension.
✦ Monitor the patient's glucose level regularly. For a diabetic patient, expect to adjust the insulin or oral antidiabetic dosage.
✦ Observe the patient for signs of folic acid deficiency, such as progressive fatigue, shortness of breath, weakness, irritability, and pallor.
✦ Monitor the results of the following tests to detect estrogen-induced abnormalities: metyrapone test, platelet count, thyroid and liver function tests, prothrombin time, and folate, triglyceride, and phospholipid levels. When any specimen is submitted, inform the laboratory that the patient is receiving estrogen. Notify the prescriber of any abnormal test results.
✦ Roll the I.M. drug vial between your palms to mix the contents completely.
✦ Give an I.M. injection deeply into a large muscle.
✦ Notify the prescriber if adverse reactions or drug interactions occur.
✦ Monitor the patient for signs and symptoms of fluid retention.
✦ If fluid retention occurs, place the patient on a low-sodium diet and restrict the fluid intake to no more than 2 qt (2 L) daily.

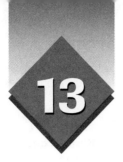

Immunomodulation drugs

Immune and inflammatory responses protect the body from invading foreign substances. These responses can be modified by four major groups of drugs, which have distinct actions.

◆ Antihistamines block the effects of histamine on target tissues.
◆ Corticosteroids suppress immune responses and reduce inflammation.
◆ Noncorticosteroid immunosuppressants prevent rejection of transplanted organs and are used to treat autoimmune diseases.
◆ Uricosurics and related drugs prevent or control the frequency of gouty arthritis attacks.

To understand the mechanisms of action of immunomodulation drugs, you need an overview of immune and inflammatory responses.

IMMUNE AND INFLAMMATORY RESPONSES

Immune and inflammatory responses protect the body from foreign substances and react to tissue injury. Usually, these responses help maintain homeostasis. Sometimes, they're harmful instead of helpful, such as when a patient undergoes organ transplantation or has an autoimmune disease. In such instances, drugs are used to suppress these responses.

The immune system is a highly complicated and regulated system. It produces two major types of response: cell-mediated and humoral responses.

Cell-mediated response

Cell-mediated response depends on the T-lymphocyte (T-cell) system. (They're called T cells because they come from the thymus.) Stem cells in the bone marrow give rise to T-cell precursors, which later are released from the thymus as mature T cells. T cells may be helper or suppressor cells. Helper T cells enhance the body's immune response; suppressor T cells inhibit it. Usually, helper T cells outnumber suppressor T cells by two to one. In a disease such as acquired immunodeficiency syndrome; however, the number of helper T cells drops to almost zero.

Reviewing cell-mediated response (*continued*)

✦ In autoimmune disease, cell-mediated response is activated by the patient's cells, which the immune system treats as foreign.

Reviewing humoral response

✦ Response depends on B-lymphocyte (B-cell) activity.
✦ B cells originate as stem-cell precursors in bone marrow.
✦ B cells respond to an antigen by differentiating into plasma cells that secrete antigen-specific antibodies.
✦ Antigen-antibody reaction activates the complement system, which causes lysis of antigen cells.

In an autoimmune disease, such as systemic lupus erythematosus or rheumatoid arthritis, the cell-mediated response is activated by the patient's cells, which his immune system treats as foreign substances.

Humoral response

The humoral response depends on B-lymphocyte (B-cell) activity. B cells are lymphocytes that originate as stem-cell precursors in the bone marrow. They respond to an antigen by differentiating into plasma cells that secrete antigen-specific antibodies. This antigen-antibody reaction activates the complement system, which causes lysis of antigenic cells.

Inflammation

Immune responses commonly result in inflammation, the local reaction of vascularized tissue to injury. When injury occurs, chemical reactions involving bradykinins, prostaglandins, and histamines result. These reactions cause vasodilation at the injury site, which increases blood flow, redness, and warmth. Capillary permeability also increases, which causes edema. Pain results from the edema and the effects of histamine and bradykinin on nerve endings. Leukocytes come to the area to remove cellular debris, which contributes to the edema and pain.

An exaggerated immune response, or hypersensitivity reaction, can occur in a sensitized individual. Reexposure to an allergen can cause such symptoms as rhinitis, wheezing, and red, tearing eyes.

ANTIHISTAMINES

Antihistamines are drugs that act as histamine-1 (H_1) receptor antagonists. In other words, they compete with histamine for binding to H_1-receptors throughout the body. However, they don't displace histamine already bound to receptors.

These drugs are used primarily to block histamine effects in an immediate (type I) hypersensitivity reaction, or allergic reaction. They're available alone or in combination products, by prescription or over the counter (OTC).

Based on their chemical structure, antihistamines are categorized into six major classes.
✦ Ethanolamines include clemastine, dimenhydrinate, diphenhydramine, and phenyltoloxamine, which is available only in combination products.
✦ Ethylenediamines include pyrilamine and tripelennamine — both of which are available only in combination products.
✦ Alkylamines include brompheniramine, chlorpheniramine, dexchlorpheniramine, and triprolidine.
✦ Phenothiazines include promethazine.
✦ Piperidines include azatadine, cetirizine, cyclizine, cyproheptadine, desloratadine, fexofenadine, loratadine, and meclizine.
✦ Miscellaneous drugs that also act as antihistamines include hydroxyzine.

Pharmacokinetics

After oral or parenteral administration, antihistamines are absorbed well. Some of these drugs can also be given rectally and are absorbed well.

Most antihistamines are distributed widely throughout the body and central nervous system (CNS), except for fexofenadine, desloratadine, and loratadine. These nonsedating antihistamines minimally penetrate the blood-brain barrier so that only a small amount of these drugs reaches the CNS, and they produce fewer adverse CNS reactions than other antihistamines.

Antihistamines are metabolized by liver enzymes and excreted in urine; only small amounts appear breast milk. Fexofenadine, mainly excreted in feces, is an exception.

Pharmacodynamics

Because antihistamines are H_1-receptor antagonists, they compete with histamine for H_1 receptors on *effector cells,* or cells that cause allergic symptoms, which blocks histamine from producing its effects. (See *How antihistamines stop an allergic response,* page 492.)

Antihistamines produce a wide range of effects. They:
+ block the action of histamine on small blood vessels.
+ decrease arteriolar dilation and tissue engorgement.
+ reduce *capillary permeability,* the leaking of plasma proteins and fluids out of the capillaries, which lessens edema.
+ inhibit most smooth-muscle responses to histamine. In particular, they block the constriction of bronchial, GI, and vascular smooth muscle.
+ relieve symptoms by affecting terminal nerve endings in the skin that flare and itch when stimulated by histamine.
+ suppress adrenal medulla stimulation, autonomic ganglia stimulation, and exocrine gland secretion, such as lacrimal and salivary secretion.

Several antihistamines have a high affinity for H_1 receptors in the brain and are used for their CNS effects. These drugs include dimenhydrinate, diphenhydramine, promethazine, and various piperidines.

Antihistamines don't affect parietal cell secretion in the stomach because they compete for H_1 receptors, not H_2 receptors.

Pharmacotherapeutics

Antihistamines are used to treat the symptoms of type I hypersensitivity reactions, such as allergic rhinitis, vasomotor rhinitis, allergic conjunctivitis, urticaria, and angioedema.

These drugs have other therapeutic uses. Many are used primarily as antiemetics to control nausea and vomiting. They can also be used as adjuncts in treating anaphylactic reactions after the serious symptoms are controlled. Diphenhydramine can help treat Parkinson's disease and drug-induced extrapyramidal reactions, such as abnormal involuntary movements. Because of its antiserotonin qualities, cyproheptadine may be used to treat Cushing's disease, serotonin-induced diarrhea, vascular cluster headaches, and anorexia nervosa.

Interactions

+ Antihistamines may block or reverse the vasopressor effects of epinephrine, which produces vasodilation, increased heart rate, and very low blood pressure.
+ Antihistamines may mask the signs and symptoms of ototoxicity caused by aminoglycosides or large doses of salicylates.
+ When used with CNS depressants, such as alcohol or tranquilizers, antihistamines may increase the sedative and respiratory depressant effects.
+ When taken with cimetidine, ciprofloxacin, clarithromycin, fluconazole, ketoconazole, itraconazole, macrolide antibiotics (such as erythromycin), or miconazole, loratadine may cause serious cardiac effects.

Adverse reactions

The most common adverse reaction to antihistamines is CNS depression, which can produce sedation and other symptoms. Occurring with usual dosages, sedation

Features of antihistamines

+ Compete with histamine for binding to histamine-1 receptor throughout the body
+ Block histamine action on small blood vessels, decrease arteriolar dilation and tissue engorgement, reduce capillary permeability, inhibit most smooth-muscle responses to histamine (especially bronchial, GI, and vascular smooth muscle), relieve symptoms in the skin, and suppress adrenal medulla stimulation, autonomic ganglia stimulation, and exocrine gland secretion
+ Are used mainly to block histamine effects in an immediate (type I) hypersensitivity reactions
+ Are also used as antiemetics and as adjuncts in treating anaphylactic reactions
+ Can be used for treating Parkinson's disease and drug-induced extrapyramidal symptoms (diphenhydramine)
+ May be used for serotonin-induced diarrhea, vascular cluster headaches, Cushing's disease, and anorexia nervosa (cyproheptadine)
+ Are available alone or in combination products, by prescription or over the counter

Understanding the action of antihistamines

✦ Antihistamines attach to H_1-receptor sites on effector cells, which are responsible for allergy symptoms
✦ By occupying these sites, antihistamines block histamine from binding to them and triggering allergic responses.

EYE ON DRUG ACTION

How antihistamines stop an allergic response

Although antihistamines can't reverse the signs and symptoms of an allergic response, they can stop the progression of the response. Here's what happens.

HISTAMINE RELEASE
When sensitized to an antigen, a mast cell reacts to repeated antigen exposure by releasing chemical mediators. One of these mediators, histamine, binds to histamine-1 (H_1) receptors on effector cells (the cells responsible for allergic symptoms). This initiates the allergic response that affects the respiratory, cardiovascular, GI, endocrine, and integumentary systems.

PREVENTION OF HISTAMINE BINDING
Antihistamines compete with histamine for H_1-receptor sites on effector cells. By attaching to these sites first, the drugs prevent more histamine from binding to effector cells.

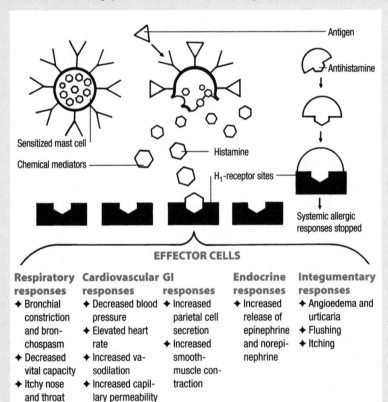

EFFECTOR CELLS

Respiratory responses
✦ Bronchial constriction and bronchospasm
✦ Decreased vital capacity
✦ Itchy nose and throat
✦ Rhinorrhea (runny nose)
✦ Sneezing

Cardiovascular responses
✦ Decreased blood pressure
✦ Elevated heart rate
✦ Increased vasodilation
✦ Increased capillary permeability

GI responses
✦ Increased parietal cell secretion
✦ Increased smooth-muscle contraction

Endocrine responses
✦ Increased release of epinephrine and norepinephrine

Integumentary responses
✦ Angioedema and urticaria
✦ Flushing
✦ Itching

can range from mild drowsiness to deep sleep. Other CNS reactions may include dizziness, lethargy, disturbed coordination, and muscle weakness. After 2 to 3 days of antihistamine therapy, these adverse reactions may disappear spontaneously. Less common reactions include CNS excitation, restlessness, insomnia, palpitations, and seizures.

The next most common adverse reactions are GI disturbances, including epigastric distress, loss of appetite, nausea, vomiting, and constipation or diarrhea. Taking the drug with meals or with milk may reduce these reactions.

The third most common reactions are anticholinergic ones, which occur especially with ethanolamines. Dry mouth, nose, and throat, and thickened bronchial secretions commonly occur. Other anticholinergic effects include urine retention and dysuria; vertigo, tinnitus, and labyrinthitis; and vision disturbances, such as diplopia and blurred vision. Cardiovascular effects, such as hypotension, hypertension, tachycardia, and arrhythmias, may also occur.

Sensitivity reactions to antihistamines aren't as common, but may include hypersensitivity, drug fever, hematologic complications, and teratogenic effects. Hypersensitivity manifested by urticaria, drug rash, and photosensitivity may occur with oral drug use, but usually results from topical application. Once a local hypersensitivity reaction occurs, topical or systemic reuse of that drug or any drug in its chemical class produces a similar reaction.

 CLINICAL ALERT Because of the wide use and ready availability of OTC antihistamines, acute poisoning (toxicity or overdose) commonly occurs, especially in children. The drugs' CNS effects pose the greatest threat and account for most of the signs and symptoms of poisoning: hallucinations, excitement, ataxia, athetosis, involuntary movements, and seizures. Another key sign of poisoning is drug fever, which is more common in children than in adults. Fixed, dilated pupils accompany other anticholinergic effects and may be followed by coma and death.

Although rare, hematologic complications include leukopenia, granulocytopenia, hemolytic anemia, thrombocytopenia, and pancytopenia.

Nursing considerations
✦ Monitor the patient for adverse reactions and drug interactions during antihistamine therapy.
✦ Decrease the dosage or use a different antihistamine if a mild adverse reaction occurs.

 CLINICAL ALERT Monitor the patient — especially a child — for signs of acute poisoning. Keep standard emergency equipment nearby. If acute poisoning occurs, stop the antihistamine and give symptomatic and supportive treatment, such as mechanical ventilation. If acute poisoning isn't recognized early, coma and death may occur.

✦ Observe the patient for signs of a hypersensitivity reaction, such as urticaria, drug rash, and photosensitivity, especially when giving a topical antihistamine.
✦ Give a standard antihistamine with meals or milk to decrease adverse GI reactions. Give a longer-acting preparation on an empty stomach or 2 hours after a meal.
✦ Monitor the patient's complete blood count (CBC) for adverse hematologic reactions to the prescribed antihistamine.
✦ Stop the antihistamine before the patient receives an allergy skin test to avoid masking abnormal results.

Adverse reactions to watch for
✦ Acute poisoning from overdose or toxicity
✦ Arrhythmias, hypertension, hypotension, tachycardia
✦ CNS depression, sedation
✦ CNS excitation, disturbed coordination, dizziness, insomnia, lethargy, muscle weakness, palpitations, restlessness, seizures
✦ Constipation, diarrhea, epigastric distress, loss of appetite, nausea, vomiting
✦ Drug fever, hematologic complications, hypersensitivity, teratogenic effects
✦ Dry mouth, nose, and throat; dysuria, urine retention; labyrinthitis, tinnitus, vertigo; thickened bronchial secretions; vision disturbances, such as blurred vision and diplopia

Teaching a patient about antihistamines

Whenever an antihistamine is prescribed, teach the patient and his family the drug's name, dose, frequency, action, and adverse effects. Also take the following actions.

✦ Review all contraindications with the patient to help prevent misuse of an over-the-counter (OTC) antihistamine. Advise against using an antihistamine if the patient is pregnant, is breast-feeding, or has a history of asthma, enlarged prostate, cardiovascular disease, hypertension, intestinal blockage, renal disease, overactive thyroid, stomach ulcer, or urinary tract blockage. Caution the patient against taking an antihistamine with an antimuscarinic, monoamine oxidase inhibitor, or a drug that can produce tinnitus or balance problems, such as aspirin, other salicylates, or aminoglycosides.

✦ Advise the patient with a severe allergy to carry identification or wear an identification band that lists the type of allergy, the usual treatment, and the prescriber's name.

✦ Review adverse central nervous system (CNS), anticholinergic, and GI reactions with the patient.

✦ Explain that the antihistamine can produce drowsiness and reduce alertness. Tell the patient that taking the drug at bedtime can minimize these symptoms, but may cause continued drowsiness in the morning. Reassure him that these effects may lessen after 2 to 3 days of use. Advise him not to drive or engage in activities that require alertness until the drug's CNS effects are known.

✦ Inform the patient that combining an antihistamine with alcohol or another CNS depressant adds to its sedative effects. Advise the patient taking an antihistamine to consult the prescriber before taking any CNS depressants, such as opioids, sedatives, barbiturates, OTC sleep aids, tranquilizers, tricyclic antidepressants, muscle relaxants, anesthetics, and alcohol.

✦ Remind the patient to keep this and other drugs out of the reach of children. Instruct him to be alert for signs of an overdose, such as clumsiness, unsteadiness, seizures, severe drowsiness, and hallucinations. Advise him to seek help immediately if an overdose is suspected.

✦ Instruct the patient to drink fluids, chew sugarless gum, or suck on sugarless candy if the antihistamine produces mouth dryness.

✦ Advise the patient to avoid exposure to the sun or to wear sunscreen, sunglasses, and a hat when in the sun.

✦ Suggest that the patient take an oral antihistamine with food or milk to minimize adverse GI reactions.

✦ Instruct the patient to take an antihistamine prescribed for motion sickness at least 30 minutes — preferably 1 to 2 hours — before traveling.

✦ Advise the patient to take a sustained-release capsule or long-acting tablet in whole form. Remind him not to break, cut, crush, or chew the drug.

✦ Instruct the patient to report adverse reactions to the prescriber because he may need a dosage change.

Key nursing actions

✦ Monitor the patient — especially a child — for evidence of acute poisoning.

✦ Watch for evidence of a hypersensitivity reaction, such as urticaria, rash, or photosensitivity, especially with a topical drug.

✦ Check CBC for adverse hematologic effects.

✦ Assess for sedation (the most common adverse reaction to antihistamines), especially when the regimen includes another CNS depressant.

✦ Give a parenteral antihistamine by deep I.M. injection, using the Z-track method to prevent subcutaneous irritation.

✦ Monitor the patient for sedation, the most common adverse reaction to antihistamines, especially when therapy also includes another CNS depressant.

✦ Take safety precautions if sedation occurs. For example, keep the bed rails up and supervise the patient's ambulation. Keep in mind that sedation and related effects may disappear spontaneously 2 to 3 days after antihistamine therapy begins.

✦ If adverse reactions or drug interactions occur or if the prescribed antihistamine is ineffective, notify the prescriber.

✦ Teach the patient and his family about the prescribed drug. (See *Teaching a patient about antihistamines*.)

CORTICOSTEROIDS

Corticosteroids suppress immune responses and reduce inflammation. They're available as natural or synthetic steroids.

Natural corticosteroids are hormones produced by the adrenal cortex; most corticosteroids are synthetic forms of these hormones. Natural and synthetic corticosteroids are classified based on their biological activities. Glucocorticoids affect carbohydrate and protein metabolism. Mineralocorticoids regulate electrolyte and water balance.

GLUCOCORTICOIDS

Most glucocorticoids are synthetic analogues of hormones secreted by the adrenal cortex. They exert anti-inflammatory, metabolic, and immunosuppressant effects.

Drugs in this class include beclomethasone, betamethasone, budesonide, cortisone, dexamethasone, hydrocortisone, methylprednisolone, prednisolone, prednisone, and triamcinolone.

Pharmacokinetics

After oral administration, glucocorticoids are absorbed well. After I.M. administration, they're absorbed completely. These drugs are bound to plasma proteins and distributed through the blood. Glucocorticoids are metabolized in the liver and excreted by the kidneys.

Pharmacodynamics

Glucocorticoids suppress hypersensitivity and immune responses through a process not entirely understood. Glucocorticoids probably inhibit immune responses by:
+ suppressing or preventing cell-mediated immune reactions
+ reducing leukocyte, monocyte, and eosinophil levels
+ decreasing immunoglobulin binding to cell surface receptors
+ inhibiting interleukin synthesis.

Glucocorticoids suppress the redness, edema, heat, and tenderness caused by the inflammatory response. They start on the cellular level by stabilizing the *lysosomal membrane,* a cell structure that contains digestive enzymes, so that it doesn't release its store of hydrolytic enzymes into the cells.

As corticosteroids, glucocorticoids prevent leakage of plasma from capillaries, suppress the migration of *polymorphonuclear leukocytes,* cells that kill and digest microorganisms, and inhibit phagocytosis.

Finally, glucocorticoids decrease antibody formation in injured or infected tissues and disrupt histamine synthesis, fibroblast development, collagen deposition, capillary dilation, and capillary permeability. (See *How glucocorticoids work,* page 496.)

Pharmacotherapeutics

Besides the use of glucocorticoids as replacement therapy for patients with adrenocortical insufficiency, these drugs are prescribed for immunosuppression and reduction of inflammation and for their effects on the blood and lymphatic systems. Topical glucocorticoids are used to treat localized inflammation.

Features of glucocorticoids

+ Are typically synthetic analogues of hormones secreted by the adrenal cortex
+ Exert anti-inflammatory, metabolic, and immunosuppressant effects (reducing the redness, edema, heat, and tenderness caused by inflammation)
+ Suppress hypersensitivity and immune responses, probably by suppressing cell-mediated immune reactions; reducing leukocyte, monocyte, and eosinophil levels; decreasing immunoglobulin binding to cell surface receptors; and inhibiting interleukin synthesis
+ Prevent plasma leakage from capillaries, suppress the migration of polymorphonuclear leukocytes, and inhibit phagocytosis
+ Decrease antibody formation in injured or infected tissues and disrupt histamine synthesis, fibroblast development, collagen deposition, capillary dilation, and capillary permeability
+ Are used as replacement therapy in adrenocortical insufficiency (for immunosuppression, reduction of inflammation, and effects on the blood and lymphatic systems)
+ Are used topically for localized inflammation

Healing actions of glucocorticoids

+ Stabilize WBC membranes
+ Reduce capillary permeability
+ Reduce WBC adhesions on capillary membranes
+ Inhibit macrophage buildup in traumatized tissue

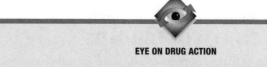

EYE ON DRUG ACTION

How glucocorticoids work

Tissue trauma normally leads to tissue irritation, edema, inflammation, and production of scar tissue. Administration of a glucocorticoid counteracts the initial effects of tissue trauma, promoting healing.

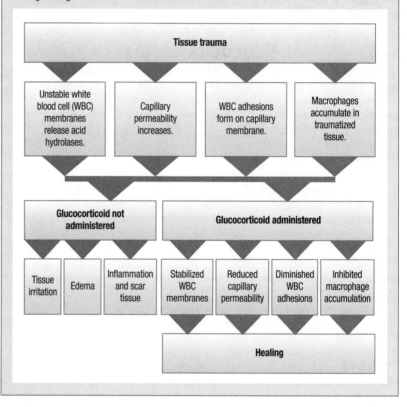

Interactions

+ Glucocorticoids can reduce the effects of aminoglutethimide, barbiturates, phenytoin, and rifampin.
+ Amphotericin B, chlorthalidone, ethacrynic acid, furosemide, and thiazide diuretics may enhance the potassium-wasting effects of a glucocorticoid.
+ Erythromycin and troleandomycin may reduce the metabolism—and increase the effects—of glucocorticoids.
+ Glucocorticoids can reduce the level and effects of a salicylate.
+ When nonsteroidal anti-inflammatory drugs or salicylates are used with glucocorticoids, the risk of peptic ulcers is increased.
+ Glucocorticoids may reduce the response to a vaccine or toxoid.
+ Estrogens and hormonal contraceptives containing estrogen can increase the effects of glucocorticoids.
+ Glucocorticoids may reduce the effects of insulin or oral antidiabetics, resulting in an increased glucose level.

WARNING

Preventing glucocorticoid effects on growth

In children, glucocorticoids can retard normal growth by affecting epiphyseal cartilage. Even small doses of glucocorticoids can inhibit — or arrest — growth by interfering with deoxyribonucleic acid synthesis and cell division.

To help prevent these effects on growth, follow these guidelines:
♦ Use only a short-acting drug (such as cortisone or hydrocortisone) or an intermediate-acting drug (such as methylprednisolone, prednisolone, prednisone, or triamcinolone).
♦ Use alternate-day therapy if an oral intermediate-acting drug is used.
♦ Closely monitor the child during glucocorticoid therapy.

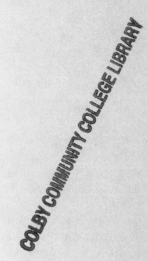

♦ Use of alcohol with a glucocorticoid can increase the risk of gastric irritation and GI ulceration.

Adverse reactions

Because systemic glucocorticoids affect nearly every body system, they can cause widespread adverse reactions, which include insomnia, increased sodium and water retention, increased potassium excretion, suppressed immune and inflammatory responses, glaucoma, osteoporosis, intestinal perforation, peptic ulcers, and impaired wound healing. Endocrine system reactions may include diabetes mellitus, hyperlipidemia, adrenal atrophy, hypothalamic-pituitary-axis suppression, cushingoid signs and symptoms (such as buffalo hump, moon face, and an elevated glucose level).

Such reactions are unlikely to occur with short-term therapy, even at high dosages. However, when glucocorticoids are given for more than a brief period, devastating reactions can occur. If long-term therapy with these drugs is needed, alternate-day therapy (a single dose given every other morning) may decrease the severity of adverse reactions. In children, the effects of glucocorticoids can be significant. (See *Preventing glucocorticoid effects on growth*.)

Reported anaphylactic reactions in patients who have received parenteral glucocorticoids may have resulted from hypersensitivity to the preservative in some parenteral formulations.

Nursing considerations
♦ Monitor the patient frequently for adverse reactions and drug interactions during therapy.

 CLINICAL ALERT Closely observe the patient for an anaphylactic reaction after glucocorticoid administration. Keep standard emergency equipment nearby.

♦ Monitor the patient's glucose level, body weight, blood pressure, CBC, blood chemistries (particularly electrolytes), and intraocular pressure. Also obtain chest and spine X-rays regularly.
♦ Monitor the patient for signs and symptoms of adrenocortical insufficiency, such as hypotension, dehydration, fatigue, hyponatremia, diarrhea, and anorexia, during and after glucocorticoid therapy.

Adverse reactions to watch for
♦ Adrenal atrophy, cushingoid effects, diabetes mellitus, hyperlipidemia, hypothalamic-pituitary-axis suppression
♦ Glaucoma
♦ Impaired wound healing, suppressed immune and inflammatory responses
♦ Increased potassium excretion, increased sodium and water retention
♦ Insomnia
♦ Intestinal perforation, peptic ulcers
♦ Osteoporosis

Identifying cushingoid signs and symptoms

Prolonged corticosteroid therapy may produce signs and symptoms of *Cushing's syndrome*—a condition marked by widespread abnormalities, including obvious fat deposits in the face, between the shoulders, and around the waist.

During corticosteroid therapy, be sure to assess the patient for the following cushingoid signs and symptoms:

- acne
- moon face
- hirsutism and masculinization
- cervicodorsal fat (buffalo hump)
- protruding abdomen
- girdle obesity
- amenorrhea
- purplish abdominal striae
- edema

- thinning and atrophy of the arms and legs
- muscle weakness or atrophy
- hypertension
- hyperglycemia
- glycosuria
- renal impairment
- mental changes, ranging from euphoria to depression
- lowered resistance to infection.

Key nursing actions

- Observe closely for anaphylactic reactions after drug administration. Keep emergency equipment nearby.
- Monitor the patient's glucose level, body weight, blood pressure, CBC, blood chemistries (particularly electrolytes), intraocular pressure, and chest and spine X-rays.
- Watch for evidence of adrenocortical insufficiency, such as hypotension, dehydration, fatigue, hyponatremia, diarrhea, and anorexia, during and after glucocorticoid therapy.
- Assess for potential stressors, such as surgery, trauma, and infections. Adjust the glucocorticoid dosage accordingly.
- Monitor for Cushing's syndrome.
- Assess for epigastric pain 1 to 3 hours after meals and for nausea, vomiting, bloody stools, hematemesis, coffee-ground emesis, decreased hemoglobin and hematocrit, and fecal occult blood.
- Watch for and report emotional changes.
- Monitor closely for signs of infection, such as delayed wound healing and an increased WBC count.

- Monitor the patient for potential stressors, such as surgery, trauma, and infections, and adjust the glucocorticoid dosage accordingly.
- Monitor the patient for Cushing's syndrome. (See *Identifying cushingoid signs and symptoms.*)
- Prevent severe GI complications by assessing the patient for epigastric pain 1 to 3 hours after meals and for nausea, vomiting, bloody stools, hematemesis, coffee-ground emesis, decreased hemoglobin and hematocrit, and fecal occult blood.
- Observe for and report any emotional changes. Suicide precautions may be needed for a severely depressed patient.
- Give the daily dosage in four equally divided doses or in one single dose in the early morning for a patient who needs short-term oral therapy. Keep in mind that early-morning administration simulates the natural circadian rhythm of corticosteroid secretion—higher in the morning, lower in the evening.
- Give alternate-day therapy to a patient who needs therapy for longer than 1 month. This minimizes the risk or severity of adverse reactions.
- Inject an I.M. glucocorticoid deeply into the gluteal muscle, and avoid using the same site for repeated injections to help prevent atrophy at injection sites. S.C. injection is usually contraindicated.
- Don't give beclomethasone via oral inhalation to a patient experiencing an acute asthmatic attack because the drug can't stop bronchospasm.
- If adverse reactions or drug interactions occur, notify the prescriber.
- Closely monitor the patient for signs of infection, such as delayed wound healing and an increased white blood cell (WBC) count, because glucocorticoids increase the susceptibility to infection.
- Handle or dress all wounds, surgical sites, tubes, and catheters with care to help prevent contamination and reduce the risk of infection.
- Apply a topical glucocorticoid in the smallest amount and lowest concentration possible.
- Teach the patient and his family about the prescribed drug. (See *Teaching a patient about glucocorticoids.*)

Teaching a patient about glucocorticoids

Whenever a systemic glucocorticoid is prescribed, teach the patient and his family the drug's name, dose, frequency, action, and adverse effects. Also take the following actions.

◆ Ensure that the patient and his family clearly understand why the systemic glucocorticoid has been prescribed and know its risks. Advise the patient who is taking the drug for more than 1 week not to stop taking it abruptly. Explain that the dosage must be decreased gradually before the drug can be stopped.

◆ Emphasize the importance of taking the drug exactly as prescribed.

◆ Review the guidelines for missed doses with the patient. In general, he should take a missed daily dose as soon as he remembers it (but not the next day — doses should never be doubled). The patient who misses one portion of a divided daily dose should take the next dose on schedule. A patient on alternate-day therapy, however, shouldn't take a missed dose, even if he remembers it that same morning. Instead, he should take the missed dose the next morning, skip a day, and then resume alternate-day therapy on the following day.

◆ Advise the patient to carry extra medication when traveling in case the trip lasts longer than expected. Also advise him not to pack the drug in a suitcase; he should carry it at all times.

◆ Instruct the patient about storage requirements.

◆ Review the signs and symptoms of adrenocortical insufficiency with the patient. Instruct him to notify the prescriber if they occur.

◆ Advise the patient to avoid alcohol, aspirin, or aspirin-containing compounds without first consulting the prescriber.

◆ Teach the patient to recognize the signs and symptoms of GI disorders and to notify the prescriber immediately if they appear.

◆ Inform the patient that the systemic glucocorticoid may cause emotional changes that should be reported to the prescriber.

◆ Instruct the patient about therapy-related dietary precautions, including adequate intake of proteins, vitamins, and calcium. High-potassium and low-sodium foods also may be prescribed. Have the patient keep a weekly weight record and report any gain over 5 lb (2.2 kg).

◆ Explain the need for the patient to keep active to prevent osteoporosis. Periodic X-rays also may be needed to monitor bone status.

◆ Instruct the patient to take an oral glucocorticoid with food or milk to decrease the risk of gastric irritation.

◆ Instruct the patient to wear a medical identification tag or to carry an identification card at all times. Also tell him to notify any health care professionals (dentists or oral surgeons, for example) about the glucocorticoid therapy before undergoing any other treatments.

◆ Help the patient reduce the risk of infection by teaching self-care practices to prevent skin injury and proper care of minor injuries.

◆ Instruct the patient to call the prescriber if he experiences signs or symptoms of infection, such as fever.

◆ Advise the patient to avoid people with infections, especially respiratory infections.

◆ Stress the importance of scrupulous oral hygiene during oral inhalation therapy, especially immediately after treatment.

◆ For a patient receiving long-term therapy, describe the possibility of appearance changes, such as fat deposits in the face, acne, hirsutism, and truncal obesity. Reassure him that these changes are therapy-related.

◆ Instruct the patient to notify the prescriber if adverse reactions occur.

◆ Teach the patient the correct way to use a beclomethasone oral inhaler: shake the inhaler well immediately before use; invert the inhaler; exhale completely; place the mouthpiece of the inhaler in the mouth and close the lips around it; while pressing the metal canister down with a finger, inhale slowly and deeply through the mouth; after holding the breath as long as possible, remove the mouthpiece and exhale as slowly as possible. Wait 1 minute (breathing normally) before inhaling again.

MINERALOCORTICOIDS

Mineralocorticoids affect electrolyte and water balance. These drugs include fludrocortisone, a synthetic analogue of hormones secreted by the adrenal cortex; and aldosterone, a natural mineralocorticoid. Because high cost and limited availability have curtailed the use of aldosterone, this section focuses on fludrocortisone.

Pharmacokinetics

After oral administration, fludrocortisone is absorbed well and distributed to all parts of the body. The drug is metabolized in the liver to inactive metabolites. It's excreted by the kidneys, primarily as inactive metabolites.

Pharmacodynamics

Fludrocortisone affects fluid and electrolyte balance by acting on the distal renal tubules to increase sodium reabsorption and potassium and hydrogen secretion.

Pharmacotherapeutics

Fludrocortisone is used as replacement therapy in patients with adrenocortical insufficiency, which reduces the secretion of glucocorticoids, mineralocorticoids, and androgens.

This mineralocorticoid may also be used to treat salt-losing congenital adrenogenital syndrome (characterized by a lack of cortisol and deficient aldosterone production) after the patient's electrolyte balance has been restored.

Interactions

Interactions with mineralocorticoids are similar to interactions with glucocorticoids.

Adverse reactions

Mineralocorticoids cause the same adverse reactions that result from systemic glucocorticoids. Although fludrocortisone doesn't cause hypersensitivity reactions, chemicals used in its preparation may do so.

Nursing considerations

✦ Regularly monitor the patient for signs and symptoms of fluid and electrolyte imbalances during mineralocorticoid therapy.
✦ Periodically monitor the patient's sodium, potassium, and calcium levels.
✦ Monitor the patient for other adverse reactions and drug interactions.
✦ If adverse reactions or drug interactions occur, notify the prescriber.
✦ Monitor the patient for signs of fluid retention by measuring his blood pressure and body weight daily, by inspecting him for edema, and by auscultating his lungs.
✦ Advise the patient to consume no more than eight 8-oz (240-ml) glasses of fluid daily.
✦ Provide a low-sodium, high-potassium diet for the patient.
✦ Teach the patient and his family about the prescribed drug. (See *Teaching a patient about mineralocorticoids.*)

NONCORTICOSTEROID IMMUNOSUPPRESSANTS

Various drugs that are used as immunosuppressants in *allograft transplantation*, transplantation between two people who aren't identical twins, are also used experimentally to treat autoimmune diseases. These noncorticosteroid immunosuppressants include anakinra, anti-thymocyte globulin (ATG) [equine], ATG (rabbit), azathioprine, basiliximab, cyclosporine, daclizumab, muromonab-CD3, mycophenolate, sirolimus, and tacrolimus.

The alkylating drug cyclophosphamide can also be used as an immunosuppressant, but is used primarily to treat cancer.

Pharmacokinetics

Different noncorticosteroid immunosuppressants take different paths through the body.

After S.C. administration, anakinra is about 95% bioavailable. When administered orally, azathioprine and mycophenolate are absorbed readily from the GI tract; cyclosporine, sirolimus, and tacrolimus undergo variable and incomplete absorption. Because ATG (equine), ATG (rabbit), basiliximab, daclizumab, and muromonab-CD3 are given I.V., they undergo no absorption.

The distribution of ATG (equine) isn't clear, but it may appear in breast milk. The distribution of azathioprine isn't understood fully. Cyclosporine and muromonab-CD3 are distributed widely throughout the body. Azathioprine and cyclosporine cross the placental barrier. Mycophenolate and sirolimus are highly bound to plasma proteins. Tacrolimus is bound to proteins and highly bound to red blood cells.

Anakinra isn't metabolized. Azathioprine and cyclosporine are metabolized in the liver. The metabolism of ATG (equine) is unknown. The metabolism of daclizumab also is unknown. However, daclizumab dosing is based on mg/kg because of a known relationship between drug clearance and body weight. Muromonab-CD3 is consumed by T cells in the blood. Mycophenolate is metabolized in the liver to mycophenolate acid, an active metabolite, and then further metabolized to an inactive metabolite. Sirolimus and tacrolimus are extensively metabolized by the mixed-function oxidase system.

Uses of noncorticosteroid immunosuppressants
✦ Are used as immunosuppressants to prevent organ rejection after transplantation
✦ Are used experimentally to treat autoimmune diseases, such as moderately to severely active rheumatoid arthritis (anakinra)

Anakinra is excreted primarily in urine. Azathioprine and ATG (equine) are excreted in urine; cyclosporine is excreted principally in bile. How muromonab-CD3 is excreted is unknown. Mycophenolate is excreted in urine and bile as an inactive metabolite. Sirolimus is excreted primarily in feces and minimally in urine. A small amount of tacrolimus is excreted unchanged in urine; 10 possible metabolites have been identified in plasma.

Pharmacodynamics

The exact mechanism of action of certain immunosuppressants hasn't been determined yet.

Anakinra blocks the biological activity of interleukin-1 (IL-1) by competitively binding to IL-1 receptors, which is expressed in various tissues and organs.

ATG (equine) may eliminate antigen-reactive T cells in the blood, alter T-cell function, or both. The actions of ATG (rabbit) may involve T-cell clearance from the circulation. The drug may also affect T-cell activation and cytotoxic activities.

Azathioprine may antagonize metabolism of the amino acid purine. By antagonizing in this way, the drug may inhibit ribonucleic acid and deoxyribonucleic acid structure and synthesis. It may also inhibit coenzyme formation and function. In patients receiving kidney allografts, azathioprine suppresses cell-mediated hypersensitivity reactions and alters antibody production.

Basiliximab and daclizumab bind specifically to and block interleukin-2 (IL-2) receptor alpha chains on the surface of T cells, preventing IL-2 from activating lymphocytes, a critical pathway in the cell-mediated response involved in allograft rejection.

Cyclosporine is thought to inhibit helper T cells and suppressor T cells.

Muromonab-CD3, a monoclonal antibody, blocks the function of T cells.

Mycophenolate inhibits the proliferative response of T and B cells, suppresses antibody formation by B cells, and may inhibit the recruitment of leukocytes into sites of inflammation and graft rejection.

Sirolimus inhibits T-cell activation and proliferation and inhibits antibody formation. Tacrolimus may inhibit T-cell activation.

Pharmacotherapeutics

Immunosuppressants are used mainly to prevent rejection in patients who undergo organ transplantation. Anakinra is used to treat moderately to severely active rheumatoid arthritis.

Interactions

Most interactions with this class of drugs involve other immunosuppressants, anti-inflammatory drugs, antibiotics, and antimicrobials.

✦ Use of anakinra with etanercept or another tumor necrosis factor blocker increases the risk of severe infection.

✦ When used with another immunosuppressant or cyclosporine, anakinra, ATG (equine), ATG (rabbit), basiliximab, daclizumab, or muromonab-CD3 increases the risk of infection and lymphoma.

✦ Allopurinol can increase the azathioprine level.

✦ Anabolic steroids, calcium channel blockers, cimetidine, erythromycin, ketoconazole, metoclopramide, and hormonal contraceptives may increase the cyclosporine level.

✦ When taken with acyclovir, aminoglycosides, and amphotericin B, cyclosporine and sirolimus can increase the risk of renal toxicity.

Actions of noncorticosteroid immunosuppressants

✦ Anakinra blocks the activity of IL-1 by competitively binding to IL-1 receptors.

✦ ATG (equine) may eliminate antigen-reactive T cells in the blood, alter T-cell function, or both.

✦ Azathioprine may antagonize the purine metabolism.

✦ Basiliximab and daclizumab bind to and block IL-2 receptor alpha chains on the surface of T cells, preventing IL-2 from activating lymphocytes.

✦ Cyclosporine may inhibit helper T cells and suppressor T cells.

✦ Muromonab-CD3 blocks the function of T cells.

✦ Mycophenolate inhibits the proliferative response of T and B cells, suppresses antibody formation by B cells, and may inhibit leukocyte recruitment to sites of inflammation and graft rejection.

✦ Sirolimus inhibits T-cell activation and proliferation and inhibits antibody formation.

✦ Tacrolimus may inhibit T-cell activation.

✦ Barbiturates, phenytoin, rifampin, sulfonamides, or trimethoprim can decrease the cyclosporine and sirolimus levels.

✦ Cyclosporine may increase the digoxin level.

✦ When used with fibrates and 3-hydroxy-3-methylglutaryl coenzyme A (HMG-CoA) reductase inhibitors, cyclosporine and sirolimus can increase the risk of rhabdomyolysis.

✦ When taken with antacids or cholestyramine, mycophenolate shows decreased absorption.

✦ When used with acyclovir, ganciclovir, or other drugs that undergo renal tubular secretion, mycophenolate increases the risk of toxicity.

✦ Use of mycophenolate with phenytoin or theophylline may increase the levels of both drugs.

✦ Probenecid or salicylates can increase the mycophenolate level.

✦ Voriconazole inhibits cytochrome P450 3A4 enzymes, which increases the sirolimus level and contraindicates combined use of these drugs. (See *Precautions for sirolimus*.)

✦ Verapamil can increase the sirolimus level.

✦ Bromocriptine, cimetidine, clarithromycin, clotrimazole, cyclosporine, danazol, diltiazem, erythromycin, fluconazole, indinavir, itraconazole, metoclopramide, nicardipine, ritonavir, or verapamil may increase the sirolimus level.

✦ Carbamazepine, phenobarbital, phenytoin, rifabutin, rifampin, or rifapentine may decrease the sirolimus or tacrolimus level.

✦ An antifungal, bromocriptine, a calcium channel blocker, cimetidine, clarithromycin, danazol, diltiazem, erythromycin, methylprednisolone, or metoclopramide may increase the tacrolimus level.

Adverse reactions

Common adverse reactions to anakinra include headache, upper respiratory tract infection, injection site reactions (erythema, ecchymosis, inflammation, and pain) and infections (cellulitis, pneumonia, and bone and joint infections).

With ATG (equine) therapy, the most common adverse reactions are fever and chills. Up to 20% of patients receiving kidney allografts experience leukopenia, thrombocytopenia, or both while receiving this drug. Early myelosuppression may also occur and force the drug to be stopped. The immunosuppressant effects of ATG (equine) may lead to local and systemic infections. Nausea, vomiting, diarrhea, stomatitis, hiccups, epigastric pain, and abdominal distention may also occur. Rash, pruritus, urticaria, and erythema have been reported in 10% to 15% of patients. Adverse cardiovascular reactions, such as hypotension, hypertension, tachy-

Adverse reactions to watch for

anakinra
✦ headache, injection site reactions, infections, upper respiratory tract infection

ATG (equine)
✦ Abdominal distention, chills, diarrhea, early myelosuppression, edema, epigastric pain, erythema, fever, hiccups, hypertension, hypotension, iliac vein obstruction, leukopenia, nausea, pruritus, pulmonary edema, rash, renal artery stenosis, stomatitis, tachycardia, thrombocytopenia, urticaria, vomiting

ATG (rabbit)
✦ Abdominal pain, chills, diarrhea, dizziness, dyspnea, fever, headache, leukopenia, nausea, systemic infections, thrombocytopenia

azathioprine
✦ Anorexia, diahrrea, esophagitis, leukopenia, macrocytic anemia, mouth ulcers, nausea, pancytopenia, steatorrhea, thrombocytopenia

basiliximab
✦ Abdominal pain, acidosis, acne, anemia, asthenia, candidiasis, constipation, cough, diarrhea, dizziness, dyspepsia, dyspnea, dysuria, fever, headache, hypercholesterolemia, hyperglycemia, hyperkalemia, hypertension, hyperuricemia, hypocalcemia, hypokalemia, hypophosphatemia, leg or peripheral edema, nausea, pharyngitis, rhinitis, surgical wound complications, tremor, upper respiratory tract infection, UTI, viral infection, vomiting, weight gain

Adverse reactions to watch for
(continued)

cyclosporine

✦ Abdominal discomfort, decreased bicarbonate level, diarrhea, gingival hyperplasia, hirsutism, hyperkalemia,hypertension, hyperuricemia, infection, nausea, nephrotoxicity, tremor, vomiting

daclizumab

✦ Acne, bleeding, blurred vision, chest pain, constipation, dehydration, diarrhea, dizziness, dyspepsia, fatigue, fever, headache, hyperglycemia, hypertension, hypotension, impaired wound healing, insomnia, lymphocele, musculoskeletal or back pain, pulmonary edema, renal damage, thrombosis, tremor

muromonab-CD3

✦ Chest pain, chills, diarrhea, dyspnea, fever, nausea, pulmonary edema, tremor, vomiting, wheezing

mycophenolate

✦ Abdominal pain, acne, anemia, asthenia, back pain, chest pain, constipation, cough, diarrhea, dyspepsia, dyspnea, edema, fever, headache, hematuria, hypercholesterolemia, hyperglycemia, hyperkalemia, hypertension, hypokalemia, hypophosphatemia, infection, leukopenia, nausea, oral candidiasis, pain, peripheral edema, thrombocytopenia, tremor, UTI, vomiting

cardia, edema, pulmonary edema, iliac vein obstruction, and renal artery stenosis, are uncommon.

Adverse reactions to ATG (rabbit) include fever, chills, thrombocytopenia, leukopenia, headache, abdominal pain, nausea, diarrhea, dyspnea, systemic infections, and dizziness.

The primary adverse reaction to azathioprine is bone marrow suppression, indicated by leukopenia, macrocytic anemia, pancytopenia, and thrombocytopenia. This may alter clotting mechanisms and cause hemorrhaging. Nausea, vomiting, anorexia, and diarrhea can occur with high dosages; mouth ulcerations, esophagitis, and steatorrhea can also occur. In a small number of patients, hepatic dysfunction has been reported. Other adverse reactions to azathioprine include alopecia, arthralgia, retinopathy, Raynaud's disease, and pulmonary edema.

Basiliximab may cause asthenia, headache, dizziness, tremor, fever, hypertension, leg or peripheral edema, rhinitis, pharyngitis, abdominal pain, candidiasis, constipation, diarrhea, dyspepsia, nausea, vomiting, dysuria, urinary tract infection (UTI), anemia, acidosis, hypercholesterolemia, hyperglycemia, hyperkalemia, hyperuricemia, hypocalcemia, hypokalemia, hypophosphatemia, weight gain, cough, dyspnea, upper respiratory tract infection, acne, surgical wound complications, and viral infection.

The most severe adverse reaction to cyclosporine is nephrotoxicity, usually characterized by increased blood urea nitrogen (BUN) and creatinine levels. More common adverse reactions include hyperkalemia, hyperuricemia, decreased bicarbonate level, hypertension, tremor, gingival hyperplasia, hirsutism, diarrhea, nausea, vomiting, abdominal discomfort, and infection. Less common reactions are gastritis, hiccups, and peptic ulcers. Occasional complaints include CNS effects (flushing, paresthesia, headache) and hepatotoxicity, which usually occurs during the first month of therapy and with high dosages. Leukopenia, thrombocytopenia, and anemia are uncommon, and hematuria and psychiatric disorders are rare. In a small number of patients receiving cyclosporine, sinusitis, gynecomastia, conjunctivitis, hearing loss, tinnitus, hyperglycemia, edema, fever, and muscle pain may occur.

Relatively common adverse reactions to daclizumab include tremor, headache, dizziness, insomnia, fever, fatigue, lymphocele, thrombosis, bleeding, hyperglycemia, musculoskeletal or back pain, acne, and impaired wound healing without infection. Other reactions may include hypertension or hypotension, pulmonary edema, chest pain, blurred vision, constipation, diarrhea, dyspepsia, renal damage, and dehydration.

Most adverse reactions to muromonab-CD3 occur during the first 2 days of therapy. The most common reactions are fever and chills. Others include dyspnea, chest pain, vomiting, wheezing, nausea, diarrhea, and tremor. Severe, potentially fatal pulmonary edema may occur in a small number of patients receiving this drug. The risk of infection with muromonab-CD3 therapy is comparable to the risk with high dosages of corticosteroids. The most common infections, with cytomegalovirus and herpes simplex virus, occur during the first 45 days of therapy.

Common adverse reactions to mycophenolate include tremor, fever, headache, asthenia, chest pain, hypertension, edema, diarrhea, constipation, nausea, dyspepsia, vomiting, oral candidiasis, abdominal pain, UTI, hematuria, anemia, leukopenia, thrombocytopenia, hypercholesterolemia, hypophosphatemia, hypokalemia, hyperkalemia, hyperglycemia, back pain, dyspnea, cough, infection, acne, pain, infection, and peripheral edema.

Sirolimus may produce headache, insomnia, tremor, anxiety, depression, asthenia, fever, hypertension, chest pain, edema, diarrhea, nausea, vomiting, constipation, abdominal pain, dyspepsia, pharyngitis, UTI, anemia, thrombocytopenia, hypercholesterolemia, hyperlipidemia, hypokalemia, weight gain, hypophosphatemia, hyperkalemia, back pain, arthralgia, dyspnea, cough, atelectasis, upper respiratory tract infection, rash, acne, and pain.

Common adverse reactions to tacrolimus include headache, tremor, insomnia, paresthesia, asthenia, fever, hypertension, peripheral edema, diarrhea or constipation, anorexia, nausea, vomiting, abdominal pain, abnormal renal function, UTI, oliguria, anemia, leukocytosis, thrombocytopenia, back pain, pleural effusion, atelectasis, dyspnea, pruritus, rash, and ascites.

All noncorticosteroid immunosuppressants can also cause hypersensitivity reactions, which range from rash and serum sickness to anaphylaxis. Azathioprine may cause hypersensitivity-induced pancreatitis.

Nursing considerations

✦ Monitor the patient frequently for adverse reactions or drug interactions. If any occur, notify the prescriber.

> **CLINICAL ALERT**
> ✦ Closely monitor the patient for hypersensitivity reactions. Keep standard emergency equipment nearby.

✦ Before giving the first dose of ATG (equine), perform an intradermal skin test to assess the patient's risk for severe systemic adverse reactions.

✦ Frequently monitor the patient's CBC (including platelet count) and liver function test results during azathioprine therapy.

✦ Frequently evaluate the patient's liver enzyme, BUN, creatinine, and bilirubin levels during cyclosporine therapy.

✦ Periodically monitor the cyclosporine level during cyclosporine therapy.

✦ Ensure that the patient starting muromonab-CD3 therapy has had a chest X-ray 24 hours before receiving the first dose; his chest must be clear of fluid.

✦ Regularly monitor the patient's T-cell assays during muromonab-CD3 therapy.

✦ If the patient has an active infection, don't start immunosuppressant therapy.

✦ Give azathioprine in divided doses after meals to reduce the risk or severity of adverse GI reactions.

✦ Mix oral cyclosporine in a glass container with milk or orange juice at room temperature to increase its palatability. Stir the mixture well with a metal spoon and administer it immediately. Then put a little more milk or orange juice in the container and have the patient drink it to receive the entire dose.

✦ Refrigerate the ATG (equine) solution if it won't be given immediately. If refrigeration time plus infusion time exceeds 12 hours, don't use the solution.

✦ Infuse the ATG (equine) solution into high-flow veins to decrease the risk of phlebitis and thrombosis. Always use an in-line filter and make sure the solution is free from particles and discoloration.

✦ Give a muromonab-CD3 I.V. bolus in less than 1 minute. Don't give it as an infusion or with other solutions.

> **CLINICAL ALERT**
> ✦ Monitor the patient for signs and symptoms of infection during immunosuppressant therapy. Keep in mind that classic signs of infection may be suppressed. However, the WBC count is still a reliable indicator.

✦ Take infection control measures, such as maintaining reverse isolation.

✦ Check for electrolyte imbalances in a patient receiving basiliximab, mycophenolate, or sirolimus.

Adverse reactions to watch for
(continued)

sirolimus

✦ Abdominal pain, acne, anemia, arthralgia, asthenia, atelectasis, anxiety, back pain, chest pain, constipation, cough, depression, diarrhea, dyspepsia, dyspnea, edema, fever, headache, hypercholesterolemia, hyperkalemia, hyperlipidemia, hypertension, hypokalemia, hypophosphatemia, insomnia nausea, pain, peripheral edema, pharyngitis, rash, thrombocytopenia, tremor, upper respiratory tract infection, UTI, vomiting, weight gain

tacrolimus

✦ Abdominal pain, abnormal renal function, anemia, anorexia, asthenia, ascites, atelectasis, back pain, constipation, diarrhea, dyspnea, fever, headache, hypertension, insomnia, leukocytosis, nausea, oliguria, paresthesia, peripheral edema, pleural effusion, pruritus, rash, thrombocytopenia, tremor, UTI, vomiting

Key nursing actions

+ Closely monitor for hypersensitivity reactions. Keep emergency equipment nearby.
+ Frequently monitor CBC (including platelet count) and liver function test results during azathioprine therapy.
+ Frequently evaluate the liver enzyme, blood urea nitrogen, creatinine, and bilirubin levels during cyclosporine therapy.
+ Periodically monitor the cyclosporine level during cyclosporine therapy.
+ Regularly monitor the T-cell assays during muromonab-CD3 therapy.
+ Monitor the patient for evidence of infection during immunosuppressant therapy.
+ Check for electrolyte imbalances during basiliximab, mycophenolate, or sirolimus therapy.

PATIENT TEACHING

Teaching a patient about noncorticosteroid immunosuppressants

Whenever a noncorticosteroid immunosuppressant is prescribed, teach the patient and his family the drug's name, dose, frequency, action, and adverse effects. Also take the following actions.

+ Thoroughly explain the therapeutic purpose of the immunosuppressant.
+ Inform the patient that infection, which can be life-threatening, is the most common hazard related to immunosuppressant therapy.
+ Emphasize that infection prevention requires scrupulous oral and personal hygiene.
+ Advise the patient to avoid crowds and people with infections.
+ Urge the patient to postpone immunizations until after therapy is stopped.
+ Urge a woman to avoid conception during therapy and for up to 4 months afterward.
+ Stress the importance of undergoing laboratory tests and periodic monitoring by the prescriber.
+ Teach the patient to take bleeding precautions if his platelet count falls below normal.
+ Instruct the patient receiving cyclosporine to notify the prescriber if paresthesia, tinnitus, or hearing loss occurs.
+ Inform the diabetic patient that hyperglycemia may occur during cyclosporine therapy. Instruct such a patient to monitor his glucose level closely and adhere to his prescribed regimen strictly.
+ Prepare the patient for drug-induced changes in appearance, such as alopecia, hirsutism, gynecomastia, and rashes.
+ Instruct the patient to notify the prescriber if adverse reactions occur.

+ Don't open or crush mycophenolate capsules. Avoid inhaling the powder in capsules or having it contact the skin or mucous membranes. If contact occurs, wash thoroughly with soap and water or rinse the eyes with water.

+ Give sirolimus consistently, without regard to food.
+ Teach the patient and his family about the prescribed drug. (See *Teaching a patient about noncorticosteroid immunosuppressants.*)

URICOSURICS AND OTHER ANTIGOUT DRUGS

Along with other antigout drugs, uricosurics are used for their anti-inflammatory actions.

URICOSURICS

The primary goal of uricosuric therapy is to prevent or control the frequency of gouty arthritis attacks, which they do by increasing uric acid excretion in urine. The two major uricosurics are probenecid and sulfinpyrazone.

Pharmacokinetics

Uricosurics are absorbed from the GI tract. Distribution of the two drugs is similar, with 75% to 95% of probenecid and 98% of sulfinpyrazone being protein-bound.

Metabolism of the drugs occurs in the liver, and excretion is primarily by the kidneys. Only small amounts of these drugs are excreted in feces.

Pharmacodynamics
Probenecid and sulfinpyrazone reduce uric acid reabsorption at the proximal convoluted tubules of the kidneys. This results in excretion of uric acid in urine, which reduces the urate level.

Pharmacotherapeutics
Both uricosurics are indicated for treating chronic gouty arthritis and *tophaceous gout,* the deposition of tophi or urate crystals under the skin and into joints. Probenecid is also used to promote uric acid excretion in patients with hyperuricemia.

Probenecid and sulfinpyrazone shouldn't be given during an acute gouty attack. If taken at that time, they prolong inflammation. Because these drugs may increase the chance of an acute gouty attack when therapy begins and whenever the urate level changes rapidly, colchicine is given during the first 3 to 6 months of uricosuric therapy.

Interactions
✦ Probenecid can significantly increase or prolong the effects of cephalosporins, penicillins, and sulfonamides.
✦ When used with probenecid, antineoplastics may increase the urate level.
✦ Probenecid can increase the aminosalicylic acid, dapsone, or methotrexate level, causing toxic reactions.
✦ Sulfinpyrazone increases the effectiveness of warfarin, increasing the risk of bleeding.
✦ Salicylates can reduce the effects of sulfinpyrazone.
✦ Sulfinpyrazone may increase the effects of oral antidiabetics, which increases the risk of hypoglycemia.

Adverse reactions
When given in therapeutic dosages, probenecid is usually tolerated well by patients. Its most common adverse effects are headache and GI distress, including anorexia, nausea, and vomiting. Other adverse reactions include flushing, dizziness, urinary frequency, sore gums, and anemia.

When given in therapeutic dosages, sulfinpyrazone is usually tolerated well. Nausea, dyspepsia, GI pain, and GI blood loss are the most common adverse reactions to sulfinpyrazone. Reactivation or aggravation of peptic ulcer disease can also occur. Other adverse reactions include dizziness, rash, vertigo, tinnitus, and edema. Blood dyscrasias, such as anemia, leukopenia, granulocytopenia, and thrombocytopenia, are rare.

Some patients taking probenecid or sulfinpyrazone may form uric acid calculi. This usually occurs at the beginning of therapy. Acute gouty attacks can also occur in some patients during the first 6 to 12 months of therapy.

In some patients, stopping sulfinpyrazone therapy has reversed renal impairment.

 CLINICAL ALERT Hypersensitivity reactions to probenecid can occur, producing such signs and symptoms as dermatitis, pruritus, fever, sweating, or hypotension. Rarely, a patient may experience an anaphylactic reaction, nephrotic syndrome, hepatic necrosis, or aplastic anemia.

Features of uricosurics
✦ Reduce uric acid reabsorption at the proximal convoluted tubules, which increases uric acid excretion in urine and reduces the urate level
✦ Have anti-inflammatory action
✦ Are used to treat chronic gouty arthritis and tophaceous gout
✦ Are also used to promote uric acid excretion with hyperuricemia (probenecid)

Adverse reactions to watch for
✦ Acute gouty attacks
✦ Uric acid calculi

probenecid
✦ Anemia
✦ Anorexia, nausea, sore gums, vomiting
✦ Dizziness, flushing
✦ Headache
✦ Hypersensitivity reactions
✦ Urinary frequency

sulfinpyrazone
✦ Dizziness, vertigo
✦ Edema
✦ GI blood loss, GI pain, dyspepsia, nausea
✦ Rash, tinnitus

Teaching a patient about uricosurics

Whenever a uricosuric is prescribed, teach the patient and his family the drug's name, dose, frequency, action, and adverse effects. Also take the following actions.

✦ Instruct the patient to take the drug exactly as prescribed and not to stop the drug without consulting the prescriber because gout symptoms may reappear.

✦ Advise the patient to notify the prescriber if GI distress persists.

✦ Instruct the patient not to take aspirin during uricosuric therapy. If an analgesic or antipyretic is needed, he should take acetaminophen.

✦ Caution the patient not to take the drug during an acute attack of gout. Explain that taking the drug during an attack will prolong the inflammation and won't relieve acute symptoms. Inform the patient that the drug usually isn't started until 2 to 3 weeks after an acute attack.

✦ Alert a diabetic patient who tests his urine glucose level with Clinitest of the possibility of false-positive test results. Recommend that he use Clinistix or another urine glucose testing product.

✦ Advise the patient not to perform activities that require alertness if dizziness or vertigo occurs.

✦ Emphasize the importance of having laboratory tests performed regularly.

✦ Instruct the patient to notify the prescriber if adverse reactions occur.

Key nursing actions

✦ Closely observe for hypersensitivity reactions to probenecid.

✦ Monitor the results of laboratory tests, including a CBC, urinalysis, and uric acid level. Also monitor renal function test results and the BUN level regularly.

✦ Urge the patient to drink ten to twelve 8-oz (240-ml) glasses of water daily to minimize uric acid calculi formation.

✦ Encourage the patient to consume a high-vegetable diet to alkalinize the urine.

✦ If anorexia, nausea, vomiting, or other adverse GI reactions occur, monitor the patient's hydration. Give an antiemetic as needed.

Nursing considerations

✦ Monitor the patient frequently for adverse reactions and drug interactions during uricosuric therapy.

 CLINICAL ALERT **Closely observe the patient for hypersensitivity reactions to probenecid. Keep standard emergency equipment nearby because anaphylaxis can occur.**

✦ Monitor the results of the patient's laboratory tests, including a CBC, urinalysis, and uric acid level. Regularly monitor his renal function test results and BUN level.

✦ Notify the prescriber if the patient has an acute gouty attack. Temporarily stop the uricosuric because it may prolong inflammation in an acute gouty attack.

✦ Give colchicine with a uricosuric to help prevent an acute attack of gouty arthritis, which can occur at the start of uricosuric therapy.

✦ Encourage the patient to drink ten to twelve 8-oz (240-ml) glasses of water daily. Maintaining a high fluid intake minimizes uric acid calculi formation.

✦ Encourage the patient to consume a high-vegetable diet to alkalinize the urine. Maintaining alkaline urine decreases the formation of uric acid calculi.

✦ If anorexia, nausea, vomiting, or other adverse GI reactions occur, monitor the patient's hydration status. Give an antiemetic as needed.

✦ Give the drug with food, milk, or an antacid to prevent GI distress, which is the most common adverse reaction to uricosurics.

✦ Teach the patient and his family about the prescribed drug. (See *Teaching a patient about uricosurics*.)

OTHER ANTIGOUT DRUGS

Allopurinol is used to prevent gouty attacks; colchicine is used to treat them.

Pharmacokinetics

When given orally, allopurinol is absorbed from the GI tract. Allopurinol and its metabolite oxypurinol are distributed throughout the body, except in the brain, where the drug level is 50% of that in the rest of the body. Allopurinol is metabolized by the liver and excreted in urine.

Upon absorption from the GI tract, colchicine is partially metabolized in the liver. The drug and its metabolites then reenter the intestinal tract through biliary secretions. After reabsorption from the intestines, colchicine is distributed to various tissues. It's excreted primarily in feces and to a lesser degree in urine.

Pharmacodynamics

Allopurinol and its metabolite oxypurinol inhibit xanthine oxidase, the enzyme responsible for uric acid production. By reducing uric acid formation, allopurinol eliminates the hazards of hyperuricuria.

Colchicine appears to reduce the inflammatory response to monosodium urate crystals deposited in joint tissues. The drug may produce its effects by inhibiting WBC migration to inflamed joints. This reduces phagocytosis and lactic acid production by WBCs, decreasing urate crystal deposits and reducing inflammation.

Pharmacotherapeutics

Allopurinol is used to manage primary gout, preventing acute gouty attacks. It can be prescribed with uricosurics when smaller dosages of each drug are indicated. It's used to:

◆ treat gout or hyperuricemia that may occur with blood abnormalities and during treatment of tumors or leukemia
◆ treat primary or secondary uric acid nephropathy (with or without symptoms of gout)
◆ treat and prevent recurrent uric acid calculi formation
◆ treat patients who respond poorly to maximum dosages of uricosurics or who can't tolerate or have allergic reactions to uricosurics.

Colchicine is used to relieve the inflammation of acute gouty arthritis attacks. If given promptly, it's especially effective in relieving pain. Also, the use of colchicine during the first several months of allopurinol, probenecid, or sulfinpyrazone therapy may prevent the acute gouty attacks that sometimes accompany the use of these drugs.

Interactions

Colchicine doesn't interact significantly with other drugs. Interactions with allopurinol, however, can be serious.
◆ Allopurinol can potentiate the effects of oral anticoagulants.
◆ Allopurinol can increase the azathioprine or mercaptopurine level, increasing the risk of toxicity.
◆ An angiotensin-converting enzyme inhibitor can increase the risk of hypersensitivity reactions to allopurinol.
◆ Allopurinol can increase the theophylline level.
◆ Together, cyclophosphamide and allopurinol increase the risk of bone marrow suppression.

Features of other antigout drugs

allopurinol
✦ Inhibits xanthine oxidase, the enzyme responsible for uric acid production
✦ Eliminates the hazards of hyperuricuria by reducing uric acid formation
✦ Is used to manage primary gout, preventing acute gouty attacks
✦ Is used to treat gout or hyperuricemia from blood abnormalities or treatment of tumors or leukemia, to treat primary or secondary uric acid nephropathy, to treat and prevent recurrent uric acid calculi formation, and to treat patients who respond poorly to maximum dosages of uricosurics

colchicine
✦ May reduce the inflammatory response to monosodium urate crystals deposited in joint tissues
✦ May inhibit WBC migration to inflamed joints, which reduces phagocytosis and lactic acid production by WBCs, decreasing urate crystal deposits and reducing inflammation
✦ Is used to relieve the pain and inflammation of acute gouty arthritis attacks

Adverse reactions to watch for

allopurinol
✦ Anemia, aplastic anemia, bone marrow suppression, granulocytopenia
✦ Diarrhea, intermittent abdominal pain, nausea, vomiting
✦ Drowsiness
✦ Maculopapular rash
✦ Peripheral neuritis

colchicine
✦ Abdominal discomfort, diarrhea, nausea, vomiting
✦ Alopecia, dermatitis, urticaria
✦ Aplastic anemia, bone marrow suppression, granulocytopenia, leukopenia, thrombocytopenia (with prolonged use)
✦ Arthralgia, chills, eosinophilia, fever, pruritus, rash
✦ GI signs and symptoms (with high I.V. dosage)
✦ Hypersensitivity reactions, such as bladder spasms, hypothyroidism, nonthrombocytopenic purpura, paralytic ileus, stomatitis
✦ Peripheral neuritis

Adverse reactions

The most common reaction to allopurinol is a maculopapular rash. Adverse GI reactions include nausea, vomiting, diarrhea, and intermittent abdominal pain. Less common reactions include granulocytopenia, anemia, aplastic anemia, and bone marrow suppression. However, these reactions usually result from use of allopurinol with any drug known to cause such reactions. Peripheral neuritis and drowsiness may also occur. Rare instances of sensitivity reactions, such as alopecia and altered liver function test results, may occur during allopurinol therapy.

The most common adverse reactions to oral colchicine include nausea, vomiting, abdominal discomfort, and diarrhea. These reactions usually occur with dosages used to achieve a therapeutic colchicine level. However, they also indicate drug toxicity, requiring colchicine to be stopped. Therapy shouldn't be resumed for 3 days; this waiting period minimizes the risk of cumulative toxicity. GI signs and symptoms can also occur when colchicine is given I.V., but these adverse reactions usually occur only when the recommended dosage is exceeded.

Other adverse reactions involving colchicine primarily affect the skin, hematologic system, and CNS. The most common skin problems include dermatitis, urticaria, and alopecia. Prolonged administration may cause bone marrow suppression and related hematologic problems, such as aplastic anemia, granulocytopenia, leukopenia, and thrombocytopenia. The only adverse CNS reaction is peripheral neuritis. Rare adverse reactions include renal damage, muscle weakness, reversible azoospermia, and an increased alkaline phosphatase level.

Colchicine produces few hypersensitivity reactions. These include bladder spasms, paralytic ileus, stomatitis, hypothyroidism, and nonthrombocytopenic purpura. Fever, chills, leukopenia, eosinophilia, arthralgia, rash, and pruritus may also occur.

Nursing considerations

✦ Monitor the patient closely for adverse reactions and drug interactions during antigout therapy.

✦ Monitor the patient's CBC, urinalysis, uric acid level, and liver and kidney function test results before beginning and periodically during antigout therapy.

✦ Auscultate the patient's bowel sounds regularly during colchicine therapy to detect paralytic ileus.

✦ Adjust the allopurinol dosage based on the serum creatinine level and a 12- or 24-hour urine creatinine level for a patient with renal impairment.

✦ Prevent colchicine extravasation into surrounding tissues. During I.V. administration, properly position the needle in the vein and check for good blood return before injecting the drug. If extravasation occurs, apply heat or cold to relieve the discomfort and notify the prescriber. Analgesics may also be given.

✦ If nausea, vomiting, diarrhea, or other adverse GI reactions occur, monitor the patient's hydration status. Notify the prescriber and give an antiemetic or antidiarrheal as needed. Stop colchicine until GI distress has subsided.

✦ Give allopurinol after meals; give oral colchicine with food or milk to decrease GI distress.

✦ Teach the patient and his family about the prescribed drug. (See *Teaching a patient about other antigout drugs.*)

Key nursing actions

✦ Monitor CBC, urinalysis, uric acid level, and liver and kidney function test results before beginning and periodically during antigout therapy.

✦ For a patient with renal impairment, adjust the allopurinol dosage based on the serum creatinine level and a 12- or 24-hour urine creatinine level.

✦ Auscultate bowel sounds regularly during colchicine therapy to detect paralytic ileus.

✦ Prevent colchicine extravasation into surrounding tissues.

✦ If nausea, vomiting, diarrhea, or other adverse GI reactions occur, monitor the patient's hydration.

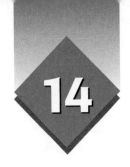

Drugs for fluid and electrolyte balance

About 60% of an adult's body is made up of water: 60% of this water is intracellular, 40% is extracellular. Food and fluid consumption and nutrient metabolism add water to the body—1,500 to 3,000 ml/day for an average adult. Normally, the fluid intake equals the fluid output, but an illness can upset this delicate balance.

Intracellular and extracellular fluid compartments have specific chemical compositions of electrolytes. The major electrolytes are potassium, sodium, calcium, magnesium, chloride, bicarbonate, and phosphorus. (See *Intracellular and extracellular electrolyte levels.*)

Electrolyte imbalances profoundly change a patient's total physiologic functioning, affecting the body's water distribution, cell function, neuromuscular activity, and acid-base balance. Such imbalances can result from any disorder or disease that alters electrolyte levels in the fluid compartments. They can also result from anorexia, drug administration, vomiting, surgery, and diagnostic tests.

Fortunately, numerous drugs can correct these imbalances and help return the body to homeostasis. Drugs commonly used for this purpose include electrolyte replacement, alkalinizing, and acidifying drugs.

ELECTROLYTE REPLACEMENT DRUGS

An *electrolyte* is a compound or element that carries an electrical charge when dissolved in water. Electrolyte replacement drugs are inorganic or organic salts that increase depleted or deficient electrolyte levels, helping to maintain homeostasis, the stability of body fluid composition, and fluid volume.

Key electrolytes include potassium, calcium, magnesium, and sodium. Potassium is the primary intracellular fluid (ICF) electrolyte; sodium, the major extracellular fluid (ECF) electrolyte. In the ICF, magnesium is also essential for homeostasis. In the ECF, calcium also plays a key role in homeostasis.

Intracellular and extracellular electrolyte levels

Blood contains intracellular fluid (ICF) in red blood cells, and extracellular fluid (ECF) in plasma. Because ICF and ECF are separated by capillary walls and cell membranes that allow different substances to permeate, these fluids contain different electrolyte levels, as shown in the chart below. For example, ICF contains about 30 times more potassium than ECF; ECF contains about 14 times more sodium than ICF.

In practice, however, you'll usually see electrolyte levels only for ECF. That's because ICF electrolyte levels aren't routinely measured. When reviewing a patient's electrolyte levels, keep in mind that normal findings vary with the laboratory and health care facility.

ELECTROLYTE	INTRACELLULAR LEVEL	EXTRACELLULAR LEVEL
Potassium	140 mEq/L	3.5 to 5 mEq/L
Sodium	10 mEq/L	135 to 145 mEq/L
Calcium	10 mEq/L	4.5 to 5.8 mEq/L
Magnesium	40 mEq/L	1.5 to 2.5 mEq/L
Chloride	4 mEq/L	100 to 108 mEq/L
Bicarbonate	10 mEq/L	24 to 28 mEq/L
Phosphorus	100 mEq/L	1.8 to 2.6 mEq/L

POTASSIUM

Potassium is the major positively charged ion, or cation, in ICF. Because the body can't store potassium, individuals must consume adequate amounts daily. If this isn't possible, they may need to be given potassium orally or I.V. To replace this electrolyte, they may receive a potassium salt, such as potassium acetate, bicarbonate, chloride, gluconate, or phosphate.

Pharmacokinetics

Oral potassium is absorbed readily from the GI tract. After absorption into the ECF, almost all of the potassium passes into the ICF. Metabolism of potassium is insignificant. The kidneys maintain a normal potassium level by excreting most of the excessive potassium intake. The remaining potassium is excreted in feces and sweat.

Pharmacodynamics

Potassium moves quickly into ICF to restore the depleted potassium level and reestablish balance. It's an essential element in determining cell membrane potential and excitability.

This electrolyte is necessary for the proper functioning of all nerve and muscle cells and for nerve impulse transmission. It's also essential for tissue growth and repair and for maintenance of acid-base balance.

Pharmacotherapeutics

With potassium, replacement therapy corrects hypokalemia. Hypokalemia commonly occurs in conditions that increase potassium excretion or depletion. Such conditions include vomiting or diarrhea (possibly related to laxative abuse or naso-

Features of potassium

+ Is the major cation in intracellular fluid (ICF)
+ Must be consumed daily because it can't be stored
+ Moves quickly into the ICF to restore the depleted level
+ Is essential in determining cell membrane potential and excitability
+ Is needed for proper functioning of nerve and muscle cells, nerve impulse transmission, tissue growth and repair, and maintenence of acid-base balance
+ Is used to correct hypokalemia, which may result from increased potassium excretion or depletion related to vomiting, diarrhea, excessive urination, some kidney diseases, cystic fibrosis, burns, excess antidiuretic hormone, alkalosis, insufficient dietary intake, or use of a potassium-depleting diuretic, glucocorticoids, I.V. amphotericin B, vitamin B_{12}, folic acid, filgrastim, or an I.V. solution that contains inadequate potassium

gastric suction), excessive urination, some kidney diseases, cystic fibrosis, burns, excess antidiuretic hormone (ADH), alkalosis, and insufficient potassium intake from starvation, anorexia nervosa, alcoholism, or clay ingestion.

Hypokalemia can also result from the use of a potassium-depleting diuretic, glucocorticoids, I.V. amphotericin B, vitamin B_{12}, folic acid, filgrastim, or an I.V. solution that doesn't contain enough potassium.

Interactions
✦ When used with potassium, a potassium-sparing diuretic (such as amiloride, spironolactone, or triamterene) or angiotensin-converting enzyme (ACE) inhibitor (such as captopril, enalapril, or lisinopril) can cause hyperkalemia.
✦ Potassium can decrease the risk of digoxin toxicity.

Adverse reactions
The use of potassium may produce hyperkalemia if the patient's potassium level isn't monitored closely. (See *Recognizing the signs and symptoms of hyperkalemia.*)

Oral potassium sometimes causes nausea, vomiting, abdominal pain, and diarrhea. Enteric-coated tablets may cause small-bowel ulceration, stenosis, hemorrhage, and obstruction. Because other formulations have largely replaced enteric-coated tablets, this adverse reaction is no longer common.

I.V. infusion of potassium can cause pain at the injection site and phlebitis. Infusion of potassium in patients with decreased urine production increases the risk of hyperkalemia.

Nursing considerations
✦ Use potassium cautiously in a patient who also receives a potassium-sparing diuretic or ACE inhibitor.
✦ Monitor the patient for adverse reactions and drug interactions during potassium therapy. Notify the prescriber if any occur.
✦ Monitor the patient's potassium level. Be particularly alert for hyperkalemia if his urine output decreases during potassium therapy.
✦ Monitor the patient regularly for signs and symptoms of hyperkalemia, such as listlessness, confusion, flaccid paralysis, paresthesia, weakness, and limb heaviness.

Adverse reactions to watch for
✦ Abdominal pain, diarrhea, nau-sea, vomiting
✦ Hyperkalemia
✦ Pain at the I.V. injection site, phlebitis
✦ Small-bowel ulceration, stenosis, hemorrhage, and obstruction (with enteric-coated tablets)

Teaching a patient about potassium

Whenever a potassium preparation is prescribed, teach the patient and his family the drug's name, dose, frequency, action, and adverse effects. Also take the following actions.

✦ Instruct the patient to take oral potassium with or after meals to minimize GI distress.
✦ Direct the patient to dissolve all powders and tablets in at least 4 oz (120 ml) of water or fruit juice, and to sip the solution slowly over 5 to 10 minutes. Also advise him to take capsules or tablets with plenty of liquid.
✦ Remind the patient not to crush or chew extended-release tablets, which will defeat the purpose of the special coating.
✦ Remind the patient that although remnants of the wax matrix may appear in his stool, the drug has been absorbed.
✦ Stress the need for periodic blood tests to measure the potassium level.
✦ Teach the patient to recognize and report to the prescriber signs or symptoms of hyperkalemia or GI distress.

CLINICAL ALERT

✦ Monitor the patient's ECG tracing for changes that suggest hyperkalemia, such as prolonged PR interval, widened QRS complex, depressed ST segment, and tall, tented T waves.

✦ Dilute an I.V. potassium preparation before infusion. Never give potassium as an I.V. bolus or I.M. injection.

✦ Give diluted I.V. potassium slowly; life-threatening hyperkalemia may result from too-rapid infusion.
✦ Don't mix I.V. potassium phosphate in a solution that contains calcium or magnesium because precipitates will occur.
✦ Inspect the patient's I.V. site regularly for signs of phlebitis. If phlebitis or pain occurs, change the I.V. site.
✦ Use liquid potassium in a cardiac patient who has esophageal compression from an enlarged left atrium or one with esophageal stasis or obstruction. In such a patient, wax matrix tablets may lodge in the esophagus and cause ulceration.
✦ Give oral potassium with or after meals to minimize GI distress.
✦ If the patient reports GI distress, perform an abdominal assessment.
✦ If nausea, vomiting, or diarrhea occurs, monitor the patient's hydration status. Give an antiemetic or antidiarrheal as needed.
✦ Teach the patient and his family about the prescribed drug. (See *Teaching a patient about potassium.*)

Key nursing actions

✦ Monitor potassium level. Be particularly alert for hyperkalemia if urine output decreases during potassium therapy.
✦ Monitor regularly for evidence of hyperkalemia, such as listlessness, confusion, flaccid paralysis, paresthesia, weakness, and limb heaviness.
✦ Monitor ECG tracings for changes that suggest hyperkalemia, such as a prolonged PR interval, widened QRS complex, depressed ST segment, and tall, tented T waves.
✦ If the patient reports GI distress, perform an abdominal assessment.
✦ If nausea, vomiting, or diarrhea occurs, monitor the patient's hydration. Give an antiemetic or antidiarrheal as needed.

SODIUM

As the major cation in ECF, sodium is necessary for many functions. Therefore, sodium replacement is needed in conditions that rapidly deplete it, such as excessive loss of GI fluids and excessive perspiration. Diuretics and tap water enemas can also deplete sodium, particularly when fluids are replaced by plain water. This electrolyte can also be lost in trauma, wound drainage, adrenal gland insufficiency, cirrhosis of the liver with ascites, syndrome of inappropriate ADH, and prolonged I.V. infusion of dextrose in water without other solutes.

Features of sodium

+ The major cation in extracellular fluid (ECF)
+ Maintains the osmotic pressure and concentration of the ECF, acid-base balance, and water balance
+ Contributes to nerve conduction, neuromuscular function, and glandular secretion
+ Is used to correct hyponatremia, which may result from excessive loss of GI fluids, excessive perspiration, diuretic use, tap water enemas, trauma, wound drainage, adrenal gland insufficiency, cirrhosis with ascites, syndrome of inappropriate ADH, and prolonged I.V. infusion of dextrose in water without other solutes
+ Is replaced with sodium chloride solution and in severe deficiency, I.V. sodium chloride

Adverse reactions to watch for

+ Hypernatremia
+ Hypokalemia
+ Pulmonary edema (with excessive speed or volume of delivery)

Key nursing actions

+ Monitor the patient's electrolyte levels.
+ Assess the patient for adverse effects.

PATIENT TEACHING

Teaching a patient about sodium

Whenever a sodium preparation is prescribed, teach the patient and his family the drug's name, dose, frequency, action, and adverse effects. Also take the following actions.
+ Stress the importance of undergoing blood tests to monitor electrolyte levels.
+ Teach the patient to recognize and report adverse reactions to the prescriber.
+ Advise the patient to inform all health care providers that he's receiving sodium replacement therapy. Explain that the risk of pulmonary edema increases when sodium is taken with a sodium-retaining drug, such as a corticosteroid.
+ Teach the patient to recognize the signs and symptoms of pulmonary edema, such as shortness of breath, difficulty breathing, cough, anxiety, wheezing, and pallor. Tell him to notify the prescriber if any of these signs or symptoms occur.

Usually, sodium is replaced in the form of sodium chloride.

Pharmacokinetics

Given orally or parenterally, sodium chloride is quickly absorbed and distributed widely throughout the body. It isn't significantly metabolized. It's eliminated primarily in urine, but also in sweat, tears, and saliva.

Pharmacodynamics

Sodium chloride solution replaces deficiencies of sodium and chloride ions in the plasma. Normally, sodium maintains the osmotic pressure and concentration of ECF, acid-base balance, and water balance. It contributes to nerve conduction and neuromuscular function. It also plays a role in glandular secretion.

Pharmacotherapeutics

Sodium chloride is used for water and electrolyte replacement in patients with hyponatremia from electrolyte loss or severe sodium chloride depletion. Severe symptomatic sodium deficiency may be treated by I.V. infusion of a solution containing sodium chloride.

Interactions

No significant interactions with sodium chloride have been reported.

Adverse reactions

Adverse reactions to sodium include pulmonary edema (if the drug is given too rapidly or in excess), hypernatremia, and hypokalemia.

Nursing considerations

+ Use sodium cautiously in a geriatric or postoperative patient or a patient with heart failure, circulatory insufficiency, renal impairment, or hypoproteinemia.
+ Monitor the patient's electrolyte levels.
+ Monitor the patient for adverse reactions. If any occur, notify the prescriber.
+ Teach the patient and his family about the prescribed drug. (See *Teaching a patient about sodium.*)

CALCIUM

Calcium is a major cation in ECF; 99% of it is stored in bone, where it can be mobilized if needed. When dietary calcium intake doesn't meet metabolic needs, calcium stores in bone are reduced.

Much extracellular calcium is bound to albumin or found in phosphate, citrate, or sulfate complexes. It represents about 47% of ionized calcium and is physiologically active.

Chronic insufficient calcium intake can result in bone demineralization. Oral and I.V. replacements use calcium salts, such as calcium carbonate, chloride, citrate, glubionate, gluceptate, gluconate, or lactate.

Pharmacokinetics

Oral calcium is absorbed readily from the duodenum and proximal jejunum. A pH of 5 to 7, parathyroid hormone, and vitamin D all aid calcium absorption.

Absorption also depends on dietary factors, such as calcium binding to fiber, phytates, and oxalates and to fatty acids, with which calcium salts form insoluble soaps.

Calcium is distributed primarily in bone and isn't significantly metabolized. Calcium salts are eliminated primarily in feces and, to a lesser degree, in urine.

Pharmacodynamics

Calcium moves quickly into ECF to restore the calcium level and reestablish balance. This electrolyte has several important roles in the body. Extracellular ionized calcium plays an essential role in normal nerve and muscle excitability. Calcium is integral to normal functioning of the heart, kidneys, and lungs. It affects the blood coagulation rate and cell membrane and capillary permeability. Calcium is a factor in neurotransmitter and hormone activity, amino acid metabolism, vitamin B_{12} absorption, and gastrin secretion. It plays a major role in normal bone and tooth formation.

Pharmacotherapeutics

Calcium is used to treat magnesium intoxication. It's also helpful in strengthening myocardial tissue after defibrillation or a poor response to epinephrine during resuscitation. Pregnancy and breast-feeding increase the calcium requirement, as do periods of bone growth during childhood and adolescence.

The major indication for I.V. calcium is acute hypocalcemia, which calls for a rapid increase in the calcium level. Conditions that create this need are tetany, cardiac arrest, vitamin D deficiency, parathyroid surgery, and alkalosis. I.V. calcium is also used to prevent a hypocalcemic reaction during exchange transfusions.

Oral calcium is commonly used to supplement a calcium-deficient diet and prevent osteoporosis. (See *Preventing osteoporosis,* page 518.) This form of calcium is also prescribed to treat chronic hypocalcemia from such conditions as chronic hypoparathyroidism, long-term glucocorticoid therapy, vitamin D deficiency, and *osteomalacia,* or bone softening.

Interactions

✦ When used with digoxin, calcium may cause arrhythmias.
✦ Calcium may reduce the response to calcium channel blockers.
✦ Calcium may inactivate tetracyclines.
✦ Calcium may decrease the amount of atenolol available to the tissues, reducing its effectiveness.

Features of calcium

✦ Is a major cation in ECF, almost completely stored in bone
✦ Affects nerve and muscle excitability, blood coagulation rate, cell membrane and capillary permeability, and the function of the heart, kidneys, and lungs
✦ Influences neurotransmitter and hormone activity, amino acid metabolism, vitamin B_{12} absorption, gastrin secretion, bone and tooth formation
✦ Is used to treat magnesium intoxication and to strengthen myocardial tissue after defibrillation or a poor response to epinephrine during resuscitation
✦ Is used I.V. to prevent hypocalcemia during exchange transfusions and to treat acute hypocalcemia, usually from tetany, cardiac arrest, vitamin D deficiency, parathyroid surgery, or alkalosis
✦ Is used orally to supplement a low-calcium diet, prevent osteoporosis, and treat chronic hypocalcemia from such conditions as chronic hypoparathyroidism, long-term glucocorticoid therapy, vitamin D deficiency, and osteomalacia

Preventing osteoporosis

As the most common bone disease, osteoporosis is a progressive loss of bone density that increases the risk of fractures. It typically develops with age, when calcium is reabsorbed from bones into the body, which weakens the bone tissue. Osteoporosis affects more women than men. About 20% of American women over age 50 have osteoporosis, and about 50% of all women over age 50 fracture a hip, wrist, or vertebra.

The use of oral calcium supplements can help women to obtain the calcium they need and prevent osteoporosis. For women, the recommended calcium intake varies with their developmental status:
+ 1,000 mg/day for nonpregnant women of childbearing age
+ 1,200 mg/day for pregnant women
+ 1,500 mg/day for breast-feeding or postmenopausal women.

Adverse reactions to watch for

+ Hypercalcemia (drowsiness, lethargy, muscle weakness, headache, constipation, metallic taste, shortened QT interval, heart block)
+ Local burning, necrosis, and tissue sloughing (with I.M. use)
+ Renal calculi (with a high calcium level)
+ Severe hypercalcemia (arrhythmias, cardiac arrest, coma)
+ Venous irritation (with I.V. use)

 CLINICAL ALERT When mixed in a solution for total parenteral nutrition (TPN), calcium may react with phosphorous to form a precipitate of insoluble calcium phosphate granules. These granules may deposit in pulmonary arterioles, leading to an embolism and possibly death. To reduce the risk of precipitation, take such measures as increasing the amino acid concentration in the TPN and using calcium gluconate rather than calcium chloride.

Adverse reactions

Calcium preparations may produce hypercalcemia if the calcium level isn't monitored closely. Early signs of hypercalcemia include drowsiness, lethargy, muscle weakness, headache, constipation, and a metallic taste in the mouth. ECG changes include a shortened QT interval and heart block. Severe hypercalcemia can cause arrhythmias, cardiac arrest and, eventually, coma. Because calcium is excreted by the kidneys, a high level can predispose patients to renal calculi.

With I.V. administration, calcium may cause venous irritation; I.M. injection may cause severe local reactions, such as burning, necrosis, and tissue sloughing.

Key nursing actions

+ Monitor the patient's calcium level.
+ Regularly assess for early signs of hypercalcemia, such as drowsiness, lethargy, muscle weakness, headache, constipation, and a metallic taste.
+ Monitor ECG tracings for changes that suggest hypercalcemia, such as a shortened QT interval, heart block, or arrhythmias.
+ Keep the patient recumbent for 15 minutes after injecting calcium.

Nursing considerations

+ Monitor the patient for adverse reactions and drug interactions.
+ Monitor the patient's calcium level.
+ Monitor the patient regularly for early signs of hypercalcemia, such as drowsiness, lethargy, muscle weakness, headache, constipation, and a metallic taste in the mouth.
+ Monitor the patient's ECG for changes that suggest hypercalcemia, such as a shortened QT interval, heart block, or arrhythmias.

 CLINICAL ALERT Give an I.V. infusion slowly to prevent a high calcium level from reaching the heart and possibly causing arrhythmias and cardiac arrest.

+ Keep the patient recumbent for 15 minutes after injecting calcium.
+ If extravasation occurs, stop the I.V. infusion. Apply warm, moist compresses to the area.

Teaching a patient about calcium

Whenever a calcium preparation is prescribed, teach the patient and his family the drug's name, dose, frequency, action, and adverse effects. Also take the following actions.
✦ Advise the patient to avoid eating large amounts of spinach, rhubarb, bran, whole grain cereals and breads, and fresh fruits and vegetables when taking calcium because these foods interfere with calcium absorption. Or, unless instructed otherwise, the patient can take calcium tablets 1 to 2 hours after eating these foods.
✦ Suggest that the patient eat foods containing vitamin D, which enhances calcium absorption.
✦ Stress the importance of returning for blood tests to monitor the calcium level.
✦ Teach the patient to recognize the signs and symptoms of hypercalcemia and to report them to the prescriber if any occur.

✦ Give the drug I.M. in an emergency, only when the I.V. route is impossible to use. If the I.M. route is used, give the injection in the gluteal muscle in an adult or in the lateral thigh in an infant or small child.
✦ Give an oral calcium supplement 1 to 2 hours after meals.
✦ If hypercalcemia occurs, notify the prescriber immediately. Keep emergency equipment nearby.
✦ Give calcium and digoxin slowly and in small amounts to avoid precipitating arrhythmias during therapy with both drugs.
✦ Teach the patient and his family about the prescribed drug. (See *Teaching a patient about calcium.*)

MAGNESIUM

After potassium, magnesium is the most abundant cation in ICF. It's essential for a variety of processes in the body.

Various disorders may deplete magnesium stores. These include malabsorption, chronic diarrhea, hyperaldosteronism, hypoparathyroidism or hyperparathyroidism, excessive release of adrenocortical hormones, and acute and chronic alcoholism. Nasogastric suctioning, prolonged therapy with diuretics or with parenteral fluids that don't contain magnesium, and therapy with such drugs as cisplatin, aminoglycosides, cyclosporine, or amphotericin B, can also deplete magnesium stores.

Parenteral magnesium replacement typically calls for magnesium sulfate. Oral replacement usually requires magnesium chloride or oxide.

Pharmacokinetics

Magnesium sulfate is distributed widely throughout the body. After I.V. administration, magnesium sulfate acts immediately; after I.M. administration, within 30 minutes. Magnesium sulfate isn't metabolized and is excreted unchanged in urine; some appears in breast milk.

Pharmacodynamics

Magnesium sulfate replenishes the key electrolyte and prevents magnesium deficiency. It also prevents or controls seizures by blocking neuromuscular transmission.

Features of magnesium

✦ Is the second most abundant cation in ICF
✦ Is essential in transmitting nerve impulses to muscles, activating the enzymes needed for carbohydrate and protein metabolism, stimulating parathyroid hormone secretion to regulate ICF calcium level, and aiding cell metabolism and sodium and potassium movement across cell membranes
✦ May be depleted by malabsorption, chronic diarrhea, hyperaldosteronism, hypoparathyroidism, hyperparathyroidism, excessive release of adrenocortical hormones, alcoholism, nasogastric suctioning, prolonged use of diuretics or of parenteral fluids that contain no magnesium, and therapy with such drugs as cisplatin, aminoglycosides, cyclosporine, or amphotericin B
✦ Is replenished preferably with magnesium sulfate
✦ As magnesium sulfate, is used to treat seizures, severe toxemia, and acute nephritis in children and to prevent and treat seizures in pregnant women with preeclampsia
✦ As magnesium oxide, is used for oral replacement therapy in mild hypomagnesemia
✦ As magnesium chloride, may be used for oral or I.V. replacement therapy

Normally, this electrolyte is essential in transmitting nerve impulses to muscles and activating the enzymes needed for carbohydrate and protein metabolism. It stimulates parathyroid hormone secretion, thus regulating the ICF calcium level. It also aids in cell metabolism and sodium and potassium movement across cell membranes.

Pharmacotherapeutics

Magnesium sulfate is the drug of choice for replacement therapy in magnesium deficiency. It's also used to treat seizures, severe toxemia, and acute nephritis in children. Magnesium sulfate is used to prevent and treat seizures in pregnant women with preeclampsia.

Magnesium oxide is used for oral replacement therapy in mild hypomagnesemia. Magnesium chloride may be used for oral or I.V. replacement therapy.

Interactions

✦ When used with digoxin, magnesium may lead to heart block.
✦ When used with alcohol, anxiolytics, antidepressants, antipsychotics, barbiturates, hypnotics, general anesthetics, and narcotics, magnesium sulfate may increase central nervous system depression.
✦ Magnesium sulfate can potentiate and prolong the neuromuscular blockade caused by succinylcholine or tubocurarine.
✦ Magnesium oxide may decrease the effects of allopurinol, antibiotics, digoxin, iron salts, penicillamine, and phenothiazines.
✦ Magnesium oxide may cause the premature release of enteric-coated drugs in the stomach.

Adverse reactions

Adverse reactions to magnesium sulfate can be life-threatening. These reactions include hypotension, circulatory collapse, flushing, depressed reflexes, and respiratory paralysis. I.M. injections of magnesium can cause pain, can induce sclerosis, and must be repeated frequently.

Nursing considerations

✦ Use parenteral magnesium cautiously in a patient with renal impairment because the risk of hypermagnesemia is increased in such a patient.
✦ For an adult, give an undiluted 50% magnesium solution by deep I.M. injection. For a child, dilute the solution to 20% or less.
✦ Keep I.V. calcium available to reverse the respiratory depression and heart block that may occur with magnesium overdose.
✦ Test the patient's knee-jerk and patellar reflexes before giving each additional dose. If absent, notify the prescriber and withhold the dose until the patient's reflexes return; otherwise, he may develop temporary respiratory failure and need cardiopulmonary resuscitation or I.V. administration of calcium.
✦ Check the magnesium level after repeated doses.
✦ Monitor the patient's fluid intake and output. His output should be 100 ml or more during the 4 hours before a dose is given.
✦ Monitor the patient's renal function.
✦ If a pregnant woman receives magnesium for toxemia within 24 hours before delivery, monitor the neonate for signs and symptoms of magnesium toxicity, including neuromuscular and respiratory depression.
✦ Teach the patient and his family about the prescribed drug. (See *Teaching a patient about magnesium*.)

Adverse reactions to watch for

✦ Circulatory collapse, depressed reflexes, flushing, hypotension, respiratory paralysis
✦ Pain, sclerosis (with I.M. injection)

Key nursing actions

✦ Keep I.V. calcium available to reverse the respiratory depression and heart block that may occur with magnesium overdose.
✦ Test the knee-jerk and patellar reflexes before giving each dose. If absent, notify the prescriber and withhold the dose until the reflexes return; this avoids temporary respiratory failure and the need for cardiopulmonary resuscitation or I.V. calcium administration.
✦ Check the magnesium level after repeated doses.
✦ Monitor fluid intake and output. Output should be 100 ml or more during the 4 hours before a dose is given.
✦ Monitor the patient's renal function.

ALKALINIZING AND ACIDIFYING DRUGS

Alkalinizing and acidifying drugs act to correct acid-base imbalances in the blood. These acid-base imbalances include metabolic acidosis and metabolic alkalosis. In metabolic acidosis, excess hydrogen ions in ECF decrease the pH level and is treated with alkalinizing drugs. In metabolic alkalosis, excess bicarbonate in ECF increases the pH level and is treated with acidifying drugs.

Alkalinizing and acidifying drugs have opposite effects. An alkalinizing drug increases the blood pH; an acidifying drug decreases it. Some of these drugs also alter the urine pH, making them useful in treating certain urinary tract infections and drug overdoses.

ALKALINIZING DRUGS

Alkalinizers are used to increase the blood pH level and treat metabolic acidosis. They include sodium salts, such as sodium acetate, bicarbonate, citrate, and lactate, as well as tromethamine. Sodium bicarbonate is also used to increase the urine pH level.

Pharmacokinetics

All alkalinizing drugs are absorbed well when given orally. Sodium bicarbonate is distributed naturally to the systemic circulation. At a pH of 7.4, about 25% of tromethamine is unionized; this portion may enter cells to neutralize acidic ions in ICF. Sodium citrate and sodium lactate are metabolized to the active ingredient, bicarbonate.

Sodium bicarbonate isn't metabolized. It's filtered and reabsorbed by the kidneys. Less than 1% of the filtered drug is excreted. Tromethamine undergoes little or no metabolism and is excreted unchanged in urine.

Pharmacodynamics

In the blood, sodium bicarbonate separates to provide bicarbonate ions that are used in the blood buffer system to decrease the hydrogen ion level and raise the blood pH level. (Buffers prevent extreme changes in the pH level by taking or giving up hydrogen ions to neutralize acids or bases.) As the bicarbonate ions are excreted in urine, the urine pH level rises. After conversion to bicarbonate, sodium citrate and lactate alkalinize the blood and urine in the same way.

Features of alkalinizing drugs

+ Increase blood pH and possibly urine pH
+ Are used to increase blood pH and treat metabolic acidosis
+ Are also used to raise urine pH level to help remove certain substances, such as phenobarbital, after an overdose
+ Sodium bicarbonate separates to provide bicarbonate ions used in the blood buffer system to decrease the hydrogen ion level and raise the blood pH
+ Tromethamine combines with hydrogen ions to alkalinize the blood and then the combination is excreted in urine

Tromethamine acts by combining with hydrogen ions to alkalinize the blood; the resulting tromethamine–hydrogen ion complex is excreted in urine.

Pharmacotherapeutics

Usually, alkalinizing drugs are used to treat metabolic acidosis. Other uses include raising the urine pH to help remove certain substances, such as phenobarbital, after an overdose.

Interactions

✦ Sodium bicarbonate, citrate, and lactate may increase the excretion — and reduce the effects — of ketoconazole, lithium, or a salicylate.
✦ Sodium bicarbonate, citrate, and lactate may reduce the excretion — and increase the effects — of an amphetamine, pseudoephedrine, or quinidine.
✦ An alkalinizing drug can reduce the antibacterial effects of methenamine.
✦ When taken with milk, sodium bicarbonate may cause hypercalcemia, alkalosis, and possibly renal calculi.

Adverse reactions

The most severe adverse reaction to I.V. sodium bicarbonate is overdose, which leads to metabolic alkalosis as evidenced by hyperirritability, tetany, or both. In a patient with diabetic ketoacidosis, rapid administration of sodium bicarbonate can correct acidosis too quickly and may cause cerebral dysfunction, tissue hypoxia, and lactic acidosis. The high sodium content of this drug may cause water retention and edema in some patients, especially those with renal impairment, heart failure, or other disorders that can cause fluid imbalance. administration of I.V. sodium bicarbonate can cause extravasation that may result in tissue sloughing, ulceration, and necrosis.

Oral sodium bicarbonate may produce gastric distention and flatulence as the drug combines with hydrochloric acid in the stomach to release carbon dioxide. Shohl's solution, which produces less gastric upset than sodium bicarbonate, usually is preferred for this reason.

Typically, sodium citrate produces few adverse reactions. However, an overdose may cause metabolic alkalosis or tetany or may aggravate existing cardiac disease by decreasing the calcium level. Oral sodium citrate can have a laxative effect.

Sodium lactate also produces few adverse reactions, except for metabolic alkalosis (from overdose) and extravasation. Because the sodium content is high, this drug may cause water retention and edema in a patient whose ability to excrete sodium is impaired, particularly by renal impairment or heart failure.

Adverse reactions to tromethamine may be mild, such as phlebitis or irritation at the injection site, or severe, such as hypoglycemia, respiratory depression (especially in a patient who already has depressed respirations or is receiving a drug that depresses respirations), extravasation, and hyperkalemia. In a patient with renal impairment, this renally excreted drug may accumulate to a toxic level. In a severely ill neonate, hypertonic tromethamine given through the umbilical vein can cause hepatic necrosis. Because of these adverse reactions, tromethamine use shouldn't exceed 24 hours for most patients.

Nursing considerations

✦ Monitor the patient for adverse reactions and drug interactions during alkalinizing drug therapy. If the patient reports GI distress, use a different alkalinizing drug because this reaction can lead to noncompliance and subsequent acute acidosis.

Teaching a patient about alkalinizing drugs

Whenever an alkalinizing drug is prescribed, teach the patient and his family its name, dose, frequency, action, and adverse effects. Also take these actions.
✦ Advise the patient that prolonged therapy with sodium bicarbonate tablets can cause GI distress and flatulence, which he should report to the prescriber.
✦ Teach the patient to recognize the signs of fluid retention, such as ankle swelling and increasing tightness of rings on the fingers. Emphasize the importance of immediately reporting these signs to the prescriber.
✦ Inform the patient with diabetes that tromethamine can cause hypoglycemia. Encourage him to monitor his glucose level closely.
✦ Teach the patient how to prepare and administer Shohl's solution to improve its taste and minimize its laxative effects.
✦ Instruct the patient to notify the prescriber if adverse reactions occur.
✦ Advise the patient to avoid milk while taking sodium bicarbonate in order to avoid milk-alkali syndrome, hypercalcemia, or renal calculi production.

✦ Regularly monitor the patient's pH and bicarbonate level to evaluate the effectiveness of therapy and to detect problems.
✦ If sodium bicarbonate is used to alkalinize a patient's urine, frequently monitor his urine pH.
✦ Inspect the I.V. site regularly for extravasation in a patient receiving sodium bicarbonate, sodium lactate, or tromethamine. Also check the site for phlebitis or irritation in a patient receiving tromethamine.
✦ Treat extravasation by elevating the affected limb, applying warm compresses, and giving lidocaine.
✦ Monitor the patient for signs and symptoms of overdose with the alkalinizing drug.

 CLINICAL ALERT
✦ Give sodium bicarbonate slowly to a patient with diabetic ketoacidosis because cerebral dysfunction, tissue hypoxia, and lactic acidosis can occur.
✦ Monitor for signs of fluid retention, such as crackles, peripheral edema, and jugular venous distention, in a patient receiving sodium bicarbonate or sodium lactate. The high sodium content of these drugs may cause fluid retention, especially in a patient with renal disease or heart failure.

✦ Don't give tromethamine for more than 24 hours. This limitation helps prevent severe adverse reactions.
✦ Dilute Shohl's solution with 2 to 3 oz (60 to 90 ml) of water before administration, refrigerate it to improve the taste, and give it after meals to minimize its laxative effects.
✦ Notify the prescriber if adverse reactions or drug interactions occur.
✦ Teach the patient and his family about the prescribed drug. (See *Teaching a patient about alkalinizing drugs*.)

Key nursing actions
✦ Monitor pH and bicarbonate level regularly to evaluate the drug's effectiveness and detect problems.
✦ If sodium bicarbonate is used to alkalinize the urine, monitor urine pH frequently.
✦ Monitor for evidence of overdose.
✦ Watch for evidence of fluid retention, such as crackles, peripheral edema, and jugular venous distention, in a patient receiving sodium bicarbonate or sodium lactate.

ACIDIFYING DRUGS

Two acidifying drugs are used to correct metabolic alkalosis: ammonium chloride and hydrochloric acid. Ammonium chloride also serves as a urinary acidifier, as does ascorbic acid.

Pharmacokinetics

The action of most acidifying drugs is immediate.

Oral ammonium chloride is absorbed completely in 3 to 6 hours. It's metabolized in the liver to form urea, which is excreted by the kidneys, and hydrochloric acid, the acidifying drug.

After I.V. administration, hydrochloric acid is broken down into hydrogen and chloride ions. The hydrogen ions are used as the acidifying drug.

Oral ascorbic acid usually is absorbed well, distributed widely in body tissues, and metabolized in the liver. Its metabolites are excreted in urine, along with excess ascorbic acid, which is excreted unchanged.

Pharmacodynamics

Acidifying drugs have several actions. Ammonium chloride lowers the pH after being metabolized to urea and to hydrochloric acid, which provides hydrogen ions to acidify the blood or urine. Hydrochloric acid lowers the pH directly by acidifying the blood with hydrogen ions. Ascorbic acid directly acidifies the urine, which provides hydrogen ions and lowers the urine pH.

Pharmacotherapeutics

A patient with metabolic alkalosis requires therapy with an acidifying drug that provides hydrogen ions. Such a patient may also need chloride ion therapy. Although the patient can receive both in a hydrochloric acid infusion, this infusion is difficult to prepare, and an overdose can produce severe adverse reactions.

Most patients receive both types of ions in oral or parenteral doses of ammonium chloride, a safer drug that's easy to prepare.

Interactions

+ Use of ammonium chloride with spironolactone may cause increased systemic acidosis.

Adverse reactions

Acidifying drugs usually produce mild adverse reactions, such as GI distress. However, overdose can occur, especially with parenteral administration, and may lead to acidosis.

Oral ammonium chloride may cause nausea, vomiting, anorexia, and thirst. Large dosages may cause metabolic acidosis and loss of electrolytes, especially potassium. Rapid I.V. administration may cause pain and irritation at the infusion site. Ammonium toxicity may also occur, producing twitching and hyperreflexia.

With hydrochloric acid administration, metabolic acidosis may occur with an overdose.

In high dosages, ascorbic acid can produce GI distress, such as nausea, vomiting, diarrhea, and abdominal cramps, and flushing, headache, and insomnia. In a patient with glucose-6-phosphate dehydrogenase (G6PD) deficiency, hemolytic anemia may develop after administration of a high dose of ascorbic acid.

Teaching a patient about acidifying drugs

Whenever an acidifying drug is prescribed, teach the patient and his family the drug's name, dose, frequency, action, and adverse effects. Also take the following actions.
◆ Instruct the patient to take ascorbic acid or oral ammonium chloride exactly as prescribed, to report severe adverse GI reactions, and to monitor his urine pH regularly.
◆ Instruct the patient to withhold the next ammonium chloride dose and notify the prescriber if twitching occurs because twitching may indicate ammonium toxicity.
◆ Advise the patient to request a prescription for a mild analgesic if headache results from high-dosage ascorbic acid therapy.
◆ If the patient reports insomnia, suggest relaxation techniques, such as a warm bath or reading before bedtime. If these techniques are ineffective, advise him to request a prescription for a hypnotic.
◆ Advise the patient to notify the prescriber if adverse reactions occur.

Nursing considerations

◆ Monitor the patient for adverse reactions and drug interactions.
◆ Monitor the patient for signs and symptoms of metabolic acidosis. Review his laboratory test results for alterations in his arterial blood pH, bicarbonate, chloride, and potassium levels.
◆ Observe for signs and symptoms of ammonium toxicity in a patient receiving ammonium chloride. If any appear, withhold the drug, notify the prescriber immediately, and switch the patient to a different acidifying drug.
◆ Monitor the patient for signs and symptoms of hypokalemia during therapy with large dosages of ammonium chloride. If any occur, notify the prescriber. Determine electrolyte levels and start therapy to correct the imbalance.
◆ Monitor the complete blood count for a patient with G6PD deficiency who receives high doses of ascorbic acid. Particularly note changes that suggest hemolytic anemia.
◆ Administer an I.V. acidifying drug slowly to prevent pain or irritation at the infusion site as well as other adverse reactions.
◆ Teach the patient and his family about the prescribed drug. (See *Teaching a patient about acidifying drugs.*)

Key nursing actions

◆ Monitor for evidence of metabolic acidosis. Review laboratory test results for alterations in arterial blood pH and bicarbonate, chloride, and potassium levels.
◆ Watch for evidence of ammonium toxicity during ammonium chloride therapy. If it appears, withhold the drug, notify the prescriber immediately, and switch the patient to a different acidifying drug.
◆ Assess for evidence of hypokalemia during therapy with large amounts of ammonium chloride. If it occurs, notify the prescriber, check electrolyte levels, and start therapy to correct the imbalance.
◆ Check the complete blood count for a patient with glucose-6-phosphate dehydrogenase deficiency who receives high doses of ascorbic acid. Note changes that suggest hemolytic anemia.

Essentials of dosage calculations

As a nurse, you commonly have to perform drug and I.V. fluid calculations. That's why you need to understand drug weights and measures and know how to convert between systems and measures, compute drug dosages, perform special calculations, and make dosage adjustments for children.

SYSTEMS OF DRUG WEIGHTS AND MEASURES

The two most common systems of measurement used to prescribe drugs are the metric and the household systems. These are so widely used that most brands of medication cups for liquid measurements are calibrated in both systems. A third system, the apothecaries' system, is no longer popular, but occasionally may be encountered in practice. Other special systems of measurement are used for selected drugs.

METRIC SYSTEM

The metric system is the international system of measurement, the most widely used system, and the system used by the U.S. Pharmacopeia. This system offers many advantages. It enables accurate calculations of small drug dosages. It uses Arabic numerals, which are commonly used by prescribers worldwide. Plus, it's used by most manufacturers to calibrate newly developed drugs.

The metric system includes units for liquid and solid measures. These measurements offer relative ease of conversion within the metric system. (See *Metric measures.*)

Reviewing the metric system

+ Is the international system of measurement
+ Is the most widely used system of measurement
+ Is the measurement system used by the U.S. Pharmacopeia
+ Allows accurate calculation of small drug dosages
+ Uses Arabic numerals, which are commonly used by prescribers worldwide
+ Is used by most manufacturers to calibrate new drugs

Metric measures

Metric weight equivalents

1 kilogram (kg or Kg)	= 1,000 grams (g or gm)
1 gram	= 1,000 milligrams (mg)
1 milligram	= 1,000 micrograms (mcg)
0.6 g	= 600 mg
0.3 g	= 300 mg
0.1 g	= 100 mg
0.06 g	= 60 mg
0.03 g	= 30 mg
0.015 g	= 15 mg
0.001 g	= 1 mg

Metric volume equivalents

1 liter (l or L)	= 1,000 milliliters (ml)
1 milliliter	= 1,000 microliters (mcl)

Metric weight conversions

Household	Metric
1 ounce	= 30 grams
1 pound	= 453.6 grams
2.2 pounds	= 1 kilogram

Metric volume conversions

Household	Metric
1 teaspoon (tsp)	= 5 ml
1 tablespoon (T or tbs)	= 15 ml
2 tablespoons	= 30 ml
8 ounces	= 240 ml
1 pint (pt)	= 473 ml
1 quart (qt)	= 946 ml
1 gallon (gal)	= 3,785 ml

Liquid measures

In the metric system, one liter (L) is about equal to 1 quart in the household system. Liters commonly are used for ordering and administering I.V. solutions. Milliliters (ml) typically are used for parenteral and some oral drugs.

Solid measures

The gram (g) is the basis for solid measures or units of weight in the metric system. Drugs commonly are ordered in grams (g), milligrams (mg), or micrograms (mcg). 1 mg equals 1/1000 of a g; 1 mcg equals 1/1000 of a mg. Body weight usually is recorded in kilograms (kg). 1 kg equals 1,000 g.

The following sample drug orders use the metric system:
+ 30 ml milk of magnesia by mouth (P.O.) at bedtime (h.s.)
+ Ancef 1 g I.V. every (q) 6 hours
+ Lanoxin 0.125 mg P.O. daily.

HOUSEHOLD SYSTEM

Most foods, recipes, over-the-counter drugs, and home remedies use the household system. Prescribers use this system less commonly than the metric system for ordering drugs. However, your knowledge of household measures may be useful in some situations.

Liquid measures

Liquid measurements in the household system include the teaspoon (tsp) and the tablespoon (tbs). For drug purposes, these measurements have been standardized to 5 milliliters and 15 milliliters, respectively. Using these standardized amounts, for example, 3 tsp equal 1 tbs, and 6 tsp equal 1 ounce (oz). Patients who need to measure doses by teaspoon or tablespoon should use a calibrated device to make sure they receive exactly the prescribed amount. They shouldn't use an ordinary household teaspoon to measure a tsp of a drug because the amount is likely to be inaccurate. Household teaspoon sizes vary from 4 to 6 ml or more.

Reviewing the household system

+ Is used for most foods, recipes, over-the-counter drugs, and home remedies
+ Is used less often than the metric system among prescribers
+ Has the liquid measurements teaspoon (tsp) and tablespoon (tbs)
+ Is standardized for drug measurement to 5 ml for 1 tsp and 15 ml for 1 tbs
+ Should be measured using a calibrated device for liquids and not an ordinary household spoon

The following sample drug orders use the household system:

✦ 2 tsp Bactrim P.O. twice daily (b.i.d.)

✦ Riopan 2 tbs P.O. 1 hour before meals (a.c.) and h.s.

APOTHECARIES' SYSTEM

Two features distinguish the apothecaries' system from other systems: the use of Roman numerals and the placement of the unit of measurement before the Roman numeral. For example, a measurement of 5 grains would be written as *grains V*.

In the apothecaries' system, equivalents among the various units of measure are close approximations of one another. By contrast, equivalents in the metric system are exact. When using apothecaries' equivalents for calculations and conversions, the calculations aren't precise but fall within acceptable standards.

The apothecaries' system is the only system of measurement that uses symbols and abbreviations to represent units of measure. Although this system is infrequently used in healthcare, you must be able to read dosages that were written in it and convert them to the metric system.

Liquid measures

The smallest unit of liquid measurement in the apothecaries' system is the minim, which is about the size of a drop of water. Fifteen to sixteen minims equal about 1 ml.

Solid measures

The grain (gr) is the smallest solid measure or unit of weight in the apothecaries' system. It equals about 60 mg. One dram equals about 60 gr.

The following sample drug order uses the apothecaries' system:

✦ Tylenol gr X P.O. q 4 hours as needed (p.r.n.) for headache.

SPECIAL SYSTEMS

For some drugs, you'll need to use a special system of measurement developed by the drug manufacturer. Three of the most common special systems are units, international units, and milliequivalents.

Units

Once commonly abbreviated "U," units should no longer be abbreviated because this can contribute to serious drug errors. Insulin is one of several drugs measured in units. Although many types of insulin exist, all are measured in units. The international standard of U-100 insulin means that 1 ml of insulin solution contains 100 units of insulin, regardless of type. The anticoagulant heparin is also measured in units. So are several antibiotics, which are available in liquid, solid, and powder forms for oral or parenteral use.

The unit isn't a standard measure. That's why different drugs measured in units may have no relationship to one another in quality or activity. That's also why each drug manufacturer provides specific information about measuring each drug that's given in units.

The following sample drug orders use units:

✦ 14 units NPH insulin S.C. this a.m.

✦ heparin 5,000 units S.C. q 12 hours.

✦ nystatin 200,000 units P.O. q 6 hours.

Reviewing the apothecaries' system

✦ Is used infrequently in health care

✦ Uses symbols and abbreviations to represent units of measure

✦ Has as its smallest liquid unit the minim, about the size of one drop

✦ Has as its smallest solid measure the grain, about 60 mg

✦ Is distinguished by use of Roman numerals and placement of the unit of measurement before the Roman numeral

✦ Uses equivalents among units of measure that are close approximations of one another

✦ Provides calculations and conversions that aren't precise but are within acceptable standards

Reviewing units

✦ Aren't standard measures

✦ Don't relate drugs by quality or activity

✦ Should be spelled out because abbreviation as U can cause serious drug errors

✦ Measure drugs, such as insulin, heparin, certain antibiotics

International units

International units are used to measure biologicals, such as vitamins, enzymes, and hormones. For instance, the activity of calcitonin, a synthetic hormone used to regulate calcium, is expressed in international units. Once commonly abbreviated "IU," international units should no longer be abbreviated so that the abbreviation is not mistaken for "I.V."

The following sample drug orders use international units:

✦ 100 international units calcitonin (salmon) S.C. daily
✦ 8 international units somatropin S.C. three times per week.

Milliequivalents

Electrolytes may be measured in milliequivalents (mEq). Drug manufacturers provide information about the number of metric units needed to provide a prescribed number of milliequivalents. Potassium chloride (KCl), for example, is usually ordered in milliequivalents.

The following sample drug orders use milliequivalents:

✦ 30 mEq KCl P.O. b.i.d.
✦ 1 L dextrose 5% in normal saline solution with 40 mEq KCl to be run at 125 ml/hour.

CONVERSIONS BETWEEN MEASUREMENT SYSTEMS

Sometimes you need to convert from one measurement system to another, particularly when a drug is prescribed in one system but only available in another system. To perform conversion calculations, you need to know the equivalents for the different measurement systems.

For a simple conversion, you may be able to use the standard equivalent. (See *Metric measures*, page 527.) For a more complex conversion, you may employ the equivalent and the fraction method, which is the most commonly used technique for converting between measurement systems.

FRACTION METHOD

For measurement conversions, the fraction method involves an equation consisting of two fractions. Set up the first fraction by placing the ordered dosage over the unknown (x) units of the available dosage.

For example, say a prescriber orders 7.5 ml of acetaminophen elixir to be given by mouth. To find the equivalent in teaspoons, first set up a fraction in which the milliliter dosage represents the ordered dosage and the teaspoon dosage represents the unknown available dosage:

$$\frac{7.5 \text{ ml}}{x \text{ tsp}}$$

Then set up the second fraction, which appears on the right side of the equation. This fraction consists of the standard equivalents between the ordered and the available measures. Because milliliters must be converted to teaspoons, the right side of the equation appears as:

$$\frac{5 \text{ ml}}{1 \text{ tsp}}$$

The same unit of measure should appear in the numerator of both fractions. Likewise, the same unit of measure should appear in both denominators. The entire equation should appear as:

$$\frac{7.5 \text{ ml}}{x \text{ tsp}} = \frac{5 \text{ ml}}{1 \text{ tsp}}$$

To solve for x, cross multiply.

$$x \text{ tsp} \times 5 \text{ ml} = 7.5 \text{ ml} \times 1 \text{ tsp}$$

$$x \text{ tsp} = \frac{7.5 \text{ ml} \times 1 \text{ tsp}}{5 \text{ ml}}$$

$$x \text{ tsp} = \frac{7.5 \times 1 \text{ tsp}}{5}$$

$$x \text{ tsp} = 1.5 \text{ tsp}$$

The patient should receive 1.5 tsp of acetaminophen elixir.

COMPUTATION OF DRUG DOSAGES

After verifying a drug order, you can compute the drug dosage. In this two-step process, first determine whether the ordered drug is available in units of the same measurement system. If it's not, convert the ordered drug measurement to the system used for the available drug, as previously described.

If the ordered units of measurement are available, move to step two: Calculate how much of the available dosage form should be given. For example, if the prescribed dose is 250 mg, determine the quantity of tablets (tab), powder, or liquid that equals 250 mg. To determine that quantity, use the fraction, ratio, or desired-available method or dimensional analysis.

FRACTION METHOD

When using the fraction method to compute a drug dosage, write an equation consisting of two fractions. First, set up a fraction showing the number of units to be given over x, which represents the quantity of the dosage form.

On the other side of the equation, set up a fraction showing the number of units of the drug in its dosage form over the quantity of dosage forms that supply that number of units. The number of units and the quantity of dosage forms are specific for each drug. In most cases, the stated quantity equals 1. Information on the drug label should supply the details you need to form the second fraction.

For example, if the number of units to be given equals 250 mg, the first fraction in the equation is:

$$\frac{250 \text{ mg}}{x \text{ tab}}$$

The drug label states that each tablet contains 125 mg. So the second fraction is:

$$\frac{125 \text{ mg}}{1 \text{ tab}}$$

Note that the same units of measure appear in the numerators and the same units appear in the denominators. However, the units of measure in the denominators differ from the units in the numerators.

Steps in computing a drug dosage

◆ Verify the drug order.
◆ Determine whether the ordered drug is available in the ordered units.
◆ If not, convert the ordered units to the available units, using equivalents and the fraction method.
◆ If the ordered units are available, calculate how much of the available dosage form to give, using the fraction, ratio, or desired-available method or dimensional analysis.

Steps in the fraction method

◆ Write an equation consisting of two fractions separated by an equals sign.
◆ On the left, write the fraction to show ordered units over x, which represents the quantity of the dosage form.
◆ On the right, write the fraction to show drug units over the quantity of dosage forms that supply that number of units (from the drug label).
◆ Solve for x.

The entire equation should appear as:

$$\frac{250 \text{ mg}}{x \text{ tab}} = \frac{125 \text{ mg}}{1 \text{ tab}}$$

Solving for x determines the quantity of the dosage form, which is 2 tablets in this example.

RATIO METHOD

To use the ratio method, write the amount of the drug to be given and the quantity of the dose (x) as a ratio. Using the above example, you'd write:

$$250 \text{ mg} : x \text{ tab}$$

Next, complete the equation by forming a second ratio with the number of units in each tablet (or appropriate dosage form), which is listed on the manufacturer's label. Again using the example from above, the entire equation is:

$$250 \text{ mg} : x \text{ tab} :: 125 \text{ mg} : 1 \text{ tab}$$

To solve for x, set up an equation in which the product of the means (inner portions of the ratio) equals the product of the extremes (outer portions).

$$x \text{ tab} \times 125 \text{ mg} = 250 \text{ mg} \times 1 \text{ tab}$$

$$x \text{ tab} = \frac{250 \text{ mg} \times 1 \text{ tab}}{125 \text{ mg}}$$

$$x = 2 \text{ tab}$$

The patient should receive 2 tablets.

DESIRED-AVAILABLE METHOD

Also called the dose over on-hand (D/H) method, the desired-available method lets you convert ordered units into available units and compute the drug dosage all in one step. The desired-available equation appears as:

$$x \text{ quantity to give} = \frac{\text{ordered units}}{1} \times \text{conversion fraction} \times \frac{\text{quantity of dosage form}}{\text{stated quantity of drug within each dosage form}}$$

For example, suppose you receive an order for gr X of a drug. The drug is available only in 300-mg tablets. To determine the number of tablets to give the patient, substitute gr X (the ordered number of units) for the first element of the equation. Then use the conversion fraction as the second portion of the formula. The conversion fraction is:

$$\frac{60 \text{ mg}}{1 \text{ gr}}$$

The measure in the denominator must be the same as the measure in the ordered units. Because the order specified gr X, grains appears in the denominator of the conversion fraction.

Steps in the ratio method

+ Write the amount of the drug to be given and the quantity of the dose *(x)* as a ratio.
+ Form a second ratio with the number of units in each dosage form (from the drug label).
+ Solve for *x* by making the product of the means (inner elements) equal the product of the extremes (outer elements).

Reviewing the desired-available method

+ Is also called the dose over on-hand (D/H) method
+ Lets you convert ordered units into available units and compute the dosage in one step
+ Uses only one equation, but it's a more elaborate one than that used in the fraction or ratio method

The third element of the equation shows the dosage form over the stated drug quantity for that dosage form. Because the drug is available in 300-mg tablets, the fraction is:

$$\frac{1 \text{ tab}}{300 \text{ mg}}$$

The dosage form (in this case, tablets) should always appear in the numerator, and the quantity of drug in each dosage form should always appear in the denominator. The completed equation is:

$$x \text{ tab} = 10 \text{ gr} \times \frac{60 \text{ mg}}{1 \text{ gr}} \times \frac{1 \text{ tab}}{300 \text{ mg}}$$

Solving for x shows that the patient should receive 2 tablets.

The desired-available method has the advantage of using only one equation. However, it requires you to memorize a more elaborate equation than the one used in the fraction or ratio methods. Relying on your memory of a more complicated equation may increase the chance of error.

DIMENSIONAL ANALYSIS

A variation of the ratio method, dimensional analysis (also called factor analysis or factor labeling) eliminates the need to memorize formulas and requires only one equation to determine the answer. To compare the two methods at a glance, read the following problem and solutions.

Suppose a prescriber orders 0.25 g of streptomycin sulfate I.M. The vial reads 2 ml = 1 g. How many milliliters should you give?

Dimensional analysis

$$\frac{0.25 \text{ g}}{1} \times \frac{2 \text{ ml}}{1\text{g}} = 0.5 \text{ ml}$$

Ratio method

$$1 \text{ g} : 2 \text{ ml} :: 0.25 \text{ g} : x \text{ ml}$$

$$x = 2 \times 0.25$$

$$x = 0.5 \text{ ml}$$

When using dimensional analysis, you arrange a series of ratios, called factors, in a single (although sometimes lengthy) fractional equation. Each factor, written as a fraction, consists of two quantities and their related units of measurement. For instance, if 1,000 ml of a drug should be given over 8 hours, the relationship between 1,000 ml and 8 hours is expressed by the fraction

$$\frac{1,000 \text{ ml}}{8 \text{ hours}}$$

When a problem includes a quantity and a unit of measurement that are unrelated to any other factor in the problem, they serve as the numerator of the fraction, and 1 (implied) becomes the denominator.

Some mathematical problems contain all of the information needed to identify the factors, set up the equation, and find the solution. Other problems require the use of a conversion factor. Conversion factors are equivalents (for example, 1 g = 1,000 mg) that you can memorize or obtain from a conversion chart. (See *Metric*

Reviewing dimensional analysis

+ Is a variation of the ratio method
+ Is also called factor analysis or factor labeling
+ Eliminates the need to memorize formulas
+ Requires only one equation to find the answer
+ Involves arranging a series of ratios, called factors, in a single fractional equation, with each fraction consisting of two quantities and their related units of measurement
+ Names factors given in the problem and the conversion factors needed to solve the problem as *knowns;* names the quantity of the answer *unknown.*
+ Requires setting up the equation by working backward, beginning with the unit of measurement of the answer

measures, page 527.) Because the two quantities and units of measurement are equivalent, they can serve as the numerator or the denominator; thus, the conversion factor 1 g = 1,000 mg can be written in fraction form as

$$\frac{1{,}000 \text{ mg}}{1\text{g}} \quad \text{or} \quad \frac{1 \text{ g}}{1{,}000 \text{ mg}}$$

The factors given in the problem plus the conversion factors needed to solve the problem are called *knowns.* The quantity of the answer, of course, is *unknown.* When setting up an equation in dimensional analysis, work backward, beginning with the unit of measurement of the answer. After plotting all the knowns, find the solution by following this sequence:

✦ Cancel similar quantities and units of measurement.
✦ Multiply the numerators.
✦ Multiply the denominators.
✦ Divide the numerator by the denominator.

Mastering dimensional analysis can take practice, but you may find your efforts well rewarded. To understand more fully how dimensional analysis works, review the following problem and the steps taken to solve it.

A prescriber orders gr X of a drug. The pharmacy supplies the drug in 300-mg tablets (tab). How many tablets should you administer?

✦ Write down the unit of measurement of the answer, followed by an "equal to" symbol.

$$\text{tab} =$$

✦ Search the problem for the quantity with the same unit of measurement. (If one doesn't exist, use a conversion factor.) Place this quantity in the numerator and its related quantity and unit of measurement in the denominator.

$$\text{tab} = \frac{1 \text{ tab}}{300 \text{ mg}}$$

✦ Separate the first factor from the next with a multiplication symbol.

$$\text{tab} = \frac{1 \text{ tab}}{300 \text{ mg}} \times$$

✦ Place the unit of measurement of the denominator of the first factor in the numerator of the second factor. Then search the problem for the quantity with the same unit of measurement (if one doesn't exist, as in this example, use a conversion factor). Now place this quantity in the numerator and its related quantity and unit of measurement in the denominator, and follow with a multiplication symbol. Repeat this step until all known factors are included in the equation.

$$\text{tab} = \frac{1 \text{ tab}}{300 \text{ mg}} \times \frac{60 \text{ mg}}{1 \text{ gr}} \times \frac{10 \text{ gr}}{1}$$

✦ Treat the equation as a large fraction. First, cancel similar units of measurement in the numerator and the denominator. (What remains should be what you began with—the unit of measurement of the answer. If not, recheck your equation to find and correct the error.) Next, multiply the numerators and then the denominators. Finally, divide the numerator by the denominator.

$$\text{tab} = \frac{1 \text{ tab}}{300 \text{ \cancel{mg}}} \times \frac{60 \text{ \cancel{mg}}}{1 \text{ \cancel{gr}}} \times \frac{10 \text{ \cancel{gr}}}{1}$$

$$= \frac{60 \times 10 \text{ tab}}{300}$$

$$= \frac{600 \text{ tab}}{300}$$

$$= 2 \text{ tab}$$

For more practice, study the following examples, which use dimensional analysis to solve various mathematical problems common to dosage calculations and drug administration.

1. A patient weighs 140 lb. What is his weight in kg?

Unit of measurement of the answer: kg

$$\text{1st factor (conversion factor): } \frac{1 \text{ kg}}{2.2 \text{ lb}}$$

$$\text{2nd factor: } \frac{140 \text{ lb}}{1}$$

$$\text{kg} = \frac{1 \text{ kg}}{2.2 \text{ lb}} \times 140 \text{ lb}$$

$$= \frac{140 \text{ lb}}{2.2 \text{ lb}}$$

$$= 63.6 \text{ kg}$$

2. A prescriber orders 75 mg of a drug. The pharmacy stocks a multidose vial containing 100 mg/ml. How many milliliters should you administer?

Unit of measurement of the answer: ml

$$\text{1st factor: } \frac{1 \text{ ml}}{100 \text{ mg}}$$

$$\text{2nd factor: } \frac{75 \text{ mg}}{1}$$

$$\text{ml} = \frac{1 \text{ ml}}{100 \text{ mg}} \times \frac{75 \text{ mg}}{1}$$

$$= \frac{75 \text{ ml}}{100}$$

$$x = 0.75 \text{ ml}$$

3. A prescriber orders 1 tsp of a cough elixir. The pharmacist sends up a bottle whose label reads 1 ml = 50 mg. How many milligrams should you administer?

Unit of measurement of the answer: mg

$$\text{1st factor: } \frac{50 \text{ mg}}{1 \text{ ml}}$$

$$\text{2nd factor (conversion factor): } \frac{5 \text{ ml}}{1 \text{ tsp}}$$

$$\text{3rd factor: } \frac{1 \text{ tsp}}{1}$$

$$mg = \frac{50 \text{ mg}}{1 \text{ ml}} \times \frac{5 \text{ ml}}{1 \text{ tsp}} \times \frac{1 \text{ tsp}}{1}$$

$$= \frac{50 \text{ mg} \times 5}{1}$$

$$= 250 \text{ mg}$$

4. A prescriber orders 1,000 ml of an I.V. solution to be administered over 8 hours. The I.V. tubing delivers 15 drops (gtt)/ml/minute (min). What is the infusion rate in gtt/minute?

Unit of measurement of the answer: gtt/minute

$$\text{1st factor: } \frac{15 \text{ gtt}}{1 \text{ ml}}$$

$$\text{2nd factor: } \frac{1,000 \text{ ml}}{8 \text{ hr}}$$

$$\text{3rd factor (conversion factor): } \frac{1 \text{ hr}}{60 \text{ min}}$$

$$\text{gtt/minute} = \frac{15 \text{ gtt}}{1 \text{ ml}} \times \frac{1,000 \text{ ml}}{8 \text{ hr}} \times \frac{1 \text{ hr}}{60 \text{ min}}$$

$$= \frac{15 \text{ gtt} \times 1,000 \times 1}{1 \times 8 \times 60 \text{ min}}$$

$$= \frac{15,000 \text{ gtt}}{480 \text{ min}}$$

$$= 31.3 \text{ or } 31 \text{ gtt/min}$$

5. A prescriber orders 10,000 units of heparin added to 500 ml of dextrose 5% in water (D_5W) at 1,200 units/hour. How many drops per minute should you administer if the I.V. tubing delivers 10 gtt/ml?

Unit of measurement of the answer: gtt/minute

$$\text{1st factor: } \frac{10 \text{ gtt}}{1 \text{ ml}}$$

$$\text{2nd factor: } \frac{500 \text{ ml}}{10,000 \text{ units}}$$

$$\text{3rd factor: } \frac{1,200 \text{ units}}{1 \text{ hour}}$$

$$\text{4th factor (conversion factor): } \frac{1 \text{ hr}}{60 \text{ min}}$$

$$\text{gtt/minute} = \frac{10 \text{ gtt}}{1 \text{ ml}} \times \frac{500 \text{ ml}}{10,000 \text{ units}} \times \frac{1,200 \text{ units}}{1 \text{ hr}} \times \frac{1 \text{ hr}}{60 \text{ min}}$$

$$= \frac{10 \text{ gtt} \times 500 \times 1{,}200}{10{,}000 \times 60 \text{ min}}$$

$$= \frac{6{,}000{,}000 \text{ gtt}}{600{,}000 \text{ min}}$$

$$= 10 \text{ gtt/min}$$

SPECIAL COMPUTATIONS

You can use the fraction, ratio, and desired-available methods and dimensional analysis to compute drug dosages when the ordered drug and the available form of the drug occur in the same units of measure. You can also use these methods when the quantity of a particular dosage form differs from the units in which the dosage form is given.

For example, if a patient is to receive 1,000 mg of a drug available in liquid form and measured in milligrams, with 100 mg contained in 6 ml, how many milliliters should the patient receive? Because the ordered and the available dosages are in milligrams, you don't need to make conversions first. Rather, you can simply use the fraction method to determine the number of milliliters the patient should receive, which is 60 ml in this case.

Because the drug is to be given in ounces, you should determine the number of ounces using a conversion method. For the fraction method of conversion, the equation would appear as:

$$\frac{60 \text{ ml}}{x \text{ oz}} = \frac{30 \text{ ml}}{1 \text{ oz}}$$

Solving for x shows that the patient should receive 2 oz of the drug.

To use the desired-available method, change the order of the elements in the equation to correspond with the situation. The revised equation is:

$$\frac{x}{\text{quantity to give}} = \frac{\text{ordered units}}{1} \times \frac{\text{quantity of dosage form}}{\text{stated quantity of drug within each dosage form}} \times \text{conversion fraction}$$

Placing the given information into the equation results in:

$$x \text{ oz} = \frac{1{,}000 \text{ mg}}{1} \times \frac{6 \text{ ml}}{100 \text{ mg}} \times \frac{1 \text{ oz}}{30 \text{ ml}}$$

Solving for x shows that the patient should receive 2 oz of the drug.

INEXACT NATURE OF DOSAGE COMPUTATIONS

Converting drug measurements from one system to another and then determining the amount of a dosage form to give can easily produce inexact dosages. A rounding error during computation or discrepancies in the dosage may occur, depending on the conversion standard used in calculation. Or, you may determine a precise amount to be given, only to find that administering that amount is impossible. For example, precise computations may indicate that a patient should receive 0.97 tablet. Administering such an amount is impossible.

To help avoid calculation errors and discrepancies between theoretical and real dosages, follow this general rule: *No more than a 10% variation should exist between the dosage ordered and the dosage to be given.* Following this simple rule, if your calculations show that a patient should receive 0.97 tablet, you can safely give 1 tablet.

COMPUTING PARENTERAL DOSAGES

The methods for computing oral drug dosages can also be used for parenteral dosages. The following example shows how to determine a parenteral drug dosage. Suppose a prescriber orders 75 mg of Demerol. The package label reads: meperidine (Demerol), 100 mg/ml. Using the fraction method to determine the number of milliliters the patient should receive, the equation is:

$$\frac{75 \text{ mg}}{x \text{ ml}} = \frac{100 \text{ mg}}{1 \text{ ml}}$$

To solve for *x*, cross multiply:

$$x \text{ ml} \times 100 \text{ mg} = 75 \text{ mg} \times 1 \text{ ml}$$

$$x \text{ ml} = \frac{75 \; \cancel{\text{mg}} \times 1 \text{ ml}}{100 \; \cancel{\text{mg}}}$$

$$x \text{ ml} = \frac{75 \text{ ml}}{100}$$

$$x = 0.75 \text{ ml}$$

The patient should receive 0.75 ml.

RECONSTITUTING POWDERS FOR INJECTION

Although a pharmacist usually reconstitutes powders for parenteral use, nurses sometimes perform this function by following the directions on the drug label. To do this, first consult the drug label. The label gives the total quantity of drug in the vial or ampule, the amount and type of diluent to be added to the powder, and the strength and expiration date of the resulting solution. When you add diluent to a powder, the powder increases the fluid volume. That's why the label calls for less diluent than the total volume of the prepared solution. For example, a label may say to add 1.7 ml of diluent to a vial of powdered drug to obtain a 2-ml total volume of prepared solution.

Next, determine the amount of solution to administer, using the manufacturer's information about the concentration of the solution. For example, if you want to administer 500 mg of a drug and the concentration of the prepared solution is 1 g (1,000 mg)/10 ml, use the following equation:

$$\frac{500 \text{ mg}}{x \text{ ml}} = \frac{1,000 \text{ mg}}{10 \text{ ml}}$$

The patient should receive 5 ml of the prepared solution.

I.V. DRIP RATES AND FLOW RATES

Before you can calculate I.V. drip rates and flow rates, make sure you know the difference between them. The drip rate refers to the number of drops of solution to be

Reminders about reconstitution

✦ The label gives the total quantity of drug in the vial or ampule, the amount and type of diluent to be added to the powder, and the strength and expiration date of the resulting solution.

✦ When you add diluent to a powder, the powder increases the fluid volume. That's why the label calls for less diluent than the total volume of the prepared solution.

Reviewing drip rate and flow rate

✦ Drip rate is the number of drops of solution to be infused per minute.

✦ Flow rate is the number of milliliters of fluid to be infused over 1 hour.

infused per minute. The flow rate refers to the number of milliliters of fluid to be infused over 1 hour.

To calculate an I.V. drip rate, first set up a fraction showing the volume of solution to be delivered over the number of minutes in which that volume should be infused. For example, if a patient should receive 100 ml of solution in 1 hour, the fraction is:

$$\frac{100 \text{ ml}}{60 \text{ min}}$$

Next, multiply the fraction by the drip factor (the number of drops contained in 1 ml) to determine the drip rate. The drip factor varies among different I.V. sets and should appear on the package that contains the I.V. tubing administration set. Following the manufacturer's directions for drip factor is a crucial step. Standard administration sets have drip factors of 10, 15, or 20 gtt/ml. A microdrip (minidrip) set has a drip factor of 60 gtt/ml. (See *Drip factors and flow rates.*)

Use the following equation to determine the drip rate of an I.V. solution:

$$\text{gtt/min} = \frac{\text{total no. of ml}}{\text{total no. of min}} \times \text{drip factor}$$

The equation applies to I.V. solutions that infuse over many hours or to small-volume infusions, such as those used for antibiotics, usually given in less than 1 hour. For example, if an order requires 1,000 ml of 5% dextrose in normal saline solution to infuse over 12 hours and if the administration set delivers 15 gtt/ml, what should the drip rate be?

$$x \text{ gtt/min} = \frac{1,000 \text{ ml}}{720 \text{ min}} \times 15 \text{ gtt/ml}$$

$$x \text{ gtt/min} = 20.83 \text{ gtt/min}$$

The drip rate can be rounded to 21 gtt/minute.

You'll calculate flow rates when working with I.V. infusion pumps to set the number of milliliters to be delivered in 1 hour. To perform this calculation, you need to know the total volume (in milliliters) to be infused and the amount of time required for the infusion. Use the following equation:

$$\text{flow rate} = \frac{\text{total volume ordered}}{\text{number of hours}}$$

Quick methods for calculating drip rates

Quicker methods exist for computing I.V. solution administration rates. To administer an I.V. solution with a microdrip set, adjust the flow rate (number of milliliters per hour) to equal the drip rate (number of drops per minute). To do this, divide the flow rate by 60 minutes and then multiply by the drip factor, which also equals 60. Because the flow rate and the drip factor are equal, the two arithmetic operations cancel each other out. For example, if the ordered flow rate were 125 ml/hour, the equation would be:

$$\text{Drip rate (125)} = \frac{125 \text{ ml}}{60 \text{ min}} \times 60$$

Rather than spend time calculating the equation, you can simply use the number assigned to the flow rate as the drip rate.

Drip factors and flow rates

When calculating the flow rate of I.V. solutions, remember that the number of drops required to deliver 1 ml varies with the type of administration set you're using. To calculate the drip rate, you must know the calibration of the drip rate for each specific manufacturer's product. As a quick guide, refer to the table below. Use this formula to calculate specific drip rates:

$$\frac{\text{volume of infusion (in ml)}}{\text{time of infusion (in minutes)}} \times \text{drip factor (in drops/ml)} = \text{drops/minutes}$$

	ORDERED VOLUME					
	500 ml/24 hour or 21 ml/hour	1,000 ml/24 hour or 42 ml/hour	1,000 ml/20hour or 50 ml/hour	1,000 ml/10 hour or 100 ml/hour	1,000 ml/8 hour or 125 ml/hour	1,000 ml/6 hour or 166 ml/hour
INDICATION	DROPS/MINUTES TO INFUSE					
Macrodrip **10**	3	7	8	17	21	28
15	5	11	13	25	31	42
20	7	14	17	34	42	56
Microdrip **60**	21	42	50	100	125	166

For I.V. administration sets that deliver 15 gtt/ml, divide the flow rate by 4 to get the drip rate. For sets with a drip factor of 10 gtt/ml, divide the flow rate by 6 to find the drip rate.

CRITICAL CARE CALCULATIONS

On the critical care unit, many drugs are used to treat acute, life-threatening problems. This means that you must be able to perform calculations swiftly and accurately, prepare and infuse the drug, and then observe the patient closely to evaluate its effectiveness. Before administering a critical care drug, you must calculate: the drug's concentration in an I.V. solution, the flow rate needed to deliver the desired dose, and the required dosage.

Calculating concentration

To calculate the drug's concentration, use the following formula:

$$\text{concentration in mg/ml} = \text{mg of drug/ml of fluid}$$

To express the concentration in mcg/ml, multiply the answer by 1,000.

Reminders for critical care calculations

♦ On a critical care unit, many drugs are used to treat acute, life-threatening problems.

♦ You must be able to calculate swiftly and accurately, prepare and infuse the drug, and observe the patient closely to evaluate the drug's effectiveness.

♦ Before giving a critical care drug, calculate its concentration in an I.V. solution, the flow rate needed to deliver the desired dose, and the required dosage.

Calculating flow rate

To determine the I.V. flow rate per minute, use the following formula:

$$\frac{\text{dose/min}}{x\ \text{ml/min}} = \frac{\text{concentration of solution}}{1\ \text{ml of fluid}}$$

To calculate the hourly flow rate, first multiply the ordered dose, given in milligrams or micrograms per minute, by 60 minutes to determine the hourly dose. Then use the following equation to compute the hourly flow rate:

$$\frac{\text{hourly dose}}{x\ \text{ml/min}} = \frac{\text{concentration of solution}}{1\ \text{ml of fluid}}$$

Calculating dosage

To determine the dosage in milligrams per kilogram of body weight per minute, first determine the concentration of the solution in milligrams per milliliter. (If a drug is ordered in micrograms, convert milligrams to micrograms by multiplying by 1,000.) To determine the dose in milligrams per hour, multiply the hourly flow rate by the concentration, using this formula:

$$\text{dose in mg/hr} = \text{hourly flow rate} \times \text{concentration}$$

Then calculate the dose in milligrams per minute. Divide the hourly dose by 60 minutes:

$$\text{dose in mg/min} = \frac{\text{dose in mg/hr}}{60\ \text{min}}$$

Divide the dose per minute by the patient's weight, using the following formula:

$$\text{mg/kg/min} = \frac{\text{mg/min}}{\text{patient's weight in kg}}$$

Finally, make sure that the drug is being given within a safe and therapeutic range. Compare the amount in milligrams per kilogram per minute to the safe range shown in a drug reference book.

The following examples show how to calculate an I.V. flow rate using the different formulas.

Example 1

A patient has frequent runs of ventricular tachycardia that subside after 10 to 12 beats. The prescriber orders 2 g (2,000 mg) of lidocaine in 500 ml of D_5W to infuse at 2 mg/minute. What's the flow rate in milliliters per minute? In milliliters per hour?

First, find the concentration of the solution by setting up a proportion with the unknown concentration in one fraction and the ordered dose in the other fraction:

$$\frac{x\ \text{mg}}{\text{ml}} = \frac{2{,}000\ \text{mg}}{500\ \text{ml}}$$

Cross multiply the fractions:

$$x\ \text{mg} \times 500\ \text{ml} = 2{,}000\ \text{mg} \times 1\ \text{ml}$$

Solve for x by dividing each side of the equation by 500 ml and canceling units that appear in both the numerator and denominator:

$$\frac{x\ \text{mg} \times \cancel{500\ \text{ml}}}{500\ \text{ml}} = \frac{2{,}000\ \text{mg} \times 1\ \cancel{\text{ml}}}{500\ \cancel{\text{ml}}}$$

$$x = \frac{2{,}000 \text{ mg}}{500}$$

$$x = 4 \text{ mg}$$

The concentration of the solution is 4 mg/ml. Next, calculate the flow rate per minute needed to deliver the ordered dose of 2 mg/minute. To do this, set up a proportion with the unknown flow rate per minute in one fraction and the concentration of the solution in the other fraction:

$$\frac{2 \text{ mg}}{x \text{ ml}} = \frac{4 \text{ mg}}{1 \text{ ml}}$$

Cross multiply the fractions:

$$x \text{ ml} \times 4 \text{ mg} = 1 \text{ ml} \times 2 \text{ mg}$$

Solve for x by dividing each side of the equation by 4 mg and canceling units that appear in both the numerator and denominator:

$$\frac{x \text{ ml} \times 4 \text{ \sout{mg}}}{4 \text{ \sout{mg}}} = \frac{1 \text{ ml} \times 2 \text{ \sout{mg}}}{4 \text{ \sout{mg}}}$$

$$x = \frac{2 \text{ ml}}{4}$$

$$x = 0.5 \text{ ml}$$

The patient should receive 0.5 ml/minute of lidocaine. Because lidocaine must be given with an infusion pump, compute the hourly flow rate. Set up a proportion with the unknown flow rate per hour in one fraction and the flow rate per minute in the other fraction:

$$\frac{x \text{ ml}}{60 \text{ min}} = \frac{0.5 \text{ ml}}{1 \text{ min}}$$

Cross multiply the fractions:

$$x \text{ ml} \times 1 \text{ min} = 0.5 \text{ ml} \times 60 \text{ min}$$

Solve for x by dividing each side of the equation by 1 minute and canceling units that appear in the numerator and denominator:

$$\frac{x \text{ ml} \times 1 \text{ \sout{min}}}{1 \text{ \sout{min}}} = \frac{0.5 \text{ ml} \times 60 \text{ \sout{min}}}{1 \text{ \sout{min}}}$$

$$x = 30 \text{ ml}$$

Set the infusion pump to deliver 30 ml/hour.

Example 2

A 200-lb patient is scheduled to receive an I.V. infusion of dobutamine at 10 mcg/kg/minute. The package insert says to dilute 250 mg of the drug in 50 ml of D_5W. Because the drug vial contains 20 ml of solution, the total to be infused is 70 ml (50 ml of D_5W plus 20 ml of solution). How many micrograms of the drug should the patient receive each minute? Each hour?

First, compute the patient's weight in kilograms. To do this, set up a proportion with the weight in pounds and the unknown weight in kilograms in one fraction and the number of pounds per kilogram in the other fraction:

$$\frac{200 \text{ lb}}{x \text{ kg}} = \frac{2.2 \text{ lb}}{1 \text{ kg}}$$

Cross multiply the fractions:

$$x \text{ kg} \times 2.2 \text{ lb} = 1 \text{ kg} \times 200 \text{ lb}$$

Solve for x by dividing each side of the equation by 2.2 lb and canceling units that appear in the numerator and denominator.

$$\frac{x \text{ kg} \times \cancel{2.2 \text{ lb}}}{\cancel{2.2 \text{ lb}}} = \frac{1 \text{ kg} \times 200 \cancel{\text{ lb}}}{2.2 \cancel{\text{ lb}}}$$

$$x = \frac{200 \text{ kg}}{2.2}$$

$$x = 90.9 \text{ kg}$$

The patient weighs 90.9 kg. Next, determine the dose in micrograms per minute by setting up a proportion with the patient's weight in kilograms and the unknown dose in micrograms (mcg) per minute in one fraction and the known dose in micrograms per kilogram per minute in the other fraction:

$$\frac{90.9 \text{ kg}}{x \text{ mcg/min}} = \frac{1 \text{ kg}}{10 \text{ mcg/min}}$$

Cross multiply the fractions:

$$x \text{ mcg/min} \times 1 \text{ kg} = 10 \text{ mcg/min} \times 90.9 \text{ kg}$$

Solve for x by dividing each side of the equation by 1 kg and canceling units that appear in the numerator and denominator:

$$\frac{x \text{ mcg/min} \times \cancel{1 \text{ kg}}}{\cancel{1 \text{ kg}}} = \frac{10 \text{ mcg/min} \times 90.9 \cancel{\text{ kg}}}{1 \cancel{\text{ kg}}}$$

$$x = 909 \text{ mcg/min}$$

The patient should receive 909 mcg of dobutamine every minute. Finally, determine the hourly dose by multiplying the dose per minute by 60:

$$909 \text{ mcg/min} \times 60 \text{ min/hr} = 54{,}540 \text{ mcg/hr}$$

The patient should receive 54,540 mcg of dobutamine every hour.

Reminders about pediatric dosages

+ For children, dosage calculations should be based on dosage range per kilogram of body weight or on body surface area.
+ Other methods aren't recommended because they're less accurate.

PEDIATRIC DOSAGE CONSIDERATIONS

To determine the correct pediatric dosage of a drug, prescribers, pharmacists, and nurses usually use two computation methods. One is based on weight in kilograms. The other uses the child's body surface area. (See *Using a pediatric nomogram, p. 543.*) Other methods are less accurate and not recommended.

DOSAGE RANGE PER KILOGRAM OF BODY WEIGHT

Many pharmaceutical companies provide information on the safe dosage ranges for drugs given to children. Usually, the companies provide the dosage ranges in milligrams per kilogram of body weight and, in many cases, give similar information

LIFESPAN

Using a pediatric nomogram

Body surface area (BSA) is critical when calculating dosages for children and when using extremely potent drugs that need to be given in precise amounts. The nomogram shown here lets you plot the patient's height and weight to determine his BSA. Here's how it works:

✦ Locate the patient's height in the left column of the nomogram and his weight in the right column.

✦ Use a ruler to draw a straight line connecting the two points. The point where the line intersects the surface area column indicates the patient's BSA in square meters.

✦ For an average-sized child, use the simplified nomogram in the box. Just find the child's weight in pounds on the left side of the scale, and then read the corresponding BSA on the right side.

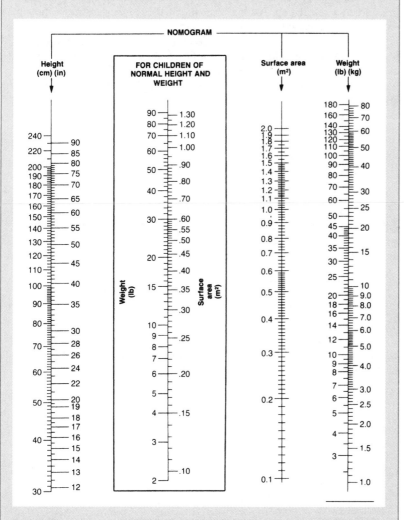

Reprinted from Behrman: *Nelson Textbook of Pediatrics*, 17th edition, Copyright 2003, with permission from Elsevier.

for adult dosage ranges. The following example and explanation show how to calculate the safe pediatric dosage range for a drug, using the company's suggested safe dosage range provided in milligrams per kilogram.

For a child, the prescriber orders a drug with a suggested dosage range of 10 to 12 mg/kg of body weight daily. The child weighs 12 kg. What is the safe daily dosage range for the child?

You must calculate the lower and upper limits of the dosage range provided by the manufacturer. First, calculate the dosage based on 10 mg/kg of body weight. Then, calculate the dosage based on 12 mg/kg of body weight. The answers represent the lower and upper limits of the daily dosage range, expressed in mg/kg of the child's weight.

BODY SURFACE AREA

Dosage computations based on the child's body surface area may provide a safer, more accurate calculation. That's because the child's body surface area is thought to parallel his organ growth and maturation and metabolic rate.

To determine a child's body surface area, use a three-column chart called a nomogram. Mark the child's height in the first column and his weight in the third column. Then draw a line between the two marks. The point at which the line intersects the vertical scale in the second column is the child's estimated body surface area in square meters.

To calculate the child's approximate dose, use his body surface area measurement in the following equation:

$$\frac{\text{body surface area of child}}{\text{average adult body surface area (1.73 m}^2)} \times \text{average adult dose} = \text{child's dose}$$

The following example illustrates how to use this equation. Suppose the nomogram shows that a 25-lb (11.3-kg) child who is 33 inches (84 cm) tall has a body surface area of 0.52 m^2. To determine this child's dose of a drug with an average adult dose of 100 mg, the equation is:

$$\frac{0.52 \text{ mg}^2}{1.73 \text{ m}^2} \times 100 \text{ mg} = 30.06 \text{ mg (child's dose)}$$

The child should receive 30 mg of the drug.

Keep in mind that many facilities have guidelines that determine acceptable calculation methods for pediatric dosages. If you work with children, be sure to familiarize yourself with your facility's policies about pediatric dosages.

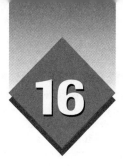

Drug administration

You may give drugs by many routes, including topical, oral, buccal, sublingual (S.L.), ophthalmic, otic, respiratory, nasogastric (NG), vaginal, rectal, subcutaneous (S.C.), I.M., and I.V. No matter which route you use, however, you'll need to follow an established set of precautions to make sure you give the right drug in the right dose to the right patient at the right time and by the right route. These precautions include checking the order and medication administration record, checking the label, confirming the patient's identity, following standard safety procedures, and responding to patient questions.

CHECK THE ORDER

Make sure you have a written order for every drug given. Verbal orders should be signed by the prescriber within the time specified by your facility. If your facility has a computerized order system, it may allow prescribers to order drugs electronically from the pharmacy. The computer, which may indicate whether the pharmacy has the drug, triggers the pharmacy staff to fill the prescription. A computerized order may also generate a patient record on which you can document drug administration. In fact, you may be able to document the administration on the computer.

Computer systems offer several advantages over paper systems. For instance, drugs may arrive on the unit or floor more quickly. Documentation is quicker and easier. Prescribers can see at a glance which drugs have been given. Errors no longer result from poor handwriting (although typing mistakes may occur). Finally, computerized records are easier to store than paper records.

CHECK THE MEDICATION RECORD

Check the order on the patient's medication administration record against the prescriber's order.

Reminders about drug administration

- ✦ Drugs may be given by many routes, including topical, oral, buccal, S.L., ophthalmic, otic, respiratory, NG, vaginal, rectal, S.C., I.M., and I.V.
- ✦ For all routes, follow a routine set of precautions to make sure you give the right drug and the right dose to the right patient at the right time and by the right route.
- ✦ Make sure you have a written order for every drug.
- ✦ Before giving a drug, check the label three times to make sure you're giving the prescribed drug and the prescribed dose.
- ✦ Confirm the patient's identity by asking his full name and checking the name and medical record number on his wristband against the medication administration record.

CHECK THE LABEL

Before giving a drug, check its label three times to make sure you're giving the prescribed drug and the prescribed dose. First, check the label when you take the container from the shelf or drawer. Next, check the label right before pouring the drug into the medication cup or drawing it into the syringe. Finally, check the label again before returning the container to the shelf or drawer. For a unit-dose drug, open the container at the patient's bedside. Then check the label for the third time immediately after pouring the drug and again before discarding the wrapper.

Don't give a drug from a poorly labeled or unlabeled container. Also, don't attempt to label a drug or to reinforce a label; a pharmacist must perform these actions.

CONFIRM THE PATIENT'S IDENTITY

Before giving the drug, ask the patient his full name, and confirm his identity by checking his name and medical record number on his patient identification wristband against the medication administration record. Don't rely on information that can vary during a hospital stay, such as a room or bed number. Check again that you have the correct drug, and make sure the patient has no allergy to it.

If the patient has drug allergies, check to make sure the chart and medication administration record are labeled accordingly and that the patient is wearing an allergy wristband identifying the allergen.

FOLLOW SAFETY PROCEDURES

Whenever you give a drug, follow these safety procedures:
✦ Never give a drug poured or prepared by someone else.
✦ Never allow the drug cart or tray out of your sight once you've prepared a dose.
✦ Never leave a drug at a patient's bedside.
✦ Never return unwrapped or prepared drugs to stock containers. Instead, dispose of them and notify the pharmacy.
✦ Keep the drug cart locked at all times.
✦ Follow standard precautions, as appropriate.

RESPOND TO QUESTIONS

If the patient questions you about his drug or dosage, check his medication administration record again. If the drug you're giving is correct, reassure the patient. Explain any changes in his drug or dosage. Also, teach him, as appropriate, about possible adverse reactions and ask him to report anything that he feels may be an adverse reaction.

TOPICAL ADMINISTRATION

Topical drugs, such as patches, lotions, and ointments, are applied directly to the skin. They're commonly used for local, rather than systemic, effects. Keep in mind, however, that certain types of topical drugs—known as transdermal drugs—are meant to enter the patient's bloodstream and exert a systemic effect after you apply them.

Reviewing topical drugs

✦ May be in patches, lotions, and ointments
✦ Commonly used for local, rather than systemic, effects
✦ Are meant to enter the bloodstream and exert a systemic effect (transdermal drugs)

EQUIPMENT AND PREPARATION

Check the chart and the medication administration record. Gather the prescribed drug, sterile tongue blades, gloves, sterile gloves for open lesions, sterile 4″ × 4″ gauze pads, transparent semipermeable dressing, adhesive tape, normal saline solution, cotton-tipped applicators, cotton gloves, and linen savers, if needed.

IMPLEMENTATION

✦ Confirm the patient's identity by asking his full name and checking the name and medical record number on his wristband.
✦ Explain the procedure to the patient because, after discharge, he may have to apply the drug by himself.
✦ Premedicate the patient with an analgesic if the procedure is uncomfortable. Give the analgesic time to take effect.
✦ Wash your hands to reduce the risk of cross-contamination, and put on gloves.
✦ Help the patient to a comfortable position, and expose the area to be treated. Make sure his skin or mucous membrane is intact (unless the drug has been prescribed to treat a skin lesion). Drug application to broken or abraded skin may cause unwanted systemic absorption and further irritation.
✦ If needed, clean debris from the skin. Change your gloves if they become soiled.

To apply paste, cream, or ointment

✦ Open the container. Place the cap upside down to avoid contaminating its inner surface.
✦ Remove a tongue blade from its sterile wrapper, and cover one end of it with the drug from the tube or jar. Then transfer the drug from the tongue blade to your gloved hand.
✦ Apply the drug to the affected area with long, smooth strokes that follow the direction of hair growth. This technique avoids forcing drug into hair follicles, which can cause irritation and lead to folliculitis. Avoid excessive pressure when applying the drug because it could abrade the skin or cause the patient discomfort.
✦ When applying the drug to the patient's face, use cotton-tipped applicators for small areas, such as under the eyes. For larger areas, use a sterile gauze pad.
✦ To prevent contamination of the drug, use a new sterile tongue blade each time you remove the drug from the container.
✦ Remove and discard your gloves, and wash your hands.

To apply transdermal ointment

✦ Choose the application site—usually a dry, hairless spot on the patient's chest or upper arm.
✦ To promote absorption, wash the site with soap and warm water. Dry it thoroughly.
✦ Put on gloves.
✦ If the patient has a previously applied drug strip at another site, remove it and wash this area to clear away any drug residue.
✦ If the area you choose is hairy, clip excess hair rather than shaving it; shaving causes irritation, which the drug may worsen.
✦ Squeeze the prescribed amount of ointment onto the application strip or measuring paper. Don't get the ointment on your skin.
✦ Apply the strip, drug side down, directly to the patient's skin.
✦ Maneuver the strip slightly to spread a thin layer of ointment over a 3″ (8-cm) area, but don't rub the ointment into the skin.

Applying paste, cream, or ointment

✦ Use long, smooth strokes.
✦ Follow the direction of hair growth.
✦ Use cotton-tipped applicators for small areas on the face, such as under the eyes.
✦ Use sterile gauze pads for larger areas on the face.

◆ Secure the application strip to the patient's skin by covering it with a semipermeable dressing or plastic wrap.
◆ Tape the covering securely in place.
◆ If required by your facility's policy, label the strip with the date, time, and your initials.
◆ Remove your gloves and wash your hands.

To apply a transdermal patch
◆ Wash your hands and put on gloves
◆ Remove the old patch.
◆ Choose a dry, hairless application site.
◆ As with transdermal ointment, clip (don't shave) hair from the chosen site. Wash the area with warm water and soap, and dry it thoroughly.
◆ Open the drug package and remove the patch.
◆ Without touching the adhesive surface, remove the clear plastic backing.
◆ Apply the patch to the site without touching the adhesive.
◆ If required by your facility's policy, label the patch with the date, time, and your initials.

To remove ointment
◆ Wash your hands and put on gloves.
◆ Gently swab ointment from the patient's skin, using a sterile $4'' \times 4''$ gauze pad saturated with normal saline solution.
◆ Don't wipe too hard because you could irritate the skin.
◆ Remove and discard your gloves, and wash your hands.

NURSING CONSIDERATIONS
◆ To prevent skin irritation from drug accumulation, never apply a drug without first removing previous applications.
◆ Always wear gloves to prevent absorption by your skin.
◆ Don't apply ointment to the eyelids or ear canal. The ointment may congeal and occlude the tear duct or ear canal.
◆ Frequently inspect the treated area for allergic or other adverse reactions.
◆ Don't apply a topical drug to scarred or callused skin because this type of skin may impair absorption.

 CLINICAL ALERT Don't place a defibrillator paddle on a transdermal patch. The aluminum on the patch can cause electrical arcing during defibrillation, resulting in smoke and thermal burns. If a patient has a patch on a standard paddle site, remove the patch before applying the paddle.

ORAL ADMINISTRATION
Because oral drug administration is usually the safest, most convenient, and least expensive method, most drugs are given by this route. Drugs for oral administration come in many forms: tablets, enteric-coated tablets, capsules, syrups, elixirs, oils, liquids, suspensions, powders, and granules. Some require special preparation before administration, such as mixing with juice to make them more palatable.

Oral drugs sometimes are prescribed in higher dosages than their parenteral equivalents because, after absorption through the gastrointestinal (GI) system, they're broken down by the liver before they reach the systemic circulation.

Key nursing actions for topical drugs
◆ To prevent skin irritation from drug accumulation, don't apply a drug without first removing previous applications.
◆ Always wear gloves to prevent absorption by your skin.
◆ Don't apply ointment to the eyelids or ear canal because it could congeal and occlude the tear duct or ear canal.
◆ Inspect the treated area frequently for allergic or other adverse reactions.
◆ Don't apply a topical drug to scarred or callused skin because it may impair absorption.

Reviewing oral drugs
◆ May be in tablet, enteric-coated tablet, capsule, syrup, elixir, oil, liquid, suspension, powder, or granule form
◆ May need special preparation before administration, such as mixing with juice, to increase palatability
◆ May be prescribed in higher dosages than parenteral equivalents because, after GI absorption, they're broken down by the liver before they reach the systemic circulation

EQUIPMENT AND PREPARATION

Check the chart and the medication administration record. Gather the prescribed drug and medication cup. If needed, gather a mortar and pestle for crushing pills and an appropriate vehicle, such as jelly or applesauce for crushed pills or juice, water, or milk for liquid drugs. These variations commonly are used for children or geriatric patients.

IMPLEMENTATION

+ Wash your hands.
+ Confirm the patient's identity by asking his full name and checking the name and medical record number on his wristband.
+ Assess the patient's condition, including level of consciousness and vital signs, as needed. Changes in the patient's condition may warrant withholding the drug.
+ Give the patient the drug. If appropriate, crush the drug to facilitate swallowing or mix it with an appropriate vehicle or liquid to aid swallowing, minimize adverse reactions, or promote absorption.
+ Stay with the patient until he has swallowed the drug. If he seems confused or disoriented, check his mouth to make sure he swallowed it. Return and reassess the patient's response within 1 hour after giving the drug.

NURSING CONSIDERATIONS

+ To avoid damaging or staining the patient's teeth, give acid or iron preparations through a straw. To help make an unpleasant-tasting liquid more palatable, also give it through a straw because the liquid contacts fewer taste buds.
+ If the patient can't swallow a whole tablet or capsule, ask the pharmacist if the drug is available in liquid form or if it can be given by another route. If not, ask the pharmacist if the tablet can be crushed or if capsules can be opened and mixed with food.
+ Don't crush sustained-action drugs, buccal tablets, S.L. tablets, or enteric-coated drugs.

BUCCAL AND SUBLINGUAL ADMINISTRATION

Certain drugs are given buccally (between the cheek and teeth) or sublingually (under the tongue) to bypass the GI tract and promote absorption into the bloodstream. Erythrityl tetranitrate is an example of a drug given buccally. Drugs given by the S.L. route include ergotamine tartrate, erythrityl tetranitrate, isoproterenol hydrochloride, isosorbide dinitrate, and nitroglycerin. With either administration method, observe the patient carefully to make sure he doesn't swallow the drug or develop mucosal irritation.

EQUIPMENT AND PREPARATION

Check the chart and the medication administration record. Gather the prescribed drug, medication cup, and gloves.

Key nursing actions for oral drugs

+ Stay with the patient until he has swallowed the drug. If he seems confused or disoriented, check his mouth to make sure he swallowed it. Return and reassess the patient's response within 1 hour after giving the drug.
+ To avoid damaging or staining the patient's teeth, give acid or iron preparations through a straw.
+ To help make a bad-tasting liquid more palatable, give it through a straw.
+ If the patient can't swallow a whole tablet or capsule, find out if it's available as a liquid, if it can be given by another route, or if a tablet can be crushed or a capsule can be opened and mixed with food.
+ Don't crush sustained-action drugs, buccal tablets, S.L. tablets, or enteric-coated drugs.

Reviewing buccal and sublingual drugs

✦ In buccal administration, the drug is placed between the cheek and teeth.

✦ In sublingual administration, the drug is placed under the tongue.

✦ Theses routes are intended to bypass the GI tract and promote absorption into the bloodstream.

Key nursing actions for buccal and sublingual drugs

✦ Assess the patient to make sure he doesn't swallow the drug or develop mucosal irritation.

✦ Tell the patient to keep the drug in place until it dissolves completely to ensure absorption.

✦ Caution the patient against chewing the tablet or touching it with his tongue to prevent accidental swallowing.

✦ Tell the patient not to smoke before the drug has dissolved because nicotine constricts vessels, which slows absorption.

Giving buccal and sublingual drugs

Proper placement of buccal and sublingual (S.L.) tablets is the key to effective therapy with these drugs. For buccal administration, place the tablet in the patient's buccal pouch, between his cheek and teeth, as shown in the top illustration. For S.L. administration, place it under his tongue, as shown in the bottom illustration.

BUCCAL DRUG PLACEMENT

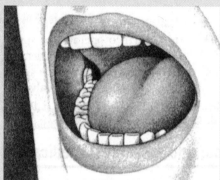

S.L. DRUG PLACEMENT

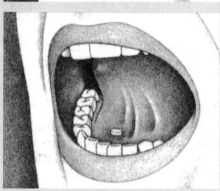

IMPLEMENTATION

✦ Wash your hands. Put on gloves if you'll be placing the drug into the patient's mouth.

✦ Confirm the patient's identity by asking his full name and checking the name and medical record number on his wristband.

✦ Place the tablet in the patient's mouth, as indicated. (See *Giving buccal and sublingual drugs.*)

✦ Remove and discard your gloves, and wash your hands.

✦ Instruct the patient to keep the drug in place until it dissolves completely to ensure absorption. Caution the patient against chewing the tablet or touching it with his tongue to prevent accidental swallowing.

✦ Tell the patient not to smoke before the drug has dissolved because nicotine constricts vessels, which slows absorption.

NURSING CONSIDERATIONS

✦ Don't give the patient liquids until the buccal tablet is absorbed, which can take up to 1 hour.

✦ If the patient has angina, tell him to wet the nitroglycerin tablet with saliva and keep it under his tongue until it's fully absorbed.

✦ Make sure a patient with angina knows how to take the drug, how many doses to take, and when to call for emergency help.

OPHTHALMIC ADMINISTRATION

Ophthalmic drugs—drops or ointments—serve diagnostic and therapeutic purposes. During an ophthalmic examination, drugs can be used to anesthetize the eye, dilate the pupil, and stain the cornea to identify anomalies. Therapeutic uses include eye lubrication and treatment of conditions such as glaucoma and infections.

EQUIPMENT AND PREPARATION

Check the chart and the medication administration record. Gather the prescribed ophthalmic drug, sterile cotton balls, gloves, warm water or normal saline solution, sterile gauze pads, and facial tissue. An eye dressing may also be used.

Make sure the drug is labeled for ophthalmic use. Then check the expiration date. Remember to date the container after the first use.

Inspect the ocular solution for cloudiness, discoloration, and precipitation, although some drugs are suspensions and normally appear cloudy. Don't use a solution that appears abnormal.

IMPLEMENTATION

✦ Make sure you know which eye to treat because different drugs or doses may be ordered for each eye.

✦ Confirm the patient's identity by asking his full name and checking the name and medical record number on his wristband.

✦ Put on gloves.

✦ If the patient has an eye dressing, remove it by pulling it down and away from his forehead. Avoid contaminating your hands. Don't apply pressure to the area around the eyes.

✦ To remove exudates or meibomian gland secretions, clean around the eye with sterile cotton balls or sterile gauze pads moistened with warm water or normal saline solution. Have the patient close his eyes; then gently wipe the eyelids from the inner to the outer canthus. Use a fresh cotton ball or gauze pad for each stroke, and use a different cotton ball or pad for each eye.

✦ Have the patient sit or lie in the supine position. Instruct him to tilt his head back and toward his affected eye so that any excess drug can flow away from the tear duct, minimizing systemic absorption through the nasal mucosa.

✦ Remove the dropper cap from the drug container, and draw the drug into the dropper. Or, if the bottle has a dropper tip, remove the cap and hold or place it upside down to prevent contamination.

✦ Before instilling eyedrops, instruct the patient to look up and away. This moves the cornea away from the lower lid and minimizes the risk of touching it with the dropper.

Reviewing ophthalmic drugs

✦ Are usually drops or ointments

✦ May serve diagnostic or therapeutic purposes

✦ Can be used to anesthetize the eye, dilate the pupil, and stain the cornea to identify anomalies during ophthalmic examination

✦ May be used for eye lubrication and conditions such as glaucoma and infections

Applying eye ointment

To apply eye ointment, squeeze a small ribbon of drug on the edge of the conjunctival sac from the inner to the outer canthus. Cut off the ribbon by turning the tube. Don't touch the eye with the tip of the tube.

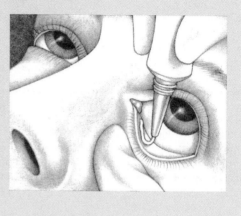

Key nursing actions for ophthalmic drugs

- Know which eye to treat because different drugs or doses may be ordered for each eye.
- After instilling eyedrops, tell the patient to close his eyes gently, without squeezing the lids shut, and then to blink.
- After applying ointment, tell the patient to close his eyes gently, without squeezing the lids shut, and to roll his eyes behind closed lids to help distribute the drug over the eyeball.
- When giving a drug that may be absorbed systemically, gently press your thumb on the inner canthus for 1 to 2 minutes after instillation while the patient closes his eyes. Avoid applying pressure around the eye.
- To keep the drug container sterile, don't put the cap down after opening the container, and never touch the tip of the dropper or bottle to the eye area.

To instill eyedrops

- Steady the hand that's holding the dropper by resting it against the patient's forehead. With your other hand, gently pull down the lower lid of the affected eye, and instill the drops in the conjunctival sac. Never instill eyedrops directly onto the eyeball.
- When teaching a geriatric patient how to instill eyedrops, keep in mind that he may have difficulty sensing drops in the eye. Suggest chilling the drug slightly because cold drops should be easier to feel when they enter the eye.

To apply eye ointment

- Squeeze a small ribbon of drug on the conjunctival sac. (See *Applying eye ointment.*)

To complete ophthalmic administration

- After instilling eyedrops or applying ointment, instruct the patient to close his eyes gently, without squeezing the lids shut. If you instilled drops, tell the patient to blink. If you applied ointment, tell him to roll his eyes behind closed lids to help distribute the drug over the eyeball.
- Use a clean tissue to remove any excess drug that leaks from the eye. Use a fresh tissue for each eye to prevent cross-contamination.
- Apply a new eye dressing, if needed.
- Remove and discard your gloves. Wash your hands.

NURSING CONSIDERATIONS

- When giving an ophthalmic drug that may be absorbed systemically, gently press your thumb on the inner canthus for 1 to 2 minutes after instillation while the patient closes his eyes. Avoid applying pressure around the eye.
- To maintain the drug container's sterility, don't put the cap down after opening the container, and never touch the tip of the dropper or bottle to the eye area. Discard any solution remaining in the dropper before returning it to the bottle. If the dropper or bottle tip has become contaminated, discard it and use another sterile dropper. Never share eyedrops from patient to patient.

OTIC ADMINISTRATION

Eardrops may be instilled to treat infection and inflammation, to soften cerumen for later removal, to produce local anesthesia, or to facilitate removal of an insect trapped in the ear.

EQUIPMENT AND PREPARATION

Check the chart and the medication administration record. Gather the prescribed eardrops, gloves, a light, and facial tissue or cotton-tipped applicators. Cotton balls and a bowl of warm water may be needed as well.

First, warm the drug to body temperature in the bowl of warm water, or carry the drug in your pocket for 30 minutes before administration. If needed, test the temperature of the drug by placing a drop on your wrist. (If the drug is too hot, it may burn the patient's eardrum.) To avoid injuring the ear canal, check the dropper before use to make sure it's not chipped or cracked.

IMPLEMENTATION

✦ Wash your hands and put on clean gloves.
✦ Confirm the patient's identity by asking his full name and checking the name and medical record number on his wristband.
✦ Have the patient lie on the side opposite the affected ear.
✦ Straighten the patient's ear canal. (See *Adjusting eardrop administration for children,* page 554.)
✦ Using a light, examine the ear canal for drainage. If you see drainage, gently clean the canal with the tissue or cotton-tipped applicators because drainage can reduce the drug's effectiveness. Never insert an applicator past the point where you can see it.
✦ Compare the label on the eardrops to the order on the patient's medication administration record. Check the label again while drawing the drug into the dropper. Check the label for the final time before returning the eardrops to the shelf or drawer.
✦ Straighten the patient's ear canal once again, and instill the ordered number of drops. To avoid patient discomfort, aim the dropper so that the drops fall against the sides of the ear canal, not on the eardrum. Hold the ear canal in position until you see the drug disappear down the canal. Then release the ear.
✦ Instruct the patient to remain on his side for 5 to 10 minutes to allow the drug to run down into the ear canal.
✦ Tuck a cotton ball with a small amount of petroleum jelly on it (if ordered) loosely into the opening of the ear canal to prevent the drug from leaking out. Be careful not to insert it too deeply into the canal because doing so may prevent drainage of secretions and increase pressure on the eardrum.
✦ Clean and dry the outer ear.
✦ If indicated, repeat the procedure in the other ear after 5 to 10 minutes.
✦ Help the patient into a comfortable position.
✦ Remove your gloves and wash your hands.

NURSING CONSIDERATIONS

✦ Be especially gentle because some conditions make the normally tender ear canal even more sensitive.

Key nursing actions for otic drugs

✦ Instill eardrops to treat infection and inflammation, to soften cerumen for later removal, to produce local anesthesia, or to facilitate removal of an insect trapped in the ear.
✦ Instruct the patient to remain on his side for 5 to 10 minutes to allow the drug to run down into the ear canal.
✦ Be especially gentle because some conditions make the normally tender ear canal even more sensitive.
✦ To prevent injury to the eardrum, never insert a cotton-tipped applicator into the ear canal past the point where you can see the tip.

Adjusting eardrop administration for children

Although you need to straighten the ear canal when giving eardrops to any patient, adjust your technique based on the patient's age. For an adult or a child age 3 or older, pull the auricle up and back. For an infant or child under age 3, gently pull the auricle down and back, as shown. At this age, the ear canal is straighter and needs less manipulation.

Also, if the child struggles, gently rest the hand holding the dropper against his head to secure a safe position before giving the eardrops. This helps avoid damaging the ear canal with the dropper.

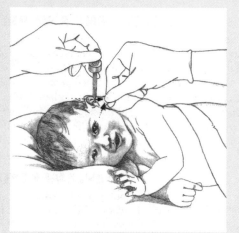

✦ To prevent injury to the eardrum, never insert a cotton-tipped applicator into the ear canal past the point where you can see the tip.

✦ After instilling eardrops to soften cerumen, irrigate the ear to promote its removal. If the patient has vertigo, keep the side rails of his bed up and assist him as needed during the procedure. Also, move slowly and unhurriedly to avoid worsening his vertigo.

✦ If needed, teach the patient to instill the eardrops correctly so that he can continue treatment at home. Review the procedure and let the patient try it himself while you observe.

Reviewing inhaled drugs

✦ Handheld oropharyngeal inhalers deliver topical drugs to the respiratory tract, producing local and systemic effects.

✦ Devices include the metered-dose inhaler and the turbo-inhaler.

✦ The mucosal lining of the respiratory tract absorbs inhalants almost immediately.

RESPIRATORY ADMINISTRATION

Handheld oropharyngeal inhalers include the metered-dose inhaler and the turbo-inhaler. These devices deliver topical drugs to the respiratory tract, producing local and systemic effects. The mucosal lining of the respiratory tract absorbs the inhalant almost immediately. Examples of inhalants are bronchodilators, which improve airway patency and promote mucous drainage, and mucolytics, which liquefy tenacious bronchial secretions.

EQUIPMENT AND PREPARATION

Check the chart and the medication administration record. Gather the metered-dose inhaler or turbo-inhaler, prescribed drug, and normal saline solution.

Preparing a metered-dose inhaler

Before using a metered-dose inhaler, shake the inhaler bottle. Then remove the cap and insert the stem of the bottle into the small hole on the flattened portion of the mouthpiece, as shown here.

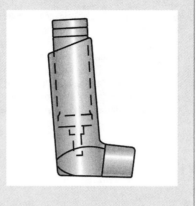

IMPLEMENTATION

◆ Confirm the patient's identity by asking his full name and checking the name and medical record number on his wristband.

To use a metered-dose inhaler

◆ Prepare the inhaler. (See *Preparing a metered-dose inhaler.*)
◆ Place the inhaler about 1″ (2.5 cm) in front of the patient's open mouth.
◆ Tell the patient to exhale.
◆ If you're using a spacer, which can make the inhaler more effective, tell the patient to place the spacer's mouthpiece in his mouth and to press his lips firmly around it.
◆ As you push the bottle down against the mouthpiece, instruct the patient to inhale slowly through his mouth and to continue inhaling until his lungs feel full. Compress the bottle against the mouthpiece only once.
◆ Remove the inhaler and tell the patient to hold his breath for several seconds. Then instruct him to exhale slowly through pursed lips to keep distal bronchioles open and allow increased drug absorption and diffusion.
◆ Have the patient gargle with normal saline solution or water to remove the drug from his mouth and the back of his throat. This step helps prevent oral fungal infections. Warn the patient not to swallow after gargling, but rather to spit out the liquid.

To use a turbo-inhaler

◆ Prepare the inhaler. (See *Preparing a turbo-inhaler,* page 556.)
◆ Holding the inhaler with the mouthpiece at the bottom, slide the sleeve all the way down and then up again to puncture the capsule and release the drug. Do this only once.
◆ Have the patient exhale completely and tilt his head back. Instruct him to place the mouthpiece in his mouth, close his lips around it, and inhale once. Tell him to hold his breath for several seconds.
◆ Remove the inhaler from the patient's mouth, and tell him to exhale as much air as possible.

Preparing a turbo-inhaler

To prepare a turbo-inhaler, hold the mouthpiece in one hand. With the other hand, slide the sleeve away from the mouthpiece as far as possible, as shown here.

Next, unscrew the tip of the mouthpiece by turning it counterclockwise. Press the colored portion of the drug capsule into the propeller stem of the mouthpiece. Then screw the inhaler together again.

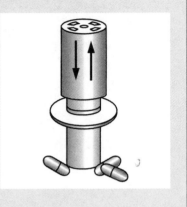

Key nursing actions for inhaled drugs

+ If the patient must receive a bronchodilator and a corticosteroid, give the bronchodilator first so his air passages can open fully before you give the corticosteroid.
+ Teach the patient how to use the inhaler so he can continue treatments after discharge, if needed.
+ Be aware that some oral respiratory drugs may cause restlessness, palpitations, nervousness, and other systemic effects. They can also cause hypersensitivity reactions, such as rash, urticaria, or bronchospasm.

+ Repeat the procedure until the patient has inhaled all the drug in the device.
+ Have the patient gargle with normal saline solution, if desired.

NURSING CONSIDERATIONS

+ Teach the patient how to use the inhaler so he can continue treatments after discharge, if needed. Explain that overdosage can cause the drug to lose its effectiveness. Tell him to record the date and time of each inhalation and his response.
+ Be aware that some oral respiratory drugs may cause restlessness, palpitations, nervousness, and other systemic effects. They can also cause hypersensitivity reactions, such as rash, urticaria, or bronchospasm.
+ Give oral respiratory drugs cautiously to patients with heart disease because these drugs may potentiate coronary insufficiency, arrhythmias, or hypertension. If paradoxical bronchospasm occurs, discontinue the drug and call the prescriber to order another drug.
+ If the patient must receive a bronchodilator and a corticosteroid, give the bronchodilator first so his air passages can open fully before you give the corticosteroid.
+ Instruct the patient to keep an extra inhaler handy.
+ Instruct the patient to discard the inhaler after taking the prescribed number of doses and to then start a new inhaler.

Reviewing nasogastric drugs

+ An NG tube provides an alternate means of nourishment for patients who can't eat normally.
+ An NG tube also allows direct instillation of drugs into the GI system.

NASOGASTRIC ADMINISTRATION

Besides providing an alternate means of nourishment for patients who can't eat normally, an NG tube allows direct instillation of drugs into the GI system.

EQUIPMENT AND PREPARATION

Check the chart and the medication administration record. Gather equipment for use at the bedside, including the prescribed drug, a towel or linen-saver pad, 50- or 60-ml piston-type catheter-tip syringe, feeding tubing, two 4″ × 4″ gauze pads, stethoscope, gloves, diluent (juice, water, or a nutritional supplement), cup for mix-

Giving a drug via nasogastric tube

To administer a drug by the naso-gastric (NG) route, hold the NG tube upright at a level slightly above the patient's nose. Then open the clamp and pour the drug in slowly and steadily, as shown here. To keep air from entering the patient's stomach, hold the tube at a slight angle and add more drug before the syringe empties.

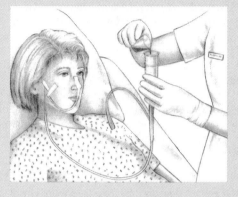

ing drug and fluid, spoon, 50-ml cup of water, and rubber band. Pill-crushing equipment and a clamp (if not already attached to the tube) may also be needed.

Make sure that liquids are at room temperature to avoid abdominal cramping. Also ensure that the cup, syringe, spoon, and gauze are clean.

IMPLEMENTATION

✦ Wash your hands and put on gloves.
✦ Confirm the patient's identity by asking his full name and checking the name and medical record number on his wristband.
✦ Unpin the tube from the patient's gown. To avoid soiling the sheets during the procedure, fold back the bed linens and drape the patient's chest with a towel or linen-saver pad.
✦ Help the patient into Fowler's position, if his condition allows.
✦ After unclamping the tube, auscultate the patient's abdomen about 3″ (7.5 cm) below the sternum as you gently insert 10 ml of air into the tube with the 50- or 60-ml syringe. You should hear the air bubble entering the stomach. Gently draw back on the piston of the syringe. The appearance of gastric contents suggests that the tube is patent and in the stomach.
✦ If no gastric contents appear or if you meet resistance, the tube may be lying against the gastric mucosa. Withdraw the tube slightly or turn the patient to free it.
✦ Clamp the tube, detach the syringe, and lay the end of the tube on the 4″ × 4″ gauze pad.
✦ If the drug is in tablet form, crush it before mixing it with the diluent. Make sure the particles are small enough to pass through the eyes at the distal end of the tube. Keep in mind that some drugs (extended-release, enteric-coated, or S.L. drugs, for example) shouldn't be crushed. If you aren't sure, ask the pharmacist. Also, check to see if the drug comes in liquid form or if a capsule form may be opened and the contents poured into a diluent. Pour liquid drugs into the diluent and stir well.
✦ Reattach the syringe, without the piston, to the end of the tube. Then give the drug through the attached syringe. (See *Giving a drug via nasogastric tube.*)

Key nursing actions for nasogastric drugs

✦ Make sure that liquids are at room temperature to avoid ab-dominal cramping.
✦ If the drug is in tablet form, crush it before mixing it with the diluent. Make sure the particles are small enough to pass through the eyes at the distal end of the tube.
✦ Keep in mind that some drugs (extended-release, enteric-coated, or S.L. drugs, for exam-ple) shouldn't be crushed. If you aren't sure, ask the pharmacist.
✦ If you must give a tube feeding as well as instill a drug, give the drug first to make sure the pa-tient receives it all.

✦ If the drug flows smoothly, slowly give the entire dose. If it doesn't flow, it may be too thick. If so, dilute it with water. If you suspect that tube placement is inhibiting flow, stop the procedure and reevaluate the placement.

✦ Watch the patient's reaction. Stop immediately if you see signs of discomfort.

✦ As the last of the drug flows out of the syringe, start to irrigate the tube by adding 30 to 50 ml of water (15 to 30 ml for a child). Irrigation clears the drug from the tube and reduces the risk of clogging.

✦ When the water stops flowing, clamp the tube. Detach the syringe and discard it properly.

✦ Fasten the tube to the patient's gown and make the patient comfortable.

✦ Leave the patient in Fowler's position or on her right side with her head partially elevated for at least 30 minutes to promote flow and prevent esophageal reflux.

✦ Remove and discard your gloves, and wash your hands.

NURSING CONSIDERATIONS

✦ If you must give a tube feeding as well as instill a drug, give the drug first to make sure the patient receives it all.

✦ Certain drugs, such as Dilantin, bind with tube feedings, decreasing the drug's availability. Stop the tube feeding for 2 hours before and after the dose, according to your facility's policy.

✦ If residual stomach contents exceed 150 ml, withhold the drug and feeding, and notify the prescriber. Excessive stomach contents may indicate intestinal obstruction or paralytic ileus.

✦ Never crush enteric-coated, buccal, S.L., or sustained-release drugs.

✦ If the NG tube is on suction, turn it off for 20 to 30 minutes after giving a drug.

VAGINAL ADMINISTRATION

Vaginal drugs can be inserted as topical treatment for infection, particularly *Trichomonas vaginalis* infection and vaginal candidiasis or inflammation. Suppositories melt when they contact the vaginal mucosa, and the drug diffuses topically.

Vaginal drugs usually come with a disposable applicator that enables drug placement in the anterior and posterior fornices. Vaginal administration is most effective when the patient can remain lying down afterward to retain the drug.

EQUIPMENT AND PREPARATION

Check the chart and the medication administration record. Gather the prescribed drug and applicator (if needed), gloves, water-soluble lubricant, and a small sanitary pad.

IMPLEMENTATION

✦ If possible, plan to give vaginal drugs at bedtime when the patient is recumbent.

✦ Confirm the patient's identity by asking her full name and checking the name and medical record number on her wristband.

✦ Wash your hands, explain the procedure to the patient, and provide privacy.

✦ Ask the patient to void.

✦ Ask the patient if she would rather insert the drug herself. If so, provide appropriate instructions. If not, proceed with the following steps.

Reviewing vaginal drugs

✦ Can be inserted as topical treatment for infection, particularly *Trichomonas vaginalis* infection and vaginal candidiasis or inflammation

✦ Usually come with a disposable applicator that enables drug placement in the anterior and posterior fornices

✦ Are most effective when the patient can remain lying down afterward to retain the drug

✦ Melt when they contact the vaginal mucosa, and the drug diffuses topically (suppositories)

Giving a vaginal drug

After cleaning the perineum, keep the patient's labia separated. Then insert the suppository or vaginal applicator about 3" to 4" (7.5 to 10 cm) into her vagina, as shown here. Fully depress the plunger on the vaginal applicator to release the entire dose.

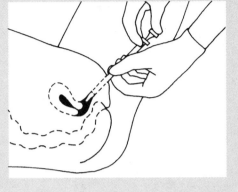

✦ Help the patient into the lithotomy position. Drape her, exposing only her perineum.
✦ Remove the suppository from the wrapper and lubricate it with water-soluble lubricant.
✦ Put on gloves, and expose the vagina by spreading the labia. If you see discharge, wash the area with several cotton balls soaked in warm, soapy water. Clean each side of the perineum and then the center, using a fresh cotton ball for each stroke. Then insert the prescribed drug. (See *Giving a vaginal drug.*)
✦ After insertion, wash the applicator with soap and warm water, and store or discard it, as appropriate. Label it so it will be used only for one patient.
✦ Remove and discard your gloves.
✦ To keep the drug from soiling the patient's clothing and bedding, provide a sanitary pad.
✦ Help the patient return to a comfortable position, and tell her to stay in bed as much as possible for the next several hours.
✦ Wash your hands thoroughly.

NURSING CONSIDERATIONS

✦ Refrigerate vaginal suppositories that melt at room temperature.
✦ If possible, teach the patient how to insert the vaginal drug because she may have to give it to herself after discharge. Give her instructions in writing if possible.
✦ Instruct the patient not to insert a tampon after inserting a vaginal drug because it will absorb the drug and decrease its effectiveness.

RECTAL ADMINISTRATION

A rectal suppository is a small, solid, medicated mass, usually cone shaped, with a cocoa butter or glycerin base. It may be inserted to stimulate peristalsis and defecation or to relieve pain, vomiting, and local irritation. An ointment is a semisolid drug used to produce local effects. It may be applied externally to the anus or internally to the rectum.

Key nursing actions for vaginal drugs

✦ Refrigerate suppositories that melt at room temperature.
✦ Teach the patient how to insert the drug if she'll have to do so after discharge. Give her written instructions if possible.
✦ Instruct the patient not to insert a tampon after the drug because the tampon will absorb the drug and decrease its effectiveness.

Reviewing rectal drugs

✦ A rectal suppository is a small, solid, medicated mass, usually cone shaped, with a cocoa butter or glycerin base. It may be inserted to stimulate peristalsis and defecation or to relieve pain, vomiting, and local irritation.

✦ An ointment is a semisolid drug used to produce local effects. It may be applied externally to the anus or internally to the rectum.

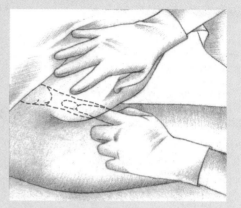

Inserting a rectal suppository

Using the index finger of your dominant hand, insert the rectal suppository—tapered end first—about 3" (7.5 cm) until you feel it pass the patient's internal anal sphincter, as shown. Direct the tapered end of the suppository toward the side of the rectum so that it contacts the membranes.

EQUIPMENT AND PREPARATION

Check the chart and the medication administration record. Gather the rectal suppository or tube of ointment and applicator, 4" × 4" gauze pads, gloves, and a water-soluble lubricant. A bedpan may also be needed.

Store rectal suppositories in the refrigerator until needed to prevent softening and possibly decreased drug effectiveness. A softened suppository is also difficult to handle and insert. To harden it again, hold the suppository (in its wrapper) under cold running water.

IMPLEMENTATION

✦ Confirm the patient's identity by asking his full name and checking the name and medical record number on his wristband.

✦ Wash your hands.

To insert a rectal suppository

✦ Place the patient on his left side in Sims' position. Drape him with the bedcovers, exposing only his buttocks.

✦ Put on gloves. Unwrap the suppository and lubricate it with water-soluble lubricant.

✦ Lift the patient's upper buttock with your nondominant hand to expose the anus.

✦ Instruct the patient to take several deep breaths through his mouth to relax the anal sphincter and reduce anxiety. When he's relatively relaxed, insert the suppository. (See *Inserting a rectal suppository*.)

✦ Encourage the patient to lie quietly and, if applicable, to retain the suppository for the correct length of time. Press on his anus with a gauze pad, if needed, until the urge to defecate passes.

✦ Remove and discard your gloves, then wash your hands.

To apply an ointment

✦ Wash your hands.

◆ For external application, don gloves and use a gauze pad to spread the drug over the anal area. For internal application, attach the applicator to the tube of ointment, and coat the applicator with water-soluble lubricant.

◆ Expect to use about 1″ (2.5 cm) of ointment. To gauge how much pressure to use during application, try squeezing a small amount from the tube before you attach the applicator.

◆ Lift the patient's upper buttock with your nondominant hand to expose the anus.

◆ Tell the patient to take several deep breaths through his mouth to relax the anal sphincter and reduce discomfort during insertion. Then gently insert the applicator, directing it toward the umbilicus.

◆ Squeeze the tube to eject the drug.

◆ Remove the applicator and place a folded 4″ × 4″ gauze pad between the patient's buttocks to absorb excess ointment.

◆ Disassemble the tube and applicator and recap the tube. Clean the applicator with soap and warm water. Remove and discard your gloves. Then wash your hands thoroughly.

NURSING CONSIDERATIONS

◆ Because the intake of food and fluid stimulates peristalsis, a suppository for relieving constipation should be inserted about 30 minutes before mealtime to help soften the stool and promote defecation. A medicated retention suppository should be inserted between meals.

◆ Tell the patient not to expel the suppository. If retaining it is difficult, put him on a bedpan.

◆ Make sure that the patient's call button is handy, and watch for his signal because he may be unable to suppress the urge to defecate.

◆ Inform the patient that the suppository may discolor his next bowel movement.

SUBCUTANEOUS ADMINISTRATION

Injection of a drug into S.C. tissue allows slower, more sustained administration than an I.M. injection. Drugs and solutions delivered by this route are injected through a relatively short needle using meticulous sterile technique.

EQUIPMENT AND PREPARATION

Check the chart and the medication administration record. Gather gloves, the prescribed drug, a needle of appropriate gauge and length, 1- to 3-ml syringe, and alcohol pads. Other materials may include an antiseptic cleanser, filter needle, insulin syringe, and insulin pump.

Inspect the drug to make sure it's not cloudy and is free of precipitates. Wash your hands and put on gloves.

For single-dose ampules

Wrap the neck of the ampule in an alcohol pad and snap off the top. If desired, attach a filter needle to the needle and withdraw the drug. Tap the syringe to clear air from it. Cover the needle with the needle sheath by placing the sheath on the counter or drug cart and sliding the needle into the sheath. Before discarding the ampule, check the label against the patient's medication administration record.

Reviewing subcutaneous injection

✦ Allows slower, more sustained administration than I.M. injection
✦ Uses a relatively short needle and requires meticulous sterile technique

Selecting a subcutaneous injection site

To select an appropriate injection site, consider the available areas for subcutaneous (S.C.) injection. These areas offer sites on the abdomen, upper arms, thighs, shoulders, and lower back, as shown here. Also consider the patient's site rotation pattern and plan to use the next available injection site. This promotes drug absorption and helps prevent adverse reactions.

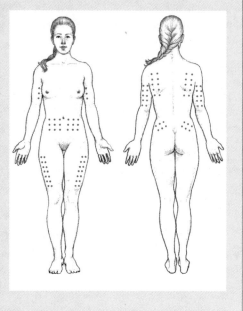

Discard the filter needle and the ampule. Attach the appropriate needle to the syringe.

For single-dose or multidose vials

Reconstitute powdered drugs according to the instructions on the label. Clean the rubber stopper on the vial with an alcohol pad. Pull the syringe plunger back until the volume of air in the syringe equals the volume of drug to be withdrawn from the vial. Insert the needle into the vial. Inject the air, invert the vial, and keep the bevel tip of the needle below the level of the solution as you withdraw the prescribed amount of drug.

Tap the syringe to clear air from it. Cover the needle with the needle sheath by placing the sheath on the counter or drug cart and sliding the needle into the sheath.

Check the drug label against the patient's medication administration record before returning the multidose vial to the shelf or drawer or before discarding the single-dose vial.

IMPLEMENTATION

✦ Confirm the patient's identity by asking his full name and checking the name and medical record number on his wristband.
✦ Choose an injection site and tell the patient where you'll be giving the injection. (See *Selecting a subcutaneous injection site.*)
✦ Put on gloves. Position and drape the patient if needed.
✦ Clean the injection site with an alcohol pad. Loosen the protective needle sheath.

Injecting a subcutaneous drug

While pinching up the patient's skin with your nondominant hand, hold the syringe in your dominant hand and grip the needle sheath with the free fingers of your nondominant hand. Pull the sheath back to uncover the needle, but don't touch the needle. Position the needle with its bevel up.

Tell the patient he'll feel a prick as you insert the needle. Do so quickly, in one motion, at a 45- or 90-degree angle, as shown at right. The needle length and the angle you use depend on the amount of S.C. tissue at the site. Some drugs, such as heparin, should always be injected at a 90-degree angle.

Release the skin to avoid injecting the drug into compressed tissue and irritating the nerves. Pull the plunger back slightly to check for blood return. If blood appears, withdraw the needle, prepare another syringe, and repeat the procedure. If no blood appears, slowly inject the drug.

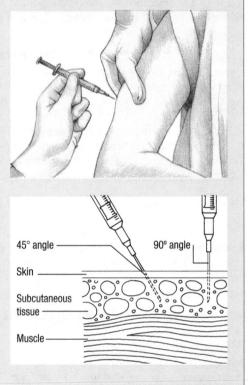

- 45° angle
- 90° angle
- Skin
- Subcutaneous tissue
- Muscle

✦ With the index finger and thumb of your nondominant hand, pinch the skin around the injection site firmly to elevate the S.C. tissue, forming a 1″ (2.5 cm) fat fold.

✦ Give the injection. (See *Injecting a subcutaneous drug*.)

✦ After injection, remove the needle at the same angle you used to insert it. Cover the site with an alcohol pad, and massage the site gently.

✦ Remove the alcohol pad and check the injection site for bleeding or bruising.

✦ Don't recap the needle. Follow your facility's policy to dispose of the injection equipment.

✦ Remove and discard your gloves. Wash your hands.

NURSING CONSIDERATIONS

✦ Don't aspirate for blood return when giving insulin or heparin. It's not necessary with insulin and may cause a hematoma with heparin.

✦ Don't massage the site after giving heparin.

 CLINICAL ALERT Repeated injections in the same site can cause lipodystrophy, a natural immune response. This adverse reaction can be minimized by rotating injection sites.

Key nursing actions for subcutaneous drugs

✦ Don't aspirate for blood return when giving insulin or heparin. It isn't necessary with insulin and may cause a hematoma with heparin.

✦ Don't massage the site after giving heparin.

✦ Don't repeat injections in the same site to minimize lipodystrophy, a natural immune response.

**Reviewing
I.M. injection**

✦ Deposits up to 5 ml of a drug deep into well-vascularized muscle for rapid systemic action and absorption
✦ Requires the use of a longer needle than an S.C injection to reach the muscle

I.M. ADMINISTRATION

You'll use I.M. injections to deposit up to 5 ml of a drug deep into well-vascularized muscle for rapid systemic action and absorption.

EQUIPMENT AND PREPARATION

Check the chart and the medication administration record. Gather the prescribed drug, diluent or filter needle (if needed), 3- to 5-ml syringe, 20G to 25G 1″ to 3″ needle, gloves, and alcohol pads.

Make sure the equipment is sterile. The needle may be packaged separately or already attached to the syringe. Needles used for I.M. injections are longer than those used for S.C. injections because they reach deep into the muscle. Needle length also depends on the injection site, the patient's size, and the amount of S.C. fat covering the muscle. A larger needle gauge accommodates viscous solutions and suspensions.

Make sure the prescribed drug is sterile. Check the drug for abnormal changes in color and clarity. If in doubt, ask the pharmacist.

Use alcohol to wipe the stopper that tops the drug vial, and draw up the prescribed amount of drug. Provide privacy and explain the procedure to the patient. Position and drape him appropriately, making sure that the site is well lit and exposed.

IMPLEMENTATION

✦ Wash your hands.
✦ Confirm the patient's identity by asking his full name and checking the name and medical record number on his wristband.
✦ Next, select an appropriate injection site. (See *Choosing an I.M. injection site.*)
✦ Loosen, but don't remove, the needle sheath.
✦ Gently tap the site to stimulate nerve endings and minimize pain.
✦ Clean the site with an alcohol pad, starting at the site and moving outward in expanding circles to about 2″ (5 cm). Allow the skin to dry because wet alcohol stings in the puncture.
✦ Put on gloves.
✦ With the thumb and index finger of your nondominant hand, gently stretch the skin.
✦ With the syringe in your dominant hand, remove the needle sheath with the free fingers of the other hand.
✦ Position the syringe perpendicular to the skin surface and a few inches from the skin. Tell the patient that he will feel a prick. Then quickly and firmly thrust the needle into the muscle.
✦ Pull back slightly on the plunger to aspirate for blood. If blood appears, the needle is in a blood vessel. Withdraw it, prepare a fresh syringe, and inject another site. If no blood appears, inject the drug slowly and steadily to let the muscle distend gradually. You should feel little or no resistance. Gently but quickly remove the needle at a 90-degree angle.
✦ Using a gloved hand, apply gentle pressure to the site with the alcohol pad. Massage the relaxed muscle, unless contraindicated, to distribute the drug and promote absorption.
✦ Inspect the site for bleeding or bruising. Apply pressure as needed.

Choosing an I.M. injection site

When reviewing sites for I.M. injection, avoid any site that looks inflamed, edematous, or irritated. Also, avoid using a site that contains moles, birthmarks, scar tissue, or other lesions. Then select an appropriate site, such as one of those shown below, and consider these guidelines:
- ✦ The dorsogluteal and ventrogluteal muscles are used most commonly for I.M. injections.
- ✦ The deltoid muscle may be used for injections of 2 ml or less.
- ✦ The vastus lateralis muscle is used most commonly in children.
- ✦ The rectus femoris may be used in infants.

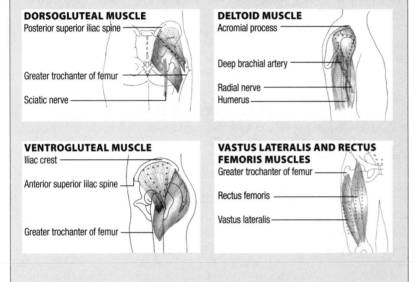

DORSOGLUTEAL MUSCLE
Posterior superior iliac spine
Greater trochanter of femur
Sciatic nerve

DELTOID MUSCLE
Acromial process
Deep brachial artery
Radial nerve
Humerus

VENTROGLUTEAL MUSCLE
Iliac crest
Anterior superior iliac spine
Greater trochanter of femur

VASTUS LATERALIS AND RECTUS FEMORIS MUSCLES
Greater trochanter of femur
Rectus femoris
Vastus lateralis

✦ Discard all equipment properly. Don't recap needles; put them in an appropriate biohazard container to avoid needle-stick injuries.
✦ Remove and discard your gloves. Wash your hands.

NURSING CONSIDERATIONS

✦ To slow absorption, some drugs are dissolved in oil. Mix them well before use.
✦ If you must inject more than 5 ml, divide the solution and inject it in two sites.
✦ If the patient must have repeated injections, consider numbing the area with ice before cleaning it.
✦ Rotate injection sites for a patient who needs repeated injections.
✦ Urge the patient to relax the muscle to reduce pain and bleeding.
✦ Never inject into the gluteal muscles of a child who has been walking for less than 1 year.
✦ Keep in mind that I.M. injections can damage local muscle cells and elevate the creatine kinase level, which can be confused with the elevated level caused by myocardial infarction. Diagnostic tests can be used to differentiate between them.

Key nursing actions for I.M. drugs

- ✦ For drugs dissolved in oil, mix well before use.
- ✦ If you must inject more than 5 ml, divide the solution and inject it in two sites.
- ✦ Rotate injection sites for a patient who needs repeated injections.
- ✦ Keep in mind that I.M. injections can damage local muscle cells and elevate the creatine kinase level, which can be confused with the elevated level caused by myocardial infarction. Diagnostic tests can be used to differentiate between them.

Reviewing I.V. bolus injection

+ Allows the drug level to peak quickly in the bloodstream
+ May be used for drugs that can't be given I.M. because they're toxic or because the patient has a reduced ability to absorb them.
+ May also be used to deliver drugs that can't be diluted
+ May be injected directly into a vein or through an existing I.V. line

Key nursing actions for I.V. bolus drugs

+ If the existing I.V. line is capped, making it an intermittent infusion device, verify patency and placement of the device before injecting the drug. Then flush the device with normal saline solution, give the drug, and follow with the appropriate flush.
+ Immediately report evidence of acute allergic reaction or anaphylaxis.
+ If extravasation occurs, stop the injection, estimate the amount of infiltration, and notify the prescriber.
+ When giving diazepam or chlordiazepoxide hydrochloride through a steel needle winged device or an I.V. line, flush with bacteriostatic water to prevent precipitation.

I.V. BOLUS ADMINISTRATION

In this method, rapid I.V. administration allows the drug level to peak quickly in the bloodstream. This method may also be used for drugs that can't be given I.M. because they're toxic or because the patient has a reduced ability to absorb them. In addition, it may be used to deliver drugs that can't be diluted. Bolus doses may be injected directly into a vein or through an existing I.V. line.

EQUIPMENT AND PREPARATION

Check the chart and the medication administration record. Gather the prescribed drug, 20G needle and syringe, diluent (if needed), tourniquet, alcohol pad, sterile 2″ × 2″ gauze pad, gloves, adhesive bandage, and tape. Other materials may include a winged device primed with normal saline solution and second syringe (and needle) filled with normal saline solution.

Draw the drug into the syringe and dilute it if needed.

IMPLEMENTATION

+ Confirm the patient's identity by asking his full name and checking the name and medical record number on his wristband.
+ Wash your hands and put on gloves.

To give a direct injection

+ Select the largest vein suitable to dilute the drug and minimize irritation.
+ Apply a tourniquet above the site to distend the vein. Clean the site with an alcohol pad, working outward in a circle.
+ If you're using the needle of the drug syringe, insert it at a 30-degree angle with the bevel up. The bevel should reach ¼″ (0.6 cm) into the vein. Insert a winged device bevel-up at a 10- to 25-degree angle. Lower the angle once you get into the vein. Advance the needle into the vein. Tape the wings in place when you see blood return, and attach the syringe containing the drug.
+ Check for blood backflow.
+ Remove the tourniquet and inject the drug at the prescribed rate.
+ Check for blood backflow to ensure that the needle remained in place and the entire injected drug entered the vein.
+ For a winged device, flush the line with normal saline solution from the second syringe to ensure complete delivery.
+ Withdraw the needle and apply pressure to the site with the sterile gauze pad for at least 3 minutes to prevent hematoma.
+ Apply an adhesive bandage when the bleeding stops.
+ Remove and discard your gloves. Wash your hands.

To inject through an existing line

+ Wash your hands and put on gloves.
+ Check the compatibility of the drug.
+ Close the flow clamp, wipe the injection port with an alcohol pad, and inject the drug as you would a direct injection.
+ Open the flow clamp and readjust the flow rate.
+ Remove and discard your gloves. Wash your hands.
+ If the drug isn't compatible with the I.V. solution, flush the line with normal saline solution or another compatible solution before and after the injection.

NURSING CONSIDERATIONS

✦ If the existing I.V. line is capped, making it an intermittent infusion device, verify patency and placement of the device before injecting the drug. Then flush the device with normal saline solution, give the drug, and follow with the appropriate flush.

✦ Immediately report signs of acute allergic reaction or anaphylaxis. If extravasation occurs, stop the injection, estimate the amount of infiltration, and notify the prescriber.

✦ When giving diazepam or chlordiazepoxide hydrochloride through a steel needle winged device or an I.V. line, flush with bacteriostatic water to prevent precipitation.

I.V. ADMINISTRATION THROUGH A SECONDARY LINE

A secondary I.V. line is a complete I.V. set connected to the lower Y-port (secondary port) of a primary line instead of to the I.V. catheter or needle. It features an I.V. container, long tubing, and either a microdrip or a macrodrip system. A secondary line can be used for continuous or intermittent drug infusion. When used continuously, it permits drug infusion and titration while the primary line maintains a constant total infusion rate.

A secondary I.V. line used only for intermittent drug administration is called a piggyback set. In this case, the primary line maintains venous access between drug doses. A piggyback set includes a small I.V. container, short tubing, and usually a macrodrip system. It connects to the primary line's upper Y-port (piggyback port).

EQUIPMENT AND PREPARATION

Check the chart and the medication administration record. Gather the prescribed I.V. drug, diluent (if needed), prescribed I.V. solution, administration set with secondary injection port, 22G 1″ needle or a needleless system, alcohol pads, 1″ (2.5 cm) adhesive tape, time tape, labels, infusion pump, extension hook, and solution for intermittent piggyback infusion.

Wash your hands. Inspect the I.V. container for cracks, leaks, or contamination. Check the drug's expiration date and its compatibility with the primary solution. Determine whether the primary line has a secondary injection port.

If needed, add the drug to the secondary I.V. solution (usually 50- to 100-ml "mini-bags" of normal saline solution or D_5W). To do so, remove any seals from the secondary container and wipe the main port with an alcohol pad. Inject the prescribed drug and agitate the solution to mix the drug. Label the I.V. mixture.

Insert the administration set spike and attach the needle or needleless system. Open the flow clamp and prime the line. Then close the flow clamp.

Some drugs come in vials for hanging directly on an I.V. pole. In this case, inject the diluent directly into the drug vial. Then spike the vial, prime the tubing, and hang the set.

IMPLEMENTATION

✦ If the drug is incompatible with the primary I.V. solution, replace the primary solution with a fluid that's compatible with both solutions. Then flush the line before starting the drug infusion.

Reviewing I.V. infusion through a secondary line

✦ Requires a complete I.V. set connected to the lower Y-port (secondary port) of a primary line instead of to the I.V. catheter or needle

✦ Features an I.V. container, long tubing, and a microdrip or macrodrip system

✦ Can be used for continuous or intermittent drug infusion

✦ Permits drug infusion and titration while the primary line maintains a constant total infusion rate (when used continuously)

✦ Is sometimes used only for intermittent drug administration (as a piggyback set) while the primary line maintains venous access between drug doses

✦ Includes a small I.V. container, short tubing, and usually a macrodrip system (piggyback set) and connects to the primary line's upper Y-port (piggyback port)

Key nursing actions for I.V. infusion through a secondary line

+ If facility policy allows, use a pump for drug infusion.
+ Place a time tape on the secondary container to help prevent an inaccurate administration rate.
+ When reusing secondary tubing, change it according to your facility's policy, usually every 48 to 72 hours.
+ Inspect the injection port for leakage with each use; change it more often if needed.
+ Except for lipids, don't piggyback a secondary I.V. line to a total parenteral nutrition line because it risks contamination.

✦ Hang the container of the secondary set and wipe the injection port of the primary line with an alcohol pad.

✦ Insert the needle or needleless system from the secondary line into the injection port, and tape it securely to the primary line.

✦ To run the container of the secondary set by itself, lower the primary set's container with an extension hook. To run both containers simultaneously, place them at the same height.

✦ Open the clamp and adjust the drip rate.

✦ For continuous infusion, set the secondary solution to the desired drip rate; then adjust the primary solution to the desired total infusion rate.

✦ For intermittent infusion, wait until the secondary solution has completely infused; then adjust the primary drip rate, as required.

✦ If the secondary solution tubing is being reused, close the clamp on the tubing and follow your facility's policy: Either remove the needle or needleless system and replace it with a new one, or leave it taped in the injection port and label it with the time it was first used.

✦ Leave the empty container in place until you replace it with a new dose of drug at the prescribed time. If the tubing won't be reused, discard it appropriately with the I.V. container.

NURSING CONSIDERATIONS

✦ If facility policy allows, use a pump for drug infusion. Place a time tape on the secondary container to help prevent an inaccurate administration rate.

✦ When reusing secondary tubing, change it according to your facility's policy, usually every 48 to 72 hours. Inspect the injection port for leakage with each use; change it more often if needed.

✦ Except for lipids, don't piggyback a secondary I.V. line to a total parenteral nutrition line because it risks contamination.

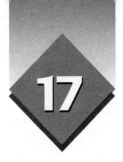

Medication errors

In the state where you practice nursing, different health care professionals may be legally permitted to prescribe, dispense, and administer drugs—such as physicians, nurse practitioners, dentists, podiatrists, and optometrists. Most commonly, however, physicians prescribe drugs, pharmacists dispense them, and nurses administer them.

That means you're almost always on the front line when it comes to patients and their drugs. It also means that you bear a major share of the responsibility for avoiding medication errors. Besides faithfully following your facility's drug administration policies, you can help prevent medication errors by studying common ones and avoiding the slip-ups that allow them to happen.

COMMON CAUSES OF ERRORS

To help you avoid medication errors, this chapter outlines some of their most common causes. These include similar names, overlooked allergies, compound errors, wrong administration routes, ambiguous abbreviations, unclear orders, color changes, and high stress levels.

SIMILAR NAMES

Drugs with similar-sounding names can be easy to confuse. What's more, even different-sounding names can look similar when written out rapidly by hand on a medication order: Soriatane and Loxitane, for example, both of which are capsules.

Any time a patient's drug order doesn't seem right for his diagnosis, call the prescriber to clarify the order. Also, be particularly alert for commonly confused names. (See *Avoiding morphine–hydromorphone mix-ups,* page 570.)

Drug names aren't the only kinds of words that are easily confused. Patient names can also cause trouble if you fail to verify each person's identity. This problem can be especially troublesome if two patients have the same first name.

Common causes of drug errors
- ✦ Similar names
- ✦ Overlooked allergies
- ✦ Compound errors
- ✦ Wrong administration routes
- ✦ Ambiguous abbreviations
- ✦ Unclear orders
- ✦ Color changes
- ✦ High stress levels

569

Reminders about similar drug names

+ Similar-sounding names can be easy to confuse.
+ Different-sounding names can look similar when written out rapidly by hand.
+ If a drug order doesn't seem right for the patient's diagnosis, call the prescriber to clarify the order.
+ Be particularly alert when dealing with drugs that are commonly confused.
+ Always verify the patient's identity; drug names aren't the only words that can be easily confused.

Reminders about drug allergies

+ Verify the patient's full name, and ask whether he has any drug allergies—even if he's in distress.
+ If a patient in distress needs or wants a drug fast, resist the urge to act first and document later. Skipping crucial assessment steps could easily lead to a drug error.
+ If you're giving ipratropium (Atrovent) aerosol by metered-dose inhaler, find out if the patient is allergic to peanuts; if so, he could have an anaphylactic reaction to the drug.

WARNING

Avoiding morphine–hydromorphone mix-ups

An order for morphine is easy to confuse with one for hydromorphone (Dilaudid). Plus, both drugs come in 4-mg prefilled syringes, which adds to the confusion. If you give morphine when the prescriber really ordered hydromorphone, the patient could develop respiratory depression or arrest.

To prevent such dangerous mix-ups, consider posting a prominent notice in your drug room that warns the staff about this common error. Or, try attaching a fluorescent sticker printed with "NOT MORPHINE" to each hydromorphone syringe.

Consider this clinical scenario. Robert Brewer, age 5, was hospitalized for measles. Robert Brinson, also age 5, was admitted after a severe asthma attack. The boys were assigned to adjacent rooms on a small pediatric unit. Each had a nonproductive cough. When Robert Brewer's nurse came to give him an expectorant, the child's mother told her that Robert had already inhaled a drug through a mask.

The nurse quickly figured out that another nurse, new to the unit, had given Robert Brinson's drug (acetylcysteine, a mucolytic) to Robert Brewer in error. Fortunately, no harmful adverse reactions occurred. Had the new nurse checked her patient's identity more carefully, however, no error would have happened in the first place.

Always check each patient's full name. Also, teach each patient (or parent) to offer an identification bracelet for inspection and to state a full name when anyone enters the room to administer a drug. Also, urge the patient to tell you if an identification bracelet falls off, is removed, or gets lost. Replace it right away.

OVERLOOKED ALLERGIES

After verifying your patient's full name, take time to check whether he has any drug allergies—even if he's in distress. Consider this real-life example.

A prescriber issued a stat order for chlorpromazine (Thorazine) for a distressed patient. By the time the nurse arrived with it, the patient had grown more distressed and was demanding relief. Unnerved by the patient's demeanor, the nurse gave the drug—without checking the patient's medication administration record or documenting the order—and the patient had an allergic reaction to it.

Any time you're in a tense situation with a patient who needs or wants a drug fast, resist the temptation to act first and document later. Skipping that crucial assessment step could easily lead to a medication error.

 CLINICAL ALERT A patient who is severely allergic to peanuts could have an anaphylactic reaction to ipratropium (Atrovent) aerosol given by metered-dose inhaler. Ask your patient or his parents whether he's allergic to peanuts before you administer this drug. If you find that he has such an allergy, you'll need to use the nasal spray and inhalation solution form of the drug. Because it doesn't contain soy lecithin, it's safe for patients who are allergic to peanuts.

COMPOUND ERRORS

Many medication errors stem from compound problems—a mistake that could have been caught at several steps along the way. For a drug to be given correctly, each health care team member must fulfill the appropriate role. The prescriber must write the order correctly and legibly. The pharmacist must evaluate whether the order is appropriate and then fill it correctly. And the nurse must evaluate whether the order is appropriate and then administer it correctly.

A breakdown at any point in this chain of events can lead to a medication error. That's why it's so important for health care team members to act as a real team, checking each other and catching any problems that arise before those problems affect the patient's health. Do your best to foster an environment in which professionals can double-check each other.

For instance, the pharmacist can help clarify the number of times a drug should be given each day. He can help you label drugs in the most appropriate way. He can remind you to always return unused drugs to the pharmacy.

You can—in fact, you must—clarify any prescriber's order that doesn't seem clear or correct. You also must correctly handle and store any multi-dose vials obtained from the pharmacist. Only administer drugs that you've prepared personally. Never give a drug that has an ambiguous label or no label at all. Here's an actual example of what could happen if you do.

A nurse placed an unlabeled cup of phenol (used in neurolytic procedures) next to a cup of guanethidine (a postganglionic-blocking drug). The nurse accidentally injected the phenol instead of the guanethidine, causing severe tissue damage to the patient's arm. The patient needed emergency surgery and developed neurologic complications.

Obviously, this was a compound error. The prescriber should have labeled each cup clearly, and the nurse shouldn't have given an unlabeled substance to a patient.

Here's another example of a compound error. In the neonatal intensive care unit, a nurse prepared and administered a dose of aminophylline to an infant. The nurse didn't have anyone else check his work. After receiving the drug, the infant developed tachycardia and other signs of theophylline toxicity. She later died. The nurse thought the order read 7.4 ml of aminophylline; instead, it read 7.4 mg.

This tragedy might have been avoided if the prescriber had written a clearer order, if the nurse had clarified the order, if a pharmacist had prepared and dispensed the drug, or if another nurse had checked the dose calculation. To help prevent such problems, many facilities prefer or require that a pharmacist prepare and dispense nonemergency parenteral doses whenever commercial unit doses aren't available.

Here's another example. A container of 5% acetic acid, used to clean tracheostomy tubing, was left near nebulization equipment in the room of a 10-month-old infant. A respiratory therapist mistook the liquid for normal saline solution and used it to dilute albuterol for the child's nebulizer treatment. During treatment, the child experienced bronchospasm, hypercapnia, dyspnea, tachypnea, and tachycardia.

Leaving dangerous chemicals near patients is extremely risky, especially when the container labels don't warn of toxicity. To prevent such problems, read the label on every drug you prepare, and never administer anything that isn't labeled or is labeled poorly.

For any patient who is discharged with prescriptions, be sure to teach him about each one. (See *Teaching a patient how to reduce medication errors*, page 572.) This helps prevent errors from being committed or compounded by the patient.

Reminders about compound errors

+ Many drug errors stem from a mistake that could have been caught at several steps along the way.
+ For a drug to be given correctly, each member of the health care team must fulfill the appropriate role.
+ The prescriber must write the order correctly and legibly.
+ The pharmacist must evaluate whether the order is appropriate and then fill it correctly.
+ The nurse must evaluate whether the order is appropriate and then administer it correctly.
+ A breakdown at any point in this chain of events can lead to an error.

Reducing drug errors through teaching

+ Teach the patient about his diagnosis and the purpose of drug therapy—including the drug name, dose, and frequency of administration.
+ Provide information in writing.
+ Make sure the patient fully understands the information you give him.
+ Help the patient set up a dosing schedule that will fit his daily activities, if possible.
+ Assess the patient's use of over-the-counter drugs and herbal and nutritional supplements.
+ Inform the patient about possible adverse effects and which should be reported to the prescriber.

Teaching a patient how to reduce medication errors

Patients are at an even higher risk than you are for making medication errors because they know so much less about drugs. That's why patient teaching is one of your crucial responsibilities in minimizing medication errors and their consequences—especially as more patients receive outpatient rather than inpatient care. To help reduce patients' medication errors, take the following actions:

+ Teach the patient about his diagnosis and the purpose of his drug therapy. Make sure he knows the name of each drug in his regimen, how much of each drug he's supposed to take, and when and how he's supposed to take it. Use an interpreter if he doesn't understand English.
+ Provide drug information in clear and legible writing for the patient to take home.
+ Also explain the drug regimen to the patient's family and others closely involved with his care and drug administration.
+ Ensure that the patient fully understands his regimen, keeping in mind that some types of therapy can be confusing for patients. For example, one patient who went home with a warfarin prescription took the 2.5-mg and 5-mg tablets at the same time rather than 2.5 mg and 5 mg on alternating days. He eventually was hospitalized with GI bleeding—a problem that might have been avoided had he better understood his dosage regimen.
+ Help the patient set up a practical, workable dosing schedule. Remember: any regimen that requires him to take more than one drug greatly increases the complexity of the therapy and the chance of confusion and medication errors.
+ Ask if your patient takes over-the-counter drugs at home in addition to his prescribed drugs. Make a special point of asking about herbal remedies and nutritional supplements. Some herbal remedies have drug-like effects and can cause or contribute to drug-related problems. What's more, these preparations aren't regulated as drugs, so their ingredients can be misrepresented, substituted, or contaminated.
+ Advise your patient about possible adverse reactions and tell him drug-related problems warrant a call to his prescriber. Encourage him to report anything about his drug therapy that concerns or worries him.

WRONG ADMINISTRATION ROUTES

Many medication errors stem at least in part from problems related to the administration route. The risk of error increases when a patient has several lines running for different purposes. Consider this example.

A nurse prepared a dose of digoxin elixir for a patient who had a central I.V. line and a jejunostomy tube. Then she mistakenly administered the drug into the central I.V. line. Fortunately, the patient had no adverse reaction. To help prevent such mix-ups in route of administration, prepare all oral drugs in a syringe that has a tip small enough to fit an abdominal tube but too big to fit a central line.

Here's another error that could have been avoided: To clear air bubbles from a 9-year-old patient's insulin drip, a nurse disconnected the tubing and raised the pump rate to 200 ml/hour to flush the bubbles through quickly. Then she reconnected the tubing and restarted the drip, but forgot to reset the rate back to 2 units/hour. The child received 50 units of insulin before the error was detected. To prevent this kind of error, never increase a drip rate to clear bubbles from a line. Instead, remove the tubing from the pump, disconnect it from the patient, and use the flow-control clamp to establish gravity flow.

AMBIGUOUS ABBREVIATIONS

Abbreviating drug names is risky, as in this example. Cancer patients with anemia may receive epoetin alfa, commonly abbreviated EPO, to stimulate red blood cell production. In one case, when a cancer patient was admitted to a hospital, the prescriber wrote, "May take own supply of EPO." However, the patient wasn't anemic. Sensing that something was wrong, the pharmacist interviewed the patient, who confirmed that he was taking "EPO"—evening primrose oil—to lower his cholesterol level. Ask all prescribers to spell out drug names.

UNCLEAR ORDERS

A patient was supposed to receive one dose of the antineoplastic lomustine to treat brain cancer. (Lomustine typically is given as a single oral dose once every 6 weeks.) The prescriber's order read, "Administer h.s." Because a nurse misinterpreted the order to mean every night, the patient received nine daily doses, developed severe thrombocytopenia and leukopenia, and died.

If you're unfamiliar with a drug, check a drug book before administering it. If a prescriber uses "h.s." but doesn't specify the frequency of administration, ask him to clarify the order. When documenting orders, note "h.s. nightly" or "h.s. one dose today."

COLOR CHANGES

In two reports, alert nurses noticed that antineoplastics prepared in the pharmacy didn't look the way they should. The first error involved a 6-year-old child who was to receive 12 mg of methotrexate intrathecally. In the pharmacy, a 1-g vial was mistakenly selected instead of a 20-mg vial, and the drug was reconstituted with 10 ml of normal saline solution. The vial containing 100 mg/ml was incorrectly labeled as containing 2 mg/ml, and 6 ml of the solution was drawn into a syringe. Although the syringe label indicated 12 mg of drug, the syringe actually contained 600 mg of drug.

When the nurse received the syringe and noted that the drug's color didn't appear right, she returned it to the pharmacy for verification. The pharmacist retrieved the vial used to prepare the dose and drew the remaining solution into another syringe. The solutions in both syringes matched, and no one noticed the vial's 1-g label. The pharmacist concluded that a manufacturing change caused the color difference.

The child received the 600-mg dose and experienced seizures 45 minutes later. A pharmacist responding to the emergency detected the error. The child received an antidote and recovered.

A similar case involved a 20-year-old patient with leukemia who received mitomycin instead of mitoxantrone. The nurse had questioned the drug's unusual bluish tint, but the pharmacist assured her that the color difference was due to a change in manufacturer. Fortunately, the patient didn't suffer any harm.

If a familiar drug seems to have an unfamiliar appearance, investigate the cause. If the pharmacist cites a manufacturing change, ask him to double-check whether he has received verification from the manufacturer. Document the appearance discrepancy, your actions, and the pharmacist's response in the patient record.

Red flags for drug errors
- Unapproved or ambiguous abbreviations
- Unclear or incomplete drug orders
- A familiar drug with an unfamiliar appearance
- High stress levels

HIGH STRESS LEVELS

A nurse-anesthetist administered the sedative midazolam (Versed) to the wrong patient. When she discovered the error, she reached for what she thought was a vial of the antidote flumazenil (Romazicon), withdrew 2.5 ml of the drug, and administered it. When the patient didn't respond, she realized she had reached for a vial of ondansetron (Zofran), an antiemetic, instead. Another practitioner assisted with proper I.V. administration of flumazenil, and the patient recovered without harm.

Committing a serious error can cause enormous stress and cloud your judgment. If you're involved in a medication error, ask another professional to administer the antidote.

Clearly, you carry a great deal of responsibility for making sure that the right patient gets the right drug in the right dose at the right time by the right route. By keeping these common errors in mind, you can minimize your risk of making them and maximize the therapeutic effects of your patients' drug regimens.

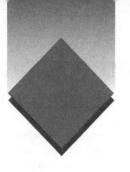

Appendices
Index

Adverse reactions misinterpreted as age-related changes

In elderly patients, adverse drug reactions can easily be misinterpreted as the typical signs and symptoms of aging. The table below, which shows possible adverse reactions for common drug classifications, can help you avoid such misinterpretations.

DRUG CLASSIFICATIONS	ADVERSE REACTIONS							
	Agitation	Anxiety	Arrhythmias	Ataxia	Changes in appetite	Confusion	Constipation	Depression
Angiotensin-converting enzyme (ACE) inhibitors						✦	✦	✦
Alpha₁ adrenergic blockers		✦					✦	✦
Antianginals	✦	✦	✦			✦		
Antiarrhythmics			✦				✦	
Anticholinergics	✦	✦	✦			✦	✦	✦
Anticonvulsants	✦		✦	✦	✦	✦	✦	✦
Antidepressants, tricyclic	✦	✦	✦	✦	✦	✦	✦	
Antidiabetics, oral								
Antihistamines						✦	✦	✦
Antilipemics							✦	
Antiparkinsonians	✦	✦		✦	✦	✦	✦	✦
Antipsychotics	✦	✦	✦	✦	✦	✦	✦	✦
Barbiturates	✦	✦	✦			✦		
Benzodiazepines	✦			✦		✦	✦	✦
Beta blockers		✦	✦					✦
Calcium channel blockers		✦	✦				✦	
Corticosteroids	✦					✦		✦
Diuretics						✦		
Nonsteroidal anti-inflammatory drugs (NSAIDs)		✦				✦	✦	✦
Opioids	✦	✦				✦	✦	✦
Skeletal muscle relaxants	✦	✦		✦		✦		
Thyroid hormones			✦		✦			

	Difficulty breathing	Disorientation	Dizziness	Drowsiness	Edema	Fatigue	Hypotension	Insomnia	Memory loss	Muscle weakness	Restlessness	Sexual dysfunction	Tremors	Urinary dysfunction	Visual changes
			✦			✦	✦	✦				✦			✦
			✦	✦	✦	✦	✦	✦				✦		✦	✦
			✦		✦	✦	✦	✦			✦	✦		✦	✦
	✦		✦		✦	✦									
		✦	✦	✦		✦	✦		✦	✦	✦			✦	✦
	✦		✦	✦	✦	✦	✦	✦					✦	✦	✦
	✦	✦	✦	✦		✦	✦	✦			✦	✦	✦	✦	✦
					✦	✦									
		✦	✦	✦		✦							✦	✦	✦
			✦			✦		✦		✦		✦		✦	✦
		✦	✦	✦		✦	✦	✦		✦			✦	✦	✦
			✦	✦		✦	✦	✦			✦	✦	✦	✦	✦
	✦	✦		✦		✦	✦				✦				
	✦	✦	✦	✦		✦		✦	✦	✦			✦	✦	✦
	✦		✦			✦	✦		✦			✦	✦	✦	✦
	✦		✦		✦	✦	✦	✦				✦		✦	✦
					✦	✦		✦		✦					✦
			✦			✦	✦			✦				✦	)
			✦	✦		✦		✦		✦					✦
	✦	✦	✦	✦		✦	✦	✦	✦		✦	✦		✦	✦
			✦	✦		✦	✦	✦					✦		
								✦					✦		

Herb-drug interactions

HERB	DRUG	POSSIBLE EFFECTS
aloe (dried juice from leaf [latex])	antiarrhythmics, digoxin	May lead to hypokalemia, which may potentiate digoxin and antiarrhythmics.
	thiazide diuretics, other potassium-wasting drugs, such as corticosteroids	May cause additive effect of potassium wasting.
	oral drugs	May decrease drug absorption because of more rapid GI transit time.
	stimulant laxatives	May increase risk of potassium loss.
bilberry	anticoagulants, antiplatelets	Decreases platelet aggregation.
	hypoglycemics, insulin	May increase insulin level, causing hypoglycemia; additive effect with antidiabetics.
capsicum	angiotensin-converting enzyme (ACE) inhibitors	May cause cough.
	anticoagulants, antiplatelets	Decreases platelet aggregation and increases fibrinolytic activity, prolonging bleeding time.
	antihypertensives	May interfere with antihypertensives by increasing catecholamine secretion.
	aspirin, nonsteroidal anti-inflammatory drugs (NSAIDs)	Stimulates GI secretions to help protect against NSAID-induced GI irritation.
	central nervous system (CNS) depressants, such as barbiturates, benzodiazepines, opioids	Increases sedative effect.
	cocaine	May increase effects of drug and risk of adverse reactions, including death. Use together includes exposure to capsicum in pepper spray.
	histamine-2 (H_2) blockers, proton-pump inhibitors	Decreases effects of the increased catecholamine secretion by herb.
	hepatically metabolized drugs	May increase hepatic metabolism of drugs by increasing glucose-6-phosphatase dehydrogenase (G6PD) and adipose lipase activity.
	monoamine oxidase (MAO) inhibitors	May decrease effectiveness because of increased acid secretion by capsicum.
	theophylline	Increases absorption of theophylline, possibly leading to higher drug level or toxicity.
chamomile	anticoagulants	Warfarin constituents in herb may enhance drug therapy and prolong bleeding time.
	drugs requiring GI absorption	May delay drug absorption.
	drugs with sedative properties, such as benzodiazepines	May cause additive effects and adverse reactions.

HERB	DRUG	POSSIBLE EFFECTS
chamomile (continued)	iron	Tannic acid content in herb may reduce iron absorption.
echinacea	hepatotoxic drugs	Hepatotoxicity may increase with drugs known to elevate liver enzyme levels.
	immunosuppressants	Herb may counteract drugs.
	warfarin	Increases bleeding time without increased international normalized ratio (INR).
evening primrose oil	anticonvulsants	Lowers seizure threshold.
	antiplatelets, anticoagulants	Increases risk of bleeding and bruising.
feverfew	anticoagulants, antiplatelets	May decrease platelet aggregation and increase fibrinolytic activity.
	methysergide	May potentiate drug.
garlic	anticoagulants, antiplatelets	Enhances platelet inhibition, leading to increased anticoagulation.
	antihyperlipidemics	May have additive lipid-lowering properties.
	antihypertensives	May cause additive hypotension.
	cyclosporine	May decrease effectiveness of drug. May induce metabolism and decrease drug level to subtherapeutic; may cause rejection.
	hormonal contraceptives	May decrease efficacy of drugs.
	insulin, other drugs causing hypoglycemia	May increase insulin level, causing hypoglycemia, an additive effect with these drugs.
	nonnucleotide reverse transcriptase inhibitors (NNRTIs)	May affect metabolism of these drugs.
	saquinavir	Decreases drug level, causing therapeutic failure and increased viral resistance.
ginger	anticoagulants, antiplatelets	Inhibits platelet aggregation by antagonizing thromboxane synthetase and enhancing prostacyclin, leading to prolonged bleeding time.
	antidiabetics	May interfere with diabetes therapy because of hypoglycemic effects.
	antihypertensives	May antagonize drug effects.
	barbiturates	May enhance drug effects.
	calcium channel blockers	May increase calcium uptake by myocardium, leading to altered drug effects.
	chemotherapy	May reduce nausea caused by chemotherapy.
	H_2 blockers, proton-pump inhibitors	May decrease effectiveness because of increased acid secretion by herb.

HERB	DRUG	POSSIBLE EFFECTS
ginkgo	anticoagulants, antiplatelets	May enhance platelet inhibition, leading to increased anticoagulation.
	anticonvulsants	May decrease effectiveness of drugs.
	drugs known to lower seizure threshold	May further reduce seizure threshold.
	insulin	Ginkgo leaf extract can alter insulin secretion and metabolism, affecting glucose level.
	thiazide diuretics	Ginkgo leaf may increase blood pressure.
ginseng	alcohol	Increases alcohol clearance, possibly by increasing activity of alcohol dehydrogenase.
	anabolic steroids, hormones	May potentiate effects of drugs. Estrogenic effects of herb may cause vaginal bleeding and breast nodules.
	antibiotics	Herb may enhance effects of some antibiotics.
	anticoagulants, antiplatelets	Decreases platelet adhesiveness.
	antidiabetics	May enhance glucose-lowering effects.
	antipsychotics	Because of CNS stimulant activity, avoid use with these drugs.
	digoxin	May falsely elevate drug level.
	furosemide	May decrease diuretic effect with this drug.
	immunosuppressants	May interfere with drug therapy.
	MAO inhibitors	Potentiates action of MAO inhibitors. May cause insomnia, headache, tremors, and hypomania.
	stimulants	May potentiate drug effects.
	warfarin	Causes antagonism of warfarin, resulting in a decreased INR.
goldenseal	antihypertensives	Large amounts of herb may interfere with blood pressure control.
	CNS depressants, such as barbiturates, benzodiazepines, opioids	Increases sedative effect.
	diuretics	Causes additive drug effect.
	general anesthetics	May potentiate hypotensive action of drugs.
	heparin	May counteract anticoagulant effect of drug.
	H$_2$ blockers, proton-pump inhibitors	May decrease effectiveness because of increased acid secretion by herb.
grapeseed	warfarin	Increases effects and INR because of tocopherol content of herb.

HERB	DRUG	POSSIBLE EFFECTS
green tea	acetaminophen, aspirin	May increase effectiveness of these drugs by as much as 40%.
	adenosine	May inhibit hemodynamic effects of drug.
	albuterol, isoproterenol, metaproterenol, terbutaline	May increase the cardiac inotropic effect of these drugs.
	clozapine	May cause acute exacerbation of psychotic symptoms.
	disulfiram	Increases risk of adverse effects of caffeine; decreases clearance and increases half-life of caffeine.
	ephedrine	Increases risk of agitation, tremors, and insomnia.
	hormonal contraceptives	Decreases clearance by 40% to 65%. Increases effects and adverse effects.
	lithium	Abrupt caffeine withdrawal increases drug level; may cause lithium tremor.
	MAO inhibitors	Large amounts of herb may precipitate hypertensive crisis.
	mexiletine	Decreases caffeine elimination by 50%. Increases effects and adverse effects.
	verapamil	Increases caffeine level by 25%; increases effects and adverse effects.
	warfarin	Causes antagonism resulting from vitamin content of herb.
hawthorn berry	cardiovascular drugs	May potentiate or interfere with conventional therapies used for congestive heart failure, hypertension, angina, and arrhythmias.
	CNS depressants	Causes additive effects.
	coronary vasodilators	Causes additive vasodilator effects when used with theophylline, caffeine, papaverine, sodium nitrate, adenosine, and epinephrine.
	digoxin	Causes additive positive inotropic effect, with potential for drug toxicity.
kava	alcohol	Potentiates depressant effect of alcohol and other CNS depressants.
	benzodiazepines	Use with these drugs may result in comalike states.
	CNS depressants or stimulants	May hinder therapy with CNS stimulants.
	hepatotoxic drugs	May increase risk of liver damage.
	levodopa	Decreases effectiveness because of dopamine antagonism by herb.

HERB	DRUG	POSSIBLE EFFECTS
licorice	antihypertensives	Decreases effect of drug therapy. Large amounts of herb cause sodium and water retention and hypertension.
	aspirin	May provide protection against aspirin-induced damage to GI mucosa.
	corticosteroids	Causes additive and enhanced effects of drugs.
	digoxin	Herb causes hypokalemia, which predisposes to drug toxicity.
	hormonal contraceptives	Increases fluid retention and potential for increased blood pressure resulting from fluid overload.
	hormones	Interferes with estrogen or antiestrogen therapy.
	insulin	Causes hypokalemia and sodium retention.
	spironolactone	Decreases effects of drug.
ma huang (ephedra)	amitriptyline	May decrease hypertensive effects of herb.
	caffeine	Increases risk of stimulatory adverse effects of ephedra and caffeine and risk of hypertension, myocardial infarction, stroke, and death.
	caffeine, CNS stimulants, theophylline	Causes additive CNS stimulation.
	dexamethasone	Increases clearance and decreases effectiveness of drug.
	digoxin	Increases risk of arrhythmias.
	hypoglycemics	Decreases drug effect because of hyperglycemia caused by herb.
	MAO inhibitors	Potentiates drugs.
	oxytocin	May cause hypertension.
	theophylline	May increase risk of stimulatory adverse effects.
melatonin	CNS depressants, such as barbiturates, benzodiazepines, opioids	Increases sedative effect.
	fluoxetine	Improves sleep in some patients with major depressive disorder.
	fluvoxamine	May significantly increase melatonin level; may decrease melatonin metabolism.
	immunosuppressants	May stimulate immune function and interfere with drug therapy.
	isoniazid	May enhance effects of drug against some *Mycobacterium* species.

HERB	DRUG	POSSIBLE EFFECTS
melatonin *(continued)*	nifedipine	May decrease effectiveness of drug; increases heart rate.
	verapamil	Increases melatonin excretion.
milk thistle	drugs causing diarrhea	Increases bile secretion and often causes loose stools. May increase effect of other drugs commonly causing diarrhea.
	hepatotoxic drugs, such as acetaminophen, butyrophenones, ethanol, phenothiazines, phenytoin	May have liver membrane-stabilization and antioxidant effects, leading to protection from liver damage.
	indinavir	May decrease trough level of drug, reducing virologic response.
nettle	anticonvulsants	May increase sedative adverse effects; may increase risk of seizure.
	anxiolytics, hypnotics, opioids	May increase sedative adverse effects.
	iron	Tannic acid content of herb may reduce iron absorption.
	warfarin	Antagonism resulting from vitamin K content of aerial parts of herb.
passion flower	CNS depressants, such as barbiturates, benzodiazepines, opioids	Increases sedative effect.
St. John's wort	5-hydroxytriptamine$_1$ (HT$_1$) agonists (triptans)	Increases risk of serotonin syndrome.
	alcohol, opioids	Enhances the sedative effect of these drugs.
	anesthetics	May prolong effect of drugs.
	barbiturates	Decreases drug-induced sleep time.
	cyclosporine	Decreases drug level below therapeutic levels, threatening transplanted organ rejection.
	digoxin	May reduce drug level, which decreases therapeutic effects.
	human immunodeficiency virus (HIV) protease inhibitors, indinavir, NNRTIs	Induces cytochrome P-450 metabolic pathway, which may decrease therapeutic effects of drugs using this pathway for metabolism. Avoid use together because of the potential for subtherapeutic antiretroviral level and insufficient virologic response that could lead to resistance or class cross-resistance.
	hormonal contraceptives	Increases breakthrough bleeding; decreases level and effectiveness of drugs.
	irinotecan	Decreases drug level by 50%.
	iron	Tannic acid content of herb may reduce iron absorption.

HERB	DRUG	POSSIBLE EFFECTS
St. John's wort *(continued)*	MAO inhibitors, nefazodone, selective serotonin reuptake inhibitors (SSRIs), trazodone	Causes additive effects with MAO inhibitors, SSRIs, and other antidepressants, potentially leading to serotonin syndrome, especially when combined with SSRIs.
	photosensitizing drugs	Increases photosensitivity.
	reserpine	Antagonizes effects of drug.
	sympathomimetic amines, such as pseudoephedrine	Causes additive effects.
	theophylline	May decrease drug level, making the drug less effective.
	warfarin	May alter INR. Reduces effectiveness of anticoagulant, requiring increased dosage of drug.
valerian	alcohol	May be risk of increased sedation.
	CNS depressants, sedative hypnotics	Enhances effects of these drugs.
	iron	Tannic acid content of herb may reduce iron absorption.

Index

i refers to an illustration; t refers to a table.

i refers to an illustration; t refers to a table.

---

i refers to an illustration; t refers to a table.

i refers to an illustration; t refers to a table.

i refers to an illustration; t refers to a table.

i refers to an illustration; t refers to a table.

i refers to an illustration; t refers to a table.